Date Due

Pathophysiology for Health Practitioners

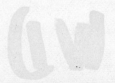

athophysiology
or Health
Practitioners

Gwen J. Stephens, Ph.D.

*Associate Professor, University of Colorado
Health Sciences Center School of Nursing, Denver
and Nurse Practitioner, Emergency Department,
Adult Walkin Clinic, University of Colorado
Hospitals, Denver*

Macmillan Publishing Co., Inc.
NEW YORK

Collier Macmillan Publishers
LONDON

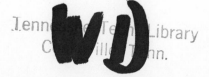

Macmillan Publishing Co., Inc.
866 Third Avenue, New York, New York 10022

Collier Macmillan Canada, Ltd.

Library of Congress Cataloging in Publication Data

Stephens, Gwen J
  Pathophysiology for health practitioners.

  Includes bibliographies and index.
  1. Physiology, Pathological.   2. Nurses.
3. Allied health personnel.   I. Title.
RB113.S73   157   79-47
ISBN 0-02-417120-4

Printing: 1 2 3 4 5 6 7 8   Year: 0 1 2 3 4 5 6

To my parents

     Esther Mae Lundquist and
     Wesley LeRoy Jones
with devotion and gratitude;

and to my three sons

     Peter, John, and Joseph
with love and pride.

Preface

Background

This book is the direct outgrowth of a group of courses which I have developed and taught during several years as a faculty member of the University of Colorado Health Sciences Center School of Nursing. One was a series of lectures on the pathophysiology, manifestations, and management of common clinical disorders for upper division students in the baccalaureate program. Another was a two-semester sequence for graduate students in the master's degree program and covered similar material to the above but in greater detail, at a more advanced level of basic knowledge and clinical application. The third course, also for graduate students, I offered in seminar format with a clinical practice component; it dealt with the pathophysiology, assessment, and management of both medical and surgical critical care states.

The fourth course, which I still teach, is a two-semester sequence, Primary Care I and II, which is the adult nurse practitioner specialty area in the Medical–Surgical Nursing Master's program. It combines some lecture material, seminar-type presentations of work-ups of their patients by the students, development of clinical protocols, and a major clinical practice component with physician and/or nurse practitioner preceptors in a variety of both in-patient and ambulatory clinical settings. The sequence covers the pathophysiology, manifestations, assessment, and management of commonly encountered acute and chronic, major and minor, clinical entities of adults. It includes the psychosocial

tion in the care of patients has added dimensions to the book's content which could have been achieved in no other way. In addition, he has patiently and conscientiously served as my preceptor in clinical practice as an adult nurse practitioner at the University of Colorado Hospitals for several years. What knowledge and competence in these functions I have, I owe largely to his teaching and example. I also wish to thank Thomas L. Kurt MD, formerly clinical faculty member of the Department of Medicine at the University of Colorado, for reading and commenting on the chapters on exercise and the heart, and cardiac arrhythmias; the contributions to this content made by his knowledge and clinical expertise in these areas is considerable.

Finally, Ann Underwood worked faithfully and competently in the preparation of the manuscript through several revisions to the finished product. I thank her warmly for her dedication and perseverance. Kay Horne also brought four of the chapters to typed first draft. I am grateful to them both.

G. J. S.

Contents

CHAPTER ONE

Disorders of Water and Solute Balance

NORMAL FLUID AND ELECTROLYTE HOMEOSTASIS

Introduction

Approximately 50–60% of the body weight is water; total body water (TBW) is 60% of the body weight in males, and about 50% in females. Total body water is distributed among a number of physiologic compartments, all of which are in equilibrium with each other. Two thirds of the TBW is in the intracellular space (intracellular fluid or ICF), and one third is in the extracellular space (extracellular fluid or ECF). One fourth of the extracellular fluid is intravascular (IVF; plasma). Serum is plasma without the fibrinogen and certain clotting factors. Interstitial fluid (ISF or extravascular ECF) is similar in composition to plasma, but with much less protein. These relationships are shown in Figure 1-1.

Electrolytes are unequally distributed between ICF and ECF across the two sides of the cell membranes. In the ICF the principal cation is potassium, and the anions are mainly phosphate, sulfate, and organic ions. Total body K^+ is about 2500 milliequivalents (meq; 1 meq is 1/1000 of the molecular weight of an ionized compound in grams divided by its valence) most of which is in the intracellular space. K^+ concentration in the ECF is only 3.8 to 5 meq/L, while in the ICF it is 150 meq/L. Sodium is the major cation, and chloride and bicarbonate the major anions, of the ECF. Total body Na^+ is about 4000 meq, most of which is in the extracellular space. Na^+ concentration in the ECF is about 143–152 meq/L; in the ICF it is about 14 meq/L. Cell membranes maintain this differential distribution of electrolytes between ICF and ECF mainly by oxygen- and energy-consuming active transport mechanisms. In addition to these ionic concentration gradients, electrical gradients also exist across most types of cell membranes, with the cell interior being electronegative to the interior by about −70 mV. Ions and their concentrations in ECF and ICF are diagrammed in Figure 1-2.

Water moves easily and rapidly across most cell membranes to and from the ICF and ECF. For this reason a change in osmotic pressure on either side of the

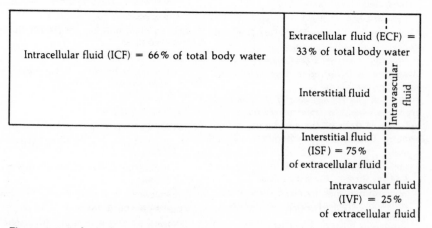

Figure 1-1. Body fluid compartments. Of the total body water, two thirds is intracellular fluid (ICF), while one third is extracellular fluid (ECF). The ECF in turn is comprised of three fourths interstitial fluid (ISF), which is extravascular ECF, while only one fourth is the intravascular fluid: the circulating blood volume.

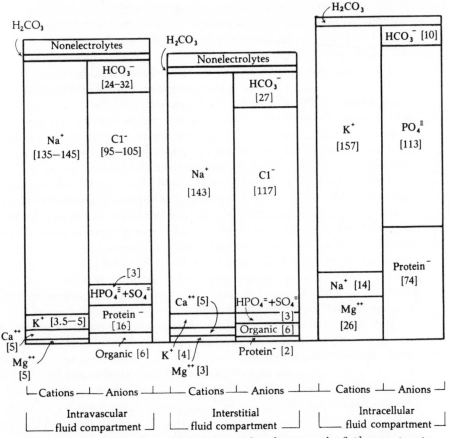

Figure 1-2. Constituents of intracellular, interstitial, and intravascular fluid compartments. The numbers in brackets refer to the approximate concentration of each component in milliequivalents per liter (meq/L).

Electrolytes		
Cations		*Anions*
Na⁺ – sodium		HCO₃⁻ – bicarbonate
K⁺ – potassium		Cl⁻ – chloride
Mg⁺⁺ – magnesium		PO₄⁼ – phosphate
Ca⁺⁺ – calcium		SO₄⁼ – sulfate
H⁺ – hydrogen		Protein anions
		Organic anions, such as acetate and lactate
Non-electrolytes		
Proteins		
H₂CO₃ – carbonic acid		

cell membrane, intracellular or extracellular, readily leads to osmotic movement of water along the osmotic gradient, into or out of the cell, until a new equilibrium is attained. On the other hand, electrolytes do not readily move across cell membranes, and when they do it is more often by some active transport mechanism rather than by passive diffusion along a concentration gradient.

The osmolarity of a solution refers to the number of osmols (the molecular weight of a substance in grams divided by the number of particles it dissociates into when in solution) of the substance per liter of the total solution, for example, plasma. The electrolytes (cations and anions) of the ICF and ECF are the principle determinants of body fluid osmolarity, and therefore of the osmotic pressure; there is a small additional component—the colloidal osmotic pressure—provided by the plasma proteins. In the normal individual plasma osmolarity is about 290 milliosmoles (1/1000 of an osmol) per liter (mosm/L). In the average individual who does not have abnormal quantities of plasma solutes, such as would be present in diabetic hyperglycemia (glucose) or uremia (urea), the plasma osmolarity can be estimated by doubling the serum sodium value in meq/L. A serum Na^+ of 142 meq/L thus yields an osmolarity of 284 mosm/L.

Although the ionic composition of ICF and ECF is quite different, the osmolarity of the two is identical; this sameness of osmotic pressure on the two sides of cell membranes is brought about by the fact that water moves readily across almost all cell membranes to equalize the osmotic pressures of the two compartments. Likewise, because of the easy and rapid movement of water between the intravascular and interstitial divisions of the ECF, osmolarity values here also are closely similar between the two; the osmotic pressure of the intravascular fluid (plasma) is slightly higher than interstitial because of the colloidal osmotic pressure contributed by the plasma proteins.

There are a number of mechanisms which operate to maintain not only normal ionic composition and osmotic concentration of body fluids, but also normal total fluid volume. Normal body fluid and electrolyte balance is the consequence of a dynamic equilibrium among oral fluid and dietary intake, and fluid and electrolyte equilibria mainly in the kidneys, but to some extent also in the lungs, skin, and gastrointestinal tract.

Physiologic Mechanisms Which Maintain Fluid Volume, Osmotic Concentration, and Ionic Composition

Water Regulation

Water Intake: Thirst and Drinking

Individual fluid intake habits, social custom, and the sensation of thirst which leads to drinking, are the main factors determining the volume of oral intake in a person with intact mental status, normal level of consciousness, and a neuromotor system that will support voluntary drinking. Neural mechanisms regulating the sensation of thirst and the motivation for oral intake are located in the hypothalamus, a portion of the upper brainstem concerned with the regulation of numerous appetitive and instinctual functions. The stimuli for thirst and drinking are two: a decrease in ECF volume and/or an increase in the osmotic pressure of the plasma.

The mechanisms by which hypovolemia activates thirst are complicated, and not all the steps are known. One factor, however, is that decreased renal perfusion, resulting from low ECF volume, stimulates the release of renin from the juxtaglomerular cells of the kidney, and the production of increased amounts of angiotensin II (Chapter 3 and Figures 3-2 and 3-3). One of the short-term effects of angiotensin II is to act on a structure called the subfornical organ located in the hypothalamus; this structure activates the neural substrates in the brain which are responsible for thirst sensations. Studies show that hypovolemia also stimulates thirst by an additional mechanism: there are low-pressure volume receptors in the atria of the heart and central veins; these apparently respond to a decrease in ECF volume by neural activation of the thirst centers.

A second major stimulus to thirst is elevated osmotic pressure of the ECF; elevated plasma osmotic concentration stimulates osmoreceptor cells, also in the hypothalamus, which activate nervous pathways causing thirst sensations. Thus the thirst–drinking processes help maintain both osmotic concentration and ECF volume within normal limits by promoting oral intake of hypotonic fluid. Sensations of thirst are also evoked by dryness of the pharyngeal mucous membranes and by hyperosmolar saliva. This explains why a patient who is fluid restricted may experience relief of thirst by sucking ice chips, a cool damp cloth, or a lemon swab, even though there is no actual oral fluid intake. The brainstem centers involved in water balance are shown in Figure 1-3.

Water Output: The Kidney and ADH

Antidiuretic hormone (ADH or arginine vasopressin) is one of the two known hormones stored by the posterior pituitary gland (neurohypophysis). ADH is synthesized by cells in the supraoptic and paraventricular nuclei of the hypothalamus, is transported along neurons connecting these nuclei with the posterior pituitary, and is stored in the latter gland for future release (Figure 1-3).

The action of ADH is on the distal nephrons and collecting ducts of the kid-

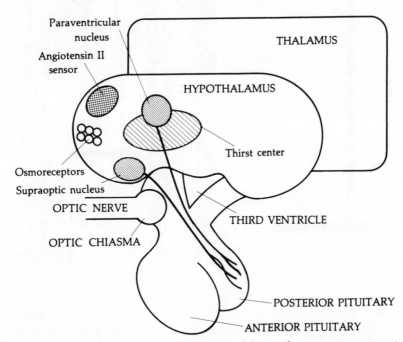

Figure 1-3. Upper brainstem areas involved in water balance. The important components of these areas are: (1) osmoreceptors that monitor the osmotic pressure of plasma; (2) the structure that responds to angiotensin II by stimulating the brainstem thirst-sensing area; (3) thirst center responding to stimuli from (1) and (2); (4) supraoptic and paraventricular nuclei that synthesize ADH; and (5) the posterior pituitary that stores and releases ADH in response to appropriate brain stimuli.

ney, where it increases the permeability of these structures to water. Under its influence water from the tubular fluid in the distal tubules and ducts moves into the hypertonic interstitium of the renal pyramids and thence into the microcirculation of the kidney, thus being returned into the ECF instead of being eliminated in the urine. Therefore the action of increased ADH secretion is to increase urine osmotic concentration and decrease urine volume. As a consequence the osmotic pressure of the plasma is decreased and ECF volume is increased by the retained water. Conversely, with low or absent ADH the urine becomes hypotonic to plasma because tubular water is retained in the ducts and then is lost in the urine, resulting in ECF water loss and increased plasma osmolarity. The relation between the kidney nephron and its blood supply that permits this exchange of water between tubular filtrate and capillary blood is shown in Figure 1-4.

As is the case with the thirst centers ADH formation and release is under the influence of both osmotic and volume factors. When osmotic pressure of the

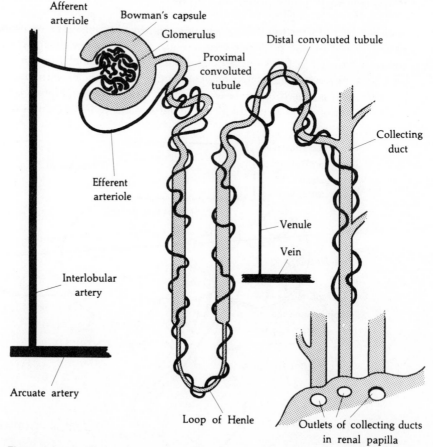

Figure 1-4. A nephron and its blood supply: the relation between the functional units of the kidney and their blood supply, the effectors for the renal regulation of water balance. Increased ADH secretion increases the permeability of the distal tubules and collecting ducts to water; the result is that more water is reabsorbed from the tubular filtrate back into peritubular blood, decreasing urine volume, increasing ECF volume, and decreasing ECF osmolarity.

ECF increases, osmoreceptors in the hypothalamus, located around the supraoptic and paraventricular nuclei (Figure 1-3), sense the increase and stimulate these nuclei to synthesize and secrete increased amounts of ADH. A decline in ECF osmotic pressure exerts an inhibitory influence on ADH formation. Very small changes in plasma osmolarity are sufficient to initiate osmoreceptor activation, though a continuous low-level release of ADH occurs to maintain ECF osmolarity close to 290 mosm/L.

Extracellular fluid volume is the other factor regulating ADH secretion. There are low-pressure sensors in the large veins, the atria of the heart, and probably in the pulmonary vasculature. These monitor the fullness of and pressure in the central venous system. With a moderate decline in circulating blood volume a decreased stimulation of the low-pressure receptors initiates decreased neural impulses from them and a stimulation of ADH release with resultant water retention. Conversely, ECF volume expansion in the normal subject suppresses the rate of ADH secretion by increasing the rate of neural firing in the low-pressure sensors. In addition, elevated angiotensin II probably stimulates the hypothalamic nuclei to produce more ADH. Figure 1-5 illustrates this relationship.

In the case of discongruent volume and osmotic stimuli, as in a hypovolemic

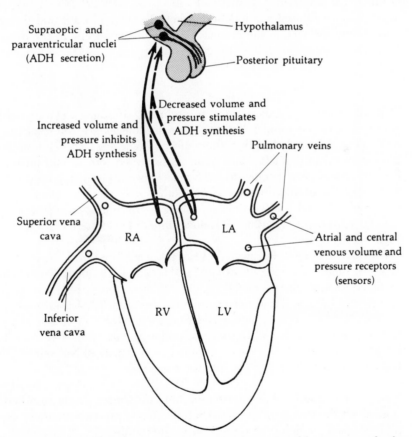

Figure 1-5. Relation between central venous pressure, monitored by pressure and volume receptors in the large veins and atria, and ADH synthesis and release. Increased volume and pressure in the central venous circuit inhibits ADH release; decreased volume and pressure stimulates it.

subject with hypoosmolar plasma (possibly in Addisonian crisis, for example) volume stimuli override osmotic stimuli, so that ADH secretion would increase to protect the patient against further hypovolemia, even at the cost of a further decline in plasma osmolarity.

Ionic Composition: The Kidney

Glomerular Filtration Rate (GFR)

This function in the normal subject is about 125 ml/min or 180 L/24 hr. Since the usual urine volume is around 1000 ml/24 hr, that means that almost 99% of the fluid filtered at the glomeruli is reabsorbed along the course of the tubules. A number of physiologic factors influence GFR, among them (1) the amount of renal blood flow; (2) the hydrostatic pressure in Bowman's space (elevated in kidney swelling or ureteral obstruction); and (3) the plasma protein concentration, which is the factor determining the colloidal osmotic pressure of the blood. In addition, in disease states such as glomerulonephritis and chronic renal failure, altered integrity of glomerular membranes and a decrease in the actual number of functional glomeruli will markedly affect overall GFR. The actual amount of any substance filtered is a function of both the overall GFR and the concentration of the substance in the plasma. Essentially everything in the plasma except the proteins filter through at the glomerulus.

Tubular Function

Depending on the location along the tubules, substances may be added to or resorbed from the tubular filtrate. Some substances are resorbed from the tubules along the whole length of the nephron; some are resorbed from it early but then secreted into it later; and some are secreted into it, and others resorbed from it, only at very specific sites. The mechanisms producing tubular transfer in and out of the tubular lumen include both active transport against a concentration gradient, and passive diffusion along a concentration gradient. The main sites for movement of various substances into or out of tubular fluid are shown in Figure 1-6.

Glucose is actively transported out of tubular filtrate in the first section of the proximal tubule; the renal threshold for this removal is about 200 mg glucose/100 ml blood; that is, glucose concentration in plasma above this level produces content in the tubular filtrate which exceeds the capacity of the tubular transport system. Na^+, K^+, PO_4^{3-}, amino acids, creatine, SO_4^{2-}, uric acid, and a number of other organic acids and organic molecules are also removed from the filtrate by active transport. The other site for active transport of Na^+ out of filtrate is at the distal renal tubule (see the following section).

Sodium Movement. Filtered sodium ions are almost totally resorbed from filtrate along the course of the renal tubule. There are two separate active transport pumps for sodium ion resorption in the tubule.

The proximal renal tubule electrogenic Na^+ pump. In the proximal tubule Na^+ diffuses passively from the filtrate into the tubular epithelial cells, but then is

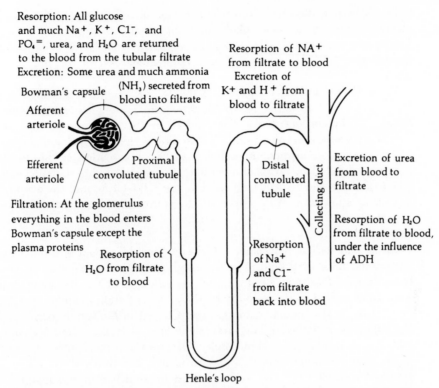

Resorption: All glucose
and much Na^+, K^+, Cl^-, and
$PO_4^=$, urea, and H_2O are returned
to the blood from the tubular filtrate
Excretion: Some urea and much ammonia
(NH_3) secreted from
blood into filtrate

Bowman's capsule

Afferent
arteriole

Efferent
arteriole

Proximal
convoluted tubule

Filtration: At the glomerulus
everything in the blood enters
Bowman's capsule except the
plasma proteins

Resorption of
H_2O from filtrate
to blood

Resorption of NA^+
from filtrate to blood
Excretion of
K^+ and H^+ from
blood to filtrate

Distal
convoluted
tubule

Collecting duct

Resorption
of Na^+
and Cl^-
from filtrate
back into blood

Excretion of urea
from blood to
filtrate

Resorption of H_2O
from filtrate to blood,
under the influence
of ADH

Henle's loop

Figure 1-6. Nephron sites of filtration of substances from the blood into the tubular filtrate; resorption from filtrate back into the blood; and excretion from blood into filtrate.

pumped actively by these cells into the peritubular interstitial fluid, where it is resorbed into the renal microvasculature and thus returned to the ECF. The high concentration of Na^+ in the interstitium around the proximal tubule raises the osmotic pressure there, and water moves from the tubular fluid into the interstitium along this osmotic gradient and is likewise returned to the ECF with the Na^+.

This sodium-resorbing mechanism is also responsible for resorption of part of the retained chloride ions. It works in the following way. As the tubular cells move the positively charged Na^+ into the renal interstitial fluid, negative charges are left behind inside the cell, and positive charges are added to the interstitial fluid. This creates an electrochemical gradient which draws chloride from the filtrate to the interstitium, where it is returned to the ECF with the Na^+ and H_2O. This mechanism is called the electrogenic sodium pump; it is inhibited by the diuretic ethacrynic acid.

The distal renal tubule cation exchange site. The second active transport system for Na^+ retention is the distal renal tubule coupled exchange pump (also called the distal renal tubule cation exchange site: DRT-CES) which transports Na^+ out of the tubule and into the interstitium in exchange for K^+ which is removed from interstitial fluid and secreted into the tubular fluid for elimination in the urine. In this case there is no net change in electrochemical gradient. Sodium and hydrogen ions also exchange in a similar way at this same site, but evidence is lacking that Na^+–H^+ exchange is an actual portion of the coupled exchange pump. It is more likely that the pump creates an electrochemical gradient favorable to Na^+–H^+ exchange, especially when K^+ concentration in the ECF is low. The ratio at which K^+ and H^+ is exchanged for Na^+ is $2K^+$ for every $1H^+$.

Three factors influence the rate of the Na^+–K^+ coupled exchange pump: (1) the amount of Na^+ delivered to the site from more proximal portions of the tubule; (2) the concentrations of K^+ and H^+ in the ECF; and (3) the concentration of aldosterone in the plasma. Aldosterone is the principal stimulating mechanism for Na^+ resorption in exchange for K^+ elimination at this locale. This pump is inhibited by ouabain (a cardiotonic drug related to digitalis) and triamterene (a drug which specifically inhibits the DRT-CES), and the action of aldosterone in stimulating it is suppressed by spironolactone, a specific aldosterone inhibitor.

Chloride and sodium movement. Chloride ions diffuse out of tubular fluid into peritubular interstitial fluid to be returned to the ECF along most of the course of the tubule. This movement is under the influence of Na^+ transport (as just described) as well as a tubule-to-interstitium concentration gradient for Cl^-. However, there is also an active transport of Cl^- out of the tubule occurring in the thick portion of the ascending limb of the loop of Henle. Here Na^+ moves out with it to maintain electrical neutrality. Of the various mechanisms for resorption of Na^+ from filtrate into the ECF, approximately two thirds of all sodium ions are resorbed with chloride ions, and one third are resorbed in exchange for K^+ and H^+.

Other factors influencing Na^+ movement. As is the case with water, about 98% of Na^+ filtered at the glomerulus is resorbed by the tubule. The fraction resorbed fluctuates to some extent with the amount filtered and with certain other factors. In general, the higher the GFR, the more is filtered and the more is resorbed. The lower the ECF volume, the less is filtered but also the more is resorbed. There is some evidence indicating that an additional factor operates along with GFR and aldosterone to modify the resorption–excretion ratios of sodium by the kidney. It has been suggested that this substance may act primarily to inhibit sodium resorption into the ECF from tubular filtrate at the proximal tubule. Research studies indicate that even when GFR and plasma aldosterone levels are held constant, an elevated ECF volume still promotes renal sodium elimination by inhibiting Na^+ resorption from filtrate into ECF. This influence has been termed natriuretic hormone or "third factor."

Water Movement. Approximately 100 L/24 hr of H_2O are filtered at the glomerulus, and 1 L/24 hr is excreted in the urine, so about 90% of the water filtered is resorbed into the ECF. The amount of water eliminated from the ECF can be varied (within limits) independently of the amount of solute excreted with it. The influence of ADH on the permeability to H_2O of the distal tubule and collecting duct is an important mechanism for this independent control of H_2O balance.

Fluid throughout the proximal tubule is isosmotic to plasma, so in this region water moves passively by osmosis out of the tubule back into the ECF along the osmotic gradient created by the active transport of solutes out of the filtrate. Three fourths of filtered water and solutes have been resorbed from tubular fluid by the time it reaches the end of the proximal tubule.

In juxtamedullary nephrons (Chapter 10) the loops of Henle dip down into the medullary pyramids and then curve back up into the cortex where the distal convoluted tubule begins. Beyond the distal tubule, the collection ducts go back down into the medullary area and drain into the renal pelvis at the apices of the pyramids (Figure 10-1). There is a graded increase in osmolarity of the interstitial tissue in the pyramid area; the osmotic pressure increases near the apices until it is much higher than that of the plasma. Since the loops of Henle curve down into this hypertonic tissue, a strong osmotic gradient is established across the loop membranes from the fluid in the lumens of the tubules to the medullary interstitium. Since the descending loop is permeable to water, water moves out of loop fluid along this osmotic gradient; this movement of water out of the tubules results in a great increase in osmotic concentration, and a large reduction in volume, of the fluid remaining in the lumens of Henle's loops.

The ascending limbs are impermeable to water, and here removal of Cl^- by active transport, accompanied by sodium ions (see above), results in a decreased osmotic pressure of tubular fluids, to about isosmotic concentration as it enters the distal tubule. At the distal tubule the cation exchange pump produces the changes in ionic composition discussed above.

Water movement at the distal tubule and collecting duct depends on the presence and concentration of ADH, as previously described. Movement of water out of the ducts, resulting in further concentration of urine, is facilitated by the high osmotic pressure of the medullary interstitium surrounding the ducts. The effect is similar to that described above for Henle's loops. Even in the total absence of ADH the distal nephron and ducts are never completely impermeable to the osmotic movement of water.

Urine osmolarity can fluctuate between 30 and 1400 mosm/L, and the specific gravity may vary from 1.010 to 1.035. Therefore the potentials of the various diluting and concentrating mechanisms described above are very great and they participate in a major fashion to the regulation of the volume and osmotic concentration of the ECF.

ABNORMALITIES OF WATER AND SOLUTE BALANCE

Deficiency of Water Relative to Solute, With or Without Volume Depletion: Dehydration, Hypernatremia, Hyperosmolar States

Causes

Inadequate Fluid Intake

Failure to replace urinary and insensible water losses—sweat from the skin, water vapor from the lungs, and about 100 ml/day in normal feces—will result in gradual dehydration. The minimal water intake required to replace urinary and insensible losses in the normal subject in an environment of usual temperature range is about 1000 ml/d. Inadequate oral fluid intake may occur because of neurologic impairment of the sensors in the upper brainstem responsible for responding to stimuli which normally cause thirst (slight increase in osmolarity of ECF or slight decline in ECF volume, as described in the previous section) so that the sensation of thirst is not experienced. Likewise, decreased levels of consciousness as in lethargy or stupor will cause a patient to fail to experience thirst sensations or, if they are experienced, may impair his ability to obtain or communicate the desire for water. In addition, altered mental status such as dementia, delirium, or psychosis may impair the behavioral response of drinking to sensations of thirst, as will muscular weakness or paralysis.

The effects of inadequate water intake occur more rapidly and are made worse by catabolic conditions such as rapid weight loss in which there is metabolic protein breakdown, or by an intake high in protein, glucose, and salt, such as tube feedings. Protein breakdown products increase the osmotic load of hydrogen ions, urea, and salt which must be removed, and therefore they make a large demand on the ECF volume for water to dilute these solutes so that they can be filtered and removed by the kidneys. Such a solute load requires large amounts of water to act as diluent and solvent for urinary solute excretion. The resulting osmotic water loss is called osmotic diuresis.

Excessive Loss of Water or Hypotonic Fluid

From the Skin.   Sweating is a significant mechanism for heat loss by evaporation of water from the skin. Hypotonic fluid loss in sweat normally is about 50 ml/h in a person at rest with normal body temperature in an environment of average temperature. With heavy muscular exercise in a warm environment fluid loss in the sweat may exceed 1000 ml/hr, however.

From the Lungs.   A marked increase in loss of water vapor from the lungs will occur in any condition in which there is hyperventilation, such as metabolic acidosis or the central neurogenic hyperventilation of brainstem trauma, both of which will be discussed in subsequent sections. Mechanical ventilation, with intubation or tracheostomy, will also induce water loss from the lungs unless adequate moisture is supplied by hydration of the airstream. Elevated body temperature greatly increases respiratory evaporation, and when combined with hyperventilation dehydration may occur rapidly. Elevation of serum sodium ion concentration above 155 meq/L seldom occurs as a result of increased water loss from lungs and intact skin alone, however, even though such insensible losses may reach several liters per day, especially if they involve combined abnormalities such as diaphoresis, fever, and marked hyperpnea.

From the Kidneys.   *Diabetes Insipidus (DI).*   Trauma, tumor, or other lesions of the hypothalamic structures concerned with ADH formation may cause inadequate synthesis and release of the hormone. The result of this deficit is decreased permeability of the distal nephrons and collecting ducts to water, so that tubular water cannot be resorbed into the ECF from the filtrate and is lost in the urine. The consequence is polyuria of an osmotically dilute, low specific gravity urine, and polydipsia, if the thirst and drinking mechanisms are intact. In the conscious person with chronic mild DI, elevated water intake will maintain the plasma at a close to normal, or perhaps a slightly hyperosmolar, water concentration. In more severe ADH deficit, where chronic replacement is required, synthetic vasopressin used as a nasal spray is usually adequate.

The danger of DI is its development in the unconscious patient who has sustained brainstem trauma, or has undergone a neurosurgical procedure such as hypophysectomy. Since a large negative water balance may develop rapidly, urinary volume and specific gravity must be carefully monitored and the losses replaced. Urine volume in such a patient who is also receiving a very low solute intake for any reason may be deceptively low. The reason for this is that low solute content of the ECF will lead to less solute being filtered at the glomeruli; tubular fluid will then be low in solute; the less solute there is in the tubular fluid, the less water will be retained and excreted with it, and this acts osmotically to restrict urinary loss. So urinary output may seem to be within normal limits, perhaps no more than 1500/24 hr, and the fact that the patient is dehydrating may not be evident from urine output alone.

A more complicated situation occurs in the patient who has sustained an upper brainstem lesion which has destroyed, or impaired circulation to, the anterior pituitary as well as the posterior pituitary and ADH-synthesizing nuclei. There may be a short period of polyuria soon after the injury, but then the DI diuresis may be greatly reduced or even absent. The reason for the lack of polyuria is the damage to the anterior pituitary, which results in the loss of its tropic hormones, especially adrenocorticotropin and thyrotropin. A marked decline in hormone output from the adrenal and thyroid glands ensues, causing a fall in glomerular filtration rate, a low serum content of organic solutes including glucose, a contracted ECF volume and a low serum Na^+, all of which will persist until there is replacement therapy with adrenal steroids and thyroxine.

Osmotic Diuresis. The hyperglycemia of severe uncontrolled diabetes mellitus causes loss of body water, dehydration, and hyperosmolarity of the plasma via several mechanisms. High plasma glucose content itself exerts a strong hyperosmolar effect. In addition, the glucose exceeds renal threshold and large amounts are excreted in the urine, taking much osmotically obligated water with it (osmotic diuresis). The water loss further concentrates plasma and leads to decline in ECF volume. Since in osmotic diuresis the urinary sodium ion concentration is less than that in the plasma (that is, the urine is hypotonic to plasma with respect to sodium in a patient having an osmotic diuresis), high levels of serum sodium (hypernatremia) develop and contribute significantly to the total hyperosmolarity of the plasma.

In such a hyperglycemic hyperosmolar patient the high glucose alone may lead to such hyperosmolarity of the plasma that the brainstem vital function centers are impaired (respiration, vasomotor control, and heart rate control) and the consciousness-maintaining functions of the brainstem reticular formation may deteriorate. The consequence is hyperosmolar coma and respiratory, cardiac, and vasomotor depression. At this point deterioration of the patient's condition may proceed rapidly in spite of treatment, in part because of hypovolemia and depressed brainstem control of vital functions. Tissue perfusion and cell oxygenation decline. Cellular hypoxia leads to anaerobic glycolysis with the production of lactate. Lactic acid contributes significantly to the hyperosmolarity, in addition to causing metabolic acidosis. Furthermore, lactic acid depresses myocardial contractility, and makes the blood vessels less responsive to catecholamines so that widespread vasodilation develops. A vicious cycle is now established, since with vasodilation and weaker cardiac pumping, tissue perfusion decreases further, lactic acid production rises more, and so on.

A controlled osmotic diuresis is often produced therapeutically in the brain-injured patient in order to lower ECF volume and draw edema fluid from the brain, since cerebral edema in these patients causes life-threatening elevated intracranial pressure, with depression of consciousness and of the brainstem control mechanisms for vital functions. Urea, mannitol, or glycerol may be used. These substances are not metabolized, but they are filtered at the glomeruli into the tubules and then not resorbed from the tubules. Hence they draw large amounts of ECF water into the tubules, which is then eliminated in the urine. Caution must be observed in their use, since renal water loss sufficient to cause severe dehydration and also plasma electrolyte abnormalities may occur if too much of these osmotic diuretics are administered.

Another cause of osmotic diuresis is high-protein tube feedings given to the obtunded or comatose patient. The result is a large plasma urea load, osmotic water loss, ECF dehydration, and hypernatremia. In such a patient the serum sodium may exceed 170 meq/L. In these often obtunded individuals, urinary output may be maintained within normal limits for a time because the osmotic diuresis obscures the fact that the high serum solute levels are producing severe dehydration and hyperosmolarity. That is, high urinary solutes draw water with them, disguising the patient's progressing dehydration and hypovolemia.

Evaporation from a Burn Surface.   The barrier to loss of water provided by the intact skin is disrupted in thermal burns, which destroy the stratum corneum. Loss of water occurs by evaporation even from areas of eschar, in addition to the moist burn surface, and, depending on the extent of the affected area and the methods of burn dressing, losses may exceed 3000 ml/24 hr. In addition there is ECF loss from extravasation and transudation into burn bullae, which also contain plasma proteins.

Consequences of Severe ECF Fluid Depletion

In all cases of water or hypotonic fluid loss a surprisingly large amount—as much as two thirds—of the total body water deficit in advanced dehydration comes from the intracellular fluid (ICF); ICF water therefore acts as a significant reservoir or buffer system operating in defense of ECF volume and osmolarity in the event of excessive water loss or inadequate intake. Since this is the case, an important aspect of patient evaluation in these conditions is the awareness that, if clinically evident dehydration and hyperosmolarity have developed, total body water deficit is already far advanced.

As the ECF becomes dehydrated and hyperosmotic with respect to the interstitial fluid (ISF), ISF water enters the capillaries along the osmotic gradient. This causes interstitial dehydration. Intracellular water then moves from the cells into the interstitial spaces and then into the intravascular compartment, because ICF became hypotonic to them as dehydration progressed. Now intracellular dehydration results. As these processes continue, when sufficient total body water depletion occurs then severe intracellular dehydration and ECF hypovolemia and hypotension develop, which is life-threatening.

Excess Accumulation of Solute: Hypernatremia and Hyperosmolarity

The conditions producing osmotic diuresis, discussed above, are ones in which there is excess ECF solute content. The actual development of intense hyperosmolarity is prevented, however, by the osmotic diuresis, which acts rapidly to remove solute. But this protective device is effective only as long as body water content is adequate to permit such removal by the kidneys. When production of the solute occurs at sustained high rates and/or total body water is inadequate to permit solute removal through diuresis, then hyperosmolarity will occur.

Hypernatremia is an increase in ECF Na^+ concentration relative to water. As is true in the conditions described in the preceding section, hypernatremia generally implies decreased body water relative to total body Na^+ content, and only seldom occurs as an absolute overall increase in total body sodium. In either case, relative or absolute hypernatremia develops, Na^+ migrates from the ECF into the ICF, and this acts as a first line of defense against the increasing osmotic pressure of the ECF. Entry of Na^+ into cells during hypernatremia not only lowers ECF Na^+ content, but elevates ICF osmotic pressure, protecting the cell interior from H_2O loss.

If the excess solute is other than Na^+, for example, glucose, lactic acid, or urea, the condition is called hyperosmolar state. In hypernatremia, of course, there is also hyperosmolarity of body fluids, since Na^+ is the principal determinant of ECF osmolarity. Occasionally hypernatremia may be the result of excess intravenous hypertonic saline or sodium bicarbonate infusion; the latter is often given after a cardiopulmonary arrest. Bicarbonate is used to combat the lactic acidemia resulting from anaerobic glycolysis during the hypoxic episode, but the excess Na^+ may cause hypernatremia.

Studies of the hyperosmolar state in critically ill patients have given useful information on the causes, complications, management, and outcomes of this condition. In such patients the abnormalities may arise as a result of either a marked loss in total body water, or a great increase in plasma solutes, or both. The solutes involved may be sodium, urea, glucose, lactate, or alcohol. Hyperosmolarity is defined as a plasma osmolarity in excess of about 350 mosm/L. The condition may develop as part of a severe progressive disease, or a complication of treatment of a serious illness. The most frequent causes are reported to be (1) renal failure (BUN above 150 mg% and creatinine above 5 mg%); (2) iatrogenic: $NaHCO_3$ IV "push," high-protein tube feedings, excessive NaCl infusions (in these causes the plasma Na^+ may be greater than 160 meq/L); (3) diabetes mellitus with hyperglycemia, with or without ketoacidosis, and an elevated BUN because of the severe osmotic diuresis (in some patients plasma glucose may be greater than 900 mg%); (4) hyperglycemia from hyperalimentation (plasma glucose may be greater than 800 mg%); (5) septic shock with the complication of renal failure resulting in a high plasma lactate and BUN; (6) dehydration from impaired mental status and level of consciousness, leading to lack of fluid intake and prerenal azotemia (Chapter 10); and (7) alcoholic stupor (blood alcohol may be greater than 400 mg%—this amount will increase plasma osmolarity by 100 mosm).

In severe hyperosmolarity, patients are comatose; most have impaired spontaneous respirations and therefore require mechanical ventilation. Most patients require nasogastric suction because of paralytic ileus. Mortality rates are reported to be high in such patients, often over 80%.

Assessment in Dehydration, Hypernatremia, and Hyperosmolarity

The signs and symptoms in this group of disorders of fluid and solute balance will vary, depending on the duration and severity of the underlying process, and the degree of accompanying ECF volume depletion. The signs and symptoms of volume depletion are rare in those processes involving simple dehydration, since fluid from the interstitial and intracellular spaces tends rapidly to enter the intravascular ECF compartment, and therefore to compensate ECF losses to a considerable extent. In mild to moderate simple dehydration there may be a decreased output of urine and it will be more concentrated, dry mouth, reduced tissue turgor, postural changes in blood pressure, and weight loss.

In more severe conditions which combine volume depletion and hyperosmolarity evidences of hypovolemia will often predominate. The signs and symptoms of ECF volume depletion are discussed in the next section.

In interpreting laboratory serum electrolyte values, it is important to recall that a serum sodium determination reflects only the sodium to water ratio, whether it is high, medium, or low, and does not give information about either total body sodium or total body water. Hypernatremia and hyperosmolarity are present when the serum Na^+ is above 145 meq/L, and the osmolarity is above 285–295 mosm/L.

Objective signs of hypernatremia and hyperosmolarity are difficult to separate from the evidences of the general systemic disorders preceding or accompanying the fluid and electrolyte abnormalities. These patients are usually already quite sick and often have multiple systemic abnormalities. In addition, it is quite difficult to distinguish the effects of hyperosmolarity per se from those of ECF volume depletion (when this is present) and from intracellular dehydration. The signs and symptoms in a critically ill patient probably relate to the latter state, and are attributable to dehydration of the neurons in the brain. Impairment of mental status and level of consciousness lead to irritability, confusion, stupor, and coma; these changes probably are caused by neuron dehydration and shrinkage, with loss of normal excitability characteristics. Brainstem vital function regulation is also impaired. During ECF hyperosmolarity, evidence indicates that neurons also accumulate intracellular solute so as to reduce the ECF to ICF osmotic gradient and minimize osmotic shrinkage of cells.

This neuron solute accumulation makes reversal of a severe hyperosmolar state in a critically ill patient somewhat precarious: when intravenous fluid is given to decrease hyperosmolarity and treat the hypovolemia, if present, water enters cells much more rapidly than excess solute can diffuse out. As ECF repletion occurs the ECF osmotic pressure declines, and the ICF spaces are now markedly hypertonic with respect to the ECF. The result is that water moves rapidly along the osmotic gradient from the ECF to the interior of the cells, causing them to swell. Seizures and cardiopulmonary arrest may occur, because the swelling alters the neuron membrane excitability characteristics, with severe disturbance to the brainstem vital function control centers and the brain motor areas. Thus, hyperosmolarity must be corrected slowly and only partially.

Prevention and Management of Dehydration, Hypernatremia, and Hyperosmolarity

Management often consists most importantly of treatment of the underlying systemic condition, while at the same time managing the fluid and electrolyte abnormality with oral fluids, where tolerated, or more usually with intravenous fluids: 5% dextrose in half normal saline or water. Since hyperosmolarity is present throughout the total body water, ICF as well as ECF, which itself is often low in volume, sometimes a surprisingly large amount of fluid is necessary to restore serum Na^+ to the normal 140 meq/L, perhaps up to 6000–8000 ml, given over a fairly extended period of time.

The most important components of assessment and management consists of prevention and early recognition. As is the case with all disturbances of fluid, electrolyte and acid–base balance; dehydration, hypernatremia, and hyperosmolarity arise in conjunction with, and as a complication of, general systemic disorders which predispose to their development. Thus prevention consists primarily in treatment of the patient's underlying disorders, recognition of the clinical situations in which such complications are most likely to develop, and anticipatory intervention directed at those components of patient management most likely, in each situation, to become the source of fluid imbalance.

Depletion of Both Water and Solute (Primarily Sodium): Hypovolemia

Causes

These disorders are the consequence of a loss of isosmotic body fluids, usually from the gastrointestinal tract, the vasculature, or the kidneys. Since the losses include Na^+, and since Na^+ is the ion which is the primary determinant of ECF volume, hypovolemia may become severe in these conditions.

Loss of Water and Solute Without Plasma Proteins (Loss of Isosmotic Fluid)

Volume depletion is the most common, and can be the most life-threatening, abnormality of fluid and electrolyte balance. It sometimes results from uncomplicated dehydration, or it may accompany hypernatremia as discussed in the preceding section, but it more often occurs in conjunction with isosmotic fluid and electrolyte losses. Renal and gastrointestinal abnormalities are the usual causes.

Gastrointestinal Secretions. Gastrointestinal secretions are produced at the rate of over 8000 ml/day, mainly in the upper digestive tract. In the normal person these fluids and electrolytes are resorbed farther on in the tract. But when they are lost from the body, as in vomiting, diarrhea, or gastric or duodenal drainage; or sequestered in the intestine, as in intestinal obstruction from strangulated hernia, a tumor, volvulus, or intussusception; or in paralytic ileus; marked decline in ECF volume will result. GI secretions are high in K^+, so hypokalemia may be a complication. If loss of the secretions are from the stomach the loss of gastric HCl may lead to a complicating metabolic alkalosis. If most are from the small intestine, including pancreatic secretions which are high in bicarbonate, a metabolic acidosis may be present.

Renal Na^+ and H_2O Loss.   *Chronic Renal Failure.*   This disorder often causes a decreased ability to retain both sodium and water because of impaired tubular resorption of both from the glomerular filtrate. The characteristic abnormality in chronic renal failure (CRF) is increased fractional excretion ratios of both Na^+ and water. This means that, although in renal failure less of both are filtered at the glomeruli, a greatly reduced percentage of what is filtered is resorbed at the tubules, and is therefore lost in the urine. This abnormality is made more severe where the patient's salt intake is for any reason restricted. Furthermore, the decline in ECF volume complicates the renal failure by causing a further decrease in renal perfusion leading to a still greater reduction in GFR, and hence a rising blood urea nitrogen (BUN) and creatinine.

Monitoring body weight and urinary Na^+ helps to avoid a worsening of uremia caused by ECF depletion. Nausea and vomiting often accompany uremia, as does decreased food and fluid intake from anorexia, and such complications deplete ECF sodium and water still more. In this combination of inadequate intake and excess loss, GFR can no longer be maintained at levels sufficient to maintain urea filtration, causing an elevation of the BUN. The increased urea, in turn, increases the solute load, contributing to an osmotic diuresis with resulting enhanced sodium and water depletion.

Diuretic Phase of Acute Renal Failure (ARF).   Following the oliguria of ARF a diuresis occurs which generally lasts for only a few days and therefore is not a serious problem provided salt intake and water intake is normal. This diuresis usually occurs on two bases: (1) during the oliguric phase salt and water are retained, and in addition excess parenteral fluids may have been administered causing an expansion of the ECF; and (2) in early recovery there is impaired ability of the tubules to resorb the sodium and water which are filtered at the glomeruli. The consequence is an increased fractional excretion ratio for both water and sodium as occurs chronically in some stages of chronic renal failure. Urinary Na^+ may be greater than 50 meq/L, indicating high rate of Na^+ loss. Excess water and Na^+ loss may occur also following a urinary tract obstruction (postobstructive nephropathy); tubular resorptive function is impaired for a time such that, following reversal of the obstruction, a similar self-limited period of diuresis may occur. During an acute rejection episode following kidney transplant a similar diuresis of water and Na^+ often develops.

Adrenal Insufficiency (Addison's Disease).   Inadequate production of mineralocorticoids, primarily aldosterone, from the adrenal cortex, leads to impairment of the kidney tubules' ability to reabsorb adequate amounts of Na^+. The Na^+ is lost in the urine, taking water with it. Adrenal insufficiency may develop acutely as in post traumatic or postburn adrenal hemorrhagic necrosis, but more often it develops insidiously from an infection or immunologic process, leading to a chronically low circulating blood volume. This chronic hypovolemia predisposes the patient to rapid development of peripheral vascular collapse in the face of trauma, surgery, infection, or other physiologic stress. Metabolic acidosis and hyperkalemia are frequent accompaniments of the low Na^+ and ECF state of aldosterone deficiency, since lack of stimulation to the DRT-CES permits excessive Na^+ loss, and a retention of the ions normally excreted in exchange for its resorption: K^+ and H^+.

Diuretics. Most diuretics impair tubular Na^+ resorption either at the distal renal tubule cation exchange site or more proximally where Na^+ is resorbed with Cl^-. Diuretics may be given for the relief of edema associated with congestive heart failure, cirrhosis, or nephrosis; and if they are continued after the interstitial fluid accumulation has been reduced to more normal levels, ECF depletion and hypovolemia may occur. Also diuretics which are given in an effort to reduce the accumulation of ascites fluid in portal hypertension may pose a similar problem, since this fluid is, for a number of reasons among which one is its high protein content, difficult to mobilize.

Thiazide diuretics are less likely to further deplete ECF sodium when levels of that ion become abnormally low than are the strong diuretics such as furosemide and ethacrynic acid, which stimulate continued sodium loss even when it is so low as to already have caused some hypovolemia and a decreased GFR.

Extreme Sweating. In moderate sweating the sweat is hypotonic not isosmotic so the consequence may be dehydration and hypernatremia. Greatly increased sweat production, however, leads to a marked increase in sodium content of sweat and therefore volume depletion may occur. The use of salt tablets during heavy exertion in a warm environment or hot weather should probably be avoided. The salt tablets produce a very high osmotic concentration in the gastrointestinal tract, which acts to draw intravascular and interstitial fluid along the osmotic gradient into the gut lumen. This may result in sudden hypovolemia and peripheral vascular collapse, especially when accompanied by peripheral vasodilation and diaphoresis, as would be characteristic physiologic responses to exercise in warm surroundings. Isosmotic fluid intake is preferable.

Sequestration of Water and Solutes, With or Without Plasma Proteins: The "Third Space"

As described earlier, total body water is distributed between the intracellular and the extracellular compartments, the latter being divided into intravascular and interstitial spaces. The concept of the "third space" evolved to encompass that group of abnormalities in which appreciable quantities of extracellular fluid are sequestered in areas or structures in which they are not normally found. If such an accumulation occurs in large amounts, and rapidly, the consequence is ECF volume contraction and hypovolemia. The initial deficit is intravascular, as is true with hypovolemia from loss of isosmotic fluid to the environment. The "third space" is therefore always an abnormal space, whether it develops rapidly as in burn wound edema, with accompanying hypovolemia; or more gradually as occurs in the ascites of cirrhosis with portal hypertension, or the interstitial edema of congestive heart failure, in which case hypovolemia is not a feature.

There are several categories of third spacing. Fluid may collect in a body cavity. In hydrothorax the fluid is often transudative (S.G. < 1.1015 and protein < 2.5 gm%). The causes may be pleural effusion from the elevated pulmonary capillary pressure of congestive heart failure, or the decreased plasma colloidal osmotic pressure of nephrosis or cirrhosis. The fluid is sometimes exudative (S.G. > 1.015 and protein > 2.7 gm%); here the causes may be tuberculosis, rheumatoid arthritis, pulmonary malignancy, pneumonia, or a pulmonary embolus which has caused infarction of a portion of the lung. In abdominal ascites the fluid is often transudative, from congestive heart failure, cirrhosis and portal hypertension, or nephrosis with marked hypoproteinemia.

A hollow viscus may be the site of third spacing; a prominent example is the intestine in mechanical intestinal obstruction or paralytic ileus.

The interstitial space is often the site of abnormal accumulations of interstititial fluid which is isosmotic and largely free of plasma proteins. This may occur in the edema of congestive heart failure, portal hypertension, or nephrosis; it results from elevated capillary hydrostatic, and decreased plasma colloidal osmotic, pressures.

Third spacing is a common occurrence in trauma edema, burns, and crushing tissue injuries. Tissue damage causes increased capillary permeability. Fluid, electrolyte, and often plasma proteins ooze out of the capillaries and accumulate in the damaged tissue. Burn bullae contains fluid that is almost identical with plasma, most of which is eventually lost from the body. But the interstitial spaces in trauma and burns sequester very large amounts of plasma from the ECF. As much as 15% of the body weight may be lost from the ECF into the ICF within a short time following a major injury, resulting in severe hypovolemia and hypotension.

Likewise, if thoracentesis or paracentesis is performed and much fluid is rapidly removed from those body areas, because of the abnormal characteristics of capillaries in the third space, or persistence of other physiologic derangements which caused the fluid to accumulate in the first place, these cavities may refill rapidly from the ECF causing hypovolemia and hypotension. Hypovolemia is less likely to occur in a patient who is edematous, since the interstitial fluid accumulation in edema readily moves into the intravascular space permitting rapid repletion of circulating blood volume.

As certain forms of third spacing resolve, the reentry of the fluid into the circulating blood may cause ECF overload. In the case of sequestration of plasma in the interstitial spaces from trauma, or collections of isosmotic transudates or interstitial edema in CHF, as capillary permeability is restored to normal by healing in the former, and capillary hydrostatic pressure declines in the latter with treatment (bed rest, oxygen, digitalis) the abnormal collections of fluid are mobilized from "third spaces" and resorbed into the circulation. The result is an increase of intravascular ECF which may be sufficient to cause intravascular overload; this hypervolemia increases venous return to the right heart and may cause left ventricular overload, elevated pulmonary capillary pressure, and pulmonary edema, especially in a patient with borderline left ventircular performance.

Acute Hypovolemia and Hypovolemic Shock

The factors regulating blood pressure may be expressed by the formula: systemic arterial pressure = cardiac output (heart rate × stroke volume) × total peripheral resistance. The interaction of these parameters involved in maintaining systemic arterial pressure within normal limits are discussed in Chapter 3. However, the formula is useful in this context: reduction in circulating blood volume brought about by marked fluid loss from the vasculature will produce a decline in venous return to the right atrium and a resulting reduction in cardiac output into the systemic circuit from the left ventricle. According to the relationship above, a decline in cardiac output without a compensatory increase in peripheral vasoconstriction will lead to a decline in blood pressure.

Causes of Hypovolemic Shock. Any one of the causes of ECF volume depletion described in preceding sections may lead to shock if not recognized and reversed before hypovolemia is well established. The consequences of hypovolemia depend to an important extent on the rapidity with which it develops; upon complicating conditions such as hypoxemia, impaired myocardial contractility, and presence of toxic agents from tissue destruction; and upon the integrity of compensatory mechanisms which operate to maintain tissue perfusion in the face of decreased circulating blood volume. The hallmark of hypovolemic shock, regardless of cause, is a significant generalized decline in tissue perfusion.

Compensatory and Correctional Responses to Hypovolemic Shock. A relatively minor rapid reduction in the circulating plasma volume, of the order of 500–1000 ml, leads to the activation of a number of both compensatory and correctional mechanisms for maintaining systemic arterial pressure, and hence tissue and organ perfusion, within normal limits. Rapidly acting *compensatory* responses to a drop in ECF are increased heart rate and peripheral vasoconstriction. These responses are mediated by the high pressure baroreceptors in the aortic arch and carotid sinuses which sense the decline in blood pressure caused by the low ECF volume; they send afferent impulses to the brainstem vasopressor area which result in generalized vasoconstriction. In addition, baroreceptor stimulation results in accelerated heart rate, by inhibiting the cardioinhibitory centers resulting, according to the formula, in increased cardiac output. Hypotension also activates the sympathetic nervous system to produce widespread adrenergic discharge, leading to increased heart rate and myocardial contractility, as well as widespread vasoconstriction. According to the relationships given in the equation above, arterial blood pressure is elevated by both increased cardiac output and increased total peripheral resistance, to compensate for the decreased volume, and to maintain tissue perfusion. These are reflex compensatory changes.

We will take a brief detour at this point. Students are sometimes confused by the statement that an increase in vasoconstriction (elevated peripheral resistance) can improve tissue perfusion. Like everything else, this is a matter of degree. The perfusion pressure in a system of fluid-filled tubes is a function of the volume of fluid, the rate of flow and the cross-sectional diameter of the system. If the volume declines, then the perfusion pressure will decline, unless the cross-sectional diameter is reduced, or the pumping force behind the fluid is increased, or both. An *excessive* degree of vasoconstriction (greatly decreased cross-sectional diameter) will of course reduce perfusion of a tissue, and in fact this does actually occur in the extreme vasoconstriction (overcompensation) sometimes ensuing as a result of profound and protracted hypovolemia and hypotension. As is well known from the clinical setting, such overcompensatory vasoconstriction will produce, for example, acute and sometimes irreversible ischemic kidney damage. But a moderate degree of generalized vasoconstriction acts to reduce the total cross-sectional diameter of the vasculature, accommodate it to the reduced circulating blood volume, and therefore increase perfusion pressure to the organs and tissues.

An early *correctional* response operating to combat hypovolemia is a largely hydrostatic one. As pressure declines in the vascular tree from isosmotic fluid loss, interstitial fluid moves readily along the lowered pressure gradient into the intravascular space. Then intracellular water moves into the interstitial spaces, equalizing fluid distribution to some extent, but causing some intracellular dehydration. Note that this fluid replacement is electrolyte, not colloid, so that in blood loss, colloid osmotic pressure of ECF is decreased, even though volume repletion in the ECF may have occurred by this mechanism.

There are several more slowly developing correctional mechanisms operating to restore normal ECF volume as a response to isosmotic intravascular fluid loss: (1) stimulation of ADH release; and (2) activation of the renin–angiotension–aldosterone system. Both of these operate to increase ECF volume, the former by improving water resorption in the distal tubule and collecting duct; and the latter by increasing distal tubule sodium ion resorption, which retains osmotically obligated water with it and expands ECF volume and maintains normal osmotic concentration. Additional slower correction of volume depletion and blood composition is attained by (1) stimulation of the renal hormone erythropoietin, which causes production of increased numbers of erythrocytes; and (2) an increased synthesis of plasma proteins by the liver, which helps to retain fluid in the vascular tree by increasing plasma colloidal osmotic pressure. These last two mechanisms are activated more commonly in whole blood, rather than ECF water and electrolyte, loss.

A more marked reduction of intravascular ECF, of about 20% (1000 ml) or more, leads to a greatly reduced venous return to the right atrium and hence a large drop in cardiac output which produces a more intense baroreceptor stimulation and exaggerated adrenergic response. Both arteriole and venule vasoconstriction occurs in a selective or differential pattern. The skin and most viscera have mainly α-adrenergic receptors, and so respond to endogenous catecholamines by vasoconstriction. Conversely, those organs with a smaller supply of α receptors, such as skeletal muscle and myocardium, undergo less vasoconstriction and therefore receive a proportionately greater blood supply. Muscle tissue has mainly β-adrenergic receptors; these respond to the endogenous catecholamines by increased rate and contractility in the case of myocardium, and vasodilation in skeletal muscles. Since the brain is not well supplied with either α or β receptors, vessel diameter there is not very responsive to sympathetic stimulation.

Secondary Abnormalities in Hypovolemic Shock.   Sympathetic adrenergic manifestations comprise a significant aspect of assessment in rapid marked hypovolemia and hypotension. The patient may become restless and anxious early in the course because of sympathetic stimulation to the brainstem reticular formation and reticular activating system. Later, as inadequate cerebral perfusion and hypoxemia develop, apathy, lethargy, and obtundation may ensue. Tachycardia, tachypnea, skin pallor, diaphoresis, and piloerection are all sympathetic adrenergic manifestations.

Because decreased renal perfusion leads to a prompt decline in GFR, oliguria, sometimes of less than 25 ml/hr, may develop. Intrarenal circulatory reflexes occur in response to the profound decline in kidney perfusion; there is abnormal blood distribution with a pale relatively bloodless cortex and congested medullary areas. Kidney impairment in which prerenal azotemia from inadequate renal blood flow progresses to acute renal failure results from prolonged severe hypoperfusion; if the hypovolemia has resulted from a condition causing hemolysis or myoglobinemia, such as muscle crush injuries, kidney damage will be increased by hemoglobin deposition in the glomerular filters and tubules (Chapter 10).

Impairment of myocardial function occurs in hypovolemia of this severity. A blood pressure of less than about 75 mmHg is inadequate to sustain coronary blood flow and results in myocardial ischemia and hypoxia. Generalized anaerobic metabolism leads to lactic acid accumulation with resulting myocardial depression. In this event cardiac output declines, lowering the already inadequate tissue perfusion—a vicious cycle as we saw already in severe osmotic diuresis. When acidosis develops, the oxygen–hemoglobin dissociation curve is shifted in the direction of increased hemoglobin affinity for oxygen, impairing hemoglobin release of oxygen to the tissues.

Perfusion to the liver is adequate early in hypovolemic shock, but later it and the whole splanchnic vascular bed develop vasocongestion and stagnant hypoxia. The liver then can no longer carry out its detoxification and other metabolic functions, so organic acids, glucose, and potassium released from the intracellular spaces enter the circulation. Hypoxic viscera, especially the pancreas, release toxic substances which further depress myocardial contractility. As cellular damage becomes more generalized, intracellular enzymes and kinins, and other vasoactive substances, are released which cause generalized vasodilation, depressed myocardial contractility, and elevated capillary permeability. The microcirculation is often further impaired by a consumption coagulopathy: disseminated intravascular coagulation (DIC), or defibrination syndrome. Eventually the intestinal mucosa loses its selective permeability and toxic substances from the lumen diffuse into the blood.

The lungs early in shock are not adversely affected beyond some ventilation–perfusion mismatch which produces a mild hypoxemia and hypocapnia (Chapters 2 and 9). However, in severe hypovolemia, especially if protracted, there is atelectasis, vasocongestion, and consolidation; the alveolar–capillary membranes are adversely affected by inadequate perfusion such that respiratory gas transport is decreased, fluid collects in the interstitial and intraalveolar spaces, lung compliance declines, and arterial hypoxemia may become extreme (below 45 mmHg PaO_2). This complication is termed adult respiratory distress syndrome, traumatic lung, or shock lung.

Patient Assessment in Hypovolemic Shock.   Evaluation of the patient in conditions where hypovolemic shock may develop consists in watching for signs of inadequate brain perfusion and the sympathetic automatic and general physiologic manifestations mentioned above: mental status and level of consciousness, skin condition, blood pressure and heart rate, and urinary output. In the critical care setting, continuous monitoring of EKG, intraarterial pressure, central venous pressure, and pulmonary capillary wedge pressure with a Swan-Ganz catheter, are technologic means of accurate patient assessment for evaluating progression of the hypovolemia; and the response to volume expansion with intravenous fluids, and to pharmalogic measures.

Management in Hypovolemic Shock.   *Ascertain and Reverse the Cause and Institute Prompt Volume Expansion.*   The interventions in acute hypovolemic shock consist in ascertaining the cause so that it can be reversed, and prompt and effective volume repletion with intravenous electrolytes, colloids, and blood. General measure include supine position to assist cerebral perfusion; relief of pain and restlessness if necessary with minimal analgesics to avoid respiratory depression; oxygen by nasal prongs; monitoring of arterial blood gases to check on metabolic acidosis, hypoxemia, and respiratory alkalosis, and to assess the possible development of pulmonary shunting. Dextrans and colloidal albumin remain longer in the circulation than crystalloids and produce a significantly greater volume expansion because of the colloidal osmotic pressure effects they exert. The central venous pressure should probably not rise above 15 cmH_2O because of the danger of left ventricular overload and pulmonary edema from elevated pulmonary capillary pressure. Posterior lung fields should be checked for bibasilar rales indicating development of this complication. This is especially important if the patient has a history of impaired myocardial contractility (congestive heart failure or borderline compensation). A Swan-Ganz catheter is useful in evaluating the balance between volume repletion and myocardial performance. Pulmonary artery diastolic and pulmonary capillary wedge pressures are taken as reflections of left ventricular end-diastolic pressure; they evaluate the completeness of left ventricle emptying and so reflect its contractility in the light of its hemodynamic load (Chapters 5 and 7).

Autonomic pharmacologic agents.   The use of autonomic pharmacologic agents in hypovolemic shock appears to be an area of some disagreement in the management of this disorder. It is certain that in hypovolemic shock the endogenous catecholamines, epinephrine and norepinephrine, are secreted in large amounts both from adrenergic nerve terminals and the adrenal medulla. The more severe and protracted the shock, probably the greater the output of these sympathetic autonomic substances.

Epinephrine is secreted by the adrenal medullae; it stimulates both α- and β-adrenergic receptors and constricts blood vessels in the skin and splanchnic areas but not vessels of the skeletal muscles. Norepinephrine, secreted both by adrenergic nerve terminals and the adrenal medullae, stimulates α receptors more than β, and constricts blood vessels in all areas.

The agents used in the clinical setting vary in their pharmacologic actions as α or β adrenergic stimulators (agonists). Pure α receptor stimulation causes generalized vasoconstriction of muscle, skin, and splanchnic–visceral areas; relaxation of intestinal musculature; and contraction of pupillodilator muscles. Pure β receptor activation results in stimulation to heart muscle rate and force of contraction, and increase in facility of cardiac impulse conduction; generalized vasodilation of skin, muscle, and splanchnic–visceral areas; and relaxation of smooth muscle in bronchi and intestine.

Methoxamine is an almost pure α-adrenergic agonist, that is, it is a sympathominetic agent with α effects which are primarily vasoconstriction.

Isoproterenol is a pure β agonist, that is, a sympathomimetic agent which is a strong vasodilator: it relaxes vascular smooth muscle; it stimulates the myocardium to increased rate and force of contraction and facilitates transmission of the cardiac impulse along the conduction pathways of the heart. A large increase in stroke volume and cardiac output is the result of these actions, since elevated cardiac output is coupled with decreased peripheral resistance to ventricular ejection (decreased afterload, Chapter 7). It probably does not elevate blood pressure.

Norepinephrine causes both α- and β-adrenergic stimulation; it constricts all blood vessels, both in the skin and skeletal muscles, and in the visceral and splanchnic circulation. It raises blood pressure. It increases the force and rate of heart muscle contraction, but minute volume does not change significantly because of the elevated peripheral resistance (increased afterload); that is, the heart is doing increased pressure work, not volume work.

Metaraminol is a substance which when injected is taken up by sympathetic nerve endings, replacing norepinephrine. Then when sympathetic nerves are activated, the new transmitter is released instead of norepinephrine. The effects are essentially those of norepinephrine but are longer lasting: vasoconstriction of skin, muscles, and splanchnic–visceral structures; increase in rate and force of heart contraction without much increase, if any, of cardiac output and elevation of blood pressure.

Some general guidelines for the use of vasoactive drugs in hypovolemic shock have been provided: (1) sparing usage of all such agents; (2) slow or inadequate response to volume expansion may be an indication for cautious trial of a vasoconstrictor; (3) vasodilators may be tried for shock in which endogenous vasoconstriction is marked, and fluid repletion has not resulted in improved clinical status; (4) vasodilators should be avoided if central venous pressure is low; if it is high then such agents may improve renal blood flow and promote diuresis, relieve too-intense peripheral vasoconstriction, and elevate blood pressure and perhaps increase cardiac output by exchanging pressure work for volume work; (5) a great danger in the use of vasoconstrictors is the increase of blood flow to the brain and heart at the expense of the kidneys, which will promote renal vasoconstriction, decreased GFR, and possibly acute renal failure. The impaired renal hemodynamics in shock may improve with the use of furosemide, which appears to promote renal vasodilation and improve renal blood flow.

Correctional Responses to Isosmotic Fluid Loss and Hypovolemia

There are several correctional mechanisms of response to depleted Na^+ and low ECF which operate to increase conservation of body sodium and water and to restore ECF volume: (1) a decline in ECF leads to decreased renal perfusion, decreased GFR, and a corresponding decline of Na^+ filtered at the glomerulus; (2) the kidney increases production of renin from the juxtaglomerular cells; this renin acts to elevate plasma antiogension II, a strong stimulus to aldosterone secretion by the adrenal cortex and therefore to Na^+ resorption at the DRT-CES; (3) "third factor"—the postulated natriuretic substance—may be suppressed; (4) the neurohypophysis releases increased amounts of ADH which increases resorption of water at the distal nephron and collecting ducts; and (5) the thirst center is stimulated to induce an increased oral fluid intake.

Patient Assessment in Isotonic Fluid Loss and Hypovolemia

History

Since most conditions of ECF depletion, as with all disorders of fluid, electrolyte, and acid–base balance, occur in conjunction with acute or chronic systemic disorders; the clinical situation and the immediate and past health history of the patient are of great importance in determining the cause of the disturbance. One needs to ascertain symptoms of an illness, such as chills and fever; symptoms of development or exacerbation of a chronic systemic disorder; prior fluid intake; symptoms which would inhibit oral intake such as severe pharyngitis, and a history of vomiting, diarrhea, or polyuria. Does the patient have a strong family history for renal disorders, and what is his own renal status? Has there been use of diuretics? Has he an endocrine abnormality such as Addison's disease or diabetes? In interviewing the patient it is important to take note of mental status and level of consciousness, such as signs of apathy, mental confusion, or drowsiness, which might indicate decreased cerebral perfusion, or point to a systemic disorder causing the ECF depletion.

Physical Examination

Palpation and inspection of the skin may reveal decreased tissue turgor, especially of the face and extremities. Postural blood pressure and pulse rate measurements should always be taken in conditions of suspected hypovolemia. A drop of blood pressure of 10 mmHg on changing from lying to sitting (or standing, if the patient is able), accompanied by increased heart rate of more than 10–20 beats per minute, indicates hypovolemia. The mechanism for this response is that the effect of gravity on blood distribution lowers perfusion pressure at the aortic arch and carotid sinus baroreceptors and initiates a reflex tachycardia. If hypovolemia is more severe there will be hypotension and tachycardia even when the patient is reclining and at rest. The eyeballs may feel soft to gentle palpation on closed lids. There may be oliguria from decreased renal perfusion. The mouth may be dry and the tongue appear fissured.

Laboratory Values

In loss of isosmotic fluid the serum Na^+ will usually be within normal limits; that is, Na^+ concentration *relative to water* in the ECF will not be low, although *total body* Na^+ would be low if it could be measured. (Similarly, in isosmotic hypervolemia, in which edema may occur, serum Na^+ is often normal or even low, although total body Na^+ content is increased.) A serum Na^+ determination gives information only as to the Na^+ concentration relative to body water. Elevated hematocrit, plasma proteins, and hemoglobin may indicate decreased plasma volume on the basis of isosmotic loss. An elevated plasma creatinine concentration is an early warning of ECF volume depletion, which is causing a decreased GRF. This value may increase even before the reduced renal perfusion has led to discernible oliguria. Urinary Na^+ determinations may be helpful in identifying the cause of an isosmotic ECF loss: if an abnormality involving the kidney is the cause, then urinary Na^+ may be above 30 meq/24 hr indicating renal failure, adrenocortical insufficiency or a diuresis; if the depletion has been caused by loss of gastrointestinal secretions or sweat, then the ECF volume contraction produces a marked renal Na^+ retention so that urinary sodium will be very low. The low urinary sodium results in the short term from a fall in GFR with reduced Na^+ filtration and increased tubular resorption; and in the longer term from stimulation to the renin–angiotensin–aldosterone system which promotes Na^+ conservation. In the nonrenal cause of isosmotic fluid loss, urinary Na^+ will be low; less than 10 meq/24 hr.

Management of Isosmotic Fluid Loss and Hypovolemia

The goal of treatment once the problem has been recognized is to remove the cause, or correct it, and to expand the ECF with oral fluid intake where indicated; or with saline, colloid, or blood, depending on the hematocrit. Monitoring during volume repletion in a seriously ill patient is often useful to determine whether rate and amount are adequate: improvement in skin turgor, mental status and level of consciousness, blood pressure and heart rate, serum creatinine, and increase in body weight are all useful indices of volume repletion. Increased urine output signals improved renal perfusion, and serum Na^+ determinations will indicate the Na^+ to H_2O ratio. Other electrolyte and acid–base abnormalities would be corrected if present, for example, the hypokalemia and alkalemia of gastric secretion loss from severe vomiting.

Deficiency of Sodium Relative to Water: Hyponatremia

Sodium is the cation in highest concentration in the ECF and therefore it is the most important factor determining osmolarity of the extracellular fluid. Since the osmotic pressure of the ECF determines the distribution of water between the ECF and ICF, serum sodium level plays a crucial role in this extracellular–intracellular water balance. Hyponatremia may be defined as a decrease in the ECF sodium–water ratio, which in the normal subject is a serum sodium concentration of about 140 meq/L. Hyponatremia may result from any process in which body water is retained in excess of sodium, as occurs in excessive ADH secretion; or in which body sodium is lost in excess of water, as in a failure of the renal tubular sodium resorption mechanisms. It should be emphasized again that any serum electrolyte measurement gives information only about the ratio between ECF levels of that electrolyte and the ECF water, not about the total body content of either water or electrolyte. Since sodium is the ion responsible for the major contribution to ECF osmolarity, hyponatremia implies hypoosmolarity, except in cases of abnormally high ECF content of another osmotically active substance such as urea, glucose, or mannitol.

Causes of Hyponatremia

Correction of Hypovolemia with Excess Hypoosmotic Fluid

Depletion of isosmotic extracellular fluid, as in the conditions discussed in the prior section, causes a marked decline in blood flow to the kidney. Such decreased renal perfusion exerts a strong inhibition of the glomerular filtration rate, which declines not only because of the decrease in ECF volume, but also because of renal vasoconstriction. This response is part of the compensatory adrenergic response to hypovolemia. However, the depressed GFR markedly impairs the kidneys' ability to eliminate a sudden water load. If then during the process of repletion of ECF following hypovolemia, a large amount of water is taken orally, or hypoosmotic fluid is administered intravenously, the urine-diluting mechanisms of the kidney are unable to eliminate excess body water rapidly enough to prevent dilution of the serum Na^+ content, and hyponatremia results.

Syndrome of Inappropriate Secretion of ADH (SIADH)

As discussed previously, the amount of ADH released from the hypothalamus is a significant factor in determining the solute–water ratio present in the urine. Excessive secretion of ADH may lead to urine osmolarity of over 900 mosm/L, indicating marked retention of water in excess of solute, particularly Na^+. That is, Na^+ is being lost in the urine in excessive amounts relative to urinary water output. The result is hyponatremia and an expanded hypoosmolar total body water. A number of theories have been advanced to account for the persistent hyponatremia in certain forms of SIADH, but at the present time the responsible mechanisms are as yet not known. It is probably of significance for theories of the cause of the continued water retention, urinary Na^+ loss, and hyponatremia of SIADH, that in this disorder plasma renin concentration is reported to be depressed and aldosterone to be within normal limits. This indicates a disruption of the usual direct correlation between renin and aldosterone levels, which may be of significance in explaining the hyponatremia of this disorder. In any event, the hypoosmotic state would be expected to suppress ADH release and stimulate the renin–angiotensin–aldosterone system for Na^+ retention, but these responses do not occur.

There are several categories of cause of SIADH. In some forms of the disorder the source of the excessive ADH is not the hypothalamic nuclei which normally synthesize and release it, but rather a malignant tumor which produces a substance indistinguishable from ADH in its action on the distal tubule and collecting ducts of the kidney. Neoplasms of the lung, pancreas, gastrointestinal tract, prostate, and lymphoid organs have all been identified as ectopic sources of arginine vasopressin or closely related substances.

Other conditions producing SIADH include a wide variety of pathologic conditions which appear to cause excess production of ADH from the normal source in the hypothalamus. Various intrathoracic disease states such as pneumonias, tuberculosis, and lung abscesses; and central nervous system disorders: head trauma, cerebral infarction, encephalitis and meningitis, brain abscess, and subarachnoid hemorrhage may all be associated with excessive synthesis and release of ADH from the hypothalamic nuclei.

It has been suggested that in certain of these intrathoracic and intracranial processes, the brainstem osmoreceptors and the intrathoracic low pressure volume receptors, become reset to lower osmotic pressure and higher volume tolerance levels. This readjustment of threshold values for the activation of corrective or compensatory processes would result in the continued output of ADH in spite of elevated total body water volume and decreased total body Na^+ which normally would have caused ADH suppression. Abnormal solute concentration in the receptor cells has been suggested as one possible mechanism for the resetting.

When it is not known whether the source of the excess ADH is ectopic or from the hypothalamic nuclei, the distinction can be made by administration of diphenylhydantoin or alcohol, both of which suppress the release of ADH from the hypothalamicohypophyseal system. A diuresis and decreased urine osmolarity in response to these agents indicates the latter as the source of the excess hormone.

A number of pharmacologic agents also stimulate excess ADH release leading to SIADH; some psychoactive drugs, some immunosuppressives and antimetabolites, and certain oral hypoglycemic agents are included in the drug-caused category. More recently clofibrate and carbemazepine have been noted to have this effect.

Other stimuli to excessive ADH release which will produce hyponatremia are those to which many hospitalized patients, especially those undergoing surgery, are exposed. Pain and trauma; emotional arousal with fear and anxiety; and certain drugs: some anesthetics, hypnotics, and narcotic analgesics, increase ECF water retention and cause hyponatremia by stimulation of ADH release.

Psychogenic Polydipsia

In some psychiatric disorders patients may take oral fluids in excess of even the normal kidneys' capacity to eliminate them. Oral intake of close to 1 L/hr is usually necessary to produce life-threatening hyponatremia from this cause. Urine specific gravity in this situation may be as low as 1.001.

Excess Water Intake by a Patient with Oliguric Chronic Renal Failure

This situation may lead to a dilution of serum and total body Na^+. The excess hypotonic fluid intake may overload the capacity of the decreased population of relatively normal nephrons to filter and remove it, leading to dilutional hyponatremia somewhat akin to that occurring in the subject with normal renal function but extraordinarily increased water intake, above. An occasional patient may force fluids with the mistaken notion that such intake will facilitate elimination of accumulated nitrogenous wastes and relieve the uremia.

Addison's Disease (Adrenocortical Insufficiency)

In Addison's disease (adrenocortical insufficiency), glucocorticoid (cortisol) and mineralocorticoid (aldosterone) deficits are present and produce abnormalities in renal handling of sodium ions and water which set the stage for the development of hyponatremia if the Addison's patient takes excess water or receives a hypotonic fluid load intravenously. Insufficient aldosterone chronically depresses tubular Na^+ resorption, both at the DRT-CES and at more proximal portions of the tubule. Therefore, as Na^+ is lost, water is lost with it, leading to a chronically contracted plasma volume, and an abnormally low GFR. The cortisol deficit not only causes chronic depression of the GFR but also appears to produce an increase in permeability of the nephron to water. Therefore, when the patient with adrenal insufficiency receives excess hypotonic fluid, the combination of a chronically depressed GFR and abnormally high permeability of the tubule to water resorption causes the water to be retained in the ECF causing hyponatremia. In addition there is some evidence that in the presence of chronic cortisol deficiency, ADH secretion is chronically excessive, perhaps because of the continuous low plasma volume. Other endocrine disorders in which SIADH may occur are hypopituitarism and myxedema.

Regardless of the cause of the hyponatremia, among the conditions discussed above and others not discussed, the subsequent osmotic and volume abnormalities which occur in these conditions are physiologically similar. As hyponatremia develops, the fluid of the interior of all cells becomes hypertonic relative to the extracellular fluid, because of progressive ECF dilution and hypoosmolarity. Since water moves much more readily across cell membranes than do solutes, including electrolytes, water enters the relatively hypertonic cell interior from the hypotonic ECF along the newly created osmotic gradient. The result is that the cells swell. In most cells this water uptake and swelling does little harm, but in the neurons of the brain, neuron swelling leads to abnormal excitability characteristics and abnormal neurologic function. The result is water intoxication. The manifestations may be altered mental status, depressed levels of consciousness, and neurologic signs.

Assessment in Hyponatremia

If the serum Na^+ remains above 120 meq/L there may be no signs or symptoms, but below this level central nervous system impairments from water intoxication comprise the outstanding manifestations and the life-threatening complications of hyponatremia. Irritability and mental confusion with personality changes may be the earliest development. As the serum Na^+ declines to about 110 meq/L neurologic signs may be seen, including neuromuscular hyperexcitability manifested as muscle twitching or even seizures, decreased deep tendon reflexes, plantar extensor responses (positive Babinski, or "upgoing toes"), and extreme motor weakness. Lethargy, stupor, and coma may presage generalized convulsions and death. It is important to note that the signs and symptoms are determined not only by the absolute serum Na^+ level, but by the rapidity with which it develops. The more rapid the decline in ECF osmolarity, the more marked the signs and symptoms, and the more life-threatening the consequences.

Blood pressure and tissue turgor are normal; edema is unusual because the excess body water is primarily intracellular rather than interstitial and intravascular. Increasing body weight may be an early sign. The urine is usually hypertonic with respect to the plasma because of continued urinary Na^+ loss. Laboratory values reveal a decreased serum Na^+ and plasma osmolarity and an elevated urinary Na^+ content. BUN and creatine are often low in patients without primary renal disorders.

Management of Hyponatremia

Treatment of patients with hyponatremia is directed at the underlying condition which has predisposed to water retention in excess of Na^+. In most cases in which the hyponatremia is mild, simple restriction of fluid intake will be adequate to control the abnormalities, particularly if this restriction is combined with increased salt intake.

Where hyponatremia is severe, and has developed rapidly, especially if there are the central nervous signs and symptoms of water intoxication, fluid intake is markedly restricted and hypertonic saline may be infused in the amount necessary to bring the serum Na^+ to above 120 meq/L. This procedure requires careful monitoring of the patient particularly where there is borderline left ventricular performance. The reason for this that if the hyponatremia is accompanied by overall water retention, the hypertonic infusion will osmotically draw water out of cells along the rising ECF–ICF osmotic gradient. This will produce a marked expansion of ECF volume, raise central venous pressure, and increase the volume workload of the left ventricle. If its contractility is impaired, elevation of pulmonary capillary pressure and development of pulmonary edema may occur. Therefore, patient assessment during correction may include evaluation of posterior lung fields for basilar rales; of central venous pressure via subclavian line (if the patient has one) or jugular venous pressure; and of respiratory rate and tidal volume. Some centers advocate the use of intravenous furosemide with hypertonic saline and potassium infusions, since it produces an increased Na^+ without expanding the ECF. This treatment requires frequent laboratory serum and urine electrolyte determinations. Where a more leisurely approach to the return of serum Na^+ to a normal range is possible, it is probably indicated because of the possible complications associated with more heroic measures.

Excess Fluid and Electrolyte (Sodium): Hypervolemia

As emphasized in prior sections, the total volume of the ECF is determined primarily by the total amount of osmotically active solute in the ECF; since Na^+ is the cation in highest concentration in the ECF therefore total body sodium content is the most important single determinant of ECF volume. For this reason physiologic, primarily renal, mechanisms which regulate total body sodium have a significant impact on the volume of the ECF. Sodium retention and excess total body sodium leads to an expanded ECF; such expansion, in turn, may produce edema. Since sodium retention leads to expanded circulating blood volume, it is appropriate to consider those conditions in which renal mechanisms for conserving sodium are activated. These are mainly abnormalities leading to decreased renal perfusion and increased resorption of sodium and water.

Causes of Hypervolemia

Conditions Resulting in Secondary Aldosteronism

Congestive Heart Failure   Congestive heart failure (Chapter 7) is characterized by a decreased cardiac output and impaired tissue perfusion because of impaired myocardial contractility. The low cardiac output leads to decreased renal perfusion, which in turn activates the secretion of renin from the juxtaglomerular cells according to mechanisms described in Chapter 3. The longer-term consequence of stimulation of the renin–angiotensin system is elevated adrenocortical output of aldosterone which causes enhanced resorption of sodium at the distal convoluted tubule cation exchange site. Water is retained with sodium, and an expanded isotonic plasma volume results.

Cirrhosis of the Liver.   This disorder (Chapter 12), often accompanied by portal hypertension, leads to sodium and water retention. Because of destroyed liver parenchyma, liver synthesis of the plasma proteins is impaired, leading to a decreased colloidal osmotic pressure (COP) of the plasma. When accompanied by portal hypertension, large amounts of ECF as well as plasma proteins are sequestered in the peritoneal cavity as ascites fluid. So there is a combination of inadequate synthesis and excessive loss of these proteins, resulting in a decline of the plasma colloidal osmotic pressure. The low plasma COP reduces the effective plasma volume and impairs renal perfusion, causing activation of the renin–angiotensin–aldosterone system. Under the stimulus of aldosterone, sodium (and water) are retained by the kidney, expanding the ECF. In liver disease, another mechanism contributing to ECF expansion may be a failure of the liver to inactivate circulating aldosterone and ADH effectively.

Nephrotic Syndrome.   This is a condition resulting from many forms of kidney disease (Chapter 10), and is characterized by proteinuria, hypoproteinema, hyperlipidemia, and interstitial edema. A chronic leakage of plasma proteins into the tubular filtrate results from abnormal filtration by damaged glomerular capillary membranes having impaired selective permeability. This protein loss lowers plasma colloidal osmotic pressure and effective renal perfusion pressure, and leads to the secretion of high levels of renin which stimulates adrenal production of aldosterone.

The three above conditions lead to secondary aldosteronism; they are often accompanied by edema formation (see following). Secondary hyperaldosteronism causes renal sodium retention, retention of water, and elevation of circulating plasma volume.

Chronic Renal Failure

In chronic renal failure, primary sodium retention is not prominent until the renal failure is far advanced, but in certain kidney diseases involving the glomeruli, sodium filtration at this site is impaired and thus Na^+ is retained in the ECF instead of entering the tubular filtrate and being eliminated in the urine. The sodium retention, in addition to expanding the ECF, promotes the development of hypertension (Chapter 3) and predisposes to congestive heart failure and cerebrovascular disease. The congestive heart failure then leads to a further decline in renal perfusion, secretion of excess aldosterone, more sodium retention, and more ECF overload.

Edema Formation

Edema often accompanies disorders in which there is excessive accumulation of Na^+ and an expanded ECF volume. It is the accumulation of interstitial fluid in abnormally large amounts. Since the ECF is in hydrostatic and osmotic equilibrium with the interstitial fluid, increasing hypervolemia, if not reversed, will lead to edema. The actual rate of filtration of ECF from the capillary into the interstitial fluid depends on the balance between filtration pressure and colloidal osmotic pressure across the capillary membrane. Although generalized systemic edema occurs in conditions of expanded ECF volume with Na^+ retention, it also occurs with local changes. The following discussion applies to both types.

Filtration pressure is equal to the hydrostatic pressure in the capillary minus the hydrostatic pressure of the interstitial fluid. Since the hydrostatic pressure (blood pressure) is greater at the arteriole end of the capillary than at the venule end, the filtration pressure decrease along the length of the capillary, but is directed outward all of the way.

Oncotic pressure is equal to the colloidal osmotic pressure of the plasma minus the colloidal osmotic pressure of the interstitial fluid, the latter value being close to zero. As blood passes through the capillary, some water and solute filters out into the interstitial spaces, but most of the protein is retained. Therefore, the colloidal osmotic pressure of capillary blood increases slightly along the length of the capillary, but the direction of the gradient is always inward, since capillary filtrate averages only 0.3% protein (interstitial fluid protein is less than 5% of that in the blood). Thus more intravascular ECF, minus the plasma proteins, enters the ISF at the arteriolar end of the capillary where filtration pressure exceeds oncotic pressure.

Toward the venular end of the capillary, the oncotic pressure exceeds the filtration pressure, so some of the ICF which oozed out earlier is returned to the intravascular ECF. The amount flowing out is overall slightly greater than the amount flowing back in. The excess is drained off by the lymphatics and returned to the circulation at the thoracic duct.

The pressure relationships between the capillary and the interstitial fluid in the various portions of the capillary are as follows. At the arteriole end of the capillary, the hydrostatic pressure is 37 mmHg. At the venule end of the capillary the hydrostatic pressure is 17 mmHg. The colloidal osmotic pressure of the blood throughout the system is about 25 mmHg (slightly higher at the venule end). Interstitial fluid pressure around the capillary is close to zero. Therefore, at the arteriolar end of the capillary, the hydrostatic force tending to push water out is 37 mmHg; the colloid osmotic force tending to retain water or pull it in is $25 + 1 = 26$. The net pressure directed outward at the arteriolar end therefore is 11 mmHg (37–26).

At the venule end of the capillary, the hydrostatic force tending to push water out is 17 mmHg and the colloid osmotic pressure tending to draw water in is $25 + 1 = 26$. So here the net pressure is 9 mmHg directed inward (25 + 1 − 17). Therefore the overall movement inward, in the normal subject, at most anatomical sites (not the lungs, see following) is greater than that outward by about 2 mmHg (11–9 mmHg). These relationships are indicated in Figure 1-7.

Elevated interstitial fluid volume is edema; it may be occult or overt, localized or general. Relatively large amounts of ECF must accumulate in the interstitial spaces before the transition occurs from occult to overt edema, detectable by physical examination as pitting edema. It is estimated that an 8–10% increase in body weight as interstitial fluid must accumulate before the latter occurs.

It should be emphasized that, whenever there is greater than normal retention of sodium, there is corresponding increase in retention of osmotically obligated

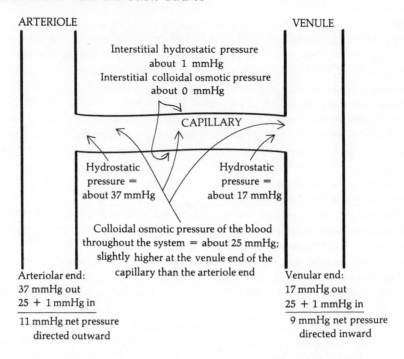

ARTERIOLE   VENULE

Interstitial hydrostatic pressure
about 1 mmHg
Interstitial colloidal osmotic pressure
about 0 mmHg

CAPILLARY

Hydrostatic
pressure =
about 37 mmHg

Hydrostatic
pressure =
about 17 mmHg

Colloidal osmotic pressure of the blood
throughout the system = about 25 mmHg;
slightly higher at the venule end of the
capillary than the arteriole end

Arteriolar end:
37 mmHg out
25 + 1 mmHg in
_____
11 mmHg net pressure
directed outward

Venular end:
17 mmHg out
25 + 1 mmHg in
_____
9 mmHg net pressure
directed inward

Overall: 11 mmHg outward
         − 9 mmHg inward
         _____
         2 mmHg net pressure directed outward

Figure 1-7. Hydrostatic and oncotic pressure relationships in systemic capillaries. At the arteriolar end of the capillary: 37 mmHg hydrostatic pressure is directed outward, and 25 mmHg oncotic pressure and 1 mmHg hydrostatic pressure is directed inward. Thus at this end of the capillary the net force is 11 mmHg directed outward. At the venular end of the capillary: 17 mmHg hydrostatic pressure is directed outward; and the same or slightly higher (because of slightly increased proportion of plasma proteins at this end) pressure is directed inward as at the arteriolar end: 25 + 1. Therefore at the venular end of the capillary the net movement of ECF is inward at a pressure of about 8 or 9 mmHg. Overall, therefore, in the systemic capillaries as a whole, the overall movement of fluid outward is slightly higher than that moving back in, because the overall pressure differential from arteriolar to venular end is 2 mmHg outwardly directed.

water, and hence overall water retention, resulting in elevated isosmotic ECF volume and pressure. Since intravascular and interstitial fluid are in equilibrium, this increased isosmotic fluid is distributed between interstitial and intravascular spaces.

Whenever edema is seen on physical examination, then an assessment of heart, kidney, and liver function is indicated, in a search for congestive failure, cirrhosis (with or without ascites), and nephrosis. In the latter two conditions especially, as mentioned above, the tendency to interstitial fluid accumulation is accentuated by decreased plasma colloidal osmotic pressure from inadequate plasma protein content, whether caused by inadequate synthesis or excessive loss. In congestive heart failure elevated central venous hydrostatic pressure results in passive venous congestion and greatly increased intracapillary pressure.

The degree of ankle edema is assessed in the ambulatory patient by firm

Table 1-1
Classification of Causes of Edema

INCREASED INTRACAPILLARY HYDROSTATIC PRESSURE
  inflammatory arteriole dilation
  venule constriction, compression, or obstruction (garters; long sitting with legs dependent and compressed by chair edge; venous thrombosis; incompetent vein valves)
  Elevated central venous pressure (congestive heart failure; increased ECF volume from secondary hyperaldosteronism from any cause: cirrhosis, nephrosis, ascites)
DECREASED PLASMA OSMOTIC PRESSURE (cirrhosis, nephrosis, protein starvation)
INCREASED CAPILLARY PERMEABILITY (vasoactive substances such as histamine and bradykinin)
INADEQUATE LYMPHATIC DRAINAGE FROM AN AREA (arm edema from destruction of lymph channels in radical mastectomy with axillary node dissection; in this situation wrapping the arm with elastic bandage effectively increases the interstitial fluid pressure which acts to promote retention of fluid within the capillaries)

thumb pressure against distal tibia or fibula, and then an estimate of the depth of the resulting depression in millimeters is made. In the bedfast patient a similar pressure is exerted over dorsal thighs, sacral area, or other dependent body parts in the systemic circuit.

Acute Pulmonary Edema

Processes Involved in Acute Pulmonary Edema

Acute hypervolemia may occur in overzealous treatment with intravenous saline infusions in patients with burns, surgical blood loss, trauma, or other causes of acute ECF volume depletion. On acute ECF overload, a common complication is acute pulmonary edema. The pulmonary vasculature is a low pressure circuit and lung interstial pressure is also low because of the delicate membranous air-filled alveolar sacs of the lung parenchyma, and an absence of connective tissue supporting structures. Pulmonary capillary hydrostatic pressure in the normal subject is much less—about 10 mmHg—than intracapillary pressures in the systemic circuit. Thus the normal 25 mmHg intravascular colloidal osmotic pressure provides a larger osmotic than hydrostatic gradient—and therefore an entirely inward-directed gradient—for maintaining the ECF within the capillaries and out of the pulmonary interstitial and intraalveolar spaces. Specifically, the values are 25 mmHg colloidal osmotic pressure directed inward minus 10 mmHg hydrostatic pressure directed outward equals 15 mmHg net inward pressure tending to retain ECF within the capillaries of the pulmonary circuit. The lymphatic system of the lungs is also proportionately much greater than in the systemic circuit, an additional safety factor in protecting pulmonary tissue from overhydration by providing an increased drainage system to remove ECF that has extravasated from the pulmonary capillaries.

However, when pulmonary capillary pressure is greatly increased by ECF overload, especially when coupled with marginal left ventricular contractility, which would cause more blood to be pumped into the lungs by the right ventricle than the left ventricle can pump out, the pressure gradient for diffusion of pulmonary capillary ECF may be reversed. When pulmonary capillary hydrostatic pressure exceeds pulmonary capillary oncotic pressure (which itself may be decreased by dilution with infused crystalloids) interstitial pulmonary edema may develop rapidly. Overhydration of the lungs leads to decreased compliance (more pressure required to move an equivalent volume of air) and hence increased work of breathing, decreased tidal volume, and larger proportion of tidal air moving over the respiratory dead space.

In the case of marginal left ventricular myocardial reserve even a slight elevation of central venous pressure produced by intravenous infusion may exceed left ventricular pumping capacity. The result will be a discrepancy between right and left heart output and elevated pulmonary capillary pressure. If the left ventricular output is less than that of the right ventricle by only 0.01 ml per contraction, more than 1000 ml will be added to pulmonary vessel volume in 24 hours. An excess of about 2 liters above normal is usually sufficient to produce clinically significant pulmonary edema.

Patient Assessment in Acute Pulmonary Edema

Important aspects consist of noting dyspnea, tachypnea, moist cough with or without frothy or blood-tinged sputum, and bibasilar fine moist rales. Measurement of central venous pressure when a subclavian line is in place, and of pulmonary capillary wedge pressures in patients having a Swan-Ganz catheter, are aids in patient evaluation. Increased pressure volume ratios for delivery of the same tidal volume in a patient on mechanical ventilation with a volume-cycled ventilator, and hypoxia and hypocapnia on arterial blood gas measurement, are indications of markedly elevated pulmonary capillary pressure. Cyanosis is a late development.

Management of Hypervolemia: Diuretics

Since most cases of hypervolemia develop as a complication of some general chronic systemic disorder, the prime considerations in treatment will be directed toward locating and if possible correcting or at least managing the basic abnormality. For this reason most aspects of treatment of hypervolemia will be discussed under the appropriate subject headings of the basic disorders elsewhere in the text. The common denominator of management in almost all these physiologic problems, however, is the administration of diuretics, and that topic will be discussed here. The principal sites of action of commonly used diuretics along the various portions of the nephron are indicated in Figure 1-8.

Most diuretics combat edema by specifically inhibiting resorption of sodium ions (and consequently of water) from the tubular filtrate, at various points along its course, back into the renal interstitium and microvasculature. Osmotic diuretics, on the other hand, act by adding to the ECF a solute which is filtered but not resorbed, such as glycerol, urea, and mannitol. The solute therefore osmotically obligates large amounts of tubular water. The consequence is delivery of an increased volume of isosmotic fluid to the loop of Henle. The Na^+ resorption mechanism here is limited and not enough Na^+ can be resorbed from the loop into the medullary interstitium to maintain its hypertonicity; instead this isosmotic tubular fluid diffuses out into the interstitial area, reduces the osmotic pressure gradient of the renal pyramids, and results in less water being resorbed from the collecting ducts. Therefore larger urine volumes are produced.

When transport of sodium ions out of the filtrate at the level of the proximal tubule back into the renal vessels is inhibited by diuretics such as the mercurials

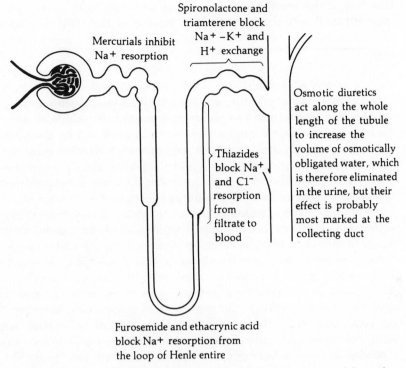

Mercurials inhibit
Na⁺ resorption

Spironolactone and
triamterene block
Na⁺ –K⁺ and
H⁺ exchange

Osmotic diuretics
act along the whole
length of the tubule
to increase the
volume of osmotically
obligated water, which
is therefore eliminated
in the urine, but their
effect is probably
most marked at the
collecting duct

Thiazides
block Na⁺
and Cl⁻
resorption
from
filtrate to
blood

Furosemide and ethacrynic acid
block Na⁺ resorption from
the loop of Henle entire

Figure 1-8. Main site of action of diuretics along the various portions of the nephron.

(which are now seldom used), the filtrate in the tubule lumen remains isosmotic and the tubular water is thus osmotically obligated to remain in the tubule instead of being resorbed. Increased tubular fluid volumes brought about in this way appear to promote a more rapid flow of tubular fluid, further dilute tubular sodium ions, and hence increase the concentration gradient against which they would have to be transported out of the tubule. Thus more remain in the tubular filtrate to be eliminated in the urine.

Acetazolamide inhibits sodium ion resorption by blocking carbonic anhydrase activity, making less H^+ available for exchange with Na^+ at the distal tubule. Thiazides inhibit sodium and chloride ion resorption at the ascending limb of Henle's loop and the proximal end of the distal tubule. Ethacrynic acid and furosemide block Na^+ resorption in the ascending limb of Henle's loop and the first part of the distal tubule. Spironolactone and triamterene prevent the exchange of Na^+ for K^+ and H^+ in the distal tubule. The former is a specific antagonist to the action of aldosterone on the distal renal tubule; the latter suppresses the DRT-CES directly, independent of any action on aldosterone. Both promote K^+ retention.

Thiazides act on the site in the tubule at which Na^+ and Cl^- are resorbed together from the tubular fluid back into the renal microcirculation. This is probably just beyond the ascending limb of Henle's loop and just before the distal convoluted tubule. Here thiazides inhibit Na^+ and Cl^- resorption from the tubule into the renal interstitium (peritubular fluid). They thus greatly increase delivery of Na^+ to the DRT-CES where Na^+ is resorbed in exchange for K^+ and H^+. The capacity of this site to resorb sodium is exceeded, hence the diuresis.

However, hypokalemia and metabolic alkalosis may be the consequence of this large stimulation to the Na^+-resorbing capacity of the DRT. Thiazides probably also act to some extent to inhibit Na^+ resorption at the ascending limb of the loop of Henle.

Assessment in thiazide administration includes monitoring serum K^+. A decline in serum K^+ concentration may lead to side effects of weakness, fatigue, and paresthesias; or may be manifested by anorexia, nausea, weakness, and lethargy. Gastrointestinal complaints in hypokalemia include nausea, epigastric distress, and abdominal cramps. Hypokalemia produced by thiazides may worsen digitalis toxicity arrhythmias. A patient with borderline renal function may have an increase in azotemia precipitated by hypovolemia caused by thiazides. The hypokalemia induced by thiazides makes their use questionable in Cushing's syndrome or adrenal steroid administration, since these states may be accompanied by low levels of serum potassium to begin with. Decreased glucose tolerance caused by thiazides is of special significance in the patient with a positive family history of diabetes mellitus, an abnormal glucose tolerance test, or overt diabetes mellitus. Increased serum uric acid may precipitate an attack of gout in a susceptible person; thiazides are weak acids like uric acid, which is secreted at the proximal tubule, and they interfere with its excretion. In gout being managed by uricosuric agents (sulfinpyrazone and probenecid), however, thiazide is not contraindicated, since it acts at a tubular level different from that at which agents blocking uric acid resorption occurs. Occasional skin rashes occur from thiazides. In chronic liver disease thiazides may predispose to the development of hepatic encephalopathy by decreasing the ability of the kidney to eliminate ammonia.

Furosemide acts on the loop of Henle to block active transport of sodium from the ascending limb. It is a sulfonamide, related to the thiazides, and has a diabetogenic effect. It is a powerful diuretic with a rapid onset and a short duration (4 hours); it may cause hypovolemia, and does cause hypokalemia. Since Na^+ and water loss may continue under the influence of furosemide, even after serum Na^+ and ECF volume is markedly decreased, peripheral vascular collapse can be induced by this agent.

Ethacrynic acid acts to inhibit the active transport of Na^+ out of proximal tubules and throughout the loop of Henle. KC1 supplements must be given because excessive amounts of Na^+ reaching the DRT-CES stimulate it to increased Na^+ resorption in exchange for K^+, and cause K^+ loss. It is potent and can be dangerous, resulting in dehydration, hypovolemia, hypotension, alkalosis, deafness, and elevated plasma uric acid. It has a rapid onset and short duration.

Spironolactone antagonizes the action of aldosterone in stimulating Na^+ resorption in exchange for K^+ and H^+ elimination at the DRT-CES and is therefore most effective when hypervolemia and edema are caused by primary or secondary hyperaldosteronism. Is is a weak diuretic usually used in association with the thiazides, and has a slowly developing effect (2–3 days). It may cause gynecomastia or hyperkalemia.

Triamterene produces sodium loss and potassium retention by direct suppression of the action of the DRT-CES, rather than by antagonism of aldosterone at that site; it is often used in combination with a thiazide and may elevate BUN with long-term use.

Potassium Ion Balance

Normal K⁺ Distribution and Regulation

Potassium is the cation responsible for intracellular osmotic pressure, is essential for maintaining nerve and muscle cell membrane excitation and conduction, and is necessary for the function of a number of metabolic enzyme systems.

The large difference in K^+ concentration between the intracellular and extracellular fluid compartments (about 30-fold greater in the ICF) tends to remain quite stable and is maintained by an active transport mechanism whereby Na^+ is extruded from the cell interior, and K^+ in the ECF is transported across the cell membrane to the interior. Because the ICF K^+ content is so large relative to that of the ECF, major fluctuations in serum K^+ brought about by various factors, including increased dietary or medicinal intake, and the movement of K^+ between cells' inside and outside, produce very minor changes in overall ICF K^+ concentration. An increase in intake of K^+ leads to rapid cellular uptake of the ion, and when renal function is normal the excess K^+ is rapidly eliminated by the kidneys. Conversely, with protracted low K^+ intake renal conservation of the ion (that is, increased resorption into the ECF from tubular filtrate) develops slowly over several days.

Serum potassium levels are influenced by a number of factors, some of which are hormonal. The most important of these is the adrenal mineralocorticoid aldosterone which acts at the distal renal tubule cation exchange site to promote sodium ion retention in exchange for K^+ and/or H^+ elimination; two K^+'s for one H^+ is the normal excretion ratio of these two ions in exchange for three Na^+ ions. Increased aldosterone secretion is promoted by any physiologic change which stimulates the kidney to release increased amounts of renin, such as salt restriction and hypovolemia or other causes of decreased renal perfusion, and by elevated serum K^+.

Increased adrenal glucocorticoids in the plasma lead to a loss of ICF K^+ into the ECF; and the gonadal anabolic hormones cause a movement of ECF K^+ into the ICF along with the increase in cell mass which they produce.

Elevation of serum H^+ concentration (acidemia) leads to an increased movement of K^+ from ICF to ECF; this apparently occurs because as serum H^+ levels increase, these ions then move into the intracellular compartment along the steepened concentration gradient. In exchange for this inward migration of H^+, an equivalent number of K^+'s move out into the plasma in order to maintain electrical neutrality across the cell membrane. A low plasma H^+ concentration (alkalemia) has the reverse effect.

Additional factors promote cellular release of K^+ into the ECF: cell damage (hypoxia, crushing tissue injury, and toxic chemical tissue damage); and the movement of cellular water from ICF to ECF which occurs during dehydration. Cells also take up some sodium ions from the ECF during the increase in ECF osmotic pressure occurring during dehydration; the Na^+ entering the cells during dehydration maintains electrical neutrality in exchange for the outmigration of positive charges carried by the K^+ leaving with the cellular water.

At the kidney, most or perhaps all of the K^+ which is filtered at the glomerulus is then resorbed from tubular fluid at the proximal convoluted tubule. K^+ excretion occurs almost entirely farther on, at the distal tubule exchange site, in exchange for the resorption of sodium ions. The rate of exchange at this site, and therefore the degree of K^+ elimination or retention, is importantly influenced by a number of factors which therefore are, in turn, instrumental in influencing plasma potassium ion concentration. The first of these has already been discussed above: plasma aldosterone content.

The second factor governing K^+ elimination at the distal convoluted tubule is the amount of sodium ion arriving at that site. When tubular resorption of Na^+ at more proximal levels of the tubule is inhibited by chemical or osmotic diuretics, then more Na^+ remains in tubular filtrate; therefore, Na^+ delivery to the DRT-CES is greatly enhanced. For this reason, more Na^+ is resorbed in exchange for more K^+ being eliminated at that site. A digression: students tend to be confused by this. If an end result of diuretic action is the stimulation of a greater rate of Na^+ *resorption* at the distal tubule, then how is it that a diuretic results in *overall* sodium—and water—loss? The answer is that the degree of inhibition of Na^+ resorption at more proximal tubular sites which some diuretics cause, is so great that the amount of Na^+ arriving at the distal tubule is enormously increased. Therefore, even though activity at the distal Na^+ resorbing site is stimulated by the increased Na^+ load, its capacity for retaining Na^+ is exceeded by the large Na^+ content of tubular fluid and the consequence is *net* Na^+ loss.

The reversed renal effect on K^+—that is, increased K^+ resorption—is produced by a greatly decreased delivery of Na^+ to the DRT-CES; this occurs, for example, in hypovolemia or dehydration. In these conditions less Na^+ is filtered at the glomerulus, because of the low GFR, so relatively more is resorbed in the more proximal portions of the tubule; therefore, less arrives at the distal site for exchange with K^+. For this reason, in hypervolemia K^+ elimination rate declines at the tubule, less is eliminated in the urine, and the concentration of K^+ in the plasma increases.

The third factor affecting Na^+–K^+ exchange at the distal tubule, and therefore serum K^+ level, is the ratio of the concentrations of serum K^+ and serum H^+. The serum content of these ions affects how much of each is filtered at the glomeruli and therefore their content in the tubular fluid. The amount of H^+ and K^+ which is filtered determines the relative amounts of each which are available at the DRT-CES to be eliminated in exchange for the resorption of Na^+. In acidemia there are large amounts of H^+ in the filtrate relative to K^+; in this case Na^+–H^+ exchange tends to exceed Na^+–K^+ exchange, resulting in elevation of plasma K^+. In alkalemia the situation is reversed: tubular fluid H^+ is low, so Na^+–K^+ exchange is preferential and serum K^+ tends to fall. This is the mechanism accounting for the fact that the patient with an acidotic process tends to be hyperkalemic, and the patient with an alkalotic process tends to develop hypokalemia (Chapter 2).

Disorders of Potassium Equilibrium

Hyperkalemia

Hyperkalemia is most frequently the result of deficient elimination of potassium ion by the kidney.

Causes of Hyperkalemia. *Adrenocortical insufficiency.* Adrenocrtical insufficiency most often occurs as a result of spontaneous atrophy of the adrenal cortex which is thought to be the result of an autoimmune process (Chapter 13). Serum K^+ is elevated even in relatively mild to moderate forms of the disorder, because of the resulting deficiency in aldosterone stimulation of the distal convoluted tubule, hyponatremia, and low ECF volume.

Renal failure. Acute or chronic anuric or oliguric renal failure causes hyperkalemia. When there is anuria the serum K^+ level may rise 0.5 meq/24 hr. This increase becomes much larger when combined with other abnormal processes such as cell destruction.

Physiologic injuries. Certain types of physiologic injuries result in the release of large amounts of intracellular contents, which are high in potassium ions, into the ECF. Hemolysis, internal bleeding, (especially from the gastrointestinal tract), burns, crushing muscle trauma, and rhabdomyolysis, which may occur after violent muscle exercise in the untrained individual, all produce hyperkalemia.

The hyperkalemia develops more rapidly and is more severe when these events are accompanied or followed by the oliguria of acute renal failure caused by a severe hypotensive episode, nephrotoxic chemicals, myoglobinemia, or other causes of kidney impairment. A further complication may be the prior presence of certain neurologic disorders or the administration of a pharmacologic agent producing paralysis by massive membrane depolarization, such as succinylcholine; as the normal transmembrane electrical potentials are abolished by this agent, large amounts of K^+ exit from the cell interior into the ECF.

Potassium supplements. Administration of potassium supplements to a patient with renal insufficiency, or who is receiving a diuretic which suppresses the DRT-CES such as spironolactone or triamterine, may cause hyperkalemia.

Acidemia. Acidemia will often cause elevated serum K^+ concentrations according to the mechanism described above which involves K^+ and H^+ redistribution, both at the level of the cell–plasma interface and at the level of the distal renal tubule exchange site.

Patient Assessment in Hyperkalemia. Subjective data such as complaints of symptoms of skeletal muscle weakness, or difficult breathing because of respiratory muscle paresis, are rare and apparently occur only at extreme levels of hyperkalemia. Higher mental functions such as mental status, level of consciousness and sensory perception appear unaffected by any K^+ elevation compatible with life. Thus reliable evidence for hypokalemia is supplied by the objective data provided by monitoring of the EKG and serum electrolyte determinations.

Elevated serum K^+ has a profound impact upon the excitation and conduction processes of the heart and will manifest as cardiac arrhythmias, heightened T waves, and a decreased P wave amplitude in moderate hyperkalemia. With increasing severity, K^+ values from about 6.5–8.5 meq/L, P-R interval prolongation and widened QRS complexes appear and may culminate in heart block, atrial asystole or ventricular fibrillation, or other ventricular arrhythmias.

Management of Hyperkalemia. The treatment of excess serum K^+, if mild, should be directed at the cause, such as reducing K^+ supplements, reversal of acidemia, stopping the K^+-sparing diuretics, or increasing mineralocorticoid replacement therapy in the patient with Addison's disease. When hyperkalemia is more severe, especially if there are accompanying manifestations of cardiac toxicity in the form of EKG abnormalities or cardiac arrhythmia, management has both short-term and long-term components. Since it is the actual level of serum K^+, rather than elevated whole body K^+ content, which is responsible for potassium toxicity, then immediate treatment consists of measures promptly to reduce serum K^+ by inducing its migration from the ECF into the ICF.

Intravenous glucose and insulin accomplish this translocation by inducing the transport of glucose from the ECF into the ICF, where it is deposited as glycogen. This transport is accompanied by an influx of K^+ into the intracellular compartment, and is brought about by insulin. Also, calcium ions (as calcium gluconate) reduces the cardiotoxic effects of K^+ excess without lowering serum K^+. In the acidemic patient, sodium bicarbonate lowers ECF pH and induces movement of intracellular H^+ along the pH gradient created by the alkali, in exchange for which K^+ moves from ECF into the ICF. Obviously sodium bicarbonate and calcium gluconate would never be given together, since calcium carbonate forms an insoluble precipitate. The therapeutic effect of these measures is evaluated by the normalization of the EKG.

The longer-term goal of reducing whole body potassium is often accomplished by administration of a sodium polystyrene sulfonate cation exchange resin (Kayexalate) by mouth, if the patient tolerates oral intake, or as a retention enema if oral intake is contraindicated. The main site of action of this compound is the large intestine, since at this site K^+ elimination is much greater than in the small intestine. Sorbitol is given with the resin, since it is a nonabsorbed compound which exerts a high osmotic pressure in the gut lumen, drawing ECF into the intestine and thus exposing more extracellular fluid to the exchange resin. This action also produces frequent liquid stools, speeding K^+ elimination from the body altogether. In the meantime, if renal function is adequate, the kidneys have responded to the increased K^+ load by a prompt increased rate of elimination. If renal function is inadequate and the patient is anuric or severely oliguric, then hemo- or peritoneal dialysis may be necessary.

Hypokalemia

Hypokalemia often indicates a severe total body K^+ deficit. It may be brought about by gastrointestinal potassium loss or by excess elimination of potassium ions from the kidneys.

Causes of Hypokalemia. *Gastrointestinal causes.* Secretions from the stomach and intestines are significantly higher in potassium—40-50 meq/L—than is the ECF, so that loss of these secretions from the body, if prolonged, will produce an abnormally low serum K^+. Vomiting, diarrhea, or upper gastrointestinal drainage are the most frequent causes. Two causes of hypokalemia in this category which patients are almost always reluctant to reveal spontaneously are laxative overuse and self-induced or psychogenic vomiting, and these should be inquired into by the health care provider when there is a low serum K^+ with no discernible cause from the patient's history or physical examination. Since stomach secretions are very high in hydrogen ion content, loss of gastric secretions will produce not only hypokalemia but also an alkalemia that lowers the serum K^+ even further; inadequate plasma H^+ is available for exchange for Na^+ resorption at the distal tubule, which means that more K^+ must be used for this purpose. Additional serious digestive tract causes of hypokalemia include starvation, malabsorption syndromes, short bowel syndrome, Crohn's disease (regional enteritis) and chronic ulcerative colitis.

Renal causes.   Hypokalemia from renal loss usually occurs under one or more of the following circumstances: osmotic or chemical diuretics; metabolic alkalosis; excess of adrenal corticosteroids; and primary or secondary hyperaldosteronism.

The diuretics which produce hypokalemia are those which result in DRT-CES stimulation because of the incresed delivery of Na^+ to the distal tubule resulting from inhibition of resorption of Na^+ at more proximal tubule regions: furosemide, ethacrynic acid, and the thiazides. Osmotic diuretics also cause marked potassium loss, especially the osmotic diuresis occurring in the hyperglycemia and ketoacidosis of uncontrolled diabetes mellitus. This condition is particularly likely to result in depletion of total body potassium. Becaue of the acidosis, H^+'s have moved into cells resulting in an outward migration of K^+'s and a deceptively high serum K^+. As ketoacidemia is ameliorated during insulin and alkali treatment, ECF pH rises, H^+'s leave cells along the now-reversed gradient, cellular reuptake of K^+ occurs, and serum K^+ drops precipitously. Thus a normal serum K^+ in an acidemic patient may be a correlate of marked depletion of total body K^+ stores. The hypokalemia of metabolic alkalosis and of the adrenal abnormalities are discussed in Chapters 2 and 13.

Patient Assessment in Hypokalemia.   In general it appears to be the case that subjective and objective data (apart from serum K^+ values) do not correlate well with those values. As is always true in disorders of fluid, electrolyte, and acid–base equilibrium, the patient's previous health history, accompanying general systemic disorders, and immediately prior health status are most helpful in determining the cause of hypokalemia. In a case where this history is unknown or uninformative, urine potassium values may be helpful in distinguishing renal from gastrointestinal causes. In general, though there are exceptions, if a hypokalemic patient has a low urinary K^+ (less than 15 meq/24 hr) then the deficits are likely to be the result of a gastrointestinal cause (the kidneys are compensatorily conserving K^+). If the patient's urine is high in K^+ (30 meq/24 hr) this indicates that the kidneys are incapable of retaining K^+, and thus a renal cause is likely. The severely hypokalemic patient receiving strong diuretics is an exception; the serum K^+ is too low to permit large renal K^+ elimination in spite of a strong stimulus to such further loss.

Patient complaints in hypokalemia may include skeletal muscle weakness, difficult breathing from respiratory muscle paresis, and abdominal distress from impaired intestinal smooth muscle motility resulting in paralytic ileus. Objectively, muscle weakness, abdominal distention, and depressed deep tendon reflexes may be evident. Such findings are more likely to occur if the hypokalemia has developed rapidly, and they appear as the serum K^+ declines to about 2.5 meq/L.

The digitalized patient tends to show cardiac arrhythmias in hypokalemia. The EKG abnormalities are characteristic: depressed S-T segment, flattened T wave, and elevated U wave.

Hypokalemia of long standing produces a renal disorder, hypokalemic nephropathy, manifested by impaired renal tubule function including impaired water resorption; the result is chronic polyuria and compensatory polydipsia.

In hypokalemia from any cause, a metabolic alkalemia may develop; the basis for this complication of hypokalemia is an inadequate amount of K^+ for exchange with Na^+ at the DRT-CES. Because of inadequate tubular K^+ to exchange for Na^+, increased H^+ elimination occurs, leading to alkalemia.

Management of Hypokalemia. Oral replacement is preferable when possible, since the slow steady absorption of K^+ from the gastrointestinal tract avoids the too-sudden influx of K^+ into the ECF, which may occur with intravenous administration. If renal function is normal, then oral potassium supplements rarely lead to a serious hyperkalemia. If intravenous infusion is necessary, it is safer when accompanied by EKG monitoring. Potassium chloride is the salt most frequently used, since many patients with hypokalemia are also low in chloride. Patients with a metabolic alkalemia, which often accompanies hypokalemia according to the mechanism discussed above, require the chloride to stop the renal processes perpetuating K^+ loss. Normally, two thirds of the Na^+ resorbed by the kidney is taken back into the ECF with chloride; the remaining one third is resorbed in exchange for K^+ or H^+. If there is inadequate serum Cl^- to accompany the resorbed Na^+, then greater amounts of K^+ and H^+ will be eliminated in exchange for Na^+. This will sustain both the hypokalemia and the alkalemia.

REFERENCES

References for Chapter 1 are included in the references at the end of Chapter 2.

CHAPTER TWO

Abnormalities of Acid-Base Equilibrium and Arterial Blood Gases

ACID–BASE REGULATION

Normal H⁺ Concentration

The normal range of plasma pH is 7.35 to 7.45. The pH of the intracellular fluid is lower than that of the ECF, probably about chemical neutrality (7.0), both because of active intracellular metabolism which produces CO_2, and differences in the intracellular buffering processes. Maintenance of ECF hydrogen ion concentration within a relatively narrow range is of great importance, since the multiple enzyme systems responsible for every aspect of cellular metabolism function optimally only within rather restricted values of the pH. The pH range compatible with life is probably not much greater than 0.7 pH unit. However, a change in pH of only one unit is equivalent to a *tenfold* change in actual concentration of hydrogen ions; pH 7.4 expresses a hydrogen ion concentration of 0.00004 meq/L, or 4×10^{-8} mol/L of H^+. Thus, the concentration of H^+ in the plasma is extremely low compared with that of the other prominent ionic constituents of plasma: K^+ of 5.0 meq/L, Na^+ of 140 meq/L, of HCO_3^- of 26 meq/L. Therefore, the latitude of tolerance for H^+ fluctuation is greater in actual meq/L of H^+ than would seem to be the case from expressing such a change in pH units.

Processes Which Defend the Normal pH Range

There are four levels of physiologic processes which operate to defend the pH of the ECF against alterations, both increase and decrease, and to maintain it within the normal limits. The immediate response to an increase or decrease in H^+ concentration is the chemical buffering of H^+ by both extracellular and intracellular buffer systems; the most important of these are the hemoglobin of red blood cells, the plasma proteins, and the carbonic acid–bicarbonate buffer system.

The second line of defense against pH change is the migration of hydrogen ions into or out of cells from the ECF, along the diffusion gradients produced by an alteration of ECF pH, in exchange for the movement of potassium ions in the opposite direction. When the pH of the ECF declines (increased amount of H^+), then the H^+ migrates into the cells along the diffusion gradient, and K^+ moves out to maintain electrical neutrality. In other words, H^+ first migrates intracellularly along a chemical gradient, and then K^+ migrates out along the newly created electrical gradient caused by the preceding H^+ movement.

The third process is that of respiratory compensation, whereby elimination of CO_2 by the lungs increases (in the case of elevated H^+ concentration) or decreases (in the case of an increased pH) appropriately to the ECF pH change. The fourth mechanism, and the last to develop in this sequence, is renal compensation: the elimination or conservation of hydrogen ions and bicarbonate ions, as appropriate to ECF pH change, by the kidney. If the ECF H$^+$ concentration rises, the kidney eliminates more H$^+$ and conserves more HCO$_3^-$. When ECF H$^+$ declines, the kidney conserves H$^+$ and eliminates HCO$_3^-$.

Types of Acid–Base Derangements

There are four major categories of process producing acid–base abnormalities: respiratory acidosis, respiratory alkalosis, metabolic acidosis, and metabolic alkalosis. The terms acidosis and alkalosis refer to abnormal *processes* which generate the *conditions* of acidemia (pH below 7.35–7.4) and alkalemia (pH above 7.4–7.45), respectively. In the discussion which follows, the terms alkalosis and acidosis refer to abnormal *processes* which generate the *states* of alkalemia and acidemia, respectively. Where an abnormal process is *compensated* so that the pH is within normal limits, although the process is still ongoing, then the terms alkalosis and acidosis are appropriate.

The H$_2$CO$_3$–HCO$_3^-$ Buffer System

The carbonic acid–bicarbonate buffer system is of central importance in an understanding of the physiologic processes involved in normal acid–base equilibrium and its abnormalities:

$$CO_2 \;+\; H_20 \;\rightleftharpoons\; H_2CO_3 \;\rightleftharpoons\; H^+ \;+\; HCO_3^-$$
$$\text{(40 mmHg)} \qquad \text{(1.2 meq/L)} \qquad \text{(pH 7.4)} \quad \text{(24 meq/L)}$$

This equation illustrates the components of the carbonic acid–bicarbonate buffer system and the dynamic relationships among them. The bidirectional arrows indicate that the reactions proceed in either direction with equal facility, depending on the concentrations of the components in each section of the equation.

In spite of the central importance of the carbonic acid–bicarbonate buffer system in acid–base regulation, it is important to be aware of two facts: (1) CO$_2$ in the blood exists as dissolved gas to a very considerably greater extent than it exists in the form of carbonic acid (H$_2$CO$_3$); and (2) most buffering in acid–base disorders, especially respiratory ones, takes place via intracellular buffering by proteins and inorganic phosphates. Probably the central importance of the H$_2$CO$_3$–HCO$_3^-$ buffer system for clinical disorders of acid–base regulation rests on the fact that it is this system which exerts the ultimate control over the rate and degree of conservation or elimination of acids and bases from the body via the lungs and kidneys, in addition to merely buffering them.

The Respiratory Component

The left side of the equation P$_{CO_2}$ + H$_2$O $\rightleftharpoons$ H$_2$CO$_3$ is the *respiratory* component. P$_{CO_2}$ is the term for the tension (or partial pressure, P) of CO$_2$ gas dissolved in the blood. This respiratory parameter is influenced and in fact controlled primarily at the lungs, by the degree of alveolar ventilation. Its value is determined by the amount of CO$_2$ eliminated by the lungs. If the P$_{CO_2}$ is above or below normal this indicates that the amount of alveolar ventilation is inadequate (hypoventilation) or excessive (hyperventilation), respectively. P_{CO_2} is regulated by pulmonary function and the brainstem reflexes controlling respiratory drive (Chapter 9).

The Renal–Metabolic Component

The right side of the equation $H_2CO_3 \rightleftharpoons H^+ + HCO_3^-$ is the *renal–metabolic* component. The carbonic acid formed by the hydration of carbon dioxide gas dissociates into hydrogen ions and bicarbonate ions. This half of the equation is regulated primarily by the kidneys, since renal glomerular filtration, and renal tubular resorption and secretion processes, regulate H^+ and HCO_3^- elimination and/or conservation. The kidney tubules excrete excess H^+ in the form of mainly NH_4^+ (ammonium ions) which account for two thirds of the H^+ elimination; and also as the titratable acids H_2SO_4 (sulfuric) and H_3PO_4 (phosphoric) which account for one third of the H^+ elimination. The kidney tubules also retain or eliminate bicarbonate ions (HCO_3^-) as needed, either with Na^+ and K^+, or in exchange for Cl^- (chloride).

The expression of base excess (B.E.) is a portion of the metabolic component of acid–base equilibrium. It is a value based on a calculation made from the laboratory determination of pH, Pa_{CO_2} and the hematocrit; it is reported as meq/L of base above or below the normal buffer base range. The addition of nonvolatile acids (i.e., not CO_2) affects the base excess; a metabolic acidemia therefore will show a negative base excess (or a base deficit), while a metabolic alkalemia will be manifested as a positive base excess. Base excess represents basic or alkaline buffer substances in the blood; these are comprised of bicarbonate, hemoglobin, and the plasma proteins.

CO_2 Content

It should be pointed out that in serum electrolyte determinations the term CO_2 content, or just CO_2, does not mean CO_2 the dissolved gas (carbon dioxide) but rather the *sum* of the hydrated CO_2 (carbonic acid)—which according to the equation has a value of 1.2 meq/L at a Pa_{CO_2} of 40 mmHg, *and* the HCO_3^- (bicarbonate), the value for which is 1.2 meq/L. Therefore, the "total CO_2 content" in a serum electrolyte determination is actually around 25.2 meq/L, and is mainly bicarbonate ion.

HCO_3^- to CO_2 Ratio

In the equation above the ratio of HCO_3^- to dissolved CO_2 gas is 20:1 (24:1.2). In other words, the ratio of base to acid is 20:1. As long as this ratio remains 20:1, then the pH is the normal 7.4, *regardless of the absolute values of the base and the acid* (within physiologic limits). All of the physiologic processes regulating acid–base balance are directed at maintaining this base–acid ratio at 20:1, because only then does the pH of the ECF remain at physiologic neutrality (7.4).

Respiratory Acidosis and Alkalosis

In the respiratory half of the equation a rise in $PaCO_2$ concentration (respiratory acidosis) as occurs, for example, in the CO_2 retention of chronic obstructive pulmonary disease, shifts the equilibrium to the right, according to the chemical law of mass action. The result is an elevation in the H^+ concentration and a fall in pH. (There is also a corresponding rise in HCO_3^- but it does not neutralize the acid effect of the increased $PaCO_2$). A decline in $PaCO_2$, as in anxiety hyperventilation (respiratory alkalosis) results in a shift of the equilibrium to the left, leading to a decrease in hydrogen ion concentration and a rise in pH.

Metabolic Acidosis and Alkalosis

At the right side of the equation, the metabolic half, a decline in plasma bicarbonate (metabolic acidosis) such as occurs in the loss of alkaline intestinal secretions from severe diarrhea, shifts the equilibrium to the right, elevating the H^+ concentration and decreasing the pH. A loss of H^+ (=rise in HCO_3^-) metabolic acidosis caused by gastric suction, for example, shifts the equation to the left, lowering the H^+ concentration and elevating the pH.

Mixed Acid–Base Disturbances

We have discussed respiratory and metabolic acidosis and alkalosis as though they were somehow isolated or mutually exclusive processes. However, such is not the case. There may be, and often is, more than one pathologic process occurring simultaneously in a patient with an acid–base abnormality. If so, they may reinforce one another. For example, a respiratory acidosis from a sedative drug overdose depression of the respiratory center, coupled with a metabolic acidosis from diabetic ketoacidosis, would be likely to result in a more severe acidemia than either process occurring alone. Likewise, respiratory alkalosis from the central neurogenic hyperventilation of brainstem trauma in a patient with metabolic alkalosis from diuretics, could be expected to produce a more severe alkalemia than either the respiratory or metabolic abnormality alone.

Similarly, there may be two metabolic processes proceeding simultaneously, for instance, the lactic acidosis of anerobic metabolism resulting from inadequate tissue perfusion on the basis of left ventricular failure, in a patient with ketoacidosis from acute alcoholism. Again, these processes would reinforce one another.

Conversely, there may be two pathologic acid–base disturbances occurring simultaneously which tend to cancel each other out, or at least moderate the pH alteration produced by either alone. An example of this ameliorating type of mixed acid–base disturbance would be respiratory alkalosis from ascent to high altitude with hyperventilation, in a patient with metabolic acidosis from the alkaline secretion loss of persistent diarrhea. In such cases where an acidosis and an alkalosis are proceeding simultaneously, the serum pH will often reveal which is the predominating or overriding process. If the pH is below physiologic neutrality (7.35–7.4) then the acidosis, whether respiratory or metabolic, is the stronger. Thus a serum pH value represents a kind of algebraic sum of whatever acid–base derangements may be present.

Correction and Compensation for Acid–Base Abnormalities

This brings us to a consideration of the normal physiologic processes operating to maintain the base:acid ratio at the normal 20:1, and therefore the ECF pH at 7.4. These normal mechanisms are *correction* and *compensation*. In *correction* of a disturbance of acid–base balance, the processes operate to eliminate the organ malfunction responsible for the abnormality and return it to normal. An example of correction is reflexly induced expulsive coughing in a patient with respiratory acidosis from bronchitis, to clear the airways of secretions and improve alveolar ventilation. In *compensation* for a disturbance of acid–base balance, however, there are physiologic adjustments in the function of the component which are not involved in the primary causative process, which operate to restore the pH toward normal. For example, in a patient with metabolic acidosis from accumulation of diabetic ketoacids, pH receptors in the brainstem respiratory center and large arteries sense the elevated H^+ concentration and initiate reflexes which increase rate and depth of respiration, more CO_2 is eliminated, and the pH is raised because *the respiratory acid is decreased to compensate for the fact that the metabolic acids are increased.* Hence, the base–acid ratio is returned to a closer approximation to the normal 20 to 1 ratio, even though the normal range of values is exceeded for both. Similarly, in the respiratory acidosis produced by chronic obstructive pulmonary disease, the kidney eventually adaptively increases its elimination of H^+ and increases its resorption and conservation of HCO_3^- to *compensate* for the increased acid load of retained CO_2. So base is retained to compensate for the increased acid; this returns the base:acid ratio to closer to the 20:1 value, and the pH is normalized, even though the absolute values of the acid and base fall outside the normal range.

It should be noted here that not only does renal compensation for respiratory acid–base disturbances occur, but also renal compensation for metabolic alkalemia or acidemia also occurs. For example, the primary process may be a metabolic alkalemia from loss of gastric acid in a patient with nasogastric suction; or the basic disturbance may be metabolic acidemia from a loss of bicarbonate through a pancreatic fistula. In these cases the kidney would compensate by decreasing or increasing, respectively, its resorption of bicarbonate and elimination of hydrogen ion, to reestablish the 20:1 base–acid ratio, and hence the pH, within more normal limits. In a sense this might be considered correction, rather than compensation, since both the derangement and the normalizing process concerns the metabolic component, rather than both respiratory and metabolic components as is the case with the classical definition of compensation. However, remedying the abnormality in the organ in which it is occurring could be thought of as the only true correction, while the examples just cited would be a *renal* metabolic compensation for a *gastrointestinal* metabolic acid–base disturbance. So this is a gray area in the terms, neither strictly a compensation as defined above, nor a true correction.

Goal of Treatment in Acid–Base Disorders

In the treatment or management of disorders of acid–base equilibrium the goal is correction of the underlying abnormality in the organ or organ system causing the disturbance, rather than just measures carried out to return the base–acid ratio, and therefore the pH, to normal range, although such a step must be taken when the acid–base alteration is life threatening. A clinical example of this situation would be a respiratory (elevated $PaCO_2$) acidemia and metabolic (elevated lactic acid) acidemia from the acute respiratory failure of flail chest. Here, intubation and mechanical ventilation are instituted promptly (correction) and sodium bicarbonate may be given intravenously (therapeutic compensation).

It should be emphasized that respiratory compensation for a metabolic acidemia or alkalemia begins quite rapidly (minutes to hours) following development of the pH derangement, whereas renal compensation for respiratory acidemia or alkalemia develops over hours to days.

Normal Arterial Blood Gas Values

The normal arterial blood gas values at sea level and at one mile of altitude are:

	Sea Level	*One Mile of Altitude*
pH	7.35–7.45	7.35–7.45
PaO_2	80–100 mmHg	65–75 mmHg
O_2sat	95% or over	92–94%
$PaCO_2$	35–45 mmHg	34–38
HCO_3^-	22–26 meq/L	22–26
B.E.	−2 to +2	−2 to +2

At one mile altitude, the PaO_2, O_2 saturation of hemoglobin, and $PaCO_2$ are all slightly lower than at sea level. Because the overall atmospheric pressure is lower, the partial pressure of oxygen in the air–gas mixture is lower, even though the *percentage* of oxygen in the air is the same 21% as at sea level. The $PaCO_2$ is lower because of the slight hypoxic drive to hyperventilation caused by the lower ambient oxygen partial pressure.

The oxygen component of arterial blood gas determinations, and its derangements, will be discussed later in this chapter.

The Major Categories of Acid-Base Disorders and the Compensatory Responses, as Indicated by ABG Determinations

The values are only approximations to indicate the directions of change.

Respiratory Acidosis

Primary derangement: elevated PCO_2; compensatory reaction: increased renal bicarbonate retention.

	Uncompensated	*Compensated*
pH	below 7.30	7.35–7.39
PCO_2	greater than 45	greater than 45
HCO_3^-	about 24	much greater than 30

Respiratory Alkalosis

Primary derangement: decreased PCO_2; compensatory reaction: increased renal bicarbonate elimination.

	Uncompensated	*Compensated*
pH	above 7.45	7.40–7.45
P_{CO_2}	less than 35	less than 35
HCO_3^-	about 24	less than 20

Metabolic Acidosis

Primary derangement: increased H^+ or decreased HCO_3^-; compensatory reaction; decreased P_{CO_2}.

	Uncompensated	*Compensated*
pH	less than 7.30	7.35–7.39
P_{CO_2}	about 40	much less than 35
HCO_3^-	less than 20	less than 20

Metabolic Alkalosis

Primary derangement: decreased H^+ or elevated HCO_3^-; compensatory reaction: elevated P_{CO_2}.

	Uncompensated	*Compensated*
pH	above 7.50	7.40–7.45
P_{CO_2}	about 40	greater than 45
HCO_3^-	greater than 30	greater than 30

Limits to Compensation

Degree and Time Limits

Three points should be emphasized concerning compensation for acid–base imbalances: (1) in general, compensatory mechanisms are seldom, by themselves, able to return the HCO_3^-:CO_2 ratio, and hence the plasma pH, to the normal value—the change is an approximation only; (2) overcompensation seldom, if ever, occurs; and (3) while respiratory compensation for metabolic acidemia or alkalemia is initiated quite promptly (within minutes to hours), renal compensation for respiratory (or gastrointestinal metabolic) acid–base derangements probably requires hours to days to develop. Therefore, in the primary respiratory derangements, the degree of renal metabolic compensation is a correlate of how long the primary disorder has persisted. That is, if the bicarbonate is close to normal and the pH abnormal, then the respiratory disturbance is of recent onset—relatively acute. If the bicarbonate is appropriately elevated or decreased (depending upon whether the primary respiratory abnormality is hypo- or hyperventilation) and the pH fairly close to the normal range, then compensation is occurring and the abnormality is of greater duration (more chronic). Since respiratory compensation for metabolic disorders takes place more rapidly, the time element is less evident.

Hypoxic Limit

The degree of hypoventilation in the compensatory respiratory response to metabolic alkalosis is limited because of the hypoxemia which results from decreased respiratory rate and tidal volume. As the alkalemia depresses the respiratory reflex centers, and alveolar ventilation declines, there comes a point where hypoxemic stimulation to these centers overrides the alkalemic depression, and the minute ventilation increases to maintain the PaO_2 of the blood at levels acceptable to the respiratory reflex receptors. Thus $PaCO_2$ will once again decline, base:acid ratio will rise above the 20:1 ratio, and pH will once again increase. The hypoxic ventilatory drive restricts compensatory $PaCO_2$ elevation to about 55 mmHg at sea level.

pH and the Direction (Acidemia or Alkalemia) of the Acid–Base Disturbance

Since, as mentioned above, the compensatory mechanisms probably never return the HCO_3^-:CO_2 ratio, and hence the pH, to completely normal values, even after the lapse of enough time for the compensatory process to be fully established, a plasma pH determination usually indicates the direction of the acid–base abnormality. Therefore, in evaluating the acid–base status of a patient from blood gas data, it is useful first to look at the pH value to determine if it is on the acidemic or alkalemic side of physiologic neutrality: pH 7.40. A pH of above 7.40 indicates that there is some primary process tending toward alkalemia; if it is below 7.40 then the reverse is indicated.

Assessing whether the disturbance is probably respiratory or metabolic in nature is aided by checking the values for the $PaCO_2$ and the HCO_3^-, and the base excess or deficit, as indicated (in very general terms) in the tables for the four primary abnormalities given above. The interpretation of mixed acid–base abnormalities is more complicated; there is no substitute for clinical experience in such interpretations, always aided, of course, by the patient's signs and symptoms, known physiologic abnormalities, past health history and treatments. Knowledge of the clinical setting as an aid to patient assessment is nowhere more essential than in disorders of fluid, electrolyte, acid–base, and blood gas equilibria.

DISORDERS OF ACID–BASE BALANCE

Respiratory Acidosis

Causes of Respiratory Acidosis: Acute and Chronic

This process results from abnormalities of pulmonary ventilation which depress the rate of CO_2 elimination from the lungs. The decrease may occur acutely (acute hypercapnia) as in flail chest, hypoventilation from depressive drug overdose, or airway obstruction from aspiration, brain trauma, and cardiopulmonary arrest. Disorders such as pulmonary embolism, pneumonia, and pulmonary edema more often lead to *hypocapnia* (respiratory alkalosis) than to hypercapnia.

The reason is that the hypoxemia caused by these abnormalities produces a strong hypoxic drive of the respiratory center reflexes. CO_2 crosses the alveolar-capillary membranes much more readily than O_2, so that the increased minute ventilation caused by the hypoxia occurring in these abnormalities leads to a decline in $Paco_2$ in spite of decreased alveolar gas exchange. In severe acute respiratory acidosis, as in asphyxiation or cardiopulmonary arrest, the resulting respiratory acidemia is worsened by an accompanying hypoxemic metabolic acidemia from the rapidly accumulating lactic acid which is produced during cellular anaerobic glycolysis.

A more gradual development and chronic persistence of respiratory acidosis results from the various forms of chronic obstructive pulmonary disease, and in Pickwickian syndrome (obesity or primary alveolar hypoventilation). In such patients acute respiratory failure is often superimposed on the chronic CO_2 retention when, for example, a patient with severe emphysema develops acute bronchitis secondary to a viral or bacterial respiratory infection.

In acute respiratory acidosis much of the early increase in H^+ concentration induced by the elevated $Paco_2$ is absorbed first by the ECF buffers and then by the ICF buffers as H^+'s move into the ICF. As $Paco_2$ rises further, the retained CO_2 shifts the reaction to the right (see equation on page 47), the H^+ increases still more and the pH declines. This is uncompensated respiratory acidemia.

In more chronically elevated $Paco_2$, the kidneys gradually increase their capacity to excrete H^+; in this process increased bicarbonate is generated and retained, resulting in some elevation of the pH. Gradually, increased renal bicarbonate resorption becomes more fully established, serum bicarbonate increases further and pH rises closer to the normal value. This process of renal compensation for respiratory acidosis requires many hours to several days.

Assessment in Respiratory Acidosis

Hypercapnia, both acute and chronic, is always accompanied by hypoxemia. For this reason subjective and objective data in patients with respiratory acidosis are always combined with the consequences of hypoxemia, and usually it is the hypoxemia itself which is responsible for many of the clinical characteristics of CO_2 retention. When the $Paco_2$ becomes greatly elevated, however, over 60 mmHg $Paco_2$, altered mental status manifested as mental confusion, and decreased levels of consciousness may develop: lethargy and obtundation. Since high $Paco_2$ produces a form of metabolic brain syndrome, asterixis (metabolic flapping hand tremor) and myoclonus (muscle jerks) may occur. Since marked hypercapnia causes considerable cerebrovascular dilation, the vascular congestion leads to elevated intracranial pressure, which may be manifested as decreased venous pulsation in the optic disc, and blurring of the disc margins—early papilledema.

The patient with chronic CO_2 retention is often acidemic, but because of the renal bicarbonate-resorbing compensatory mechanism, the pH may be within normal limits. There is some evidence that overcompensation may occur, in which case, because of the greatly elevated serum bicarbonate, the pH may be on the alkaline side (metabolic alkalemia). It is theorized that this (rare) overcompensation contributes to a worsening of the patient's blood gas abnormalities, since alkalemia produces depression of the respiratory center and hence a still lower PaO_2 and a higher $PaCO_2$. A more likely possibility when COPD patients present with alkalemia, especially those patients with cor pulmonale (right heart failure) is that, because of the systemic vascular congestion and pretibial edema, they are receiving thiazide diuretics and also may be on a salt-restricted diet. These tend to lower serum chloride. Since there is less chloride available for resorption with sodium, more H^+ (and K^+) will be eliminated in exchange for Na^+ at the DRT-CES; thus more bicarbonate is generated, and the consequence is a metabolic hypochloremic, and often hypokalemic, alkalemia.

The most important component in the assessment of respiratory acid–base abnormalities is the arterial blood gas determination, which gives information concerning every parameter necessary to the evaluation of respiratory status, as well as an index of the probable duration of the disturbance. If hypercapnia is acute, plasma bicarbonate and pH will be low; in hypercapnia of longer duration, they may be within normal limits or high.

Management of Respiratory Acidosis

The treatment in both acute and chronic hypercapnia consists first in determining the cause of the hypercapnia, and directing treatment to that abnormality which is causing the impaired alveolar ventilation. Management of the various specific abnormalities leading to respiratory acidemia will be dealt with under their respective sections (Chapter 9).

Respiratory Alkalosis

Causes of Respiratory Alkalosis

This process is caused by any situation which leads to hyperventilation and hence a lowering of the $PaCO_2$. As $PaCO_2$ declines, the equilibrium of the equation shifts to the left, producing a fall in H^+ concentration and an increased pH. The body buffer systems and the intracellular fluid supply some H^+. If the hyperventilation is maintained for any length of time the kidneys increase bicarbonate elimination, and in the chronic hyperventilation of altitude, induced by the decreased partial pressure of oxygen in the ambient air, plasma bicarbonate is often maintained at the lower levels which permit a close to normal pH. This is renal compensation for the process of respiratory alkalosis.

Acute psychogenic hyperventilation often develops in anxiety attacks. Elevated body temperature, which causes hyperpnea as an adaptive response of the central thermoregulatory mechanisms to produce cooling by evaporation from the lungs; and physical exercise, which induces hyperpnea as an adaptive response to increased oxygen demand; may produce a respiratory alkalotic process. Sudden altitude ascents; pneumonia, probably because of atelectasis and ventilation–perfusion mismatch; central neurogenic hyperventilation from brainstem trauma or lesions; mechanical ventilation set at a too-high rate and/or tidal volume; and conditions causing hypoxemia: pulmonary embolism, acute pulmonary edema, and pulmonary ventilation–perfusion mismatch, as occurs acutely in the adult respiratory distress syndrome; all induce a respiratory alkalotic process on the basis of hypoxemic hyperventilation. Metabolic acidemia induces compensatory respiratory alkalosis (see following).

Assessment in Respiratory Alkalosis

Any patient who is obviously hyperventilating should be assessed for evidence of any of the possible causative disorders listed above. The problem is complicated by the fact that an observed hyperventilation may be, instead of primary respiratory alkalosis, a respiratory compensation for metabolic acidemia. Again, ABG determinations are of great value in determining the cause, in addition to other components of clinical assessment such as the patient's history, signs and symptoms, and known disorders, physical examination, and laboratory data. In the ABG determination, if the pH is elevated and the bicarbonate low or normal the cause is probably primary hyperventilation; however, if both the pH and the plasma bicarbonate are low, there is probably respiratory compensation for a metabolic acidemia. Pulmonary edema, pulmonary embolism, pneumonia, and other disorders producing hypoxemic hyperventilation are discussed in Chapter 9.

In acute hyperventilation the patient may complain of "dizziness" or light-headedness; circumoral and extremity parasthesias consisting typically of numbness and tingling; a feeling that he is not getting enough air, which he may describe as being short of breath; and a need to sigh deeply. There may also be mental confusion, dimming or blurring of vision, and a "blackout" where there is actual loss of consciousness (Chapter 16). If hyperventilation is extreme there may be carpopedal spasms. A very low plasma CO_2 from hyperventilation induces vasoconstriction of the cerebral vasculature, reduced cerebral blood flow, and some decline in cerebral oxygen consumption. The elevated pH causes a reduction in levels of ionized calcium, which, along with the alkalemia itself, increases neuromuscular excitability. In protracted hyperventilation plasma CO_2 will be low, and bicarbonate may be less than 18 meq/L.

This action of hyperventilation in constricting cerebral vasculature is used therapeutically in patients with brain trauma, cerebral edema, and elevated intracranial pressure. The patient is placed on mechanical ventilation, the rate and tidal volume are increased deliberately, and because of the resulting reduced cerebral vascular congestion an intracranial pressure monitor may reveal a prompt decline in intracranial pressure following inception of hyperventilation, together with amelioration of the signs of cerebral edema. Although the resulting reduced cerebral blood flow to the brain may cause some cerebral hypoxia, most studies show that the benefits from the reduced cerebral edema are overriding.

Management of Anxiety Hyperventilation

This condition is most frequently seen in young persons, especially females of nervous temperament. The first task is to demonstrate to the patient the cause of the paresthesias, "dizziness," and "blackouts." If, after taking a careful history of present illness and review of systems, including other indications of tension such as muscle contraction headaches; and performing a neurological screening examination and muscle examination to determine tenderness of occiput and neck muscles, a tentative assessment of anxiety hyperventilation seems appropriate, inquiries should be directed at eliciting a recognition of the situation at home or at work which seems to the patient to be sources of tension. Often such tensions are denied. Then the patient may be asked to help you perform a little experiment. Seated in a comfortable chair, the patient should be asked to breathe deeply through the mouth while you time two or three minutes. Ask the patient in advance to signal the development of any symptoms resembling those comprising the chief complaint. Occasionally the experiment terminates with the patient lapsing briefly into a decreased level of consciousness. After cessation of the test, it is appropriate to discuss the unconscious nature and gradual insidious quality of this response to tension and the importance of recognition of early symptoms; and then to give instructions for deliberate breathholding or rebreathing in a paper bag at the onset of symptoms. Psychiatric referral may be suggested. It is always desirable to resist strongly the temptation to prescribe a tranquilizer unless the patient is willing to seek psychiatric counseling, in which case pharmacologic assistance may be given if the mental health worker deems this appropriate as part of an ongoing management regimen.

Other causes of respiratory alkalosis represent abnormal conditions which themselves require treatment and which will be discussed under their appropriate headings. Metabolic acidemia is one such cause.

Metabolic Acidosis

Causes of Metabolic Acidosis

The categories of cause of a process of metabolic acidosis are: H^+ added to the body fluids; bicarbonate lost from body fluids; or failure of the kidneys to excrete the H^+ produced as end products of cellular metabolism. Physiologic adaptive responses defending against pH change include buffer action, ion migration, and respiratory and renal compensations, as described above. Buffer systems of both the ECF and ICF: hemoglobin, plasma proteins, bicarbonate, and intracellular organic anions, absorb H^+ added to the body fluids. An H^+ load is divided about equally between the two fluid compartments, ICF and ECF. As the H^+ content of the ECF increases, H^+'s move into cells in exchange for which, to maintain electrical neutrality, K^+ and Na^+ move from ICF into the ECF. As ECF concentration of K^+ rises, renal elimination of this ion increases, unless renal function is impaired in which case hyperkalemia may develop.

The rise in H^+ concentration and/or decline in HCO_3^- shifts the equation equilibrium to the left, the base: acid 20:1 ratio declines, and pH falls. The decreased pH of the ECF stimulates the chemoreceptors of the brainstem and the large artery respiratory control mechanisms to cause hyperventilation: respiratory compensation for metabolic acidosis. The increased alveolar ventilation decreases first alveolar and then arterial PCO_2 returning the ratio, and hence the pH, to a more normal value; however, complete respiratory compensation does not occur. The increased work of breathing accompanying increased minute ventilation generates increased CO_2 which limits the pH decline that can be attained through hyperventilation; the lower limit of $PaCO_2$ is about 16–18 mmHg. A patient with already restricted pulmonary function from pulmonary fibrosis, COPD, or sedative drug depression of the respiratory center, is thus particularly susceptible to metabolic acidosis because of impairment of the respiratory compensation process.

As always, the renal compensatory response, in the form of increased elimination of NH_4^+, H_2SO_4, and H_3PO_4, takes longer to develop. This takes place by means of several mechanisms. Renal elimination of increased H_3PO_4 occurs fairly rapidly. Gradually, increased kidney output of H^+ develops via increased NH_4^+ elimination and at this time increased HCO_3^- resorption becomes well established. In the process of renal H^+ excretion, new bicarbonate is generated which aids in restoring the 20:1 $HCO_3^-:CO_2$ ratio. Again, impaired kidney function decreases the effectiveness of H^+ elimination.

H^+ Added to Body Fluids

Such addition of H^+ to the ECF may occur in any of the following abnormal processes. (1) Diabetic and alcoholic ketoacidosis, and the ketoacidosis of starvation, all result from abnormal fat metabolism. (2) Lactic acidosis develops from any condition which produces severe cellular hypoxia; oxidative cellular metabolism declines, less pyruvate enters the Krebs cycle, and instead anaerobic glycolysis forms lactic acid from the pyruvic acid. Lactic acidosis occurs in the circulatory failure accompanying severe hypovolemic, vasodilated, septic, or cardiogenic shock, or left ventricular failure. (3) Chemicals which have strong organic acids as metabolic intermediates: ethyl and methyl alcohol, salicylates, and ethylene glycol, add large numbers of H^+ to the ECF. Ammonium chloride (NH_4Cl), which is converted in the liver to urea, is also a strong H^+ donor.

Loss of HCO_3^-

Loss of HCO_3^- from loss of pancreatic and intestinal secretions, which have an HCO_3^- concentration higher than that of the ECF, may occur in pancreatic fistula and upper intestinal (duodenal) drainage. Also high intestinal obstruction acts in effect to remove bicarbonate from the ECF, since that which is secreted into the tract more proximally cannot be resorbed distally.

Impaired Renal Function

Impaired renal function, as in oliguric or anuric chronic renal failure, renders the kidney unable to eliminate the ammonium ions and resorb the bicarbonate essential to prevent metabolic acidosis; this is probably the most common cause of chronic metabolic acidosis.

Assessment in Metabolic Acidosis

The only sign reliably seen in such a patient is hyperventilation; although in chronic metabolic acidosis this may not be evident on observation, still ABGs may show a low $Paco_2$. In the metabolic acidemia of chronic renal failure the patient may experience easy fatigability, shortness of breath on exertion, anorexia, nausea, and general malaise, although to what extent these symptoms are the consequence of the acidemia or of the many other metabolic abnormalities is difficult to say.

The patient with an acute metabolic acidosis may show altered mental status, such as confusion; or decreased levels of consciousness: lethargy, stupor, or coma. However, again, such manifestations may equally be the result of the underlying systemic disorder causing the acidemia. The patient's clinical history and a knowledge of preexisting abnormalities is of great importance in assessment; ABG values, especially low pH and HCO_3^-, with a compensatory decline in $PaCO_2$, may be helpful.

The Anion Gap

In order properly to manage the underlying condition, the cause must be determined, and here the evaluation of the anion gap becomes important. Anion gap is defined as the concentration of unmeasured anions in the plasma. The measured anions are by definition Cl^- and HCO_3^-. Anions other than these normally constitute about 12 meq/L of the total anion content of the plasma.

A metabolic acidemia may develop from two categories of cause: those which do, and those which do not, lead to an increase in unmeasured anions (A^-). The concentration of unmeasured anions equals the anion gap. Figure 2-1a shows that anions other than Cl^- and HCO_3^- constitute 12 meq/L of the total about 140 meq/L anion content of the plasma; Figure 2-1b indicates that in metabolic acidosis from certain causes, bicarbonate will decrease and chloride will increase; Figure 2-1c shows the anion distribution in a metabolic acidosis from a cause which produced decreased bicarbonate without a corresponding increase of chloride (that is, an elevation in content of the unmeasured anions indicated as A^-). In the normal subject these anions are the anions of organic acids and esters, and HPO_4^{2-}, $H_2PO_4^-$ and HSO_4^-.

In calculating the anion gap the serum Cl^- and the serum HCO_3^- values in meq/L are added; this sum is subtracted from the serum Na^+ in meq/L. In the normal subject the resulting value is about 10 to 12 meq/L, and represents the negatively charged ions contained in the plasma which are neither Cl^- nor HCO_3^-. In the patient with a metabolic acidemia, the reduction in HCO_3^- concentration may be accompanied by a normal Cl^-, in which case there is an increase in the concentration of unmeasured anions; or it may be accompanied by an elevated Cl^-, in which case there is not an increase in the concentration of unmeasured anions.

If the concentration of unmeasured anions is increased, then this is evidence for the fact that H^+'s have been added to the ECF with some anion other than Cl^-. The conditions which will produce metabolic acidemia with an increased anion gap are lactic acidosis, diabetic ketoacidosis, renal failure, or toxic levels of some chemical agent such as ethyl or methyl alcohol, or the others listed above. If the concentration of unmeasured anions is not increased, i.e., there is no anion gap, then the reduction in HCO_3^- has resulted from either a loss of HCO_3^- or an addition of H^+ with Cl^-. Causes of metabolic acidosis with no anion gap are diarrhea, NH_4Cl ingestion, pancreatic juice drainage, renal tubular acidosis (these patients excrete an alkaline urine and have renal calculi), or acetazolamide intake, which suppresses renal tubular H^+ elimination by decreasing the tubular reaction: $H_2O + CO_2 \rightleftharpoons H_2CO_3$ through inhibition of the enzyme carbonic anhydrase which catalyzes it.

Prevention of Metabolic Acidosis

In many of these disorders prevention is an important aspect of health care management, especially where chronic conditions predispose the patient to acute ex-

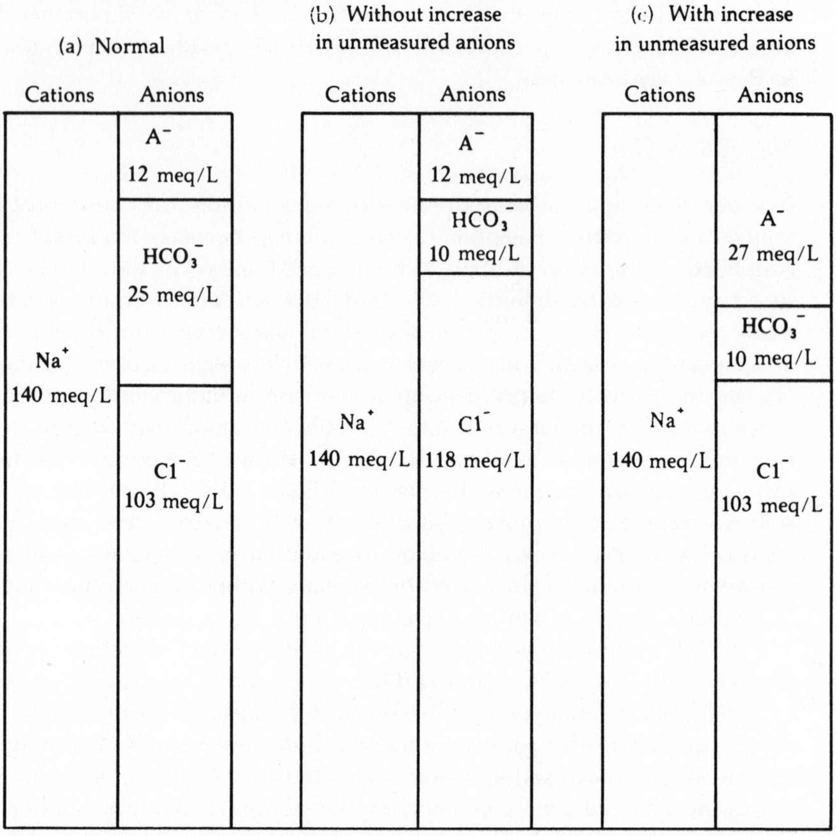

(a) Normal

(b) Without increase in unmeasured anions

(c) With increase in unmeasured anions

Cations	Anions	Cations	Anions	Cations	Anions

(a) Normal
Cations: Na^+ 140 meq/L
Anions: A^- 12 meq/L; HCO_3^- 25 meq/L; Cl^- 103 meq/L

(b) Without increase in unmeasured anions
Cations: Na^+ 140 meq/L
Anions: A^- 12 meq/L; HCO_3^- 10 meq/L; Cl^- 118 meq/L

(c) With increase in unmeasured anions
Cations: Na^+ 140 meq/L
Anions: A^- 27 meq/L; HCO_3^- 10 meq/L; Cl^- 103 meq/L

Figure 2-1. Normal serum cation and anion values, and those in metabolic acidosis, with or without an increase in unmeasured anions.

acerbations which would lead to a life-threatening metabolic acidemia. In diabetes mellitus, thorough patient education in diet, exercise, use of insulin, and faithful daily urine testing is important. Polyuria and polydipsia with craving for sweets, especially in a patient with strong family history of diabetes, should prompt testing of urine and a random blood glucose. Early recognition of hyperemesis gravidarum will help prevent damage to the fetus from the ketoacidemia of starvation. Careful management of congestive heart failure may forestall the lactic acidemia of circulatory failure.

Signs of circulatory failure in any severely ill or chronically debilitated patient need to be carefully assessed: a fall in blood pressure, mental confusion, oliguria, hypoxemia from any cause, cardiac arrhythmia, dyspnea and cyanosis, sudden elevation of temperature, a shaking chill or persistent diarrhea, are all warnings of developing complications which could produce lactic acidemia. Laboratory determinations of arterial blood gases and serum electrolytes are useful in patient assessment and early recognition of such complications. Alcoholism rehabilitation programs should be encouraged for the patient with a severe drinking problem (although, unfortunately, it is usually to no avail).

Management of Metabolic Acidosis

As in many acid–base disorders, the first consideration is controlling or reversing the underlying systemic abnormality, together with immediate measures to reverse the acidemia if it is very severe. For the ketoacidemia of diabetes, insulin and glucose intravenously is given; glucose and isotonic NaCl is used for alcoholic ketoacidemia. Lactic acidemia management consists of attempts to remedy the inadequate tissue perfusion: measures to improve myocardial contractility; fluid volume expansion; elevation of blood pressure with vasoconstrictors; or administration of vasodilators with a heart-stimulating action. If the acidemia is extreme, $NaHCO_3$ given rapidly to provide serum bicarbonate to levels of at least 20 meq/L may be necessary to return the pH to a safer value.

Since ion movement in reversal of acidemia is such that hypokalemia may occur, as discussed earlier, serum K^+ levels should be monitored as well as serum Na^+ to check for hypernatremia (iatrogenic). Another danger in intravenous $NaHCO_3$ is that the sodium may elevate ECF osmolarity, draw ICF water into the ECF, and result in hypervolemia and left ventricular failure.

In ketoacidemia and lactic acidemia, once the causative processes are controlled, the accumulated organic acid anions will be metabolized to bicarbonate, which will replenish the depleted plasma bicarbonate reserve.

A phenomenon of interest in the correction of severe metabolic acidosis is post-correction hyperventilation: a persistence of the respiratory compensation for metabolic acidemia after the pH has been returned to a more normal level with bicarbonate infusion. Bicarbonate ion, unlike CO_2, crosses the blood–brain barrier slowly. Thus, acidemia persists in the cerebrospinal fluid and brain ECF for a time after it has been reversed in the rest of the body. This stimulates brainstem respiratory reflexes to produce hyperventilation until the bicarbonate levels, and therefore the pH levels, in the brain have returned to normal; in this situation the $Paco_2$ is inappropriately low in the light of the serum pH, because of the persisting central hyperventilation.

Metabolic Alkalosis

This process results from loss of acid or excess of alkali. In either case the elevation of HCO_3^- shifts the equation equilibrium to the left, decreasing H^+ concentration and elevating pH. As always in acid–base disorders, buffer systems and ion movements between ICF and ECF operate to minimize the pH change. H^+ migrates into the ECF, and K^+ moves intracellularly. Respiratory compensation results from alkalemic depression of the respiratory control reflexes leading to decreased alveolar ventilation and an elevated $Paco_2$, though not often above about 50 mmHg because of the hypoxemia which will act to increase respiratory drive via stimulation of the arterial O_2 chemoreceptors. Later the kidneys increase H^+ retention and HCO_3^- elimination. The response occurs quite rapidly in this case and with great effectiveness, since this is the major mechanism of physiologic response to a metabolic alkalemia.

Causes of Metabolic Alkalosis

Stimulation of the Distal Renal Tubule Cation Exchange Site

Increased resorption of Na^+ from the tubular fluid in exchange for excretion of K^+ or H^+ enhances elimination of H^+ and generates HCO_3^-, which is retained with the Na^+. Therefore anything which stimulates activity at this site will tend to induce a metabolic alkalemia.

Dehydration and Hypovolemia. These are probably the most common causes of the process of metabolic alkalosis. When there is depletion of ECF volume, the normal adaptive response by the kidney is to increase the resorption of Na^+ from the tubular filtrate in order to retain isosmotic water and to reexpand the ECF. (Physiologically, the mechanisms for retaining Na^+ take precedence over those processes tending to correct the alkalemia; this is adaptive, because of the danger of circulatory collapse from hypovolemia.) Hypovolemic patients are often low in Cl^-, and for this reason there is not enough Cl^- to reabsorb with Na^+ in the proximal nephron, so that more Na^+ must be resorbed in exchange for H^+ in the distal nephron. This type of hypochloremic alkalosis usually resolves following volume expansion with isotonic saline.

Diuretics. The diuretics furosemide, ethacrynic acid, and the thiazides block the resorption of Na^+ and Cl^- in portions of the tubule proximal to the distal cation exchange site. The result is increased delivery of Na^+ and Cl^- to that site. Here, because of the high tubular content of Na^+, and because Cl^- is not retained with Na^+ at the DRT-CES, H^+ and Cl^- are eliminated in the urine and an equivalent amount of HCO_3^- is resorbed into peritubular blood. Both hypochloremia and hypokalemia make such a metabolic alkalotic process more severe.

Excess Adrenal Steroids. Glucocorticoids in Cushing's syndrome and mineralocorticoids in hyperaldosteronism stimulate this portion of the tubule.

Hypokalemia. Low K^+ in the ECF means that Na^+ must be resorbed in exchange for a greater elimination of H^+. Evidence indicates that there are additional processes involved in the alkalosis of hypokalemia which are not yet well understood.

Chronic Respiratory Acidosis

The patient with a compensated respiratory acidosis has a high plasma bicarbonate from renal compensatory bicarbonate resorption. If therapy to improve alveolar ventilation is successful, then $Paco_2$ may decline quite rapidly because of the facility with which CO_2 moves across all cell membranes. HCO_3^-, however, moves across cell membranes much more slowly, and renal elimination of the large HCO_3^- stores takes relatively long—several days. Thus as the $Paco_2$ falls, the base to acid ratio rises, and the pH increases until the excess HCO_3^- is eliminated by the kidney. The elimination is slowed by dehydration, hypochloremia, and salt restriction (because of low Na^+ filtration at the glomerulus) by the mechanisms discussed above.

Persistent Vomiting or Nasogastric Suction

Persistent vomiting or nasogastric suction may produce metabolic alkalemia. Loss of H^+ in the HCl causes a relative excess of plasma HCO_3^-; the base–acid ratio therefore increases, as does the pH. Additional processes tend to make the alkalemia more severe. Since stomach secretions are also high in chloride, ECF Cl^- concentration drops, and less is filtered at the glomeruli. Therefore, the tubular filtrate is low in available Cl^- to be resorbed back into the blood with Na^+, at the proximal portions of the nephron where Na^+ and Cl^- are resorbed together. As a result, tubular Na^+ increases. Also the higher ECF HCO_3^- produces a higher tubular HCO_3^- concentration. For these reasons, both Na^+ and HCO_3^- arrive in larger quantities at the DRT-CES than can be resorbed, and there is an initial Na^+ loss. The distal tubule responds to the loss by increasing the cation exchange site activity and more Na^+ is retained in exchange for K^+. The patient then tends to become hypokalemic; this forces Na^+ resorption in exchange for H^+ elimination, and the alkalemia worsens.

Assessment in Metabolic Alkalosis

Laboratory findings of elevated serum pH and bicarbonate in a patient with a normal or slightly elevated Pa_{CO_2}, and the presence of a disorder known to produce a metabolic alkalotic process, are the components of patient evaluation. If the patient has evidence of chronic pulmonary disease and an elevated Pa_{CO_2}, especially if receiving diuretics or adrenal steroids, then metabolic (renal) compensation for respiratory acidosis combined with excessive H^+ and K^+ loss, are the likely processes causing the elevated serum HCO_3^-. This mixed acid–base disorder tends not to result in patient complaints or physical findings on examination unless it is very severe. On occasion altered mental status and decreased levels of consciousness are seen, but such a patient may be hypoxemic and very ill, and which signs are attributable to the altered pH per se and which to the preceding and accompanying systemic disorders is a moot question.

Occasionally carpopedal spasm may occur in a patient having a low serum Ca^{2+}; Ca^{2+} is more closely bound to the plasma proteins in an alkaline pH, and the drop in ionized Ca^{2+} caused by alkalemia may be sufficient to produce tetany or a seizure. If the patient is hypokalemic, especially if digitalized, then EKG abnormalities or a cardiac arrhythmia may develop.

Management of Metabolic Alkalosis

If the alkalemia is mild it need not be considered a problem in itself and attention to the system disorders present will correct it. In dehydration, hypokalemia, and hypochloremia, isotonic saline with potassium chloride supplements may be given. Occasionally NH_4Cl (ammonium chloride) may be given intravenously, but this requires caution especially if the patient has any evidence or history of liver impairment. The rate of infusion may exceed the capacity of the liver to convert the NH_4^+ to urea, which may lead to ammonium intoxication and signs of hepatic encephalopathy (mental confusion, delirium, myoclonus, asterixis, stupor). Some hospital pharmacies do not dispense NH_4Cl for intravenous use. Arginine hydrochloride is a safer means of supplying Cl^- where K^+ or Na^+ are not needed.

A K^+ supplement, oral if possible, is used in hypokalemic metabolic alkalemia caused by diuretics. In the case of excess adrenal steroids from Cushing's or hyperaldosteronism, the basic endocrine disorder is the one which requires attention. The alkalemia from loss of gastric secretion requires management of the underlying disorder, and normal saline infusions with K^+ supplements. In persistent vomiting caused by obstructive peptic ulcer disease, severe metabolic alkalemia may develop. PUD is discussed in Chapter 11.

ARTERIAL OXYGEN TENSION (Pa_{O_2}) AND HEMOGLOBIN OXYGEN SATURATION (Sa_{O_2})

Thus far, reference to arterial blood gases has been concerned primarily with their value in assessment of the patient's acid–base status. We now consider their significance in evaluating the transport and exchange of oxygen and carbon dioxide between ambient air, alveoli, blood, and peripheral tissues. A Pa_{CO_2} determination gives information about the adequacy of alveolar ventilation; a Pa_{O_2} determination helps to assess the presence, degree, and to some extent the possible causes of, hypoxemia. The term hypoxemia refers to blood oxygen tension and saturation which is below normal, while the more general term hypoxia means a state of oxygen deficiency at the tissue level. Although some of these subjects are discussed in more detail in Chapter 9, they will be reviewed briefly here within the context of arterial blood gases.

Gaseous Exchange

The exchange of oxygen and carbon dioxide occurs at two sites: at the lung, between alveolar air and pulmonary capillary blood; and at the peripheral tissues, between systemic capillary blood and the metabolizing cells of organs and tissues.

Exchange at the Lung

The partial pressure of O_2 in the alveoli is about 100 mmHg at sea level; the O_2 tension in the venous blood entering the lung via the pulmonary artery is about 40 mmHg. Where the alveolar air and venous blood come into intimate contact at the alveolar–capillary membranes, an equalization of O_2 concentration between alveolar air and capillary blood occurs very rapidly by simple passive diffusion along the concentration gradient.

The partial pressure of CO_2 in the alveoli is about 40 mmHg; the CO_2 tension in venous blood is about 46 mmHg; as is the case with O_2, though in the opposite direction, CO_2 diffuses rapidly—more rapidly than O_2—from venous blood to alveolar air along the concentration gradient.

At the pulmonary capillaries of the lung, the exchange is influenced both by factors which affect alveolar perfusion via the pulmonary capillary circulation (cardiac output and distribution of blood flow in the lung); and by factors which affect alveolar ventilation (gas content of inspired air, air movement, and distribution in the tracherobronchial–bronchial–alveolar tree, and, questionably, diffusion across alveolar–capillary membranes).

Exchange at the Tissues

In the systemic capillaries, O_2 diffuses to metabolizing cells from the capillary blood along its concentration gradient, while CO_2 leaves the cells and enters the capillary blood, again, by simple diffusion along its concentration gradient. At the systemic capillaries, gaseous exchange is influenced by such factors as O_2 and CO_2 content of both the blood and tissues, capillary diameter and rate of blood flow, and the cardiac output. In comparing the gaseous diffusion and the transport of oxygen and carbon dioxide it is important to emphasize that the rate of carbon dioxide diffusion across all membranes is much faster than the rate of oxygen diffusion, and carbon dioxide is considerably more soluble in plasma than is oxygen.

Blood Gas Transport

Oxygen Transport

About 1% of the oxygen in arterial blood is in solution: 0.29 ml O_2/100 ml blood; this amount is a linear function of the partial pressure of oxygen (PO_2) in the gas mixture (air) with which the blood is equilibrated: 0.003 ml O_2/100 ml blood is in solution for every millimeter of mercury of partial pressure of oxygen. 99% of the oxygen in arterial blood is carried bound to hemoglobin: 19.8 ml O_2/100 ml blood. When blood is equilibrated with 100% O_2 (PO_2 = 760 mmHg at sea level) each gram of hemoglobin contains 1.34 ml of oxygen.

The amount of oxygen bound to hemoglobin (Hb) is also a function of the partial pressure of oxygen (PO_2) in the atmosphere with which Hb is equilibrated, but this relationship for Hb saturation is, unlike the oxygen in solution, not a linear function. Figure 2-2 shows Hb-O_2 dissociation curves, which illustrate the percent saturation of Hb for a series of oxygen partial pressures at three pH values.

Oxygen in the air exposed to blood dissolves in the blood according to the PO_2 of the air, and then moves rapidly along the diffusion gradient into association (binding) with Hb to yield Hb-O_2. When Hb has bound all of the O_2 which it is capable of, at that PO_2, the gradient is abolished and the Hb is fully saturated for that value of the PO_2. The Hb-O_2 affinity curves demonstrate this relationship. At each point, the oxygen in the air, the oxygen dissolved in the plasma, and the oxygen bound by the Hb, are in equilibrium.

The first thing to note about the Hb-O_2 dissociation curve is the shape of the nonlinear relationship; it is S-shaped. This sigmoid shape is the result of the fact that the more O_2 that is bound by a molecule of Hb, the more rapidly the binding of subsequent molecules will occur, up to a point. Each Hb binds four O_2 molecules and the binding of the first facilitates the binding of the second, and so on, until the fourth is bound many times more rapidly than is the first.

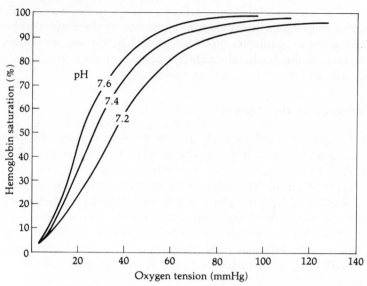

Figure 2-2. The hemoglobin—oxygen dissociation curve (see text).

The second thing to note about the curve is that the rise in the amount of O_2 bound, per increment of O_2 tension, is very rapid up to about 70 mmHg Po_2 and slow thereafter; in this steep portion of the curve a relatively small increase in Po_2 in mmHg results in a very large and rapid increase in degree of Hb-O_2 binding, and therefore in the total volume of O_2 which can be transported by the blood.

The affinity of hemoglobin for O_2 is influenced by certain factors which change the relationship between the degree of Hb-O_2 binding and the partial pressure of O_2 in the air. A change in this degree of binding, or affinity, shifts the position of the curve which relates O_2 tension in the air and in the plasma, to O_2 saturation of the Hb. A shift to the left means that the Hb has an increased oxygen affinity at each given O_2 tension, so that at that tension the Hb is more saturated and there is overall an increased blood O_2 content. But a greater affinity means that the Hb-O_2 attachment is stronger; a given level of Hb-O_2 is less effective in delivering O_2 to the tissues since the Hb gives its O_2 up less readily. Causes of a shift to the left are elevated blood pH, hypothermia, and a decrease in 2,3-diphosphoglycerate (DPG). The latter substance facilitates the release of O_2 to tissues by Hb.

A shift to the right means that at each value of the O_2 tension there is a decrease in corresponding Hb-O_2 affinity, and therefore a decreased O_2-saturation, and an overall decreased O_2 content. But, although the Hb carries less O_2 in a shift to the right, it gives up O_2 more readily to the tissues and this facilitates tissue oxygenation, even though it has taken up less O_2 at the pulmonary capillaries in the first place. Causes of a shift to the right are decreased blood pH, hypercapnea, hyperthermia, and an increase in DPG.

DPG is a normal product of cellular glycolysis which is present in large amounts in fresh erythrocytes and binds to deoxygenated Hb. Increased Hb content of this substance facilitates O_2 release from Hb. Its content in red cells falls when pH is low and rises when it is high. Exercise, increased altitude, thyroid hormones, anemia, androgens, and somatotropin (growth hormone) all increase the DPG concentration of red cells. Storage of blood, such as in a blood bank, substantially decreases DPG, so that the ability of stored blood to release O_2 to tissues is markedly impaired; this will have deleterious consequences for the hypoxemic patient who must receive transfusions of stored blood.

Oxygen delivery to tissues from the Hb of the blood in the systemic capillary circuit occurs by a process similar to, but the reverse of, that occurring at the pulmonary capillaries during O_2 uptake. Peripheral tissues have low O_2 and high CO_2 tensions, so that O_2 is released from its binding to Hb along the now-reversed gradient, and CO_2 is taken up as described below. Since Hb has a decreased affinity for O_2 in a lower pH (the Bohr effect) an increased H^+ concentration in metabolically active tissues facilitates O_2 delivery. The Hb in venous blood is 75% saturated, as opposed to the 97% saturation of arterial blood, and the O_2 content is about 15 ml/100 cc blood. So, tissues under basal conditions extract about 4.5 ml O_2 from every 100 ml blood circulating through the systemic capillaries.

Carbon Dioxide Transport

Carbon dioxide is transported in the blood in three ways: (1) A small percentage, about 5%, is carried as dissolved CO_2 gas itself, in solution in the plasma; it is this dissolved CO_2 which exerts the partial pressure (or actually tension, since it is in solution) of CO_2 in the blood. Most of the CO_2 in the blood, about 95%, is carried by the buffering systems of the erythrocytes. (2) Of this 95% about two thirds of the CO_2 is hydrated by a chemical union with H_2O; then dissociation or ionization of the resulting H_2CO_3 (carbonic acid) occurs, yielding H^+ and HCO_3^-. The resulting H^+ is carried by buffer-binding to hemoglobin. Some of the HCO_3^- leaves the red cell and enters the plasma, in exchange for Cl^- which enters the red cell; and some of the HCO_3^- remains in the red cell. (3) Of the 95% of CO_2 carried by the red cell buffer system about one third is carried as CO_2 itself, directly bound mainly to the hemoglobin of the erythrocyte, but also to other proteins. The resulting hemoglobin and protein combinations with CO_2 are called carbamino compounds.

Thus, hemoglobin is not only the principle mechanisms for oxygen transport in the blood, it is also the main means of carbon dioxide transport. The hydration of carbon dioxide, a process which occurs only very slowly without enzymic facilitation, is catalyzed by the enzyme carbonic anhydrase, present only in red cells, in gastric mucosa, and in renal tubular cells. It is this enzyme which is inhibited by acetazolamide.

Arterial Hypoxemia

Causes of Arterial Hypoxemia

Pulmonary Causes

Alveolar Hypoventilation.
This is one of the most important physiologic consequences of chronic obstructive pulmonary disease, especially of the bronchitic type. Bronchi and bron-

chioles in this disorder are narrowed because of edema, hyperemia and excessive mucus secretion. The alveolar P_{CO_2} (P_{ACO_2}) rises, and since the solubility and diffusion rate of CO_2 is so high, the arterial P_{CO_2} (P_{aCO_2}) rises to an equal level. Because of the reciprocal relationship between the levels of CO_2 and O_2 in the alveoli, a rise in alveolar CO_2 must result in a corresponding decline in alveolar O_2.

Unlike CO_2, normal arterial oxygen concentration is always 10 to 15 mmHg less than alveolar oxygen concentration because of the lower solubility and diffusibility of O_2 as compared with CO_2. An elevated P_{aCO_2} drives the respiration by stimulation of brainstem and arterial chemoreceptors to increase breathing and therefore increase alveolar ventilation; the result is a rise in P_{aO_2}. However, although theoretically hyperventilation could overcome the elevated P_{ACO_2} and decreased P_{AO_2}, the metabolic cost of such increased work of breathing, in terms of both O_2 consumption and CO_2 production, is so great that a physiologic compromise is reached whereby the patient accepts a stably elevated P_{aCO_2} and decreased P_{aO_2}—abnormal ABG values which become optimal for such a patient. It is a metabolic tradeoff. The mechanism for this equilibrium is probably an adaptation of the chemical ventilatory drives; the ventilatory stimulus exerted by an elevated P_{aCO_2} becomes attenuated and the patient comes to depend on hypoxic drive, with that also set at a lower than normal level (Chapter 9).

Ventilation and Perfusion Inequalities ($\dot{V}/\dot{Q}$ Mismatch, Venous Admixture). This occurs in both of two situations. There may be adequate capillary perfusion of poorly ventilated alveoli; or there may be inadequate capillary perfusion of adequately ventilated alveoli (Figure 9-4).

Adequate capillary perfusion of underventilated alveoli (a low $\dot{V}/\dot{Q}$ ratio). These alveoli are overperfused relative to their degree of ventilation, and this condition is an important cause of arterial hypoxemia, since it results in a return of significant amonts of underoxygenated blood to the left heart (Chapter 9).

Inadequate capillary perfusion of alveoli relative to their degree of ventilation. These alveoli are relatively underperfused (or relatively overventilated) and the result is a *high* $\dot{V}/\dot{Q}$ ratio. The consequence is as though an increased percentage of the inspired air entered respiratory deadspace, and therefore it is wasted ventilation. Such alveoli are called physiologic deadspace. This form of $\dot{V}/\dot{Q}$ mismatch is less important in producing hypoxemia than the low $\dot{V}/\dot{Q}$ ratio.

Two factors act to ameliorate the effects of $\dot{V}/\dot{Q}$ imbalance of either type. In the case of inadequately ventilated but well-perfused alveoli, the capillaries supplying these alveoli tend to respond to the low O_2 and high CO_2 which they contain by vasoconstriction, which reduces the degree of mismatch. In the case of poorly perfused but adequately ventilated alveoli, the small terminal bronchioles tend to respond to the relatively high O_2 and low CO_2 of the air in them (because there is little blood flow around the alveoli to remove the O_2 and add CO_2) by bronchoconstriction. Here again this direct adaptive response acts to reduce the discrepancy between ventilation and perfusion, and ameliorates the abnormalities of arterial blood gas values caused by ventilation–perfusion inequalities.

Intrapulmonary Shunts.   This is a more advanced, or a complete, form of the low $\dot{V}/\dot{Q}$ ratio abnormality. Some authors consider low $\dot{V}/\dot{Q}$ mismatches to be but one form of an intrapulmonary (physiologic) shunt, since their effect is to contribute blood which is underoxygenated to varying degrees, to the left heart. A shunt is defined as that portion of the cardiac output which does not exchange at all with alveolar air. A capillary shunt is a situation in which pulmonary capillaries are perfusing completely nonventilated alveoli. Such a condition results from collapsed alveoli (atelectasis) and from alveoli filled with fluid, which occurs in severe pulmonary edema and the adult respiratory distress syndrome. The normal physiologic response of pulmonary capillaries to alveolar hypoxia from nonventilation is vasoconstriction, an adaptive response, since blood then is directed away from the alveoli which are making no contribution to the oxygenation of arterial blood.

When blood in the pulmonary vein contains quantities of unoxygenated blood from shunt units, this is mixed with oxygenated blood from normal units, and the result is an overall lowering of the Pao_2. The vasoconstrictive response, where it is intact, may modify the contribution of capillary shunts to arterial hypoxemia. However, patients apparently vary in their degree of pulmonary vasoconstrictive response to nonventilated alveoli; where this adaptive response fails, then the total amount of unoxygenated pulmonary capillary blood entering the left atrium may be greatly increased, markedly lowering Pao_2.

Alveolar–Capillary Membrane Diffusion Impediments.   This type of impairment of the free equilibration of respiratory gases between alveoli and pulmonary capillary blood is proposed by some authors to be characteristic of pulmonary fibrosis, pneumonia, and interstitial pulmonary edema. It has been said to result in a slow diffusion of O_2 and CO_2 across respiratory–vascular membranes, leading to abnormalities of the arterial blood gases. However, increasingly investigators are questioning the alveolar–capillary block mechanism, and are attributing the blood gas abnormalities in these disorders to $\dot{V}/\dot{Q}$ mismatches.

It should be emphasized that in many clinical conditions causing arterial hypoxemia on a pulmonary basis, all of these abnormalities may be and probably are combined in varying degrees throughout various portions of the lungs. It should also be stressed that evaluation of the causes of inadequate arterial oxygenation must be made within the context of the other values in a blood gas determination, and in the light of the patient's total physiologic status and accompanying systemic abnormalities.

Nonpulmonary Causes of Arterial Hypoxemia

These include primarily a reduced cardiac output, and occasionally anemia. Cardiovascular causes of arterial hypoxemia are discussed in Chapters 5, 6, and 7. However, all ABG values must be considered in the light of cardiovascular status: heart rate and blood pressure; tissue and organ perfusion (urinary output, skin condition, mental status); and of the patient's metabolic rate: body temperature and motor activity. Any decrease in oxygen content of central venous blood because of cardiovascular abnormalities will contribute significantly to the arterial hypoxemia caused by the pulmonary defects cited above.

Compensatory Responses to Arterial Hypoxemia

There are a number of compensatory responses to arterial hypoxemia which may influence the values in an ABG determination. The first is the response to a decreased PaO_2 content by the chemoreceptors in the aortic arch and carotid sinuses which send afferent impulses to the brainstem respiratory control centers in the pons and medulla, to cause increased respiratory rate and depth, and hence improved alveolar ventilation. However, this response increases the work of breathing and therefore elevates O_2 consumption and CO_2 production.

A second important compensatory response to arterial hypoxemia is elevated cardiac output, the consequence of which is an increased total blood flow through tissues, which helps compensate for the decreased oxygen content. The amount of oxygen which tissues need to extract from a given volume of blood to meet their metabolic requirements is decreased because of the overall increased blood flow resulting from the elevated cardiac output. The result of the elevated blood flow is an increased oxygen content in the venous blood entering the lungs, because less O_2 was removed by the tissues. This mechanism ameliorates the effects of pulmonary shunting, because the blood enters the lungs with a higher baseline oxygen tension.

Inhalation of enriched O_2 mixtures is of course the principal therapeutic means for elevating PaO_2 by providing an increased fraction of inhaled oxygen (FIO_2) which is advantageous in that it neither increases the work of breathing nor elevates the myocardial work load, as is required by the other two compensations.

Categories of Arterial Hypoxemia Seen in ABG Determination

Hypoxemia with Hypercapnia

This condition results from inadequate alveolar ventilation and is reflected in a PaO_2 of less than 50 mmHg and a $PaCO_2$ of greater than 50 mmHg. As discussed in the section on respiratory acidosis, this abnormality may be acute and uncompensated, or chronic with renal compensation, or in transition between the two. The chronic form is typical of the abnormalities comprising chronic obstruction pulmonary disease. When acute bronchitis or pneumonia is superimposed, acute respiratory failure develops with an increase in $PaCO_2$, further decline in PaO_2, and a drop in pH worsened by lactic acidemia. When the PaO_2 is below 30 mmHg the patient is stuporous or comatose. The low pH results in decreased myocardial contractility and abnormal impulse formation in the heart, causing arrhythmias. Neurologic impairment frequently occurs. Disorders in this category may be classified as follows: (1) primary acute hypoventilation: $PaCO_2 > 50$ and pH < 7.3; (2) primary chronic hypoventilation with renal compensation: $PaCO_2 > 45$, pH ~ 7.35, HCO_3^- markedly elevated; and (3) primary metabolic alkalosis with respiratory compensation: pH > 7.45 and a low $PaCO_2$.

Hypoxemia with Hypocapnia

Acute inflammatory pulmonary disorders such as pneumonia, and atelectasis, are the most common causes; alveolar collapse and collection of secretions lead to regional impairment of alveolar ventilation. A PaO_2 of 40–80 mmHg; pH $>$

7.45, and $Paco_2$ of 30 or below may be typical values. The patient is dyspneic with a high tidal volume and respiratory rate, causing a great increase in minute volume and in work of breathing and increased movement of air over respiratory dead space. The attempt to increase Pao_2 results in a decrease in $Paco_2$ (hypoxemic hyperventilation).

Other common causes of this blood gas and respiratory pattern are the adult respiratory distress syndrome (ARDS) and an acute asthmatic attack (Chapter 9). Many cardiovascular abnormalities also produce this picture: a pleural effusion causing atelectasis, acute left ventricular failure with pulmonary edema, myocardial infarction, and pulmonary embolism (Chapters 5, 7, and 9). Some of these disorders show a shift in pH with time; early the pH will be low: respiratory alkalosis resulting from hypoxemic hyperventilation; later, as CO_2 retention, hypoxemia, and inadequate tissue perfusion develop, tissue hypoxia leads to anaerobic glycolysis, the accumulation of lactic acid, and a low pH from lactic acidemia and hypercapnia.

Hypoxemia Without Hypo- or Hypercapnia

This combination may be produced by a number of disorders of lung parenchyma, especially diffuse pulmonary fibrosis and cellular infiltration. The $Paco_2$ is often within normal limits in spite of an elevated respiratory rate and tidal volume (Chapter 9).

Guidelines for Interpretation of ABG Values

There is no substitute for clinical experience and practice with evaluating actual ABG determinations from patients for whom one knows the signs and symptoms, the systemic disorder, the present physiologic status, and the complications and treatments, and for whom there is access to other laboratory data. In general, however, using the following sequence systematically may be helpful in interpretation of ABG values.

Consider the pH first. Its direction of deviation from 7:40 will often point to the basic process, acidosis or alkalosis, because even though some compensation may have occurred if the abnormality is of some duration, it seldom returns the pH to physiologic neutrality. Even if the pH is within the normal range it will still usually point to a tendency toward alkalemia or acidemia. This, in turn, will point to either an alkalosis or an acidosis as the primary process.

Next consider the $Paco_2$, and the HCO_3^- and B.E., to see which of these respiratory or metabolic values *explains the trend seen above*. This indicates whether the primary disturbance is respiratory (altered $Paco_2$) or metabolic (abnormal HCO_3^- and B.E.). A $Paco_2 < 30-35$ mmHg indicates hyperventilation; a $Paco_2 > 45-50$ mmHg points to hypoventilation.

If the primary abnormality is in the $Paco_2$ (or HCO_3^- and B.E.), again consider the HCO_3^- and B.E. (or CO_2)—that is, the other value—to see to what extent respiratory or metabolic compensation for the primary process has occurred. This compensatory alteration will have an effect in the direction opposite to that predicted by the pH, and the reverse of that produced by the primary abnormality.

It is helpful to keep in mind that hypoxemia may produce respiratory alkalemia (via hypoxemia hyperventilation) and/or metabolic acidemia (via lactic acidosis). Evaluate the arterial oxygenation status. If the patient is receiving supplemental oxygen instead of breathing room air, and assuming ventilation–perfusion $(\dot{V}/\dot{Q})$ ratios to be reasonably normal (a large assumption in a hospitalized patient on oxygen therapy) the following relations apply:

FIO_2	Predicted Pa_{O_2}, at Sea Level
20% (room air)	100 mmHg
30	150 mmHg
40	200 mmHg
50	250 mmHg

Breathing room air of course gives the most reliable evalution of the significance of the Pa_{O_2}.

REFERENCES

Beeson PB and McDermott W, editors: *Textbook of Medicine*, 14 th ed. Philadelphia, Pa.: Saunders, 1975.

Broughton JD: Understanding blood gases. In: Hudak, C., et al, editors: *Critical Care Nursing*, 2nd ed. Philadelphia, Pa.: Lippincott, 1977.

DeGowin EL and DeGowin RL: *Bedside Diagnostic Examination*, 3rd ed. New York: Macmillan, 1976.

Filley GF, *Acid–Base and Blood Gas Regulation*. Philadelphia, Pa.: Lea and Febiger, 1971.

Frohlich ED, editor: *Pathophysiology*. Philadelphia, Pa.: Lippincott, 1976.

Fulop M, et al: Lactic acidosis in pulmonary edema due to left ventricular failure. *Ann. Intern. Med.* 79:180–185, 1973.

Ganong WF: *Review of Medical Physiology*, 8th ed. Los Altos, Calif.: Lange Medical Publications, 1977.

Guyton AC: *Textbook of Medical Physiology*, 5th ed. Philadelphia, Pa.: Saunders, 1976.

Mattar JA, et al: A study of the hyperosmolal state in critically ill patients. *Crit. Care Med.* 1:293–301, 1973.

Myers FH, Jawetz E, and Goldfien A: *Review of Medical Pharmacology*, 5th ed. Los Altos, Calif.: Lange Medical Publications 1976.

Oaks WW, editor: *Critical Care Medicine*. 28th Hahnemann Symposium. New York: Grune and Stratton, 1974.

Peterson CG: *Perspectives in Surgery*. Philadelphia, Pa.: Lea and Febiger, 1972.

Schrier RW, editor: *Pathophysiology of Renal and Electrolyte Disorders*. Boston, Mass.: Little, Brown, 1976.

Schwartz AB and Lyons H, editors: *Acid–Base and Electrolyte Balance. Normal Regulation and Clinical Disorders*. New York: Grune and Stratton, 1977.

Shapiro BA; *Clinical Application of Blood Gases*. Chicago, Ill.: Year Book Medical Publishers, 1973.

Thorn, GW, et al, editors: *Harrison's Principles of Internal Medicine*, 8th ed. New York: McGraw-Hill 1977.

Tuller MA: *Acid–Base Homeostasis and Its Disorders*. Flushing, N.Y.: Medical Examination Publishing Co., 1971.

CHAPTER THREE

Hypertension

NORMAL REGULATION OF SYSTEMIC ARTERIAL PRESSURE

The level of the systemic arterial pressure is a function of cardiac output and total peripheral resistance (SAP = COXTPR). Cardiac output, in turn, depends on the degree of vasodilation or vasoconstriction on an interaction between heart rate and stroke volume (CO = HR × SV); and total peripheral resistance depends on the degree of vasodilation or vasoconstriction in the systemic blood vessels, mainly in the arterioles. The arteries and arterioles, because of their thicker more muscular walls, make a larger contribution to peripheral resistance than the veins and venules. The latter are thinner walled, more distensible, and permit a larger increase in volume per unit change in pressure than the arteries. The arteries are called resistance vessels, since they maintain blood pressure by varying degrees of vasoconstriction; and the veins are called capacitance vessels, since they have a high capacity to store blood without much change in pressure. Thus, according to the formula above, an increase in either cardiac output or peripheral resistance, without a corresponding decline in the other value, will result in an increase in blood pressure.

Rapidly Responding Processes for Blood Pressure Regulation

Neural Regulation

Neural Influences on Cardiac Output

Neural regulation of the heart, responsible for influencing the heart rate and stroke volume, is discussed in Chapters 6 and 7. Briefly, however, the heart receives both sympathetic and parasympathetic innervation, via the cardiac and vagus nerves, respectively. The cardioinhibitory center is the motor nucleus of the vagus nerve in the medulla of the brainstem; there probably is no cardioacceleratory center, so that increases in heart rate and force of contraction are mediated mainly by inhibition of the cardioinhibitory center; but there is stimulating innervation from the adrenergic cardiac supply. Thus the cardiac output parameter in the above formula is controlled in part by neural reflexes mediated via the autonomic centers in the brainstem.

Neural Influences on Peripheral Resistance

Blood vessels, all of which are innervated except capillaries, are likewise under the control of an autonomic center in the brainstem: the vasomotor center. The vasomotor center is a diffuse group of nerve cells in the reticular formation of the medulla and is comprised of two portions: a large vasopressor area and a smaller vasodepressor area. Stimulation of the vasopressor area causes vasoconstriction, tachycardia, and elevation of blood pressure; stimulation of the vasodepressor area leads to vasodilation, bradycardia, and a decrease of blood pressure. These are not separate vasodilator and vasoconstrictor centers; both pressor and depressor effects are mediated entirely by a change in the rate of tonic firing of the vasoconstrictor efferent nerves. Thus there is but a single final effector pathway. However, excitatory fibers from the pressor area and inhibitory fibers from the depressor area do leave the vasomotor center separately and travel in different areas of the spinal cord. But they both synapse with, and control the rate of fir-

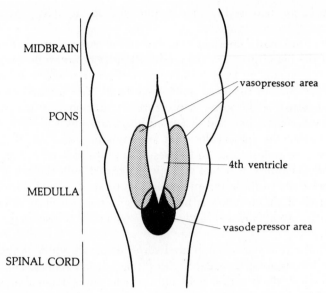

MIDBRAIN

PONS

vasopressor area

4th ventricle

MEDULLA

vasodepressor area

SPINAL CORD

Figure 3-1. Dorsal view of lower brainstem indicating approximate locations of the vasopressor and vasodepressor areas.

ing of, the vasoconstrictor nerves. Excitatory stimuli cause vasoconstriction by increasing the number of impulses in these nerves; inhibitory stimuli cause vasodilation by decreasing the number of impulses.

Aortic Arch and Carotid Sinus Baroreceptors

The vasomotor center in turn receives afferent input from, and is regulated by, a number of areas, the most important for our purposes being the arterial baroreceptors. These are high pressure sensors comprised of nerve endings in the walls of the large arteries in the neck and thorax which respond to increases and decreases in the degree of stretch on the arterial wall caused by a rise or fall of arterial pressure. The best known of these baroreceptors are those of the aortic arch and the carotid sinuses. The carotid sinus is located at the base of the internal carotid just beyond the point where it leaves the common carotid. Pressure applied to the depression below the earlobe at the angle of the jaw stimulates the carotid sinus and mimics the effect of elevated intracarotid blood pressure. An increased pressure causes an increased rate of discharge in the receptor nerve endings; afferents from the receptors travel in the glossopharyngeal and vagus cranial nerves to the vasodepressor area of the vasomotor center, and also to the cardioinhibitory center. The consequence is an inhibition—a reduced rate—of firing of the tonically active vasoconstrictor nerves, and a stimulation of the cardioinhibitory center. The results of this dual response are: vasodilation, bradycardia, a decline in cardiac output, and a fall in systemic arterial pressure.

When arterial blood pressure falls for any reason, the response is the reverse; a decline in stretch to the arterial receptor causes a decreased rate of impulses in the receptor nerve endings and in the afferents to the brainstem. This decreased stimulation removes the inhibition to the vasopressor area and decreases the rate of stimulation of the cardioinhibitory area. The effects are vasoconstriction, tachycardia, an increased cardiac output, and an elevated systemic arterial pressure.

One of the most important functions of the baroreceptor reflexes is a modification of the blood pressure change resulting from postural change. When a subject sits or stands up from reclining, the effect of gravity is to cause a decline in blood pressure in the head and upper torso. The baroreceptor firing rate declines because of the lowered pressure stimulation, and the rapid reflexly mediated vasoconstriction and increased heart rate raises perfusion pressure to the brain so that the subject does not lose consciousness. Insufficiently responsive baroreceptor reflexes may in fact result in postural hypotension, with symptoms of lightheadedness or actual syncope associated with the upright position. And oversensitivity of these receptors can also produce loss of consciousness. In this case brief, slight elevation of blood pressure may result in an overresponse and excessive vasodilation and bradycardia—essentially a vasovagal syncope (Chapter 16).

A similar but more complicated series of baroreceptor reflexes occurs in the case of the straining associated with lifting a heavy object. The Valsalva maneuver, in which the breath is held and thoracic and abdominal muscles tightly contracted, causes an elevation of intrathoracic pressure which compresses the aorta and increases pressure stimuli to the baroreceptors. The increased intrathoracic and aortic pressure, acting alone, would activate the compensatory vasodepressor and cardiodepressor reflexes and lead to a decline in arterial pressure. However, the elevated intrathoracic pressure produced by straining also compresses the large veins, leading to a decreased venous return to the right heart. The result of a low venous return is a decline in cardiac output, decreased pressure stimuli to the baroreceptors, and a decline in afferent impulses to the vasodepressor area and cardioinhibitory center. The consequence is a reflexly induced tachycardia and increased peripheral vasoconstriction; these cause a rise in blood pressure. Then when straining stops, intrathoracic pressure declines, venous return rises, and cardiac output returns to normal. Since the blood vessels are still constricted, there is a brief increase in blood pressure; this again stimulates the baroreceptors producing bradycardia and vasodilation, so that the blood pressure finally returns to baseline levels.

These are examples of the way the baroreceptor reflexes mediate the rapidly acting and brief adjustments in arterial pressure which serve the function of reducing the degree and duration of fluctuations in blood pressure occurring in the course of normal daily activities. But they are probably not an important mechanism for long-term regulation of the *mean level* of arterial pressure—only devices for reducing the range of rapid excursion about the mean. The range of pressure stimuli to which the receptors respond is about 60–160 mmHg; they are not activated by pressures much below the lower number, and at pressures above the higher one their rate of firing is maximal. However, adaptation does occur so that when the blood pressure becomes elevated by some other process to levels much higher than 160 or so, the receptors gradually decrease their firing rate within about 48 hours to baseline levels. Thus the range of pressure for stimulation becomes adjusted to the new mean, and they become reset to higher tolerance levels. This resetting is reversible with correction of the underlying abnormality at which time the blood pressure may return to its normal range.

Atrial Stretch–Volume Receptors

These are lower-pressure receptors than those in the large arteries and appear to respond to distention of the atrial walls during diastole. Their firing rate is increased by elevation of venous return. The effect on the vasomotor center of an elevated central venous pressure is similar to that of the arterial baroreceptors' response to elevated pressure in the carotids, that is, vasodilation and a decline in blood pressure. But the effect on the cardioinhibitory center is inhibition, so that tachycardia occurs, which helps to pump blood out of the great vessels and to lower central venous pressure. In this case, referring to the formula, the decline in total peripheral resistance from vasodilation is large enough to override the effect of the increased cardiac output from tachycardia, so that the net systemic effect is a decline in peripheral blood pressure. The adaptive value of the action of the atrial receptor reflex is to prevent a too large increase in central venous volume and pressure; this protects the pulmonary circuit against vascular congestion and pulmonary edema.

Based on some animal experiments, atrial receptor reflexes appear also to have two other actions which contribute to the regulation of systemic arterial pressure on a slightly longer-term basis. Atrial distention may cause reflex dilation of the renal afferent arterioles which would increase glomerular filtration rate and thus lower ECF volume; and it probably inhibits release of antidiuretic hormone from the hypothalamus. Both actions result in diuresis and a decline in extracellular fluid volume. According to the formula above, a mechanism which regulates ECF volume also regulates blood pressure.

Direct Vascular Responses

Autoregulation

This term refers to the inherent direct responsiveness of the smooth muscle layers of the arterial and arteriolar walls to elevation or decline of perfusion pressure within the vessles. When pressure of blood within the arterial lumen increases, the smooth muscle tissue is stretched; the direct response to stretch is a prompt smooth muscle constriction, producing an increase in vascular resistance to blood flow and a tendency to stabilize the amount of blood flow within normal limits. As perfusion pressure increases, the degree of arteriolar constriction increases, and hence the total peripheral resistance rises. Autoregulatory increase in vascular resistance, produced by a direct increase in vasoconstriction in response to elevated perfusion pressure, is especially prominent in the blood vessels within the kidney

An additional form of autoregulation is the increased production of vasodilator metabolites (CO_2, adenosine, and others) in active tissue; these substances act directly on local arterioles to produce vasodilation, and hence a fall in resistance, increasing the blood supply to metabolically active tissues.

Capacitance

The veins and venules constitute the storage or capacitance vessels of the circulation. Unlike the arterioles, the venules can undergo a relatively large change in volume without manifesting a marked change in pressure. In other words, veins have a greater compliance than arteries. In addition, they respond to increased volume by relaxation of the smooth muscle walls, and to decreased volume by contraction of the smooth muscle. This is an accommodative response which acts to minimize pressure changes in response to changes in circulating blood volume.

Hormonal Regulation

Angiotensin II

This hormone is produced from the action of renin from the kidney (see following) on angiotensinogen (renin substrate) formed in the liver, yielding angiotensin I; the latter is then transformed by converting enzyme, mainly in the lungs, to angiotensin II. The short-term action of angiotensin II is to cause strong arteriolar constriction, elevation of total peripheral resistance, and increase of systemic arterial pressure. To a lesser extent, constriction of the veins and venules also occurs, increasing venous return to the right heart with a consequent rise in cardiac output. The increased cardiac output, according to the formula SAP = TPR × CO, contributes to the blood pressure elevation resulting from the vasoconstriction caused by angiotensin II. This hormone has a significant role in maintaining normal blood pressure and producing rapidly responding short-term adjustment in blood pressure to both volume and vasomotor changes.

Catecholamines

Norepinephrine released from sympathetic adrenergic terminals, and norepinephrine and epinephrine secreted from the adrenal medullae, rapidly elevate systemic arterial pressure both via vasoconstriction and increased cardiac output. They are released in response to a large number of stimuli: emotions, exercise, hypoglycemia, extracellular fluid volume depletion, and others. However, except as compensatory adaptive responses to emergency situations, circulating catecholamines may not be of major significance in mediating long-term systemic arterial pressure homeostasis.

Antidiuretic Hormone (ADH; Arginine Vasopressin)

Although this hypothalamic hormone does have a direct vasoconstrictor action, its blood levels probably do not ever rise sufficiently to produce a significant elevation in total peripheral resistance. Its important action is the regulation of volume and osmolarity rather than of peripheral resistance directly. This subject is discussed in detail in Chapter 1.

Slowly Responding Processes for Blood Pressure Regulation

Renin–Angiotensin–Aldosterone System

Renin

The functional unit of the kidney is the nephron, which is comprised of a glomerulus and a renal tubule; there are about one million nephrons in each kidney

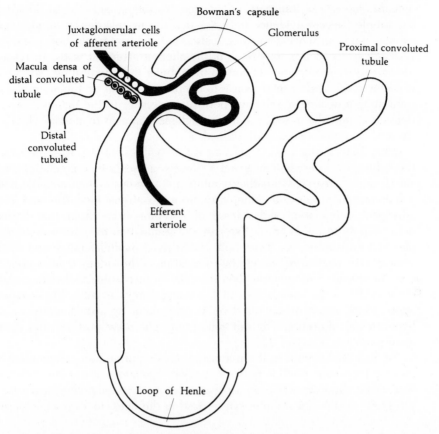

Figure 3-2. The juxtaglomerular apparatus, at the point of contact between afferent arteriole and distal tubule, made up of the juxtaglomerular cells of the afferent arteriole and the macula densa cells of the proximal portion of the distal convoluted tubule.

of the human. Each nephron contains a specialized structure, the juxtaglomerular apparatus, which includes (1) a portion of the afferent arteriole, near where it enters the glomerulus; and (2) a portion of the first (proximal) segment of the distal convoluted tubule. The afferent arteriole and the first section of the distal tubule come into close apposition at this portion of the nephron, and together form a functional unit which is intimately concerned with the sequence of processes involved in the long-term regulation of systemic arterial pressure. This functional unit is the juxtaglomerular apparatus. A group of specialized cells, the juxtaglomerular cells, surround the afferent arteriole at the point where it comes into contact with the distal tubule. The cells are specialized to act as receptors which sense the perfusion pressure in the afferent arteriole. With a decline in either circulating blood volume or systemic arterial pressure, or both, the juxtaglomerular cells respond to the stimulus of decreased perfusion pressure by synthesizing increased amounts of the renal hormone, renin, that is found within them in the form of granules, and which is released into the blood following appropriate stimulation.

The macula densa is a specialized group of cells in the first portion of the distal convoluted tubule where it touches the juxtaglomerular cells of the afferent arteriole. These cells appear to act as chemoreceptors which monitor the total amount, and rate of transport, of Na$^+$ and possibly also of Cl$^-$, at this portion of the tubule. Recent evidence indicates that the macula densa, in addition to its tubular fluid ion-sensing functions, also contains contractile fibers and directly responds to the degree of stretch of the afferent arteriolar walls. In response to an increased concentration of Na$^+$ in the tubular fluid (indicating excess Na$^+$ loss from the ECF) and/or in response to decreased stretch on the afferent arteriole (indicating a decline in effective perfusion pressure to the kidneys) the macula densa transmits the message to the juxtaglomerular cells to increase their synthesis and release of renin into the blood.

Other factors which cause an increase in synthesis and release of renin from the kidney are a decrease in serum K$^+$ levels, a decrease in circulating angiotensin II, and increased sympathetic autonomic nervous system activity: both elevated norepinephrine and epinephrine from the adrenal medullae, and increased adrenergic stimulation and release of norepinephrine from the sympathetic nerve supply to the kidneys. Sympathetic stimulation to renin secretion by the elevated catecholamines, from both the adrenal medulla source and the direct sympathetic innervation, occurs by stimulation of the kidney β-adrenergic receptors. Increased β stimulation then may act by increasing adenylate cyclase and cyclic AMP at the membranes of the juxtaglomerular cells. Physiologic alterations which result in increased renin production by juxtaglomerular cells are hypovolemia, diuretics, low salt intake, upright body posture, and decreased renal perfusion (Chapter 1).

The half-life of renin in the plasma varies around an hour, depending on the species. Its principal action in the long term regulations of systemic arterial pressure results from its action on a plasma glycoprotein, angiotensinogen (or renin substrate), which is a globulin synthesized in the liver, to form angiotensin I.

The Angiotensins

Angiotensin I is the precursor to the pressor agent angiotensin II; most of the conversion from I to II occurs under the influence of converting enzyme as blood flows through the pulmonary circuit. Angiotensin II produces vigorous constriction of arterioles, resulting in a rise of systemic arterial pressure. The degree of elevation of blood pressure produced by this substance is increased by increased serum Na$^+$ and elevated ECF volume. The half-life of angiotensin II is a few minutes; it is eliminated from the plasma by a widely distributed group of enzymes called angiotensinases; its role in short-term adjustments of systemic arterial pressure has been described in the prior section. In addition, there is evidence that it acts (1) on peripheral adrenergic neurons to enhance the synthesis and release of catecholamines; (2) on a nucleus in the hypothalamus to cause elevation of blood pressure; and (3) on upper brainstem structures to increase thirst sensations and ADH secretion.

Aldosterone

The long-term action of angiotensin II is the stimulation to the zona glomerulosa of the adrenal cortex to synthesize and release the mineralocorticoid aldosterone. There is some controversy as to whether angiotensin II itself directly stimulates

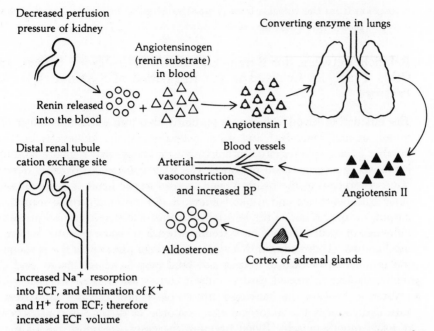

Decreased perfusion
pressure of kidney

Converting enzyme in lungs

Angiotensinogen
(renin substrate)
in blood

Renin released
into the blood

Angiotensin I

Distal renal tubule
cation exchange site

Blood vessels

Arterial
vasoconstriction
and increased BP

Angiotensin II

Aldosterone

Cortex of adrenal glands

Increased Na$^+$ resorption
into ECF, and elimination of K$^+$
and H$^+$ from ECF; therefore
increased ECF volume

Figure 3-3. Diagram of the steps involved in the activation of the renin–angiotensin I and II–aldosterone system. Stimulation of this sequence produces elevated blood pressure by two processes: the direct vasoconstrictive action of angiotensin II, and the elevated ECF volume resulting from increased renal reabsorption of Na$^+$.

aldosterone production, or whether the stimulus to the adrenal is mediated by another hormone, angiotensin III, which is formed from angiotensin II by the action of a protease enzyme. Angiotensin III has less than half the vasoconstrictor potency of angiotensin II, but is reported to be even more effective as a stimulus to adrenal aldosterone production than is angiotensin II. Some workers suggest that angiotensin III alters the cell membranes of the zona glomerulosa in such a way that they become more permeable to K$^+$, and that it is the enhanced cellular K$^+$ content itself which promotes aldosterone synthesis, rather than the amount of angiotensins present per se. Evidence for this theory is adduced to be that neither angiotensin II or III is able to stimulate aldosterone without adequate K$^+$ being present. Other effective stimuli that increase aldosterone secretion in addition to the renin–angiotensin system are ACTH from the anterior pituitary gland, a large rise in plasma K$^+$, and a large decline in plasma Na$^+$. These effects appear to operate directly on the adrenal cortex itself, without the mediation of the renin–angiotensin system.

The principal role of the renin–angiotensin system in long-term regulation of systemic arterial pressure, therefore, is in its control of aldosterone secretion, which regulates blood pressure by its effects on ECF volume. Aldosterone increases the resorption of Na$^+$ from tubular filtrate at the distal renal tubule cation exchange site, in exchange for K$^+$ or H$^+$. As Na$^+$ is resorbed, water is retained with it, and ECF volume increases. Aldosterone also elevates body Na$^+$ by increasing its resorption from sweat, gastric juice, and saliva. At the intracellular level, the action of aldosterone is to stimulate protein synthesis within cell ribosomes. The process by which increased protein synthesis leads to Na$^+$

resorption from the tubular lumen into the renal interstitium and therefore back into the blood is not known.

Relation Between the Renin–Angiotensin–Aldosterone System and Other Processes Involved in the Regulation of Systemic Arterial Pressure

The circulating blood volume, importantly determined by the effect of aldosterone in increasing Na^+ and water retention by the kidney, is but one of a number of closely integrated interacting components that regulate long-term adjustments in arterial blood pressure. The ECF volume is a primary determinant of venous return to the heart. Venous return to the heart is a significant factor, along with heart rate and stroke volume, in determining cardiac output. Cardiac output, in turn, is one of the key determinants of systemic arterial pressure. This influence of cardiac output on systemic arterial pressure operates by way of two mechanisms: (1) directly, in that systemic arterial pressure is the consequence of the interaction of cardiac output and total peripheral resistance; and (2) indirectly, in that increased cardiac output causes an increase in total peripheral resistance, because the increased arterial blood flow elevates intraarterial pressure and induces the autoregulation response of direct vasoconstriction of arteriolar smooth muscle. Blood pressure increases, therefore, as ECF volume, cardiac output, and autoregulative vasoconstriction increase.

The next step in the interaction between blood volume, cardiac output, and autoregulative vasoconstriction is that the increase in systemic arterial pressure caused by an increase in these three parameters produces an elevation of perfusion pressure to the kidney, which elevates glomerular filtration rate. An elevated GFR leads to increased urinary output. And an increased urinary output causes a decline in circulating blood volume. Decreased ECF volume causes a fall in venous return, which lowers cardiac output, which lowers blood pressure both directly and also indirectly by lowering the autoregulative component of peripheral resistance. As a result, blood pressure tends to decline toward baseline levels. This decline then decreases renal perfusion, glomerular filtration rate, and urine output. And so blood pressure is stabilized by the complex interaction among these homeostatic processes. These relationships are shown in Figure 3-4.

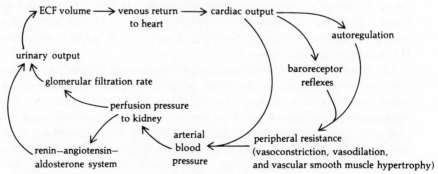

Figure 3-4. Diagram of the interaction among the various factors and processes involved in the long-term regulation of systemic arterial blood pressure.

PHYSIOLOGIC BASES OF ARTERIAL HYPERTENSION

What is the relationship between these parameters involved in the long-term regulation of the arterial blood pressure, and the disorders which are included under the heading of arterial hypertension? One conceptually useful theory attempting to account for the development and maintenance of hypertension, and which receives considerable support from research involving experimental animals as well as from some clinical studies of patients with a number of renal and/or blood pressure abnormalities, suggests that most types of protracted clinically significant hypertension is caused by factors either within the kidneys themselves, or elsewhere in the body, which lead to an impairment of normal ECF volume regulation.

In the normal intact subject, even a marked increase in ECF volume, brought about by whatever cause: increased oral intake, intravenous infusions, or whatever, causes no marked elevation of blood pressure. This is true not only because of the shorter-term adaptive changes discussed earlier which act to maintain blood pressure within normal limits, but also because well-functioning kidneys promptly respond to the increase in ECF volume with an elevation of urinary output, which lowers the ECF volume, and blood pressure, to the normal levels promptly and effectively.

However, in the case of protracted excessive intake of salt and water, or a prolonged defective elimination by the kidney of excess ECF salt and water, the rapidly responding mechanisms for the maintenance of blood pressure are unable to return the vascular volume–pressure relationships to completely normal limits in the longer term. It is only normal renal function which can accomplish this long-term adjustment by lowering the ECF volume. Since increased arterial blood pressure increases renal perfusion pressure, and hence glomerular filtration rate and urinary output, an elevation of blood pressure may be the only mechanism by which ECF volume control can be regulated under abnormal conditions (see Figure 3-4). Such abnormal conditions could be produced either by a primary renal impairment (decreased blood flow or destruction of nephrons); or an adverse effect on renal structure and function from an abnormality somewhere else in the body which produces impaired renal blood flow. Conditions which are known to produce abnormally reduced blood flow to and through the kidney include diabetes, atherosclerosis, excess catecholamines from sympathetic adrenergic overactivity, ischemic heart disease, or angiotensin II. And there are undoubtedly many such factors as yet not discovered. In addition to conditions causing impaired blood flow to and through the kidney, any abnormality that reduces the number of adequately functioning renal tubules, will also interfere with the maintenance of ECF volume within normal limits. Any additional process that produces chronic expansion of the ECF, such as a high salt intake or excess secretion of aldosterone from the adrenal cortex, would have additive effects with impaired renal blood flow and tubule destruction or malfunction to cause chronic hypertension.

In sum, it may be the case that any factor which necessitates a sustained elevation in arterial pressure in order to elevate glomerular filtration rate enough to produce a urinary output adequate to maintain ECF volume within normal limits (in the face of a given salt and water intake), predisposes to clinically significant hypertensive disease.

TYPES OF HYPERTENSION

Regardless of the ultimate or basic cause, or the initiating processes, the actual hemodynamic derangement in most patients with established hypertension is an increased total peripheral resistance, caused by excessive constriction of the smooth muscle in the walls of the small arteries and arterioles. There is evidence, however, that some patients, particularly in early stages of the disorder, may have an elevated cardiac output but a total peripheral resistance within the normal range; in some cases the increased cardiac output appears to be the result of an elevated ECF volume. However, in most patients with hypertension that is well established the cardiac output is within normal limits or may even be low, the circulating blood volume may be either normal or low, but peripheral vasoconstriction is greatly increased.

Secondary Hypertension

Patients with elevated blood pressure caused by an identifiable structural or physiologic abnormality are said to have secondary hypertension. This group comprises about 10% of all hypertensive patients, and some of the abnormalities causing secondary hypertension include the following.

Renal Ischemic Disease (Renovascular Hypertension)

There are a number of possible types of, and causes for, renal ischemic disease, not all of which have been identified. A major cause is acquired narrowing of the main renal arteries (renal artery stenosis) resulting from atherosclerosis; usually the site of stenosis is at the point of origin of one or both of the renal arteries as they leave the aorta. It is more common in males than females and is seen more often in persons older than 50. Usually there is generalized atherosclerotic vascular disease. As a result of the stenosis there is reduced blood flow to the kidney, and the ischemic kidney produces increased renin as a result of the impaired renal blood flow. Renin, released in increased amounts, leads to the production of elevated angiotensin and aldosterone via the sequence described above.

Fibromuscular dysplasia is another relatively common cause of renovascular hypertension. In this condition one or both renal arteries may be partially occluded; it develops more commonly in females than males and most often in young adults before age 40. The occlusion is progressive and is produced by a fibrous thickening of the inner layers of the renal artery, with hypertrophy of its smooth muscle layers.

There are other causes for chronically ischemic kidneys which will eventually cause renovascular hypertension; small vessel arteriosclerosis, for example, may produce patchy narrowing and occlusion of arterioles within the renal parenchyma which will lead to focal ischemic areas and localizeed hypersecretion of renin. In this form of renal vascular sclerosis, impaired function of renal tubules also occurs, causing a progressive decline in kidney function and resulting ECF expansion; this of course contributes to the development of hypertension. Angiotensin II probably not only acts systemically on all peripheral arterioles to produce vasoconstriction, but also locally within the kidney parenchyma itself to cause areas of focal arteriolar constriction. The reduced local blood flow may increase renin production, and also impair nephron function, again leading to ECF expansion.

In early renovascular hypertension, when renal ischemia has developed over a short time (as occurs, for example, in kidney trauma, renal artery emboli, and kidney infarcts) the phase of prompt elevation of blood pressure is the result of a generalized vasoconstriction caused by the increased circulating angiotensin II. This initial increase in blood pressure improves renal artery blood flow, and hence increases renal perfusion. If the causative abnormality is not corrected, then the blood pressure becomes stabilized at the increased level; this later sustained elevation of blood pressure is caused mainly by increased ECF volume resulting from increased adrenal aldosterone output, as a result of stimulation by elevated angiotensin II. This elevated ECF acts to produce a blood pressure adequate to maintain renal blood flow, GFR, and urinary output, in the face of the depressed renal perfusion.

Actually, however, the situation must be more complicated than just an activation of the renin–angiotensin–aldosterone system, because some studies seem to show that only about 50% of patients with renovascular hypertension have an elevated plasma renin activity. Other patients with renovascular hypertension have renin within the normal range, and they have a low or normal ECF volume; however, they have a generalized increased arteriolar reactivity leading to protracted vasoconstriction. It may be that plasma renin levels, ECF volume, and degree of peripheral vasoconstriction, will vary depending upon at which stage in the development of established renovascular hypertension these parameters are measured. As mentioned above, early in the development of the disease the hypertension may be on the basis of increased renin–angiotensin–aldosterone and a high ECF volume; later when the hypertension becomes established it may be maintained on the basis of excessive vasoconstriction, while the ECF volume and cardiac output have returned to normal.

A second factor in the hypertension of renal ischemic disease may relate to the fact that some studies have shown that well-perfused renal tissue, especially the medulla, secretes a systemic vasodilator substance which may be one of the prostaglandins. With decreased renal perfusion there may be a failure to synthesize the vasodilator resulting in generalized vasoconstriction and hypertension.

Renal Parenchymal Disease (Renoprival Hypertension)

Destruction of functioning renal tissue may be caused by such disases as chronic pyelonephritis, the various types of glomerulonephritis, systemic lupus erythematosus, scleroderma, diabetic nephropathy, atherosclerosis, drug and chemical nephrotoxicity, and polycystic kidney disease (Chapter 10).

Patients with a reduced total mass of normally functioning kidney tissue often show marked hypertension, especially when they have an elevated ECF volume. The elevated pressure may occur suddenly, as in acute glomerulonephritis, or develop more gradually in patients with the advanced renal damage of late stages of pyelonephritis, chronic glomerulonephritis, or polycystic disease. Such a patient cannot eliminate salt and water because of a widespread loss of functioning nephrons, and the consequence is ECF overload (hypervolemia). The elevated volume leads to increased cardiac output, autoregulative vasoconstriction, and hypertension; eventually the elevated arterial pressure may increase enough to produce a GFR adequate to elevate urinary output and equalize the output to the intake; the pressure may then stabilize at that higher level. Since nephron loss continues in patients with this type of chronic renal failure, ECF volume will continue to increase and the hypertension worsen, unless fluid and salt intake are restricted.

In general, patients with this form of hypertension tend to have a lower plasma renin and a lower cardiac output than those with renovascular hypertension, but a higher circulating blood volume. So the two groups are physiologically different in a number of respects.

The importance of Na^+ and water retention, with ECF volume expansion, as a causative factor in the hypertension of renal parenchymal destruction is attested to by the fact that lowering circulating blood volume by dialysis or diuretics (where enough renal function remains for them to be effective) reduces blood pressure in most patients with chronic renal failure. In addition, in the salt-losing nephropathy of some forms and stages of renal failure, elevated arterial pressure is not a feature. A complicating factor in hemodynamic studies of patients with end-stage renal failure is the anemia, which produces a hyperdynamic circulation with elevated cardiac output.

An interesting transition occurs in this volume-loading type of hypertension. Eventually, in the chronic situation, the elevated cardiac output drops back to the normal range, while the total peripheral resistance (systemic vasoconstriction) increases and becomes the major mechanism for the sustained elevated arterial pressure. The nature of the workload on the myocardium then changes from volume work to pressure work, which, as is discussed in Chapters 4 and 7, is more costly to the heart in terms of energy consumption and oxygen requirements.

Since it is very unlikely in all of these renal destructive disorders that nephron destruction occurs without impairment of the renal circulation, and the reverse, it is likely that these two categories of cause of hypertension are combined in many patients with elevated arterial pressure of renal cause.

Adrenocortical Hypersecretion

Glucocorticoid (Cortisol) Excess; Cushing's

Hypertension caused by disorders of the adrenal cortex is uncommon and is reported to be found in only about 2% of hypertensive patients. Excess adrenocortical secretion promotes both Na^+ retention by the kidney and increased vasomotor tone; the combination of elevated plasma volume and increased peripheral resistance is an important component of the cause of hypertension in patients with Cushing's syndrome. However, some authors consider this explanation to be inadequate and conclude that the basic processes involved in the hypertension of glucocorticoid excess remain unknown.

Primary Aldosteronism

Excessive autonomous production of aldosterone as a result of a tumor or hyperplasia of the zona glomerulosa induces Na^+ and water retention and ECF expansion, at least early in the development of the disease. Theoretically, therefore, one would predict that the hypertension in patients with primary aldosteronism would be on the basis of an expanded ECF volume and elevated cardiac output. This may well be the case at the outset and for some time thereafter. However, once the hypertension in this disorder is well established, studies show that in fact hypertension in these patients is produced primarily by an increased total peripheral resistance (that is, by vasoconstriction) and that the ECF volume is normal. This sequence repeats the same theme we have described earlier in this chapter, namely, that in early hypertension circulatory ECF volume and cardiac output are elevated; later, when the disease is established, ECF volume returns to normal, cardiac output normalizes, and the hypertension becomes sustained by excessive vasoconstriction leading to increased peripheral resistance.

Hypokalemia is a prominent feature because of stimulation of the distal renal tubule cation exchange site.

The high level of aldosterone exerts a feedback suppression on renin secretion, so that there is low plasma renin activity in these patients, unlike those with activation of the renin–angiotensin aldosterone system (secondary hyperaldosteronism) from other causes such as congestive heart failure, cirrhosis, and nephrotic syndrome, in which renin and aldosterone levels are both elevated (Chapter 1).

Pheochromocytoma

Pheochromocytoma is a tumor of the adrenal medulla, or less often of the chromaffin cells in the chain of sympathetic ganglia; the hypertension which it causes may be sustained or intermittent, and results from excess release of the catecholamines epinephrine and norepinephrine into the circulation, which produce a strong vasoconstriction, increased cardiac output, and elevated systemic arterial pressure.

Hypercalcemia; Hypothyroidism

The elevated serum Ca^{2+} of hyperparathyroidism may cause hypertension, the mechanism for which is not clear beyond the fact that hypercalcemia causes calcium deposits and lesions of both renal vasculature and renal parenchyma. Patients with hypothyroidism and myxedema are often hypertensive, but usually not severely so. The cause in this case is uncertain.

These and other endocrine disorders are discussed more fully in Chapter 13.

Secretion of an As Yet Unidentified Mineralocorticoid

It has been reported that some patients, blacks more commonly than whites, who by most criteria have essential hypertension, show a suppressed plasma renin activity, an expanded ECF volume, but no hypokalemia. The suggestion has been made that the hypervolemia and renin suppression result from production of an atypical mineralocorticoid. Spironolactone, a drug that antagonizes the Na^+-retaining action of aldosterone, may lead to a normalization of the blood pressure in such patients. Since the adrenal cortex synthesizes a number of steroids possessing varying degrees of glucocorticoid and/or mineralocorticoid activity, and which therefore can cause hypertension, this abnormality is said to possibly account for the approximately 20% of the 85% of hypertensive patients who by most criteria appear to fall within the essential or primary hypertension category, yet have certain atypical features.

Estrogen-Containing Oral Contraceptives

These drugs lead to elevated blood pressure in a significant number of females; estrogen appears to stimulate hepatic synthesis of angiotensinogen (renin substrate). Elevated plasma levels of this globulin are postulated to cause hypertension both by promoting increased angiotensin II (elevated peripheral resistance from vasoconstriction) and by fostering increased aldosterone release from the adrenal (stimulation of the distal renal tubule cation exchange site causing ECF volume expansion).

Primary (Essential, Idiopathic) Hypertension

Primary hypertension is largely asymptomatic, which complicates the problem of case finding and treatment. The patient does not seek health care for elevated blood pressure, is usually completely unaware of it, is surprised when informed of it, and often is reluctant to accept the onus of long-term medication (which may produce unpleasant side effects, and may be expensive) and life-style changes, to treat a condition which produces neither signs nor symptoms. Advice to lose weight, stop smoking, reduce dietary saturated fat and cholesterol, take up a regular exercise program, and put away the table salt shaker, may be unheeded until the inevitable signs and symptoms of blood vessel or heart damage, caused by the elevated pressure, begin to manifest themselves. The importance and effectiveness of thorough patient education and conscientious follow-up in motivating individuals to follow a therapeutic regimen has been established by many studies.

Hereditary factors are quite prominent in the disorder, as hypertension runs in families, and the incidence is higher in blacks than whites. A high salt intake appears to contribute to the development of hypertension. Psychoemotional "stress" may be implicated as a cause in some instances. Primary hypertension is probably a group of diseases, rather than a single one, which develop as a result of a derangement in one or more of the variety of processes involved in normal regulation of systemic arterial pressure discussed above, and culminates in increased vasomotor reactivity. The upper limit of normal blood pressure in a person younger than 60 is about 160/95. Essential hypertensions is rare in persons younger than 20; the onset is usually between 25 and 50 years of age, and females are affected more often than males.

Causes of Primary Hypertension

In patients with primary hypertension, which comprise probably 85 to 90% of the hypertensive population, the cause for the elevated systemic arterial pressure is not known. The elevated pressure results from increased total peripheral resistance once the disease is well established. However, studies of plasma (ECF) volume, cardiac output, and total peripheral resistance in early, borderline, or labile primary hypertension, indicate that in many cases the ECF volume is expanded, cardiac output is elevated, and the total peripheral resistance is within normal limits. However, according to the formula SAP = CO × TPR, the peripheral resistance is undeniably high *for that level of cardiac output.* Otherwise, the patient would not be hypertensive. In well-established hypertension, plasma volume is often low; and in males the higher the blood pressure, the lower the plasma volume.

Some investigators contend that there are definable subgroups of primary hypertensive patients that can be differentiated on the basis of laboratory determinations of components of the renin–angiotensin–aldosterone system, and analysis of 24-hour urinary Na^+ content. Their argument is that, since this is the system which importantly influences both ECF volume and total peripheral resistance (vasoconstriction), it must be involved in all forms of hypertension, either from the standpoint of causation or of perpetuation. A process called "renin profiling" is done in some laboratories, in which plasma renin activity, as well as angiotensin II and aldosterone content, are related to the 24-hour rate of urinary Na^+ excretion. Values for plasma renin activity fluctuate predictably in normal subjects, depending on the ratio between Na^+ intake in the diet and Na^+ output in the urine. Based on the method of renin profiling, where plasma renin activity is determined and related to Na^+ balance, these workers suggest that hypertensive patients can be subdivided into high-, normal-, and low-renin subgroups. For each of the three subgroups renin levels fluctuate within different ranges for comparable changes in urinary Na^+ excretion. About 30% of hypertensive patients are said to be in the low plasma renin group, 55% in the normal- or medium-renin group, and 15% have high plasma renin levels, for comparable levels of urinary Na^+.

These workers do not contend that renin profiling provides definite information on whether renin elevations are involved in either the cause or the perpetuation of hypertension. However, it is proposed that these subgroups have different etiologies for their hypertension, will follow different clinical courses, have different prognoses, and are optimally treated by different pharmacologic agents. All subgroups show about the same degree of left ventricular hypertrophy, but the incidence of strokes and myocardial infarctions are said by some to be highest in the high-, medium in the medium-, and lowest in the low-renin subgroups. Thus susceptibility to cardiovascular damage may appear to correlate with the renin–sodium profile. The suggestion is made on the basis of response of these three subgroups to antihypertensive pharmacologic agents, including the β-adrenergic blocking agent propranolol; the competitive inhibitor of angiotensin II, saralasin; and a converting enzyme inhibitor, SQ20881, which inhibits the enzyme that converts angiotensin I to angiotensin II; that the different subgroups might appropriately be managed with different drugs. In addition, diuretics and other standard antihypertensive agents have been evaluated for their effects in the three subgroups. The high- and most of the medium-renin patients are reported to respond with blood pressure lowering to agents which block renin production, such as propranolol. The low-renin group do not respond well to propranolol but do respond to thiazide diuretics. The suggestion is advanced that high- and most medium-renin patients are hypertensive on the basis of peripheral vasoconstriction caused by renin–angiotensin II; and most low-renin patients are hypertensive on the basis of ECF volume expansion.

More recent studies of hypertensive patients by these methods have been carried out using the converting enzyme inhibitor; results indicated that blood pressure lowering in all high-renin and many medium-renin patients occurs as a result of inhibition of conversion of angiotensin I to the powerful vasoconstrictor angiotensin II; no blood pressure lowering occurred in low-renin patients. The investigators conclude that the results indicate a significant involvement of abnormalities in the renin–angiotensin system in the disease of all high-renin and some medium-renin hypertensives.

Other investigators are convinced that hypertensive patients cannot be neatly categorized into these three divisions, but rather fall into points on a continuum; that they mostly show mixtures of plasma volume and vasoconstrictive components, with vasoconstrictive features being predominant in the majority; and that the volume–vasoconstriction characteristics may be *sequential* in the natural history of the disease in each patient rather than *constant* features dividing patients into categories. Moreover, some studies indicate that prognostic differences do not hold up for the three groups, and that treatment based on the three renin classifications is not effectual for most patients. What does appear to be confirmed, however, is that high-renin levels are characteristic of more severe forms of hypertension which carry a poorer prognosis, but it is argued that the high renin is the consequence of the basic disease process rather than its cause. Many workers conclude that renin profiling is unnecessary and of little or no value in the management of most hypertensive patients.

As concerns other theories of cause of hypertension, a number of recent studies appear to suggest that abnormalities in the content and turnover rate of the catecholamines epinephrine and norepinephrine in the central nervous system (brainstem and spinal cord) may be involved in the genesis and maintenance of human essential hypertension. Catecholamines in the peripheral circulation appear not to cross the blood–brain barrier and there are indications that the epinephrine and norepinephrine in the brain are synthesized locally, act as neurotransmitters upon α-adenergic receptors, and participate importantly in the regulation of systemic arterial blood pressure. Derangements in these central neural cardiovascular processes are proposed by some investigators to be of causal significance in clinical elevated arterial pressure.

Complications of Primary Hypertension

The complications of arterial hypertension involve (1) the effect of the elevated blood pressure itself on the blood vessels: hypertrophy of the smooth muscle of the arterial wall, sclerosis, and vasculitis; and (2) the effects of the increased workload on the myocardium, especially the left ventricle, resulting from pumping blood against an elevated arterial resistance (increased afterload): hypertrophy, dilation, and increased O_2 requirements. The vascular damage is most marked in the blood vessels of the heart, the kidney, and the brain. In early hypertension, the arteriolar narrowing from vasoconstriction is reversible (functional), but later, as smooth muscle hypertrophy and arteriosclerotic changes develop, the vascular changes probably become organic or structural and are largely irreversible.

Effects on the Heart

The response of the heart to the excessive workload imposed by years of pumping blood against the elevated resistance in the systemic circuit is first hypertrophy and then dilation as progressive left ventricular and then chronic congestive failure develop. These changes are discussed in more detail in Chapter 7. Accompanying the mechanical abnormalities and complications there is progressive myocardial ischemia and greatly elevated myocardial oxygen requirements (Chapter 4). There is some controversy as to whether the heart "outgrows" its blood supply during hypertrophy, or whether the ischemia is the result of arteriosclerosis. In either event, angina often occurs and hypertension is considered to be a significant risk factor in the cardiac deaths from accelerated coronary artery disease. Myocardial infarction and congestive heart failure are the most frequent cause of deaths from hypertensive cardiovascular disease.

Effects on the Central Nervous System

The retina, which is embryologically a portion of the brain, reveals spasm and structural narrowing of its arterioles, and progressive arteriosclerosis, with thickening of the endothelium and hypertrophy of the smooth muscle layer. The patient may complain of blurring or darkening of vision and scotomata (blind spots). On funduscopic examination there may be arteriolar narrowing relative to venular width, hemorrhages, exudates, and papilledema as shown by a decrease in sharpness of the disc margins. A-V nicking, resulting from arteriolar compression of venules at crossing points, is commonly seen in severe hypertension.

Cerebral vascular spasms, microaneurysms, and areas of infarction and hemorrhage result in a number of signs and symptoms, among them lightheadedness or giddiness, dysarthria, aphasia, and irritability, tinnitus, true vertigo if brainstem nuclei are involved, occipital morning headache often with stiff neck, and altered higher mental function such as confusion.

Effects on the Kidneys

Hypertrophy of the smooth muscle layer of the arterioles; and changes in the capillaries of the glomeruli, with the development of sclerotic lesions, thickening of the tunica intima, and hyalinization, are characteristic renal changes and lead to a decreased GFR and abnormalities of tubular concentrating and diluting functions. Nocturia, proteinuria, and microhematuria may occur. Chronic renal failure may be a later development.

In addition to the three major target areas (heart, brain, kidney) for the deleterious effects of sustained hypertension, there may be peripheral vascular abnormalities most often manifesting as intermittent claudication—ischemic pain in the leg muscles with walking, relieved by rest.

Assessment in Hypertension of Unknown Cause

History and Review of Systems

Primary hypertension is often associated with a positive family history for elevated blood pressure, strokes, myocardial infarction, and renal failure. Age of onset in primary hypertension is between 35 and 55 years of age. Secondary hypertension is more likely to develop before or after that time. The chronic use of adrenal steroids for such conditions as asthma or rheumatoid arthritis; the use of estrogen-containing oral contraceptives or estrogen for the control of menopausal symptoms; a history of repeated urinary tract infections and/or proteinuria, nocturia, polyuria, and hematuria; and a history of torso trauma, costovertebral, flank or testicular pain; all suggest the presence of hypertension secondary to steroid or renal cause.

The review of systems centers importantly on signs and symptoms referable to hypertensive vascular damage to the three prominent target areas: (1) heart: angina, palpitations, paroxysmal noctural dyspnea, orthopnea, dyspnea on exertion and decreased exercise tolerance, ankle edema, moist cough from pulmonary vascular congestion; (2) brain: headache, giddiness, vertigo, visual disturbances, tinnitus, ataxia, dysarthria, syncope; and (3) kidneys: nocturia, polyuria, proteinuria, hematuria. In addition, intermittent claudication may be one cause of decreased exercise tolerance and indicate peripheral vascular involvement. A recent marked weight gain may point to Cushing's or the development of occult edema from the fluid retention of congestive failure or early primary aldosteronism; if the weight gain represents increased body fat it may help explain a recent onset of symptoms referable to the heart, because of the combination of accelerated coronary atherosclerosis and increased workload on the myocardium.

Physical Examination

Blood pressure and pulses in both upper extremities; postural blood pressures lying, standing, and sitting; and a comparison of timing and strength of brachial and femoral pulses; are routine physical assessments in a patient with elevated blood pressure. Large fluctuations in blood pressure with positional change indicate vasomotor lability and hyperresponsiveness; marked diastolic elevation on standing occurs commonly in primary hypertension. Brachial–femoral pulse lag indicates adult aortic coarctation.

Physical examination with emphasis on the three target areas, heart, brain, and kidney, is important to evaluate the degree of impairment of these organs from hypertensive vascular damage. Examination for evidence of left ventricular or congestive heart failure is discussed in Chapter 7. Central nervous system assessment includes funduscopic and general neurologic examination, including mental status, for evidences of prior cerebral hemorrhage, infarction, hypertensive encephalopathy, or other intracerebral vascular impairment; retinal damage; elevated intracranial pressure (venous pulsations and papilledema); and cranial nerve palsies. Episodes of unilateral paresthesias or paresis; or dysarthria, ataxia and disequilibrium may indicate transient ischemic attacks possibly caused by vasospasms or platelet aggregation in combination with cerebrovascular disease (Chapter 18).

Renal status is assessed by examination for costovertebral angle tenderness, abdominal palpation for enlarged or tender kidneys, and examination of the urine for protein, red cell casts, red cells, white cells, bacteria, and glucose. Vascular assessment includes abdominal palpation and auscultation for aortic aneurysm and aortic or renal artery bruit; palpation and auscultation of the carotids and femorals for pulse strength and bruits; and palpation of peripheral pulses of the lower extremities.

Routine Laboratory Tests

Routine diagnostic tests in patients with hypertension usually include serum electrolytes, BUN and creatinine, glucose, calcium, uric acid, cholesterol, and triglycerides; electrocardiogram; chest X-ray; and urinalysis with culture. In some cases an intravenous pyelogram and urinary catecholamine determination may be appropriate. The tests are of value not only in discriminating primary from secondary hypertension but also serve the purpose of assessing target organ impairment resulting from hypertensive cardiovascular disease, and for evaluating progress during follow-up visits.

Management of Primary Hypertension

General Measures

General measures include a regimen of regular increasingly vigorous physical exercise (preceded by an EKG-monitored treadmill exercise stress test if indicated); weight-losing, low cholesterol, low refined carbohydrate diet; cessation of cigaret smoking; and restriction of salt intake. Attempts to reduce sources of psychoemotional "stress" in the individual's life circumstances may be of value. Studies show that normotensive subjects respond to psychic stress with elevated cardiac output of short duration, while primary hypertensives respond with elevated peripheral resistance of long duration, indicating sustained vascular hyperreactivity in these subjects. It is not known whether this response results from excessive sympathetic outflow from the vasopressor area, or increased vascular responsiveness to a normal neural outflow.

Pharmacologic Management

Since SAP = CO × TPR, and since, as discussed previously, the two parameters of cardiac output and total peripheral resistance are under neural (sympathetic adrenergic) and hormonal (catecholamine, angiotensin II, and aldosterone) control it would follow that pharmacologic agents which are effective in maintaining systemic arterial pressure within more normal limits would act on one or both factors; and that, in addition, agents acting directly on smooth muscle tone of arterioles would moderate the autoregulative component in hypertension.

Diuretics. These agents decrease circulating blood volume by inhibiting Na^+ and water resorption at the renal tubules. The decreased ECF causes a decline in venous return, cardiac output, and autoregulative vasoconstriction. The thiazides are most commonly used, and there is evidence that they have long-term effects in addition to the diuresis which act to reduce arterial pressure. These effects may relate to a decrease in the rigidity of arteriolar walls perhaps from a reduction in sodium and interstitial fluid content in the wall itself. The consequence would be increased flexibility and decreased total peripheral resistance. Thiazide diuretics cause a decreased glomerular filtration rate, which in turn promotes an increase in BUN and uric acid. The Na^+ and water loss induces a compensatory increase in plasma renin activity, which in turn leads to elevations of angiotensin II and aldosterone, promoting vasoconstriction and rise in ECF volume. This tends to counter the thiazide therapeutic action and is one of the reasons why other medications, such as spironolactone, which inhibit aldosterone's action, or triamterine, which directly suppresses the DRT-CES, may need to be added at some later time. An additional factor in the use of spironolactone or triamterene with thiazides relates to their K^+-sparing action. The most frequent side effects of the thiazides are hypokalemia, glucose intolerance, and hyperuricemia. The K^+ deficit is well managed by increased intake of K^+-containing foods such as bananas and oranges for patients on small thiazide doses (i.e., hydrochlorothiazide 50 mg per day); or by 20–40 meq/day of a potassium chloride liquid or powder (to be dissolved in fruit juice). At the present time, thiazide diuretics are the key component in the management of essential hypertension.

Other diuretics sometimes used in control of hypertension are furosemide and ethacrynic acid. Diuretics are discussed in more detail in Chapter 1.

Agents Which Decrease Vasomotor Tone by Direct Action on the Brainstem Autonomic Sympathetic Control Centers. Methyldopa and clonidine are two commonly used drugs in this category. Alpha-methyldopa appears to have both central and peripheral actions; the central action is to stimulate the α receptors in the brainstem vasomotor area (promoting systemic vasodilation). Peripherally, it seems to work by the following process. Dopa-decarboxylase is an enzyme which transforms dopa (dihydroxyphenylalanine) to dopamine (dihydroxyphenylethylamine), a step in the biosynthesis of norepinephrine. Alpha-methyldopa serves as a competitive substrate for the enzyme when it is present in adequate amounts in biosynthetic areas. The enzyme converts it to alpha-methylnorepinephrine which is then stored in the synaptic vesicles just as is the normal norepinephrine. In other words, alpha methylnorepinephrine becomes a substitute or false neurotransmitter, which not only displaces the normal neurotransmitter norepinephrine, but has the pharmacologic property of being a central nervous system α-adrenergic stimulator (agonist). Brainstem α receptors are reported to be the receptors for activation of a pathway which inhibits pressor responses from the vasomotor area of the medulla. Therefore, stimulation of them leads to a decline in total peripheral resistance. Note that in contrast with the *central* action of α-adrenergic receptors, which is reported to be blocking of brainstem vasoconstrictor impulses, the action of *peripheral* α-adrenergic receptors is to produce vasoconstriction, and therefore increased peripheral resistance, in blood vessels of the viscera, skeletal muscles, and skin. Clonidine appears to function in a similar manner to alpha-methyldopa. Both drugs may have side effects of weakness, fatigue, psychic depression, and sedation. In addition, the sudden withdrawal of clonidine may produce a severe blood pressure overshoot and lead to a hypertensive crisis.

Ganglionic Blockers. These drugs interfere with synaptic transmission between pre- and postganglionic fibers of both the parasympathetic and sympathetic divisions of the autonomic nervous system. Because of the parasympathetic blockade they produce the side effects of impaired micturition, paralytic ileus, erectile, and ejaculatory impotence, and decreased visual accommodation. These drugs are not used in routine management of the ambulatory hypertensive but only parenterally in hypertensive crises when a large rapid decline in blood pressure is desirable. A major effect is depression of the reflex vasoconstrictor compensatory response to upright position. Pentolinium, mecamylamine, and trimethaphan are three drugs of this class. They are infrequently used.

Agents Which Interfere with Release of Norepinephrine from Adrenergic Terminals. Norepinephrine is synthesized in the sequence: phenylalanine → tyrosine → dopa → dopamine → norepinephrine. Most synthesis takes place at the sites of storage of norepinephrine: the sympathetic adrenergic nerves; these nerves also readily take up already synthesized norepinephrine. Storage is within synaptic vesicles and cytoplasm of the adrenergic terminals. At the arrival of the nerve action potential, norepinephrine is released into the synaptic cleft, diffuses to the postsynaptic neuron membrane, and combines with both α- and β-adrenergic receptors, resulting in the α-adrenergic response of vasoconstriction, and the β-adrenergic responses of increased heart rate (chronotropic) and force of contraction (inotropic). Most of the synaptic norepinephrine is then taken back up by the presynaptic terminals and re-stored in the granular vesicles. This reuptake is a very significant process in terminating the action of the catecholamines.

In addition, excess norepinephrine entering the circulating blood is broken down by the enzyme catechol-*o*-methyl transferase (COMT) produced by the liver and kidneys. Excess norepinephrine within the nerve fibers themselves is inactivated by the enzyme monoamine oxidase (MAO). During and following sympathetic neural discharge of norepinephrine and epinephrine, significant amounts of these catecholamines enter the circulation and may produce diffuse systemic effects of sympathetic activation. Their levels can be assayed both in blood and urine, although overall amounts are small because of the effectiveness of nerve terminal reuptake and the degradation by MAO and COMT.

Reserpine interferes with the storage of dopamine and norepinephrine within the synaptic vesicles; it blocks the movement of both substances from axoplasm to vesicle. The norepinephrine which is not stored is metabolically degraded by COMT. The result is catecholamine depletion and a decrease in all adrenergically mediated functions: tonic vasoconstriction, heart rate and force of contraction, brain activation, and adrenal medullary responses. The side effects are the consequences of parasympathetic activity relatively unopposed by compensatory sympathetic action, and include gastrointestinal hypermotility and hypersecretion, nasal congestion and vasomotor rhinitis, depressed sexual functions, and depressed mood and altered mental status, most marked in the elderly. Some studies have shown increased incidence of breast malignancy in females correlated with long-term reserpine use.

Guanethidine has an action similar to reserpine in blocking norepinephrine storage in synaptic vesicles, but it also impairs the release from the nerve terminals of what little is stored. It promotes the accumulation of blood in the veins and venules (capacitance vessels) in addition to decreasing the vasomotor responses of arteries and arterioles. Reflex vasomotor adjustments are impaired, and the result is postural hypotension. Its use is also associated with retrograde (into the urinary bladder) ejaculation in males which may have marked psychic repercussions. It does not appear to deplete norepinephrine from the brain, so mood depression is not a marked side effect. Guanethidine should not be used in conjunction with amphetamine or tricyclic antidepressants as the latter impair its effectiveness by blocking its transport into the action site within the adrenergic terminal, and may even lead to a hypertensive crisis.

Propranolol blocks those sympathetic adrenergic effects mediated by β-adrenergic receptors. Thus it reduces heart rate and force of contraction and lowers cardiac output; it reduces the release of renin from juxtaglomerular cells of the kidney mediated by β receptors—this acts to reduce angiotensin II and aldosterone production. So it has the three-pronged action of lowering cardiac output, reducing angiotensin-mediated vasoconstrictive peripheral resistance, and reducing stimulation to Na^+ resorption by the distal renal tubule. There is also evidence that central nervous system influences are involved in some of its effects; that is, it may block β receptors in the brain itself, as well as peripherally, inhibiting centrally mediated vasoconstriction. It is often used in conjunction with direct vascular smooth muscle relaxing agents and with diuretics. Side effects are bronchospasm in asthmatic patients, bradycardia, and a marked decrease in myocardial contractility which may precipitate left ventricular failure and pulmonary edema in patients with borderline cardiac performance.

Direct Vascular Smooth Muscle Relaxants.   The most frequently used of these vasodilators is hydralazine. Its action is more marked on the resistance than the capacitance vessels, and so postural effects are less a problem; its vasodilator effects are not mediated via inhibition of the sympathetic nervous system, so sympathetic reflexes are unimpaired. However, this fact accounts for one of the more common adverse responses to hydralazine, namely, a compensatory increase in heart rate and cardiac output. This occurs as an adrenergically mediated reflex response of the arterial baroreceptors to the decline in peripheral resistance produced by the widespread vasodilation. The tachycardia is particularly deleterious to the patient whose hypertension is accompanied by myocardial ischemia from coronary artery disease; tachycardia increases myocardial oxygen requirements and decreases diastolic filling time, which causes a decline in coronary artery perfusion. In addition, the generalized vasodilation may increase renal production of renin, with the consequences described above which tend to negate the therapeutic effects. Thus hydralizine is often combined with propranolol and diuretics which tend to counteract the undesirable compensatory responses to direct vasodilation. A side effect of hydralazine is the occasional development of a syndrome resembling systemic lupus erythematosus, including serum antinuclear antibodies; the syndrome generally resolves when the drug is stopped.

Prazosin is one of a newer class of antihypertensive agents having a direct relaxing action on vascular smooth muscle, producing peripheral vasodilation and a decrease in total peripheral resistance, although the precise mechanism of action is not yet established. It appears not to act as an adrenergic blocking agent or to interfere with sympathetic adrenergic function. It is said not to depress cardiac output. Other direct-acting vasodilators are nitroprusside and diazoxide. Both may be used intravenously for very rapid blood pressure lowering in hypertensive crises; the former has a much briefer duration of action than the latter. They both elevate plasma renin activity.

Malignant Hypertension (Accelerated, Necrotizing Hypertension)

This serious complication develops in about 5% of hypertensive patients with primary or any form of secondary hypertension. It often evolves abruptly with rapid marked elevation of both systolic and diastolic pressures that precedes the onset of signs and symptoms by a brief interval. In a patient with compromised ventricular performance or organic heart disease the severe burden imposed by the rapidly and severely elevated peripheral resistance may lead to decompensation and congestive heart failure which may yield deceptively low blood pressure values. Manifestations of malignant hypertension include altered mental status with confusion; decreased level of consciousness with stupor or coma; local or generalized seizures; scotomata or amaurosis; transient neurologic signs such as plantar extensor reflexes, hemiparesis or hemiplegia, or aphasia; and visual blurring, vomiting, and severe headache. Abnormalities in the optic fundi may include hemorrhages, exudates, narrowed tortuous arterioles, and papilledema.

Pathologic changes accompanying malignant hypertension are most marked in the brain and the kidney. Cerebral edema and brain swelling, with petechial hemorrhages and small infarctions, are common findings at postmortem examination. Arterioles show hypertrophy and a necrotizing arteriolitis of the inner layers, with severe vasospasm. The cause of these changes is suggested to be exaggerated autoregulative vasoconstriction in response to the elevated blood pressure. It is postulated that later the capacity for autoregulation is lost, leading to marked increase of cerebral blood flow, cerebral edema, and elevated intracranial pressure.

In the kidney there is hyperplasia and hypertrophy of layers of the arteriolar wall, and fibrinoid necrosis. Both glomerular and tubular function become impaired; the results are oliguria or anuria, hematuria and proteinuria, and retention of water, Na^+, K^+, and H^+, which expands the ECF and worsens the hypertension.

Some of the abnormalities are reversible if the condition is recognized promptly and treatment begun with rapidly acting vasodilators (see above); however, there is a risk of a too rapid and vigorous decrease in blood pressure. Since the patient is acclimated to an elevated blood pressure, a too abrupt decline to too low values may cause cerebral ischemia and infarction. This is particularly a danger in the elderly patient with cerebral atherosclerosis.

The important aspect of management is prevention by careful control of the hypertension. Causes of death in malignant hypertension are cerebral hemorrhage and/or infarction, renal failure, and congestive heart failure.

REFERENCES

Alderman MH, editor: *Hypertension. The Nurse's Role in Ambulatory Care.* New York: Springer, 1977.

Beeson PB and McDermott W, editors: *Textbook of Medicine*, 14th ed. Philadelphia, Pa.: Saunders, 1975.

Case DB, et al: Possible role of renin in hypertension as suggested by renin-sodium profiling and inhibition of converting enzyme. *N. Engl. J. Med.* 296:641–646, 1977.

Coleman TG et al: Feedback mechanisms of arterial pressure control. *Contrib. Nephrol.* 8:5–12, 1977.

Frohlich ED, editor: *Pathophysiology*. Philadelphia, Pa.: Lippincott, 1976.

Ganong WF: *Review of Medical Physiology*, 8th ed. Los Altos, Calif.: Lange Medical Publications, 1977.

Guyton AC: *Textbook of Medical Physiology,* 5th ed. Philadelphia, Pa.: Saunders, 1976.

Hansson L and Werkö L: Beta-adrenergic blockade in hypertension. *Am. Heart J.* 93:394–402, 1977.

Hilton SM: Central nervous mechanisms of blood pressure control. *Contrib. Nephrol.* 8:13–17, 1977.

Kaplan NM: Renin profiles. The unfulfilled promises. *JAMA* 238(7):611–613, 15 Aug. 1977.

Laragh JH: Hypertension update: Constellations of subsets—the importance of the renin axis for understanding and treatment. In: Mason DT, editor: *Advances in Heart Disease.* New York: Grune & Stratton, 1977.

Ledingham JM et al.: The role of the kidney in hypertension. *Contrib. Nephrol.* 8:37–43, 1977.

Liebau H and Brod J: *Mechanisms and Recent Advances in Therapy of Hypertension.* Basel: S. Karger, 1977.

Saran RK, et al: 3-Methoxy-4-hydroxyphenylglycol in cerebrospinal fluid and vanillylmandelic acid in urine of humans with hypertension. *Science* 200:317–318, 1978.

Starke K et al.: Mechanism of action of antihypertensive agents. *Contrib. Nephrol.* 8:151–161, 1977.

Steptoe A: Psychological methods in treatment of hypertension: A review. *Br. Heart J.* 39:587–593, 1977.

Thorn GW et al, editors: *Harrison's Principles of Internal Medicine,* 8th ed. New York: McGraw-Hill, 1977.

Zanchetti AS: Neural regulation of renin release. *Circulation* 56:691–698, 1977.

CHAPTER FOUR

Myocardial Ischemia

BLOOD SUPPLY TO THE MYOCARDIUM

Myocardial Blood Flow

The two coronary arteries, right and left, arise from dilations at the base of the ascending aorta; the dilations are the aortic sinuses and they lie behind the cusps of the aortic valve. The arteries extend forward, one on each side of the pulmonary artery. The left main coronary artery passes to the anterior intraventricular sulcus and divides into the circumflex, which continues around the left side of the heart to its posterior surface, and the left anterior descending artery, which passes caudally along the anterior interventricular groove. The right coronary artery extends along the atrioventricular sulcus to the posterior aspect of the heart; at the interventricular groove it divides into the posterior descending artery and the anterior marginal artery, which traverses the right border of the heart.

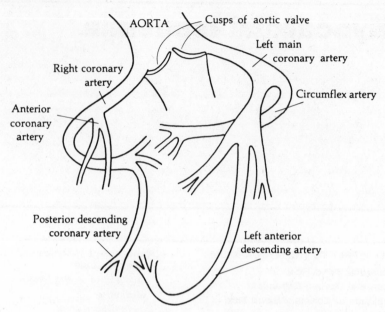

AORTA — Cusps of aortic valve

Left main coronary artery

Right coronary artery

Circumflex artery

Anterior coronary artery

Posterior descending coronary artery

Left anterior descending artery

Figure 4-1. Main arteries of the coronary blood supply (see text).

The venous drainage system of the myocardium has two divisions. The superficial system lies along and superficial to the main arteries and empties into the anterior cardiac veins and the coronary sinus. The sinus lies in the atrioventricular groove at the posterior aspect of the heart and drains directly into the right atrium. This drainage system receives blood flow mainly from the left ventricle. The deep venous drainage system receives venous blood from the remainder of the heart; it is comprised principally of minute thin-walled sinusoids, which empty directly into the heart chambers. In addition there are connections from both coronary arterioles and venules directly into the heart chambers.

During cardiac systole left ventricular systolic pressure is somewhat higher than intraaortic systolic pressure; the consequence of this is that blood flow through the coronary arterial system during myocardial contraction is greatly reduced because of increased coronary intravascular resistance resulting from muscle compression of the vessels. This systolic decrease in coronary flow applies more to the left ventricle than the right ventricle. Thus coronary blood flow and myocardial perfusion occur mainly during diastole, particularly in subendocardial areas of the left ventricle, because this is the period in the cardiac cycle when coronary intravascular resistance is the lowest.

Because of the cyclic nature of coronary artery blood flow, there are certain physiologic alterations which tend to reduce myocardial perfusion and oxygen supply in the normal subject, and therefore imperil myocardial oxygenation to an even greater extent in the subject with coronary artery atherosclerosis. The first is tachycardia, which reduces diastolic filling time. The second is hypotension (either because of hypovolemia or systemic vasodilation), which reduces venous return and hence cardiac output and intraaortic pressure. The third is reduced aortic diastolic pressure (from a number of causes: aortic valve incompetence, elevated intrathoracic pressure, or congestive heart failure). These conditions, tachycardia, hypotension, and low aortic diastolic pressure, produce decreased coronary artery blood flow and hence reduce myocardial oxygenation.

Myocardial Oxygen Extraction

In the normal person at rest, about 4 ml of oxygen/100 ml of arterial blood is extracted by noncardiac muscle tissue. Therefore, a reserve of about 8–10 ml oxygen/100 ml blood is present and potentially available for extraction and use by skeletal muscle when physical activity increases during exercise. During vigorous exertion in a healthy subject, extraction of oxygen from arterial blood by peripheral tissue increases to over 12 ml oxygen/100 ml blood. Thus, this oxygen reserve provides for a two- to threefold increase in oxygen consumption by skeletal muscle tissue.

The situation in heart muscle, however, is quite different. The oxygen content of coronary sinus blood is the lowest from any vein draining a major organ, even at absolute rest. This low oxygen content of venous blood coming from the myocardium varies only slightly under all conditions of myocardial work; the reason for this is that heart muscle, unlike skeletal muscle, maximally extracts oxygen from the arterial blood perfusing it even at complete rest. Therefore in the myocardium there is little or no oxygen extraction reserve. For this reason myocardial requirements for increased oxygen consumption during times of elevated heart and systemic demand (for example, during exercise) must be met primarily by mechanisms which increase total blood flow in the coronary arteries, mainly through decreased coronary artery resistance by coronary artery vasodilation. Increased coronary blood flow is mediated primarily by increase in caliber (vasodilation) of the smaller arterioles within the myocardium and to a lesser extent by dilation of the large and medium-sized coronary arteries on the surface of the heart. It is in these larger superficial arteries lying on the heart surface that spotty as well as generalized narrowing from atherosclerosis occurs, and not in the smaller vessels within the heart substance itself.

Regulation of Coronary Blood Flow

The physiologic processes resulting in elevated blood flow in the coronary arteries are several. (1) At the onset of increased physical activity, venous return to the heart, myocardial contractility, and heart rate all increase. The result is elevated cardiac output and possibly increased perfusion pressure in the aorta, which would tend to elevate coronary artery flow. (However, there is some question as to whether aortic perfusion pressure does in fact increase during the elevated cardiac output correlated with exercise.) (2) When the oxygen need of heart muscle increases above the O_2 supply immediately available, because of increased heart muscle work, then a brief relative local hypoxia occurs, which results in the production of metabolites, one of which is adenosine diphosphate. These metabolites are direct coronary artery vasodilators and cause an increase in coronary caliber and blood flow. (3) The increased sympathetic adrenergic neural stimuli at the onset of exercise (Chapter 8) lead to increased myocardial norepinephrine content, and the increased circulating levels of catecholamines from systemic adrenergic terminals and the adrenal medulla produce an increase in the rate and force of heart muscle contraction—the well-known positive chronotropic and inotropic effects. With increased myocardial work, more vasodilator metabolites are produced which directly dilate coronary arteries. In addition, the coronary arterioles themselves contain both α- and β-adrenergic receptors in their walls; the latter probably mediate direct coronary vasodilation and an increase in perfusion pressure to the myocardium (although the exact relation between α and β influences on coronary artery caliber in the intact subject is still controversial).

Ischemic Heart Disease

Probably over 5 million persons in the United States are victims of coronary heart disease; it is the leading cause of death in males over 35 years old, in all persons over 45, and is second only to hypertension as the most common cardiovascular disease. However, there has been a decline in the death rate from ischemic heart disease in the years from 1970 to 1978; between 1940 to 1960 the mortality rate from this disorder increased steadily, plateaued between 1960 and 1967, and then gradually decreased. There is no certain explanation for this decline, but evidence suggests that earlier discovery and better control of hypertension, lowering of serum cholesterol by dietary precautions, increased physical exercise, and a decline in cigaret smoking among older persons are contributory factors.

Inadequate oxygenation of the myocardium is the consequence of an inability of the coronary circulation to increase its rate and amount of blood flow to meet oxygen requirements of the heart muscle; the usual cause is structural narrowing of the lumen of large and medium-sized coronary vessels produced by atherosclerosis. This process apparently begins very early in life, may be completely silent for many years, but nevertheless gradually produces destruction of heart muscle via hypoxic cell death, resulting in a progressive decline in the adequacy of myocardial performance. The consequences of chronic myocardial ischemia from coronary artery atherosclerosis are sudden death from ventricular fibrillation, acute myocardial infarction, gradual development of left ventricular functional impairment and congestive heart failure (coronary artery cardiomyopathy), cardiac arrhythmias, and subjective symptoms of angina pectoris and decreased exercise tolerance.

Coronary Artery Atherosclerosis

The Process

Atherosclerosis does not produce symptoms until it is far advanced, and, in the case of ischemic heart disease, announces its presence by one of the signs or symptoms listed above, or is discovered by electrocardiographic abnormalities in an exercise test. It appears to be what is called a multifactorial disease—that is, it is associated with a number of causes, or at least is correlated with certain risk factors which appear to predispose to the development of atherosclerotic lesions and arteriolar lumen narrowing. The most significant and well-established risk factors are being a male, hypercholesterolemia, hypertension, and cigaret smoking; other risk factors which appear to be related to incidence and severity are lack of regular vigorous physical exercise, obesity, diabetes mellitus, and a positive family history of atherosclerotic cardiovascular disease, implying genetic predisposition. These risk factors have been shown by many clinical studies, particularly the Framingham study, to correlate with development of myocardial ischemia, and are thus of prognostic importance.

Atherosclerotic plaques may originate with the fatty streak, a lipid material accumulation which is found at autopsy in the aorta and carotid arteries of infants dying of other causes. By adolescence this material appears in the cerebral and coronary arteries. Fibrous plaques, characterized by the presence of connective tissue proteins, proliferations of arterial smooth muscle cells, and lipid deposits, appear to evolve from the fatty streak in early and mid-adult life. This developmental sequence has been observed in subjects from cultures having a high incidence of atherosclerotic coronary and cerebral disease, such as the United States and Finland. Complicated plaques are a later development and show such degenerative changes as calcification, increased lipid accumulation, ulceration, bleeding, and clot formation. Lesions occur in the epicardial portions of the main coronary arteries, in the left system more than the right, and involvement is usually diffuse rather than localized.

There are two main theories to account for the development of atherosclerotic plaques. The first is based primarily on the studies of atherosclerotic lesions in the arteries of experimental animals, and postulates that plaques form in response to chronically recurring injury to the thin endothelial lining of arterial walls. Many types of recurring damage to arterial linings lead to the development of abnormalities in these structures: mechanical trauma, immune reactions, platelet aggregation, clot initiation, hypoxia from a high blood content of carbon monoxide (such as occurs in the blood of cigaret smokers and freeway com-

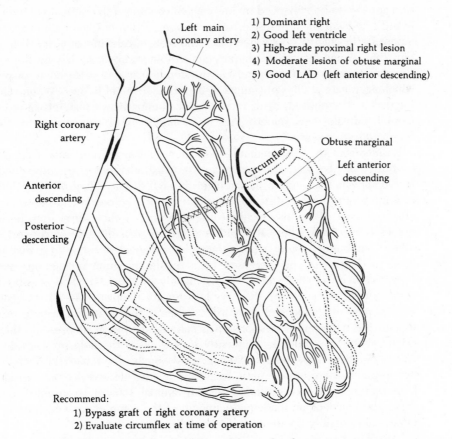

1) Dominant right
2) Good left ventricle
3) High-grade proximal right lesion
4) Moderate lesion of obtuse marginal
5) Good LAD (left anterior descending)

Left main coronary artery

Right coronary artery

Obtuse marginal

Left anterior descending

Circumflex

Anterior descending

Posterior descending

Recommend:
1) Bypass graft of right coronary artery
2) Evaluate circumflex at time of operation

Figure 4-2. Graphic representation of the results of a coronary arteriogram.

muters) and apparently from chronic hyperlipidemia itself. High blood pressure is thought also to be a major cause of chronic trauma to endothelial linings.

This theory goes on to state that once the delicate endothelial layer is disrupted, the consequence will be the passage of large molecules in the plasma, such as plasma lipoproteins, through to the smooth muscle cells of the arterial wall. Blood lipids and lipid substances such as cholesterol are carried in the blood by a group of complex molecules called lipoproteins. There are four main types of plasma lipoproteins; they are classified on the basis of their size and density. The low-density lipoproteins (LDL) carry most of the cholesterol in the blood. Certain cells normally have on their surfaces specific receptors for LDL; interaction of LDL with these receptors appears to be a first step in metabolic breakdown of LDL which leads to the suppression of cellular synthesis of cholesterol. If the receptors are abnormal then these steps do not occur, and as a consequence LDL and cholesterol levels in the blood may rise markedly. Most body cells synthesize cholesterol, and there are various specific genetic and biochemical processes which regulate endogenous cholesterol production; abnormalities in this regulation may contribute to the hypercholesterolemia which, combined with improper dietary habits and insufficient physical exercise, may damage endothelial linings and contribute to the formation of atheromata.

Some studies indicate that LDL promotes the proliferation of smooth muscle cells in arterial walls, thus hastening the development of atheromata; smooth muscle cells in tissue culture do in fact take up large amounts of LDL. This process appears to be enhanced by low oxygen content of the perfusing medium, offering a basis for the atherosclerosis-promoting action of cigaret smoking. Carbon monoxide in cigaret smoke decreases the oxygen-carrying capacity of hemoglobin, thus promoting arterial hypoxemia. Another substance having the capacity to promote arterial smooth muscle proliferation is one released from platelets which aggregate at sites of trauma to endothelial vessel linings. When release of this factor is abolished, as in reduction or elimination of platelets in an experimental animal, then smooth muscle proliferation in response to endothelial trauma does not occur.

Results from the Framingham study show that as an individual's plasma concentration of LDL rises, the risk of a myocardial infarction rises correspondingly. It also appears that higher plasma levels of high-density lipoproteins (HDL) may in some way protect against the development of atheromata and hence coronary artery disease. HDL may facilitate the transport of cholesterol from peripheral tissues to the liver where it is either excreted with the bile or converted into other compounds. Some studies have been reported suggesting that plasma levels of HDL may be increased by a regular program of vigorous exercise. Elevated levels of cholesterol, carried mainly by the LDL, and possibly triglycerides (carried mainly by the very-low-density lipoproteins—VLDL) correlate with increased incidence of myocardial ischemia and infarction in both sexes, although the triglyceride relationship is somewhat unclear at present. Infarction occurs about four times as frequently in patients with cholesterol levels above 250 mg% than those below 220 mg%. Although about one third of cases of hyperlipidemia are on a genetic basis, the major causative factors appear to be high dietary intake of saturated (mainly animal source) fat, refined carbohydrates, and alcohol; an inadequate amount of the complex carbohydrate of vegetables; and possibly a sedentary life style.

A major question remains to be answered: will lowering the plasma cholesterol levels by dietary and/or pharmacologic means promote the regression or resorption of atherosclerotic deposits from individuals in which this process is already established? Studies with laboratory animals, including primates, indicate that it may, but this remains to be demonstrated in the human.

The other hypothesis attempting to account for the generation of atherosclerotic deposits on arterial linings states that the formation of plaques is analogous to the development of a benign tumor and that the smooth muscle cells forming each plaque is a clone from a single cell which underwent unregulated proliferation. This is a newer theory and less research has accumulated to test and amplify it. Supporters of the monoclonal hypothesis state that cigaret smoking may promote atherogenesis on the basis of the known fact that constituents of cigaret smoke contain a number of chemicals which produce cell mutations, and hence could alter the genetic constitution of smooth muscle cells in a way which would promote uncontrolled growth.

Although many of the studies of myocardial ischemia and its risk factors have been based on a subject population under age 65, most ischemic heart disease occurs in age groups above 65 and accounts for about half the deaths in this elderly group. These individuals appear to have a different relationship to some of the risk factors which apply to younger age groups. Cigaret smoking and concentration of plasma LDL do not correlate as closely with incidence of heart ischemia and infarction in the elderly as does hypertension; the lower an older individual's blood pressure, the less the likelihood of heart disease. In addition, diabetes mellitus is highly correlated with heart disease in females. Also electrocardiographic abnormalities appear to offer better prediction of risk from heart attacks in the older than in the younger years.

Atherosclerotic coronary artery disease is a silent and insidious disorder, and thus its presence is not evident until a critical decline in blood flow to the myocardium produces the symptom of angina pectoris or the signs of arrhythmia and/or electrocardiographic abnormalities on an exercise stress test. However, since ischemic heart disease is so well correlated with hyperlipidemia in persons younger than age 65, all persons older than 25 should have a serum cholesterol and triglyceride determination made on blood drawn before the morning meal. A cholesterol value over 250 mg% or triglyceride value over 200 mg% is abnormal and indicates the need for further evaluation of weight gain, smoking, dietary habits, regular exercise programs, alcohol intake, diabetes mellitus, or hypothyroidism. Family history of strokes, diabetes, heart attacks, sudden death, and obesity should be explored and considered as magnification factors for other risk factors if present. The use of birth control pills and postmenopausal estrogens constitutes a further risk factor for females. Recognition and control of hypertension is an important component of prophylaxis. However, because of the early beginnings of atherosclerotic heart disease in populations of the heavily industrialized countries, prevention should be directed at health habits beginning in early childhood, especially dietary but also increased exercise and no smoking.

The Consequences

As discussed above, increased blood flow through the coronary arteries brought about by a decline in their resistance by vasodilation is the mechanism by which blood, and hence oxygen, supply to the myocardium is increased in order to meet the metabolic requirements of increased workload. This vasodilation occurs primarily not in the large arteries but in the smaller arterioles. However, it is the medium-sized and large arteries in which the larger atheromatous deposits occur. This luminal narrowing (decreased internal diameter) produces a chronically depressed level of flow in the arteries at all times. Although the decreased flow may be adequate to sustain the metabolic needs of the myocardium at rest, it may not be so at the onset of physical exertion or at times of emotional stress.

A partial obstruction in a large coronary artery or main branch leads to a chronic dilation of the smaller arteries and arterioles beyond the narrowing as a compensatory response to the decreased perfusion pressure through them. This may be a direct effect of local hypoxia and hypercapnia, or due to the accumulation of vasodilator metabolites from inadequately oxygenated myocardium. Whatever the mechanism, the consequence is that these arterioles are only slightly capable of further vasodilation in response to increased myocardial oxygen requirement. At such times then, the discrepancy between heart muscle need and coronary capacity to meet the need by vasodilation and increased blood flow, eventually becomes great enough to produce signs and symptoms of myocardial ischemia: angina pectoris, and the impairments of impulse formation, conduction, and muscle contractility, resulting from ischemia.

Blood leaving the venous drainage system of the heart during an ischemic period shows increased content of lactate and hydrogen ions, indicating anaerobic metabolism, and increased potassium ion content, indicating K^+ efflux from hypoxic cells. Such cells, because of membrane abnormalities induced by hypoxia, can no longer adequately regulate differential transmembrane ionic concentrations. Electrocardiograms reveal changes in electrical polarization signaled by inverted T waves and/or displaced (depressed in effort angina, elevated in variant angina) S-T segments. Another significant consequence of ischemia of heart cell membranes is the electrical instability which produces arrhythmias, often premature ventricular contractions and ventricular tachycardia and fibrillation.

Ventricular performance declines in poorly perfused myocardium as indicated by an increase in left ventricular end-diastolic volume and pressure, a decreased systolic ejection fraction, an increased presystolic time with decreased systolic ejection period, and a decreased systolic elevation in ventricular pressure development as a function of time (Chapter 7).

Angina Pectoris

Types

Angina is a deep, dull, slow substernal sensation of distress often described by patients experiencing it as tightness, pressure, squeezing or heaviness, and seldom characterized as sharp, stabbing or rapid. Its duration is usually about 3 to 10 minutes. It is precipitated by increased physical exertion or emotional arousal, and is relieved by rest or sublingual nitroglycerine. The pain may radiate to the left shoulder, down the ulnar aspect of the left arm, or into the left neck or jaw. It is sometimes accompanied by shortness of breath, nausea, paresthesias of the hands (numbness or tingling) and sweating. In a given patient the pain tends to produce a characteristic symptom complex, recurs in a characteristic daily temporal pattern (often more readily triggered in the morning) and made worse by heavy meals, cold air, and effort involving isometric exertion of the upper arms such as handgrips. The latter effect is brought about by a greatly increased peripheral arterial resistance and elevated blood pressure caused by upper extremity muscle tension; this increases afterload on the heart and results in increased work and oxygen need because of the requirement to pump against elevated aortic pressure. The greater frequency of anginal attacks following a meal is due to the elevated cardiac output occurring postprandially because of splanchnic vasodilation and increased blood flow to the viscera.

Complaints of the chest pain resulting from myocardial ischemia must be carefully evaluated to distinguish them from the discomfort of hiatal hernia with gastroesophageal reflux, peptic ulcer disease, intercostal myositis, costochondritis, cholelithiasis, cervical degenerative joint disease with foraminal narrowing and nerve root encroachment, pleurisy, and pericarditis.

Although the above is a characteristic picture of angina in many patients, there is a wide range of variation. Particularly in the elderly patient the symptoms may be confined to a sensation of heaviness in the hands and arms, sudden onset of shortness of breath, nausea, weakness, or epigastric distress. Prinzmetal's or variant angina occurs often at rest, the pain is frequently very severe, and is often accompanied by cardiac arrythmias. Angiographic studies indicate that Prinzmetal's angina often results from coronary artery spasms superimposed on widespread diffuse atherosclerotic narrowing of smaller coronary arteries. Decubitus angina occurs at night after the patient has been lying down for a time, or may awaken him from sleep. The processes involved in this condition appear to result from a redistribution of intravascular and interstitial body fluid. Lying down increases the blood volume in the thoracic cavity; venous return of blood to the right heart is increased because of the reduced pull of gravity which produces pooling of blood in the lower extremities. A longer term effect of lying down is that, because of the postural change, the capillary hydrostatic pressure in the lower body is reduced, and fluid which entered the interstitial spaces under the effects of gravity now reenters the circulation and expands the blood volume. In both cases the elevated venous return produces an increased workload on the myocardium. Sitting up will lower intrathoracic blood volume and provide some relief as it does in paroxysmal noctural dyspnea. In some patients nocturnal angina occurs as a consequence of the profound fluctuations in autonomic activity which occurs in all persons during rapid eye movement (REM, dreaming) sleep. Heart rate and blood pressure sometimes rise to very high levels causing increased myocardial work load and oxygen requirements. In addition, REM mentation often contains emotionally disturbing content (Chapter 15).

Cause

The processes responsible for the heart pain of myocardial ischemia are postulated by some workers to be the release of vaso- and neuroactive compounds—histamine, serotonin, and bradykinin—from platelets, red cells, and myocardial cells injured by hypoxia. Other investigators believe that the release of lactate produced by anaerobic glycolysis during hypoxia, and hydrogen and potassium ions released from cells whose membranes are no longer able to maintain their selective permeability because of hypoxia, are important stimulators of the free nerve endings which comprise pain receptors. These substances may directly stimulate the pain receptors (nociceptors) which are free nerve endings distributed among myocardial cells. The heart is supplied with sensory afferents which form both superficial and deep plexuses and leave the heart via sensory fibers of the thoracic cardiac nerves. These terminate in the upper several thoracic ganglia; presynaptic fibers then run from the ganglia and enter the cord at the upper five thoracic segments. Dermatomes one through five also supply the pericardium and ulnar surface of the arm. Both the autonomic and somatic fibers converge on the same pool of neurons in the spinal cord. This convergence is held to be the mechanism accounting for the familiar pattern of visceral (heart) to somatic (precordium and arm) radiation occurring in the pain of angina pectoris, and is illustrated diagrammatically in Figure 4-3.

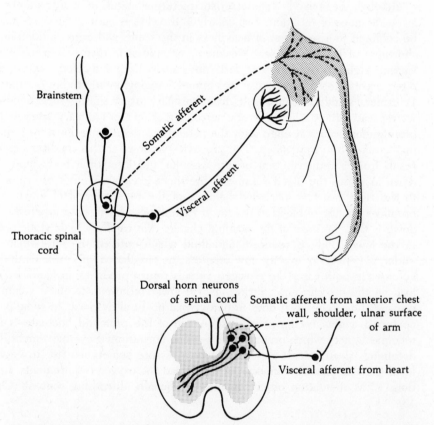

Figure 4-3. Diagram illustrating the principle of convergence in the spinal cord adduced as an explanation for the nature of ischemic heart pain. Visceral afferent (sensory) pain fibers from the heart converge on the same groups of neurons in the dorsal horn of the spinal cord which also receive sensory afferents from the anterior chest wall and arm. When the visceral pain fibers from the heart are stimulated by myocardial ischemia the impulses arrive at the same neurons in the cord receiving afferent pain fibers from the arm and chest. Activation of this common pool of neurons results in projection by the brain of the pain to the area of the body supplied by these somatic fibers.

Diagnosis of Ischemic Heart Disease

Two of the most clinically useful components of assessment of myocardial ischemia with angina pectoris are a careful history revealing the classical features of angina, above; and the relief of chest pain within 1 to 3 minutes after sublingual nitroglycerine. Confirmation should then be obtained by means of an exercise stress electrocardiogram taken during and following treadmill or bicycle ergometer exertion (Chapter 8). Physical examination as well as the electrocardiogram of a patient with a chief complaint of angina may be entirely within normal limits between attacks. During chest pain the patient may be anxious, diaphoretic, in evident discomfort, and often will have an elevated heart rate and blood pressure. An S_4 and apical systolic murmur may be heard. The EKG at this time may show T wave and S-T segment abnormalities, especially depression of the latter, although in variant angina elevation often occurs.

Exercising Testing

Exercise testing is often useful and, if properly conducted, may be a safe diagnostic tool for identifying ischemic heart disease, assessing its severity, and evaluating its impairment of and threat to the patient. Because of the importance of the relation between physical exercise and heart disease this topic is discussed in detail in Chapter 8.

Coronary Arteriography

Coronary arteriography is a method for diagnosis of the presence, location and severity of coronary atherosclerotic obstruction. Because of its invasiveness there are significant complications and fatalities, particularly in laboratories where the frequency of the procedure is low and the staff therefore less experienced. The degree of coronary narrowing necessary to produce significant myocardial ischemia during exercise is controversial. Based on pathology evaluation of autopsy material correlated with prior angiograms, the evidence indicates that arteriograms and their interpretation tend to underestimate the actual degree of anatomic narrowing. Some studies report that if there is less than 50% obstruction, flow rates (even at high myocardial oxygen requirements) show little decline, and that 75% obstruction lowers flow by only about one third.

Newer Noninvasive Methods: Myocardial Perfusion Scintigraphy

Imaging of the myocardium following intravenous injection of radioactive pharmaceutical agents is coming into increasing prominence as a procedure for detecting ischemic, that is, inadequately perfused, areas of heart muscle. Imaging with radionuclides is accomplished by injecting the compound, which is actively taken up by myocardial cells, and then detecting the pattern of photons emitted from areas of the heart with a scintillation camera. Photon density and distribution is recorded and reproduced by a computer and yields images of the heart muscle.

Thallium-201 is a radionuclide that exchanges readily with the intracellular K^+ of heart muscle; following intravenous injection thallium-201 has about a 75%

extraction by heart muscle and shows a distribution within myocardium that has been demonstrated to correlate with coronary blood flow. In ischemic areas of heart muscle, less radionuclide is taken up by poorly perfused cells, and a resulting "cold spot" appears in the myocardial scintigram. Therefore, failure of uptake is correlated with impaired myocardial perfusion, perhaps because during ischemia, and therefore hypoxia, there is impairment of the $Na^+–K^+$ (or thallium) membrane pump of heart muscle cells. In areas of prior infarction, "cold spots"—areas of decreased uptake—also are present, but chronically so; while ischemic cold spots often develop during exercise testing, but the resting perfusion scintiscan may be normal.

Several studies have reported that the correlation between thallium-201 defects in the scintiscan, and coronary artery lesions demonstrated by angiography, on the one hand; and with abnormal EKG-exercise stress testing, on the other; are good and that, in addition, thallium-201 scintigraphy adds to the diagnostic specificity and sensitivity of the exercise stress test.

Management of Myocardial Ischemia and Angina Pectoris

Modification of Risk Factors

Of the postulated risk factors for the initiation and progression of coronary artery disease, the three which appear to be most directly involved are cigaret smoking, elevated serum cholesterol level, and blood pressure. Additional ones are obesity and a sedentary life style. Thus, risk factor modification would include cessation of smoking, reduction of hyperlipidemia, discovery and control of hypertension, reducing to lean body weight, and a schedule of regular, gradually increasing dynamic exercise. The place of exercise in the diagnosis and management of ischemic heart disease, and its possible role in prevention, is discussed fully in Chapter 8. However, briefly at this point, it should be emphasized that exercise conditioning is of prime significance in the management of angina. Its long-term action is primarily that of reducing peripheral circulatory requirements rather than altering myocardial blood supply and performance. Angina patients given physical exercise training may improve exercise capacity as much as 50% in a program of regular increasingly vigorous exercise training. Preliminary treadmill testing is advisable.

Risk factor modification in the prevention and management of ischemic heart disease is based on the assumption that, since certain risk factors appear to be correlated with the occurrence and progression of coronary artery disease, elimination or modification of these will delay its development and perhaps alter the course of the disorder once it has become symptomatic. Some of the many studies which have been conducted to test these hypotheses have yielded so far largely equivocal results (except in the case of cigaret smoking). Newer, well-designed, and controlled clinical studies are under way to evaluate the impact of elimination or reduction of several risk factors, not only upon the course of established coronary artery disease, but upon the development of it in as yet asymptomatic but coronary-prone populations.

Of the three most prominent risk factors it has been unequivocally demonstrated only that stopping cigaret smoking will significantly reduce the risks of developing the disease, and the incidence and severity of the acute complications of it: myocardial infarction, serious cardiac arrhythmias, and sudden death. These data apply primarily to younger and middle-aged men. Cigaret smoking appears to be less well correlated with complications of coronary artery disease in the older age group; in these individuals hypertension appears to be the major risk factor for ischemic heart disease and infarction.

Cigaret smoking as a risk factor in ischemic heart disease occupies a unique place for two reasons: it is the only one which has been proven to significantly correlate with morbidity and mortality of this disorder; and it is the only one of the three in the category of major risk factors over which the individual has direct and total control, without intervention by a health professional and without medication or other diagnostic or therapeutic manipulations. Smoking appears to magnify or act as a multiplier for the adverse effects of the other proposed risk factors; studies indicate that elimination of other risk factors appear to be of only modest, if any, value provided smoking is continued. Patients who have stopped smoking have a gradually declining likelihood of developing the complications of ischemic heart disease, including cardiac death, and within a few years have a no higher death rate than patients who have never smoked. Thus the often-heard excuse, it's too late to do anything about it now, is not true except possibly in the elderly population. The risk of death from coronary heart disease in men under 65 who stopped smoking is one half that of those who continue. And patients who stop smoking after a myocardial infarction have one half the reinfarctions and cardiovascular mortality of those who do not.

The physiologic processes by which cigaret smoke increases morbidity and mortality from ischemic heart disease may be twofold: it may increase the atherosclerotic processes in the coronary arteries (as well as elsewhere, of course)—that is, contribute to the chronic progression of the disease; and it may precipitate an infarction in patients with coronary arteries narrowed sufficiently by the chronic atherosclerotic process—that is, cause acute changes which reduce myocardial oxygenation below the critical level. As described earlier, it is proposed that an important mechanism by which smoking accelerates atherosclerosis is by producing hypoxia of endothelial linings of blood vessels, by the binding of hemoglobin with carbon monoxide; this binding not only reduces hemoglobin oxygen-carrying capacity, but inhibits the release to cells of oxygen which is carried. Precipitation of infarction may occur by the combined actions of reducing oxygen delivery to the myocardium, increasing platelet aggregation, and producing adrenergic stimuli to heart muscle. Increased release of norepinephrine within the heart increases the electrical instability of heart muscle cells resulting in ectopic impulse formation and propagation, and cardiac arrhythmias. In addition sympathetic adrenergic discharge has been shown to increase coronary vascular resistance and decrease coronary blood flow.

It has been shown in normal individuals (1) that smoking induces a marked acceleration in heart rate and increase in systemic arterial pressure; (2) that these elevations are followed promptly by a rise in plasma norepinephrine, indicating that the hemodynamic changes may result from norepinephrine release by adrenergic nerve terminals directly into tissues, rather than systemically; and (3) that the heart rate and blood pressure elevating effects of smoking can be blocked by β-adrenergic antagonists. In addition to the probable decreases in oxygen delivery to the myocardium produced by smoking via the mechanisms described above, the elevated heart rate and blood pressure increase workload on the myocardium and therefore increase myocardial oxygen requirements. Since coronary atherosclerosis results in a discrepancy between heart muscle oxygen need and ability of the coronary circulation to meet the need, smoking appears to operate in such a way that the discrepancy is increased.

A recent study of mortality in a long-term follow-up of 4000 men and women, which compared cigaret smokers with nonsmokers, has revealed that the smoker to nonsmoker mortality ratios for ischemic heart disease were 4.7 (males) and 3.6 (females). The death rate from all causes adjusted for age was 9.02 per 1000 person-years in smokers, 3.79 in ex-smokers and 3.45 in nonsmokers. A number of variables which could possibly explain the smoking-mortality relation (such as genetic or psychoemotional factors) was evaluated. The data failed to support the contention that the smoking-increased mortality relation is secondary to some mediating third factor.

Modification of life style in minor respects is also an important component of management in ischemic heart disease. Wearing a ski-type face mask in cold weather, eating small meals, avoiding emotional tension, and slowing down the rate at which ordinary angina-inducing activities are performed, usually help patients to reduce the frequency and severity of their chest pains.

Medication

Nitroglycerine

Nitroglycerine is the cornerstone of pharmacologic management in angina; it may be taken sublingually either at onset of angina or prophylactically before performing tasks or encountering stresses which the patient has learned from experience will induce chest pain. The prophylactic effect lasts about 30 minutes. The dosage is 0.3–0.6 mg sublingually; it is rapidly absorbed into the capillary circulation from the mucous membranes, and when it does not actually prevent or stop the pain it will often decrease the severity and duration. Some patients experience pounding headache as a side effect; trials of various doses may lead to a separation of a lower dose which is still effective for the angina from the slightly higher one usually necessary to produce the unpleasant sensations of fullness or throbbing in the head. The relief of pain usually occurs in 1 to 3 minutes. If there is no relief after 5 minutes, a second tablet may be taken. If after another 5 minutes the pain still persists, it is probably wise for the patient to be seen in a hospital emergency room. If a third tablet is taken with no relief, and the pain has lasted more than 20 minutes, prompt medical evaluation would be indicated, particularly if the persistence and severity is a new development for a given patient.

Nitroglycerine is a powerful dilator of vascular smooth muscle; in normal coronary arteries it produces decreased coronary vascular resistance by vasodilation and increased coronary blood flow. However, especially in patients with considerable coronary atherosclerotic narrowing, the major amelioration of symptoms probably results from widespread systemic vasodilation of both arteries and especially veins. This action of nitroglycerine leads to pooling of blood in the veins and hence decreased venous return to the right heart, with lowered ventricular diastolic volume and pressure (decreased preload), as well as a decline in systemic arterial resistance and pressure, and decreased stroke work with a resultant drop in afterload on the heart. The consequence of both of these actions is decreased myocardial oxygen requirement because of decreased myocardial workload: less blood to pump and less resistance to pump it against. In addition, recent studies have shown that nitroglycerine induces vasodilation and increased blood flow in the coronary arteries themselves and in the collateral circulation of the heart, and increased flow to areas of ischemic myocardium.

When patients first begin a trial of nitroglycerine they should be encouraged initially to test their responses to its effects while lying or sitting down if possible, since the rapid widespread vasodilation may lower cerebral perfusion so rapidly that syncope may occur if they are standing.

Organic Nitrates

Drugs such as isosorbide dinitrate are widely used, but in the past there has been some controversy as to their objective effectiveness and the degree to which such effectiveness is in fact of long duration. It appears to be considerably less effective in the relief of anginal pain than nitroglycerine, but some studies have shown increased time intervals between attacks with its use, particularly when patients start using it regularly, and at large doses. Sublingual isosorbide may also be used prophylactically before exercise. Its duration of effect is only about 30 minutes, but some patients appear to have beneficial effects for an hour or two.

The effects of both oral isosorbide dinitrate, and nitroglycerine ointment applied to the skin, on some of the factors which influence myocardial oxygen requirements (such as systemic arterial pressure and left ventricular size) indicate that isosorbide dinitrate 20 mg taken orally, or the ointment application to the skin in doses of 12–40 mg, produces in some patients lowered wall tension, decreased ventricular and diastolic pressure, decline in systolic blood pressure, and no elevation in heart rate, throughout 4 hours of study; all of these actions contribute to a prolonged decline in myocardial oxygen requirements.

Some studies have indicated, however, that with repeated use tolerance to its vasodilating effects develops and that eventually little or no therapeutic benefit results. There is also some evidence that with the use of these organic nitrates, cross-tolerance to the action of nitroglycerine may develop, reducing the effectiveness of the latter in the management of an acute attack of angina. Some patients with angina report a several-hour (about 5) antianginal effect from high-dose oral isosorbide during exercise testing. With chronic (about 5 to 6 months) use of the drug at doses averaging 29 mg 3–4 times per day, as assessed by exercise tests on a bicycle ergometer, some tolerance to its blood pressure lowering and heart rate elevating effects develops; however, there appears to be little reported decline in the subjective antianginal effects of either oral isosorbide or sublingual nitroglycerine in this situation.

The issue of development of tolerance raises the corresponding one of development of dependence with chronic use of high dose nitrates; in view of this possibility caution should be exercised in weaning angina patients from chronic high dose nitrate use if this is indicated; the drugs should be tapered gradually rather than withdrawn rapidly in order to avoid reactive vasoconstriction, elevated systemic arterial pressure, and consequent increase in heart afterload which could result in greatly increased myocardial oxygen requirements and worsened myocardial ischemia. Such a response could also be accompanied by reactive coronary vasospasm, thus critically lowering myocardial blood supply.

Beta Adrenergic Blocking Agents

Propranolol blocks the stimulation of the β-adrenergic receptors, producing a decreased heart rate, and lowered myocardial contractility, cardiac output and oxygen consumption. Its effects are more marked during muscular exercise than at rest because most of the cardiovascular changes during physical exertion are mediated by the catecholamines norepinephrine and epinephrine, and their effects are antagonized and prevented by propranolol. Therefore it is most useful in frequent exertional angina. The heart rate decline is mediated by a suppression of sympathetic influences on the heart and by a direct increase in rate of diastolic depolarization of pacemaker tissue. Conduction in atrioventricular junctional tissues is also slowed, and direct decrease in ventricular contraction rate occurs. The β blocking action also depresses contractility perhaps by interfering with the intracellular β-adrenergic system (Chapter 7). It reduces the number and severity of anginal attacks and increases exercise tolerance on treadmill stress testing. It appears to have no effect on the coronary circulation itself, but lowers myocardial oxygen requirements by lowering oxygen consumption. It is particularly useful in hypertensive patients with angina, and also produces marked relief in unstable angina.

Patients with angina who also have hypertrophied and dilated hearts and congestive heart failure become a management problem in that propranolol is likely to decrease myocardial contractility to the point where the congestive failure is markedly worsened, with elevated left ventricular end-diastolic volume and pressure, elevated pulmonary capillary pressure, and interstitial and intraalveolar pulmonary edema. In the case of a worsening of signs and symptoms of congestive heart failure, and a heart rate slow enough to produce impaired circulation, propranolol may have to be discontinued. Contraindications to the use of propranolol include significant obstructive airway disease (especially asthma), possibly insulin-dependent diabetes, a high degree of heart block, or sick sinus syndrome (Chapter 6). Undesirable side effects are weakness and lack of energy, bronchospasm and dyspnea, gastrointestinal disturbances, and sexual impotence in the male. Reduction of dosage may control the side effects. Propranolol should never be suddenly withdrawn, since unstable angina, myocardial infarction, or sudden death may occur.

Digitalis and Diuretics

These are useful drugs in patients having angina complicated by an enlarged heart and congestive heart failure. Digitalis decreases heart size by increasing systolic ejection fraction and lowering left ventricular end-diastolic volume. Although it increases O_2 consumption in many cases, this effect appears to be offset by the decrease in end-diastolic volume and hence wall stress which it induces. The resulting decrease in wall tension lowers oxygen requirement of the myocardium. Diuretics, by decreasing ECF volume, have a similar effect: a lowering of venous return, reduced end-diastolic volume and pressure, and decreased wall tension.

Other drugs which may be helpful in the medical management of angina are those which decrease peripheral vascular resistance: prazosin and hydralazine (Chapter 3).

Aortocoronary Bypass

In this procedure a section of saphenous vein is grafted between the aorta and a segment of a coronary artery distal to an occlusive lesion in a major coronary vessel: the left main, the left anterior descending, the circumflex, or the right coronary artery. Depending on the status of the vessels as revealed by coronary arteriography and evaluation at the time of operation, one to four vessel bypass grafts may be performed. On occasion the mammary artery may be joined to a coronary artery distal to an obstructive lesion in addition to a bypass graft. The goals of the operation are increased life expectancy; reduction in the cardiovascular morbidity resulting from ischemic heart disease (myocardial infarction, congestive heart failure); improved left ventricular function; and enhanced quality of life, including increased exercise tolerance and relief of symptoms. Of these goals, the attainment of relief from anginal pain in the majority of patients has been the only clearly demonstrated consequence at the time of this writing, although in patients with left main coronary artery lesions there has been some indication of improved survival with the bypass procedure. The relief of chest pain has appeared to correlate with increased coronary blood flow after grafting, as demonstrated on coronary angiograms; other factors which are probably responsible for amelioration of angina in some patients are intra- and postoperative small infarctions in the ischemic myocardium responsible for the chest pain, and the well-known placebo effects of surgical procedures. Postoperative hemodynamic studies in patients who have undergone the bypass operation have so far failed to demonstrate improved left ventricular function.

The place of aortocoronary bypass surgery in the treatment of ischemic heart disease continues to be controversial. The major reason for this disagreement has been the lack of prospective, well-controlled studies involving a large number of patients; comparable as to risk factors, degree of vessel involvement and quality of left ventricular function, and divided into subgroups based on these factors; randomized into medical and surgical treatment groups; and receiving standardized long-term follow-up. If the relief of anginal symptoms is the major, or perhaps sole, benefit, then the basis for recommending the operation to the patient with coronary artery disease presenting a picture of chronic stable angina, becomes very tenuous indeed. This is particularly true as methods of conservative management such as those involving exercise conditioning programs and pharmacologic measures, evolve.

The question of studying subgroupings of patients with comparable risk factors, degree of vessel involvement, and grading of left ventricular function, in relation to surgical versus medical management, is a highly significant one; since there may be subgroups of patients based on various clinical, anatomic and physiologic criteria, who would demonstrate perhaps significantly better response to a bypass operation, or conversely who not only would not benefit from surgery but indeed could be actually adversely affected by it. A large prospective randomized study of the consequences of medical versus surgical management of coronary artery disease is being sponsored by the National Institutes of Health, but at the time of this writing data are not yet available.

The Veterans' Administration Study

The Veterans Administration cooperative study, involving 1015 carefully screened patients, comparing medical with surgical treatment in patients with chronic stable angina, is probably the first reported well-controlled prospective randomized trial which incorporated into the study design a large patient population; with adequate clinical and physiologic baseline data to ensure close compatability of patients in medical and surgical groups; and to permit objectively identified and comparable subgroups of patients allocated to each treatment modality; with long-term follow-up and evaluation protocols.

The study was designed to compare the effects of surgical treatment (single or multiple bypass operation) and medical treatment (short- and long-acting vasodilators, diuretics, digitalis, and β-adrenergic blocking agents) on overall survival time; incidence of myocardial infarction; congestive heart failure; acute coronary ischemic episodes; and quality of life as assessed by the number of days of hospitalization, the results of exercise testing, the frequency and severity of angina, and subjective exercise tolerance in various subgroups of patients.

Subgroup of Patients with Significant Left Main Coronary Artery Lesions

This subgroup of patients numbered 124, showed on arteriography a luminal diameter reduction of the left main coronary artery of 50% or more, had severe angina, and electrocardiographic abnormalities characteristic of ischemic heart disease. Patients were all males, aged about 53, and were entirely comparable in both medical and surgical groups with respect to duration of angina, prior history of myocardial infarction, hypertension, congestive heart failure and other clinical characteristics. Left ventricular function, as concerns heart enlargement by chest X-ray and ventriculogram, left ventricular end-diastolic pressure (LVEDP), systolic ejection fraction and contractile abnormalities, was comparable in medical and surgical groups.

Cumulative survival rates through 30 months of study revealed that 85% of surgical and 65% of medical patients survived. The proportion of patients having myocardial infarctions, congestive heart failure, angina, and episodes of acute coronary insufficiency was significantly higher in the medical treatment group than in the surgical treatment group.

Subgroup of Patients without Significant Left Main Coronary Artery Lesions

A preliminary report of these 596 patients, 310 randomized into a medical management group and 296 into a coronary artery bypass surgery group, indicates that at 3 years of follow-up 87% of the medical and 88% of the surgical group had survived. Baseline clinical and physiologic parameters in the two groups were closely identical except for serum cholesterol, which was significantly higher in the medical group. Subgroups were formed by separating the medical and surgical groups into patients with one-, two-, and three-vessel disease and with or without abnormal left ventricular function. There was no significant difference in survival between any of the medical as compared with the corresponding surgical subgroups. Preliminary evaluation of data concerning presence of ventricular arrhythmias with continuous EKG monitoring, and results of exercise stress testing, shows no difference between comparable subgroups in medical versus surgical treatment categories. Both operative mortality and graft patency data in this study are comparable to those reported in the contemporary literature according to some authorities, while others consider that the mortality rates of the VA surgical groups were excessively high. This study is continuing; data concerning cardiovascular morbidity and quality of life; and electrocardiographic, angiographic, and clinical characteristics among the subgroups are not available at the time of this writing.

Results

Overall mortality in the medically treated group at 2½ years is 13%; the highest risk subgroup (excluding the patients with left main lesions in which the 2½ year mortality is 35%) is that of patients with 3-vessel disease and some abnormality of left ventricular function: 17% at 2½ years. Data comparing survival in subgroups of patients with lesions producing 50–75% decrease in coronary blood flow, with lesions causing 76% or above reduction in flow are not yet available. The subgroup of patients with single vessel disease show low 2-year mortality of about 5%.

The investigators emphasize that a finding of major significance in this study is the favorable mortality rate of medically managed patients who receive regular follow-up and a carefully monitored treatment regimen, as compared with patients having the bypass operation. A study comparing cost effectiveness of medical and surgical management of patients with ischemic heart disease (without significant left main artery lesions) would also be of value.

It is of importance to point out that in all other studies comparing medical with surgical management of coronary artery disease, the data for patients with significant left main artery lesions has been included, instead of being separated out as a clinically and physiologically distinct subgroup, as was done in this study. Failing to exclude that subgroup, which has been demonstrated in this study to have an improved survival with surgical over medical treatment, would help account for the reports of improved life expectancy in pooled groups of bypass surgery patients over the conservatively managed ones which have appeared in some other studies.

Controversy

The publication of these data from the VA study has elicited considerable controversy concerning various aspects of the study itself. Those who believe the study to be flawed in a number of ways emphasize that the surgical results, both with respect to mortality and subsequent graft patency, are inferior to those of a number of specialized centers; the high surgical mortality and low graft patency would tend to foster the impression that there is no difference between surgical and medical management as concerns outcome (excluding patients with significant left main coronary occlusion). Another concern expressed is that the mean number of grafts per patient: 1.9, done in the study is lower than the number done in other centers: 2.5; which would be likely to result in poorer myocardial revascularization and therefore poorer survival.

The fact remains, however, that no matter how laudable the results of the coronary artery bypass procedure may be as reported from specialized centers, with respect to mortality, myocardial performance, quality of life, and other parameters; nevertheless it is the case that all reported studies that have compared concurrent trials of medical and surgical management of ischemic heart disease have concluded that (aside from the relief of angina, and excepting patients with left main occlusion) the surgical procedure offers no improvement of survival over medical management. In addition, it is reported that a study comparing the results of surgical versus medical management in unstable angina, sponsored by the NIH and conducted in specialized centers, likewise indicated no significant differences in survival in surgically as compared with medically treated patients. The enormous cost of the operation, said to be at least $15,000, as compared with a medical regimen, would seem to require controlled and objectively verified significant improvement in survival, to bring the cost–benefit ratio into an acceptable range for patients without left main coronary artery disease or angina of incapacitating severity.

A recent interim report of a small prospective, randomized study suggests that coronary artery bypass surgery has no influence on the likelihood of myocardial infarction or death, but does appear to lead to greater functional improvement and less unstable angina, as compared with medical management.

REFERENCES

Beeson PB and McDermott W, editors: *Textbook of Medicine*, 14th ed. Philadelphia, Pa.: Saunders, 1975.

Borhani NO: Primary prevention of coronary heart disease: a critique. *Am. J. Cardiol.* 40:251–259, 1977.

Botvinick EH et al: Thallium-201 myocardial perfusion scintigraphy for the clinical clarification of normal, abnormal and equivocal electrocardiographic stress tests. *Am. J. Cardiol.* 41:43–51, 1978.

Cryer PE, et al: Smoking, catecholamines, and coronary heart disease. *Cardiovasc. Med.* 2:471–474, 1977.

Danahy DT and Aronow WS: Hemodynamics and antianginal effects of high dose oral isosorbide dinitrate after chronic use. *Circulation* 56:205–212, 1977.

Danahy DT, et al: Sustained hemodynamic and antianginal effect of high dose oral isosorbide dinitrate. *Circulation* 55:381–387, 1977.

Del Bianco PL et al: Heart pain. *Adv. Neurol.* 4:375–381, 1974.

Detre K, et al: Veterans Administration cooperative study of surgery for coronary arterial occlusive disease. III Methods and baseline characteristics, including experience with medical treatment. *Am. J. Cardiol.* 40:212–224, 1977.

Friedman GD et al: Mortality in Middle-aged Smokers and Nonsmokers. *N. Engl. J. Med.* 300:213–217, 1979.

Frohlich ED, editor: *Pathophysiology*. Philadelphia, Pa.: Lippincott, 1976.

Ganong WF *Review of Medical Physiology*, 8th ed. Los Altos, Calif.: Lange Medical Publications, 1977.

Guyton AC. *Textbook of Medical Physiology*, 5th ed. Philadelphia, Pa.: Saunders, 1976.

Hardarson T, et al: Prolonged salutary effects of isosorbide dinitrate and nitroglycerin ointment on regional left ventricular function. *Am. J. Cardiol.* 40:90–99, 1977.

Kannel, WB: Some lessons in cardiovascular epidemiology from Framingham. *Am. J. Cardiol.* 37:269–272, 1976.

Klocke FJ, guest editor: Symposium on coronary circulation. In: Yu PN and Goodwin JF, editors. *Progress in Cardiology*, Vol. 5. Philadelphia, Pa.: Lea & Febiger, 1976, Chapters 1–6.

Kloster, FE, et al: Coronary bypass for stable angina. A prospective randomized study. *N. Engl. J. Med.* 300:149–157, 1979.

Lefer AM, et al., editors: *Pathophysiology and Therapeutics of Myocardial Ischemia*. New York: Spectrum, 1977.

Murphy ML, et al: Treatment of chronic stable angina. A preliminary report of survival data of the randomized veterans administration cooperative study. *N. Engl. J. Med.* 297:621–627, 1977.

Parisi AF, et al: Noninvasive cardiac diagnosis. *N. Engl. J. Med.* 296:316–320, 1977 (Part 1); 368–373, 1977 (Part 2); 427–431, 1977 (Part 3).

Rackley CE, et al.: Hemodynamic effects of sublingual and oral long-acting nitrates. In: Mason DT, editor. *Advances in Heart Disease*. New York: Grune & Stratton, 1977.

Richtsmeier TE and Preston TA: Drug management of stable angina pectoris. *Postgrad. Med.* 62:91–100, 1977.

Ross R and Harker L: Hyperlipidemia and atherosclerosis. *Science* 193:1094–1100, 1976.

Schade J, et al.: A comparison of the response to arm and leg work in patients with ischemic heart disease. *Am. Heart J.* 94:203–208, 1977.

Special correspondence: A debate on coronary bypass. *N. Engl. J. Med.* 297:1464—1470, 1977.

Takaro T, et al.: The VA cooperative randomized study of surgery for coronary arterial occlusive disease. II. Subgroup with significant left main lesions. Circulation Supp. 3. *Cardiovasc. Surg. 1975* 54:107–117, 1976.

Thorn GW, et al., editors: *Harrison's Principles of Internal Medicine*, 8th ed. New York: McGraw-Hill, 1977.

Williams, DO, et al.: The role of the coronary collateral circulation in acute and chronic coronary artery disease. In: Mason DT, editor: *Advances in Heart Disease*. New York: Grune & Stratton, 1977.

Myocardial Infarction

INTRODUCTION

It is reported that each year approximately one million persons either have their first myocardial infarction or die of a sudden cardiac event, probably ventricular fibrillation from myocardial ischemia. Less than half the patients with acute infarction live to be dismissed from the hospital, and of those about one tenth die acutely from cardiac cause within the first postinfarction year. Thus, ischemic heart disease with infarction is a major cause of mortality and morbidity in the United States.

Acute myocardial infarction (AMI) is the development of a necrotic area of heart muscle tissue; it usually results from ischemia, caused by a critical drop in perfusion pressure across a segment of coronary artery which has been narrowed by atherosclerosis. The artery may or may not become actually occluded. Infarction may occur without occlusion when, for example, a decline in systemic arterial pressure caused by hypovolemia, systemic vasodilation, decreased cardiac output, or hypotension from some other cause, or temporary platelet aggregation in a coronary artery produce a reversible decline in perfusion of a segment of myocardium. Recent evidence suggests that spasm of a coronary artery at the site of an atherosclerotic narrowing may be the cause of a critical pressure drop across the artery sufficient to cause infarction.

Conversely, actual occlusion may occur in cases where thrombus formation, subintimal bleeding at the site of an atheromatous lesion, or instability of a large plaque, produces obstruction. Evidence appears to support the conclusion that coronary occlusion by a thrombus is a significant cause of AMI. In addition, it is proposed that, as a result of an earlier coronary thrombotic lesion, emboli of platelet and fibrin aggregates are released from the affected area and cause obstructions within smaller distal coronary vessels resulting in multiple small infarctions. It may be that these subsidiary necrotic areas become foci of hyperirritability that produce ectopic arrhythmias and predispose to sudden cardiac death (Chapter 6).

In an AMI, the wedge of myocardium distal to the acute pressure drop or occlusion, as the case may be, undergoes ischemic hypoxia, and tissue death ensues in a central area of tissue supplied by the affected vessel. A variably sized zone of myocardium around the actual infarcted tissue undergoes decreased perfusion to a degree sufficient to impair its metabolism and contractility, but not enough to produce outright necrosis. The fate of this corona of tissue in a sense hangs in the balance, and depending on early recognition and treatment, the development of complications such as arrythmias and/or cardiogenic shock, and the nature and extent of the underlying disease process in the heart; the zone may go on to ischemic necrosis, thus increasing infarction size; or to recovery, the latter course decreasing the amount of nonviable tissue which will become nonfunctional and undergo scar formation.

The size and location of the infarct depend upon a number of factors which include the area supplied by the affected vessel and the degree of collateral circulation to the area. The most common site of obstruction is the left anterior descending artery, which supplies the anterior left ventricle. Obstruction of the circumflex artery produces anterolateral infarction, and right coronary artery occlusion affects the lower posterior portion of the left ventricle. Left main coronary artery obstruction is correlated with more widespread infarction, more profound hemodynamic consequences, and a poorer prognosis, corresponding with the larger distribution of its branches.

INITIAL PATIENT ASSESSMENT IN MYOCARDIAL INFARCTION

Subjective

Pain is the most frequent and severe symptom. It is of the protopathic type (Chapter 19) as is angina, but is more severe and of longer duration, and is not relieved by nitroglycerine. It is described as a deep, crushing, heavy, or squeezing pain localized in the central chest and epigastrium, and it often radiates to arms, hands, neck, and jaw, especially on the left. The patient often experiences profound weakness, apprehension, nausea, sensations of lightheadedness, and extreme restlessness, the latter contrasting with the desire for immobility manifested by the patient with typical angina. It may or may not have its onset with exertion but it is unrelieved by rest. There are occasions (about 10%) where pain is not marked; this more often occurs in the elderly and/or diabetic patient where the chief complaint may be weakness; decreased level of consciousness; or altered mental status such as confusion from decreased cerebral perfusion; palpitations; or shortness or breath with moist cough from elevated pulmonary capillary pressure and pulmonary edema, indicating left ventricular overload and early failure.

Objective

Physical Examination

The patient is usually in evident acute distress and may manifest ashen skin color, diaphoresis and cool extremities. The heart rate may be slow, rapid, regular, or irregular. The precordium is quiet and the heart sounds may be indistinctly heard. An S_3 and/or S_4 may be audible. When the infarction is extensive and myocardial contractility impaired, bibasilar rales may be present in the posterior lung fields. Hypotension may be present, and jugular venous pressure may be elevated as indicated by distension of the neck veins. With marked hypotension, urinary output will be low or the patient may be anuric. A less severe infarction may be correlated with a normal or near-normal physical examination.

Laboratory

On arterial blood gas measurement the PaO_2 may be low, and the $PaCO_2$ also low because of hyperventilation caused by anxiety and/or hypoxemia. Chest X-ray may show an enlarged heart (if the patient had prior heart disease) and increased vascular markings indicating pulmonary venous congestion. Within the first 24–48 hours serum enzyme determinations are helpful not only in the diagnosis of myocardial infarction but in assessment of its size, especially in the case of creatinine phosphokinase (CPK) which, with aspartate amino transferase: AST (formerly called glutamic oxaloacetic transaminase: GOT), rises rapidly and falls within 3 to 4 days; and lactic dehydrogenase (LDH) (a value which is nonspecific for MI) which becomes elevated at 3 to 5 days and returns to baseline after about 10 days. The appearance of these normally intracellular metabolic enzymes in the serum results from their release from necrotic cardiac cells which were destroyed by the acute ischemic hypoxia.

The Electrocardiogram

EKG changes in acute myocardial infarction often do not correlate well with the severity of the infarction or the extent of the circulatory abnormalities caused by it. The three main EKG abnormalities in infarction are (1) elevation of the ST segment; (2) the new development of Q waves, or, if they were previously present, their increasing prominence; and (3) the inversion of the T wave. These changes tend to follow an orderly sequence of appearance and development. Often the first changes, occurring within the initial hours of the infarction, are elevation of the ST segment with heightening of the T wave. The time of development of Q waves is more variable; they may appear quite early or not for several days; they generally persist indefinitely. The ST segment usually returns to the normal baseline, and as it does the T wave develops a gradually increasing inversion which may persist for weeks; then usually the inversion becomes shallower and eventually the T waves resume their normal configuration. Thus in the evolution of EKG changes in myocardial infarction the ST segment changes are earliest to develop and resolve; the T changes are more protracted and slower to disappear; and the Q waves generally remain as a permanent change. It is the Q wave changes which are correlated with the actual infarction itself, and which remain as an electrical correlate of the anatomic myocardial scar.

In an acute myocardial infarction, progressive, evolving day to day changes are characteristic. The nature of the EKG abnormalities depends on the anatomic location of the infarcted area within the heart. Different changes occur in the various leads, and these are related to the portions of the heart which are involved in the processes of ischemia and necrosis. Q waves appear to be associated with transmural infarctions, while isolated ST segment and T wave alterations correlate more with subendocardial ones.

Early Recognition of Myocardial Infarction

Self-assessment by the patient with symptomatic ischemic heart disease is probably the most important component of the presentation in myocardial infarction. There is often a long delay between the onset of symptoms and the decision of the patient to obtain help for and evaluation of chest pain. Part of this delay may be prompted by fear and denial, but part may be the result of lack of knowledge of the meaning of more severe and prolonged pain which is unrelieved by previously effective measures such as rest and nitroglycerine. Early recognition of the infarction is of prime importance. Education of the patient with angina as to the significance of a change in the frequency, intensity, timing, and precipitating factors for chest pain, and the need to seek prompt evaluation of such change, is a crucial responsibility of all health professionals. Since preservation of the zone of ischemic myocardium at risk of infarcting, which surrounds the necrotic area, is an important component in the early management of the patient with myocardial infarction; and since measures to prevent extension of this zone depend upon early recognition and intervention; therefore teaching the angina patient the early warning signs of infarction, and the danger of delay, is of great significance.

Studies have shown, and the literature emphasizes, that the eventual size of the infarct can be influenced by treatment in the early phases, and depends upon the disparity between blood supply to the affected heart muscle, and its oxygen requirements. Any factor which elevates myocardial oxygen consumption, in the face of a restricted blood supply, may act to enlarge the ischemic area and push it in the direction of necrosis. Relief of pain and anxiety; early recognition and treatment of arrhythmias; oxygen administration; and lowering the work load and hence metabolic oxygen requirements of the myocardium by other means detailed below, appear to operate to minimize the size of the infarction.

CHANGES IN CORONARY BLOOD FLOW WHICH PRECIPITATE THE INFARCTION

The sequence of abnormal changes in a coronary artery immediately preceding myocardial infarction are not known. Evidence indicates that there are probably several mechanisms which in some cases act alone, and in other cases act in concert, to produce the critical drop in perfusion pressure along a segment of coronary artery sufficient to result in necrosis of the myocardium supplied by that artery.

It appears certain that in some patients ischemia of a degree to produce infarction and even left ventricular aneurysm occurs in the absence of organic obstruction; this has been confirmed by necropsy studies. In addition, normal arteriograms may be seen in patients following earlier documented infarctions. This appears to occur more often in young, apparently healthy men; the cause is not known, although spasm of coronary arteries, aggregations of platelets to produce temporary obstructions which later disperse, and coronary artery embolism have been suggested as causes. Coronary artery spasm has been identified as the basis of the severe myocardial ischemia in patients with variant (Prinzmetal's) angina; in these patients the spasm may be superimposed on an artery with atherosclerotic lesions, or may occur in arteries which appear structurally normal.

Patients with documented myocardial infarction, studied angiographically within a few hours after the onset of symptoms and found to have what appeared to be total obstruction of the related coronary vessel, have been discovered in some cases to have a combination of organic obstruction and artery spasm. Injection of nitroglycerine into the artery may result in widening of the lumen and blood flow into the portions of the vessel beyond what initially appeared to be a total occlusion; this indicates that spasm superimposed on atheromatous narrowing may produce complete occlusion—a combination of structural and functional factors interacting to cause the pressure drop of sufficient magnitude to result in tissue necrosis beyond the lesion. It is likely that an additional factor, platelet aggregation, is involved with the other two factors (spasm and atheromata) in producing temporary obstruction sufficient to cause infarction. Both structural abnormalities of the vessel lining such as atheromatous lesions, and neurohormonal influences, such as the release of catecholamines from sympathetic adrenergic nerve terminals, can initiate platelet aggregation. Such aggregates then release vasoactive substances (prostaglandins, serotonin, and others) which cause arterial spasm. Thus in some patients, atherosclerosis and arterial constriction can combine to produce complete obstruction in an artery severely narrowed but not organically occluded by atherosclerosis. The injected nitroglycerine reveals the reversible functional component. Whether this is the mechanism which produces the infarction in these patients, or whether this phenomenon is a solely postinfarction one, is not yet known.

Such studies suggest the possibility that at least in some patients a coronary artery thrombosis may in fact be the consequence, rather than the original precipitating event, in an infarction. Evidence from other investigations which support this possibility include the following: (1) radioactive fibrinogen injected at the time of early onset of signs and symptoms of an infarction becomes incorporated into thrombi detected subsequently, indicating that the infarction preceded thrombus formation; (2) histologic studies of the age of thrombi within a coronary artery, compared with studies of the age of the associated infarction, sometimes indicate that the infarct is older; (3) thrombi are often not found in patients with sudden death from myocardial ischemia, but the frequency of thrombi increases with increasing time between infarction and death.

CIRCULATORY CONSEQUENCES OF ACUTE MYOCARDIAL INFARCTION: DECREASED STROKE VOLUME AND CARDIAC OUTPUT

AMI often results in a decrease in stroke volume and cardiac output through a number of abnormalities resulting directly from the infarction (see following). The reduced stroke volume, in turn, induces a number of reflex compensatory alterations in the circulation which help to maintain an adequate cardiac output in the face of the decreased stroke volume. The compensatory reflex changes are primarily autonomic adrenergic ones: elevated heart rate and peripheral vasoconstriction. When these compensatory responses fail, for whatever reason, or are inadequate to sustain cardiac output, then cardiogenic shock may be the result. Probably the most frequent reason for inability of the compensatory responses to sustain cardiac output is the large size of the infarction. That is, myocardial contractility is so impaired that no possible degree of reflex elevation of heart rate and increased peripheral vasoconstriction can compensate for the depressed stroke volume. In many—probably most—patients with AMI, the cardiac output is within, or close to, normal limits because the infarct is not massive and the circulatory mechanisms that compensate for the reduced stroke volume are adequate to sustain cardiac output. However, there are some patients in whom adequate cardiac output is not maintained, or is marginally maintained only with the aid of special assessment and management procedures (see following).

Causes of Reduced Stroke Volume and Cardiac Output in AMI

Loss of Functional Myocardium

The main cause of a depressed stroke volume in infarction is the actual loss of functional myocardium produced by the ischemic necrosis itself; therefore the size of the infarction, but also its location, are important determinants of the degree of fall in stroke volume resulting from an infarction. Other factors equal, the larger the infarction, the greater the reduction in stroke volume.

Depressed Myocardial Contractility

A second and important cause of lowered stroke volume is depressed contractility of noninfarcted myocardium. The area of actual necrosis is surrounded by a zone of ischemic myocardium that is at risk of extension of ischemic necrosis because of impaired blood flow, but is yet salvageable. This zone shows impaired force of contraction because of ischemic hypoxia, and therefore contributes to lowering the stroke volume.

Even the normal myocardium has a reduced contractile performance. Factors which contribute to this impairment are systemic hypoxemia from impaired alveolar ventilation, decreased blood flow in the coronary arteries as a direct result of low stroke volume, and probably chemical myocardial depressant factors released by the necrotic tissue. Both systemic hypoxemia and poor myocardial perfusion promote anaerobic cellular metabolism which results in the production of lactic acid. This substance is known to cause direct depression of heart muscle force of contraction.

Cardiac Arrhythmias

This is a major factor contributing to impaired stroke volume and cardiac output in AMI. A lack of coordination between atrial and ventricular contractions results in a loss of the atrial contribution to ventricular diastolic filling. This lack of the atrial "booster-pump" action decreases ventricular end-diastolic volume. According to the Frank-Starling principle, by which force of contraction is directly proportional to the degree of stretch on heart muscle fibers at the onset of contraction, lowered ventricular filling results in lowered stroke volume.

A lack of coordination and synchrony of contraction between the two ventricles also reduces stroke volume; normally both ventricles contract simultaneously. When they do not, because of an aberrant route of conduction of the cardiac impulse, there is a slower buildup of *pressure* per unit time during systole, a decline in the *rate* of systolic ejection, and a decrease in *force* of ejection.

Abnormalities of rate, as well as abnormalities of rhythm, cause reduced stroke volume and cardiac output. Tachycardia reduces diastolic filling time, which lowers stroke volume by the Frank-Starling principle; and tachycardia causes reduced perfusion of the coronary arteries, which occurs mainly during diastole. As diastole is shortened, myocardial perfusion, and hence oxygenation, falls and contractility is thereby impaired.

Bradycardia can also lower cardiac output markedly; because the stroke volume is reduced in AMI, an adequate cardiac output is dependent upon adequate heart rate (CO = SV × HR); therefore, with bradycardia the major compensatory mechanism for depressed stroke volume is eliminated.

Decreased Compliance of Ventricular Myocardium

In AMI there is often decreased compliance in the infarcted area, in the ischemic zone surrounding it, and even in the remaining myocardium. Compliance is the term for the relationship between change in pressure and change in volume ($\Delta P/\Delta V$); normal compliance in an organ such as the heart implies that for a given change of pressure within the chambers (reduced pressure in diastole, increased pressure in systole) there will be a corresponding change in volume (increasing volume during diastolic filling; decreasing volume during systolic ejection). A decreased compliance means that there has to be a much greater change in pressure to produce a given change of volume. The abnormalities in heart muscle after AMI often lead to altered compliance so that the normal pressure-volume relationship no longer exists. If the heart is unable to generate the pressure changes required to produce adequate diastolic filling and systolic ejection then stroke volume will decline accordingly.

Effective Hypovolemia

Effective hypovolemia refers to a decreased intravascular volume *relative to* the total cross-sectional diameter of the vascular tree, and therefore can be caused by either absolute loss of intravascular volume (=true hypovolemia) or increased cross-sectional diameter of the blood vessels (=peripheral vasodilation). The latter is sometimes called low peripheral resistance shock. In either case effective hypovolemia leads to hypotension and inadequate venous return to the right heart. Actual or true hypovolemia in AMI may be caused by loss of fluid through vomiting, diarrhea, diaphoresis or diuretics; or inadequte fluid intake.

An additional little-recognized cause of actual hypovolemia in AMI may be extravasation of fluid from the capillaries into the interstitial spaces induced by the strong vasoconstriction (caused by adrenergic stimulation) occurring as a compensatory response to the reduced stroke volume of AMI. Therapeutically administered vasoconstrictor agents produce a similar effect.

Peripheral vasodilation in AMI may be the result of the vasodilating effect of analgesics, the failure of brainstem compensatory vasoconstrictive reflexes which normally serve to counteract low cardiac output states, or the pooling of blood in venous capacitance (storage) circuits from strong vagal reflexes set off by the AMI. Regardless of the cause, the results are similar: impaired venous return to the heart, reduced ventricular diastolic filling, inadequate stretch on the heart muscle fibers and reduced stroke volume (Frank-Starling principle).

Consequences of Reduced Stroke Volume and Cardiac Output in AMI

Hypotension

Systemic arterial blood pressure is a product of the cardiac output and the total peripheral resistance: SAP = CO × TPR; if cardiac output declines then arterial pressure will fall unless there is a compensatory increase in peripheral resistance through reflex vasoconstriction.

"Backward" Heart Failure

This is an old term which is still of value in spite of our current recognition of the fact that "backward" and "forward" heart failure are but two faces of the same coin. Backward failure essentially is pulmonary vascular congestion and results from the stronger right ventricle pumping more blood into the lungs than the failing left ventricle can pump out. The symptom is shortness of breath, and the signs are dyspnea, a fall in PaO_2, bibasilar pulmonary rales, and left ventricular dilation and increased vascular markings on chest X-ray.

Sequence of Changes Leading to Pulmonary Vascular Congestion

We have seen that decreased myocardial contractility causes a decreased stroke volume. That is, of the total quantity of blood in the left ventricle at the end of diastolic filling, when stroke volume is reduced then less is put out at the next contraction; in other words, there is a reduced *systolic ejection fraction.*

Now, if the percentage of blood in the ventricle put out at systole is reduced, then obviously the amount remaining in the ventricle at the end of the systole is increased; that is, left ventricular end-systolic volume is increased. This contributes to an increased *afterload* (Chapter 7). Then after the next diastolic filling, left ventricle end-diastolic volume is increased still more. When ventricular volume rises, then ventricular pressures must rise, and as these changes occur, the left ventricle dilates.

After a certain degree of left ventricular dilation has been reached, filling of the left heart from the lungs is progressively impaired because of the large volume and high pressure in the left ventricle; and blood then accumulates in the pulmonary circuit behind the failing ventricle. Left atrial volume and pressure

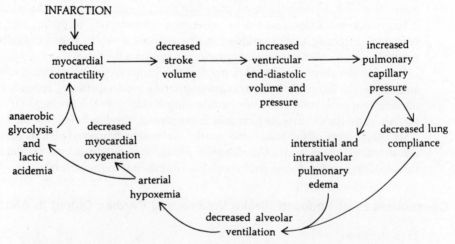

Figure 5-1. Sequence of physiologic abnormalities developing after an AMI which lead to "backward" heart failure, pulmonary vascular congestion, and further impairment of myocardial contractility.

increase, pulmonary vein volume and pressure increase, and ultimately pulmonary capillary volume and pressure increase. The pulmonary capillaries become engorged and dilated and are unable to retain their fluid which oozes out and produces first interstitial and then intraalveolar pulmonary edema.

Consequences of Pulmonary Vascular Congestion

The increased fluid in the lungs has a number of adverse effects which lead to deterioration in the patient's condition and may promote cardiogenic shock.

Decreased Lung Compliance   This is a direct consequence of pulmonary vascular engorgement; it necessitates a greater change in intrathoracic pressure to produce a normal tidal volume. Fluid-filled lungs are difficult to inflate and deflate; they respond poorly to chest wall movements during the respiratory cycle. If in the normal lung -25 cmH$_2$O pressure produces a tidal volume of 800 ml, then in pulmonary congestion the decreased compliance may necessitate -50 cmH$_2$O pressure or more to maintain an acceptable tidal volume. In addition, because of the extravasated fluid, there is less room for air and so tidal volume may be reduced even below that resulting from the decreased compliance.

The increased pressure change required to move air, caused by the decreased compliance, necessitates a greatly increased work of breathing to produce adequate alveolar ventilation. This is exhausting for the patient, and increases O$_2$ consumption and CO$_2$ production. So the patient makes a compromise and this is tachypnea. Because the lungs are hard to move, he settles for a decreased tidal volume and an increased respiratory rate, because this makes a lesser work demand on the respiratory muscles and therefore requires lower energy consumption. But tachypnea has a profound physiologic disadvantage in spite of its energy conservation, and that is that an increasing percentage of the minute ventilation goes back and forth over anatomic dead space (nasopharynx, trachea, bronchi, and bronchioles) where no gaseous exchange occurs. Anatomic deadspace is about 150 ml in normal adults. In a respiratory pattern of large tidal volume and low respiratory rate, a relatively small quantity of the minute ventilation is wasted ventilation—that is, air which cannot exchange with the blood. But in a respiratory pattern of a small tidal volume and rapid rate, which is tachypnea, a proportionately much larger percentage of the minute ventilation is wasted. The consequence is impaired alveolar ventilation, decreased oxygenation of pulmonary capillary blood and systemic hypoxemia (Chapters 2 and 9).

Pulmonary Shunting (Ventilation Perfusion Mismatch, Venous Admixture)   The excess fluid in the pulmonary capillary bed has a second major deleterious effect. Because of pulmonary edema fluid in and around the alveoli, their ventilation is impaired. But they are still adequately perfused. Adequately perfused but poorly ventilated alveolar–capillary units act as a right to left shunt; they add underoxygenated blood to the left heart to be mixed with adequately oxygenated blood from normal alveolar–capillary units, and the result is arterial desaturation of blood to be pumped out into the arterial circuit. As a consequence of this ventilation-perfusion $(\dot{V}/\dot{Q})$ mismatch the PaO$_2$ and O$_2$ saturation will decline (Chapters 2 and 9). As a result, the arterial hypoxemia feeds back to threaten the zone of ischemic myocardium around the infarct, to lower myocardial contractility, and to further depress stroke volume and coronary artery perfusion; this decreases myocardial perfusion and a vicious cycle is established (Figure 5-1).

Bronchospasm

Edema fluid in the small airways directly induces bronchospasm which decreases cross-sectional diameter of the small airways, increases airway resistance, increases work of breathing, and further reduces alveolar ventilation and PaO_2.

"Forward" Heart Failure

This venerable but still useful term can be defined as inadequate tissue and organ perfusion resulting from a depressed cardiac output. The signs and symptoms are manifested in four areas: (1) the brain: restlessness and anxiety, mental confusion, "dizziness," disorientation, obtundation; (2) the kidney: oliguria (less than 20–30 ml/hr), prerenal azotemia, anuria, acute renal failure (Chapter 10); (3) the viscera: abdominal distress, nausea, vomiting, ileus, distention, decreased bowel sounds; and (4) the skin: pallor, cyanosis, cold, and clamminess.

Inadequate peripheral perfusion in AMI has as its most serious consequence decreased coronary artery perfusion. Adequate coronary artery blood flow is directly dependent on two factors: adequate diastolic filling time, as discussed above (tachycardia), and adequate diastolic filling pressure, specifically an adequate aortic diastolic pressure. When cardiac output is low, aortic diastolic pressure falls and with it, coronary artery perfusion pressure. So the head of pressure in the aorta during diastole declines below a critical level, and worsening myocardial ischemia results which may extend the infarct and which further depresses contractility and output. Again, this comprises a downward spiral toward cardiogenic shock (Figure 5-2).

Anaerobic metabolism in other organs and tissues promotes production of lactic acid, a direct depressant to myocardial contractility. Normal arterial lactate levels are in the range of 1.5 meq/L; in AMI, with developing or established cardiogenic shock, arterial lactate may increase to more than 8 meq/L; studies have shown a direct correlation between blood lactate and mortality rate in AMI, with mortality being 90% or above where lactate reaches these higher levels.

Reflex Compensatory Responses to the Decreased Stroke Volume and Cardiac Output of AMI

These are the reactions alluded to above which function to help maintain adequate cardiac output in the face of a depressed stroke volume.

Elevated Left Ventricular End-Diastolic Volume and Pressure (LVEDV and P)

Although this is not a reflex compensatory response to decreased cardiac output in the same sense that the adrenergic responses are, nevertheless increased LVEDV acts as a compensatory mechanism for decreased stroke volume. The

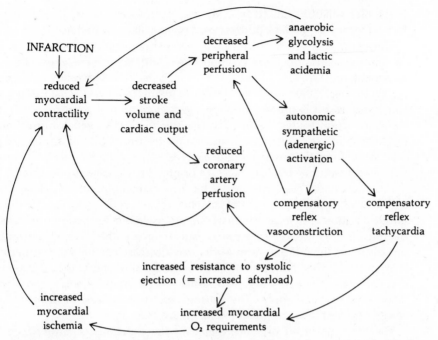

Figure 5-2. Sequence of physiologic abnormalities developing after an AMI which lead to "forward" heart failure, decreased peripheral and coronary artery perfusion, and further impairment of myocardial contractility.

increased ventricular volume resulting from incomplete ventricular emptying distends the ventricle, stretching the myocardial fibers and putting more tension on them. The increased fiber length at the onset of the next systole results in a greater force of contraction, according to the Frank-Starling relationship, and therefore a greater stroke volume and cardiac output. However, this compensatory-like response has the unfortunate consequence of increasing myocardial oxygen consumption; the greater the ventricular volume, and the stress on the wall of the ventricle (one component of afterload), caused by an abnormally increased volume, the greater the myocardial oxygen consumption, and hence oxygen requirements.

Brainstem Sympathetic Adrenergic Reflexes

The decreased cardiac output and arterial pressure resulting from the abnormalities caused by AMI, discussed above, lead to a decreased perfusion pressure to the baroreceptors of the aortic arch and carotid sinus. When pressure on these sensors falls, they relay afferent neural impulses to the vasomotor and cardiac control centers in the brainstem. The result is a massive discharge of autonomic sympathetic (adrenergic) nerve terminals, release of norepinephrine from them, and release of norepinephrine and epinephrine from the adrenal medullae. The consequences are elevated heart rate (which increases cardiac output), increased force of myocardial contraction (which elevates stroke volume), and increased peripheral vasoconstriction (which elevates blood pressure, increases venous return and improves perfusion of the brain and heart). These compensatory responses to the abnormalities caused by AMI are adaptive and aid in maintaining circulatory adequacy in the face of decreased myocardial performance.

However, as is the case with many compensatory physiologic responses, they contain the seeds of potential complications and may have adverse effects if they are excessively strong or maintained for long periods. The reflex vasoconstriction is selective and differential, involving the kidneys in direct renal vasoconstriction which may result in prerenal azotemia and acute tubular necrosis (ATN). Visceral vasoconstriction leads to reduced splanchnic blood flow which causes ileus, may produce an intestinal infarction, and stimulates the release of myocardial depressant factor from the intestine and pancreas. The systemic effect of generalized vasoconstriction also tends to increase production of lactate by peripheral tissues.

Although these responses are helpful in maintaining arterial blood pressure and cardiac output, the action of catecholamines on the heart can be deleterious in the situation of myocardial infarction and ischemia in that both increased contractility and elevated heart rate greatly increase the oxygen consumption of myocardium. In addition, tachycardia may decrease coronary artery perfusion by shortening diastolic filling time. This combination of effects may worsen myocardial ischemia by increasing myocardial oxygen requirements and decreasing myocardial oxygen supply. The causes and consequences of the compensatory adrenergic responses are included in Figure 5-2.

The elevated blood pressure increases the resistance against which the left ventricle must eject blood. That is, it increases the *afterload* on the heart, which increases its oxygen requirements, may depress systolic ejection fraction, and cause a further increase in left ventricular end diastolic volume (the *preload*), leading to dilation of the ventricle and increased wall tension. All of these changes may promote myocardial ischemia and extension of the infarct.

Although the reflex adrenergic discharge, with resulting vasoconstriction and elevated peripheral vascular resistance, is a frequent compensatory response to the low cardiac output state in AMI, some workers report that in as many as half AMI patients, overall peripheral resistance may be normal or even low. The mechanisms accounting for this may be a central failure of the brainstem reflex vasoconstrictor response, or a peripheral failure of blood vessels to constrict in response to the elevated catecholamines.

RELATIONSHIP OF THE CORONARY COLLATERAL CIRCULATION TO MYOCARDIAL ISCHEMIA AND INFARCTION

Patients with coronary atherosclerotic heart disease have been shown to have an often well-developed myocardial collateral circulation; evidence indicates that these auxiliary vessels are congenitally present—that is, they are *potential* channels of flow which develop embryologically and then are further developed into functional collateral vessels during the progression of coronary atherosclerotic disease. There is a direct relationship between the extent of the coronary artery disease and the degree of collateralization, and there is a progressive increase in auxiliary vessels correlated with one, two, and three vessel disease. That the vessels do not appear to provide a protective effect against ischemia and infarction is shown by an increasing degree of ischemic change on the electrocardiogram (abnormal Q waves indicating prior infarctions) as a function of increasing number of collaterals. Also left ventricular performance, as assessed by cardiac index (CI) and LVEDP does not differ significantly in patients with or without collaterals. And the longer the duration of coronary artery disease, the greater the number of collaterals.

However, angiographic analyses of the extent of collaterals *in patients with AMI* indicates that patients without adequate collateral development show greater impairment of cardiac index (CI), LVEDP, and systolic ejection fraction (SEF) than patients with a well established auxiliary myocardial circulation. Cardiogenic shock is said to occur *only* in patients without collaterals, and the majority of this group does not survive. There are few in-hospital deaths in the group with well developed auxiliary flow.

CLASSIFICATION OF PATIENTS WITH MYOCARDIAL INFARCTION, BASED ON HEMODYNAMIC AND VENTILATORY ABNORMALITIES

It has been recognized for some time that patients with AMI do not present a uniform group of circulatory and ventilatory abnormalities, but rather may be categorized into groups and subgroups based upon a number of variables including: left ventricular end-diastolic pressure (LVEDP); cardiac index (CI), and arterial oxygen tension (PaO_2); and the physical findings of pulmonary vascular congestion (bibasilar lung rales) and decreased perfusion of peripheral tissues: brain (altered mental status and decreased level of consciousness); kidney (oliguria below 20–30 ml/hr); and skin (cold, pale, clammy). Studies have shown, moreover, that various combinations and degrees of circulatory and ventilatory impairment appear to correlate with in-hospital mortality rate. Since physiologic derangements and mortality differ in the various groups, it seems reasonable to suppose that a different treatment would be appropriate for each of the categories.

Classification Based on Signs and Symptoms of Congestive Heart Failure

One long-established system of classification groups patients with AMI into four categories based on the signs and symptoms of congestive heart failure, especially left ventricular failure, which they manifest. *Class I patients* show essentially normal heart function and a PaO_2 within normal limits, but left ventricular diastolic pressure (LVDP) ranges between 12 and 20 mmHg (normal values are 10–12 mmHg); however, there are no signs of pulmonary vascular congestion. In-hospital mortality is 0 to 5%. *Class II patients* have mild left ventricular failure as indicated by decreased intensity of the heart sounds, an audible S_3 and bibasilar rales. There is often a sinus tachycardia which helps compensate for the decreased stroke volume, but the cardiac output remains below normal in spite of the elevated heart rate. Left ventricular diastolic pressure (LVDP) is elevated and the PaO_2 is below normal. Blood pressure is normal or low and peripheral vascular resistance is elevated. In-hospital mortality for these patients is 10 to 20%. *Class III patients* have pulmonary edema, LVDP of 25 mmHg or above, severe tachycardia and a markedly lowered stroke volume and low cardiac output. Blood pressure is normal or low, and the PaO_2 is low. In-hospital mortality is 30–45%. *Class IV patients* are those with cardiogenic shock, who manifest hypotension (blood pressure below 80–90 mmHg), signs of decreased perfusion of peripheral tissues (cold clammy skin with peripheral cyanosis, oliguria), tachycardia, a PaO_2 below 44 mmHg, and a greatly decreased stroke volume and cardiac output. Lactic acidemia is often present because of the increased cellular anaerobic glycolysis resulting from generalized hypoxemia. Over 40% of ventricular tissue may be nonfuctional. This is the picture characteristic of the massive myocardial infarction, and hospital mortality may be 85% or above.

Determination of Cardiac Index (CI), Pulmonary Artery Diastolic Pressure (PADP), and Pulmonary Capillary Wedge Pressure (PCWP)

The use of more advanced procedures to study the hemodynamic alterations resulting from AMI have led to more specific, more detailed criteria for classification of patients into groups based on their circulatory abnormalities.

The Swan-Ganz Flow-Directed Balloon Catheter

This may be used for determining both the cardiac index and the pressure gradients between the right ventricle and the left ventricle. The catheter consists of four components in parallel. The first is a lumen which connects with a small inflatable balloon near the tip; the second is a lumen with a pressure sensor at the tip, just beyond the balloon, for measuring pressures within the right ventricle and the pulmonary artery and its branches; the third is a lumen with a temperature sensor at the tip of the catheter; and the fourth is a lumen with its opening 30 cm from the tip.

The catheter is inserted into a vein in the right brachial region and advanced toward the heart from the point of insertion through the brachial, axillary or subclavian veins; into the superior vena cava, the right atrium, the right ventricle, and finally through the pulmonic valve into the pulmonary artery; and, when indicated, into one of the branches of the pulmonary artery. Since this is the direction of blood flow through the right heart, inflation of the balloon during advancement of the catheter provides a directional flow guidance for proper positioning. Figure 5-3 shows the heart with the catheter in place. There are characteristic phasic pressure changes in the right atrium, ventricle, and pulmonary artery as a function of the mechanical phases of the cardiac contraction cycle.

Measurement of Intracardiac and Pulmonary Vascular Pressures

The pressure sensor in the catheter tip provides the measurement of the typical pressures in these central vascular structures; the pressures are amplified and displayed on a cathode ray tube screen, so that location of the catheter tip can be assessed during its placement. The normal range of pressures is: right atrial, 0–8 mmHg (mean about 2.5); right ventricle end-diastolic, 1–8 mmHg (mean about 4.0); pulmonary artery systolic, about 22 mmHg; and pulmonary artery end-diastolic, about 8 mmHg (with a range of 4–12 mmHg). Mean pulmonary artery pressure is about 13 mmHg. These are the pressures which can be measured as the catheter is advanced through the heart and into the pulmonary artery. They are shown in tabular form in Table 5-1.

When the catheter is advanced into a branch of the pulmonary artery, and the balloon is inflated to occlude the artery, the head of pressure from the surge of

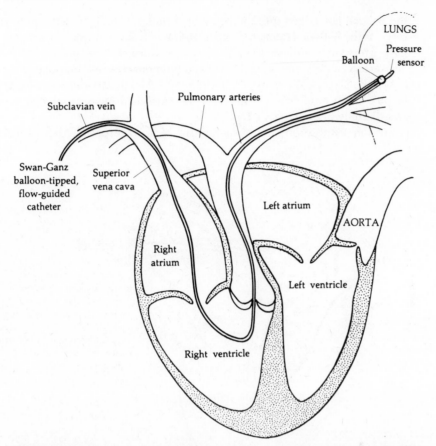

Figure 5-3. Diagram of the heart showing Swan-Ganz balloon-tipped, flow-guided catheter entering the right atrium from the subclavian vein and superior vena cava, passing through the tricuspid valve, right ventricle, and pulmonary artery, to enter a branch of that artery. When the balloon is inflated, the pressure sensor measures pressure in the pulmonary capillary circuit, which is in equilibrium with left atrial and left ventricular end-diastolic pressures. The components of the catheter that permit the measurement of cardiac index by the thermal dilution method are not shown.

blood from the right ventricle during systole is blocked by the balloon. What the tip of the catheter measures with the balloon inflated, therefore, is the pressure in the pulmonary vasculature *ahead* of the balloon—that is, the pulmonary capillary pressure (called the pulmonary capillary wedge pressure—PCWP—because

Table 5-1
Normal Right Atrial, Ventricular, Pulmonary Artery and Pulmonary Capillary Wedge Pressures

Site	Pressure Range, mmHg	$\bar{X}$ Pressure, mmHg
Right atrium	0–8.0	2.5
Right ventricle		14.0
end-diastolic	1.0–8.0	4.0
systolic	23.0	
Pulmonary artery		
end-diastolic	4.0–12.0	13.0
systolic	22.0	
Pulmonary capillary wedge	4.0–12.0	8.0

the balloon is wedged into, and briefly occludes, a branch of the pulmonary artery). If the balloon is deflated and withdrawn a few centimeters into the pulmonary artery, it then measures the phasic pressure changes in that vessel: pulmonary artery systolic pressure (PASP) and pulmonary artery end-diastolic pressure (PAEDP). The PCWP is in equilibrium with the left atrial pressure (LAP). LAP, in turn, is in equilibrium with, and therefore is a measure of, left ventricular end-diastolic pressure: LVEDP.

For the purposes of clinical monitoring of heart (especially left ventricle) per-

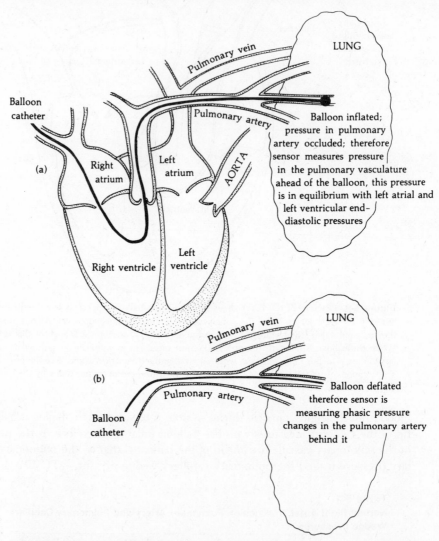

Figure 5-4. Flow-directed balloon catheter in place in the pulmonary artery. (a). The balloon is inflated; therefore the branch of the pulmonary artery in which it lies is occluded, and the pressure sensor in the catheter tip is measuring the pressure in the pulmonary vasculature ahead of the balloon. This pressure is the pulmonary capillary wedge pressure and is in equilibrium with left atrial, and left ventricular end-diastolic pressures. (b) The balloon is deflated; therefore the branch of the pulmonary artery in which it lies is open, and the pressure sensor in the catheter tip is measuring the phasic pressure changes in the right ventricle and pulmonary artery.

formance in severe AMI, PAEDP is considered to be equivalent to PCWP; the values are approximately the same (8 mmHg) with about the same range (4–12 mmHg). Also the measurement of PAEDP is often substituted for PCWP because the balloon does not need to be inflated. (However, in the complication of acute pulmonary embolism, PAEDP—balloon deflated—may be elevated above PCWP—balloon inflated). If left ventricular failure is present, LVEDV and P will increase because of inadequate ventricular emptying. The increased volumes and pressures will be gradually transmitted retrogradely to the left atrium, the pulmonary veins, the pulmonary capillaries, and ultimately the pulmonary artery, elevating diastolic pressure in that vessel.

If right ventricle failure develops, right ventricular end-diastolic volume and pressure (RVEDV and P) will increase above the normal 4 mmHg (range about 1–8); this will in turn cause a rise in right atrial pressure above the normal about 2.5 mmHg (range about 0–8 mmHg), and an elevation of central venous pressure (CVP). Conversely, in hypovolemia right atrial and central venous pressures will be low.

Therefore, PAEDP and PCWP reflect changes in performance of the left side of the heart, while RVEDP, RAP and CVP reflect changes in the right side of the heat.

A number of pathologic changes within the heart and pulmonary vasculature, such as mitral stenosis and pulmonary hypertension, will alter the pressure relationships among the various components of the central circulation outlined above. But these are complications which we will not consider. In general, for purposes of patient assessment in the clinical situation in severe myocardial infarction, the above relationships are valid unless there is underlying chronic valvular or pulmonary vascular disease.

Measurement of Cardiac Index (CI)

This value is derived from the measurement of the cardiac output and body surface according to the equation

$$\text{cardiac index} = \frac{\text{stroke volume} \times \text{heart rate}}{\text{body surface in m}^2}$$

The cardiac output may be measured by any of a number of methods. The one involving the Swan-Ganz catheter is the thermal dilution method. A small amount of cool intravenous 5% dextrose in water is injected into the right atrium through the proximal opening of the catheter; there is a resulting change in temperature of the blood reaching the thermistor tip of the catheter lying within the pulmonary artery. The rate of increase in temperature as the bolus of injected fluid passes the thermistor tip of the catheter is proportional to the cardiac output from the right ventricle, which under most conditions is equal to the cardiac output from the left ventricle. Normal cardiac output is 4.8 L/min. Cardiac index relates cardiac output to body size, and is expressed as liters per minute per square meter of body surface. If this value is below about 1.8, cardiogenic shock is assumed to be present. If the value is below 2.2, cardiac output may be inadequate to sustain sufficient perfusion to vital organs. Normal range of cardiac index is about 2.5 to 3.5.

Classification of Circulatory Abnormalities in Patients with AMI, Based on Measurement of Cardiac Index and Left Ventricular End-Diastolic Pressure; Management Correlates

Patients with Normal or Near-Normal Circulation

According to some studies, about 14% of patients with AMI may show essentially normal CI (2.5–3.0) and LVEDP (below 18). This suggests a relatively small infarction with maintenance of adequate cardiac output and reflex compensatory responses of a degree sufficient to maintain organ perfusion and prevent pulmonary congestion. Mortality rate is stated to be around 6%.

Patients with Hypovolemia

In these patients the CI may be below 2.2 and the LVEDP is often lower than 8 mmHg. The low LVEDP results in an inadequate preload on myocardial fibers. The ventricle is not sufficiently filled to put enough initial stretch on the contractile fibers so that they are capable of maximal shortening, according to the Frank-Starling relationship. Systolic arterial pressure may be low and there are signs of inadequate organ perfusion: cold extremities; altered mental status and decreased level of consciousness; and oliguria. There are no signs of left ventricular failure: bibasilar lung rales or dyspnea. In this situation, because of the hypovolemia, venous return to the right heart is reduced, and pressure and volume of blood entering the left atrium is insufficient to distend the left ventricle enough to elicit maximal contractility (the Frank-Starling relationship). Cardiac output is reported to be maximal at left ventricular filling pressures of 15–20 mmHg.

A low LVEDP in the presence of arterial hypotension tends to indicate hypovolemia and may be secondary to vomiting, diaphoresis, inadequate fluid intake, excess diuretics, or loss of intravascular fluid into the interstitial spaces because of intense peripheral vasoconstriction (either endogenous compensatory or exogenous from excess administered vasopressor agents). In some patients, a low circulating blood volume may result from pooling of blood in the venous capacitance vessels caused by strong parasympathetic (vagal) circulatory reflexes. In others, relative hypovolemia may result from peripheral vasodilation caused by morphine or meperidine.

The decline in cardiac output in cases of effective hypovolemia lowers perfusion pressure in the aorta, and coronary artery blood flow falls. Thus myocardial oxygen supply declines and with it, contractility. This further decreases cardiac output. A vicious cycle is established in this way which may contribute to enlarging the zone of infarction. Because of the impaired myocardial contractility occurring in this sequence, the cardiac output may undergo progressive decline and require an expansion of the ECF to move the myocardial fibers to a higher initial length point on the Starling curve, in order to elicit the elevated contractility response and an improved stroke volume. The added fluid increases venous return, elevates LVEDP, puts increased tension on the contractile fibers, improves contractility and increases cardiac output. Pulmonary capillary wedge pressure may increase to 20 mmHg with careful monitoring for signs of pulmonary vascular congestion and edema. It is sometimes necessary to risk some hypervolemia and borderline pulmonary edema, by slightly overloading the left ventricle and pulmonary circuit, in order to maintain the optimal venous return to the right heart required to elicit maximal contractility.

Expansion of circulating blood volume with intravenous infusions will increase venous return to the right heart, increase diastolic filling of the left ventricle, put increased tension on the fibers (elevate preload) and result in better contractility and a greater stroke volume. The result of the improved cardiac output is often a clearing of the signs of inadequate peripheral perfusion. A fluid tolerance test may be appropriate in patients of this group. In a patient with a Swan-Ganz catheter, if the PCWP or PAEDP is less than about 15 mmHg, 100 ml increments of fluid may be given over short intervals, with monitoring of arterial pressure, PCWP, and clinical signs of the adequacy of organ perfusion. For patients without the catheter, CVP and clinical signs of adequate perfusion are assessed. Elevated pulmonary capillary pressure of a degree sufficient to threaten pulmonary vascular congestion seldom occurs if the PCWP does not increase over 18–20 mmHg. Moderate to severe pulmonary congestion may occur at 20–30 mmHg PCWP, and over 30 mmHg will often lead to overt pulmonary edema, dyspnea, pulmonary rales, and alveolar hypoventilation. These values are only generalizations, and large differences occur from one patient to another in the correlation between PCWP and signs and symptoms of left ventricle overload and pulmonary edema.

This group of AMI patients demonstrating reduced tissue and organ perfusion on the basis of hypovolemia of whatever cause is reported to have an in-hospital mortality rate of about 18%.

Patients with Evidence of Pulmonary Congestion, Without Signs or Symptoms of Inadequate Organ Perfusion

These individuals tend to show an elevated PCWP of over 18 mmHg, correlated with dyspnea and pulmonary rales, but the CI may be within normal limits. Management in this group may be administration of a diuretic such as the rapidly acting furosemide. In addition to its diuretic action it improves renal blood flow and hence increases glomerular filtration rate, and also increases the storage of blood in the venous capacitance vessels, thus lowering effective circulating ECF volume by two actions. There is disagreement as to whether patients in this category should be treated with digitalis. The drug may improve myocardial contractility, and thus decrease pulmonary vascular congestion by pumping more blood out of the lung circuit, but it increases myocardial oxygen requirements and therefore may increase the size of the infarct. Mortality rate in this group is reported to be about 25%.

Patients with Both Pulmonary Vascular Congestion and Inadequate Organ Perfusion

These patients have both a low CI (below about 2.2) and a high LVEDP (over 18–20 mmHg) and these values are correlated with the clinical signs of dyspnea and pulmonary rales (backward failure) and oliguria, decreased levels of consciousness, and cold clammy skin (forward failure). Some authors suggest that a pharmacologic agent which produces peripheral vasodilation, and hence decreases afterload, is an appropriate component of management for these patients. Nitroglycerine, nitroprusside (although this is reported to increase myocardial oxyten requirements) or the α adrenergic blocking agent phentolamine have been used. Since the resistance against which the impaired left ventricle has to pump blood is an important determinant of the stroke volume, decreasing the peripheral resistance with vasodilators should increase the stroke volume. This would result in a lower LVEDV and P, and a lower wall tension in the ventricle. Afterload is an important determinant of myocardial oxygen requirements; the greater the afterload, the higher the myocardial oxygen demand. Peripheral resistance and ventricle wall tension are the two major determinants of afterload. Therefore, theoretically at least, vasodilators should not only increase cardiac output but decrease myocardial oxygen need. The mortality rate for these patients is reported to be slightly under 60%.

Patients Classified as Having Cardiogenic Shock

The criteria for this assessment are a CI of 1.8 or below, a LVEDP of over 18 mmHg, pulmonary rales and dyspnea, and increasingly severe impairment of organ and tissue perfusion. Though the preload (LVEDP and V) is very high, the stroke volume is very low, indicating that the Frank-Starling fiber length–force of contraction relation is greatly impaired. The use of a positive inotropic agent such as norepinephrine or dopamine is considered by some workers to be the major management approach, while others hold that these agents have the deleterious action on the heart of increasing oxygen requirements. The latter suggest the use of peripheral vasodilators or vasodilators in conjunction with inotropic agents.

Some reports have divided the group of patients with cardiogenic shock into subgroups for which the suggested appropriate treatment varies with the underlying abnormality. One subgroup may have a major arterial obstruction, and emergency coronary artery bypass surgery could possibly be helpful in carefully selected patients. Another subgroup may have mechanical defects resulting from the infarction such as mitral regurgitation, ventricular septal rupture, papillary muscle malfunction, or a large ventricular aneurysm. Emergency or post-stabilization operations to correct the defects have been proposed and carried out in some of these patients. Such patients may be stabilized for a few days with the balloon pump and vasodilators and then studied angiographically or by a newer noninvasive method, and then considered for remedial surgery. In subjects who are not candidates for operative intervention, vasodilators in conjunction with mechanical circulatory assist devices such as intraaortic balloon counterpulsation or noninvasive methods such as the external counterpulsation device have been proposed.

In-hospital mortality for the cardiogenic shock group as a whole is reported to be 70–90% depending on management regimen. In a subgroup of patients unresponsive to vasodilators, who show a progressive decline in arterial pressure below 80 mmHg, mortality rate is close to 100%. Dopamine or norepinephrine may be tried in these patients, but because of the massive loss of functional myocardium, both short and longer term prognosis is extremely poor.

Some authors report a small group of usually young AMI patients with elevated cardiac index and hypertension, and a normal or slightly low PCWP. Sedation and the β blocking agent propranolol have been recommended in order to attempt to reduce myocardial oxygen requirements and prevent extension of the infarct into the ischemic zone.

COMPLICATIONS OF MYOCARDIAL INFARCTION

Complications include arrhythmias, acute congestive heart failure, cardiogenic shock, and cerebral infarction. Arrhythmias are a very frequent development in myocardial infarction, and ventricular fibrillation is the most common cause of death. Rate and rhythm abnormalities are discussed in Chapter 6.

The cause of cerebrovascular accidents in acute MI is a fall in perfusion pressure to a portion of the brain induced by the hypotension often accompanying an MI. In this case the patient's cerebral vasculature is already often markedly narrowed by atherosclerosis, and a hypotensive episode is sufficient to produce the critical fall in perfusion pressure across a narrowed vessel in the brain sufficient to produce ischemic hypoxia and tissue necrosis. A second or less frequent cause of cerebral infarction in MI is vascular occlusion resulting from an embolus originating from a mural thrombus.

Cardiogenic shock is the principle cause of death in myocardial infarction patients who reach the hospital. The physiologic changes in heart muscle produced by ischemic hypoxia and necrosis, as well as the decreased pumping action of the heart resulting from decreased functioning muscle mass, cause impaired contractility. The left ventricle is the most often and most severely affected, and there is a good correlation between the severity of the heart failure, the magnitude of the infarction, and the prognosis of the patient. Impaired myocardial contractility results in poor left ventricular systolic emptying; since less blood is ejected per contraction, left ventricular filling pressure and diastolic volume increase. The pressure in the capillaries of the pulmonary circuit behind the failing left ventricle increases, and interstitial and intraalveolar pulmonary edema develop. This causes an increase in pressure in the pulmonary artery and an increased workload on the right ventricle; eventually it too may fail. Essentially, then, the complications of AMI included under acute heart failure and cardiogenic shock, represent an accentuation of the circulatory abnormalities occurring in uncomplicated AMI; this accentuation in most cases is the consequence of the larger extent of the myocardial damage.

GENERAL PRINCIPLES IN THE MANAGEMENT OF ACUTE HEART FAILURE AND CARDIOGENIC SHOCK

Some degree of heart failure occurs in upwards of half of patients with myocardial infarction; it is manifested by pulmonary rales, an audible S_3, pulmonary venous congestion on chest X-ray, and (in patients monitored with the Swan-Ganz flow-guided balloon catheter) an elevated pulmonary capillary wedge pressure which correlates with left ventricular end-diastolic pressure. The treatment of mild failure is a diuretic to reduce ECF volume and pulmonary capillary pressure and lessen the workload of the myocardium, especially the left ventricle.

In the situation where the wedge pressure is below 12 mmHg, the cause of the shock syndrome may be hypovolemia from overuse of diuretics following an episode of pulmonary edema, from vomiting and diaphoresis, from inadequate fluid intake, or from vasodilation caused by morphine or other pain medication. Fluid challenges in 100 ml increments may be given with close monitoring of left ventricular filling pressure; if the blood pressure rises with little or no increase in wedge pressure, hypovolemia is present, and fluid repletion will improve left ventricular performance. If the pulmonary capillary wedge pressure rises too much too abruptly, then hypovolemia is probably not contributing to the shock syndrome and the patient may develop pulmonary edema from left ventricular failure if too much fluid is given.

Vasoconstrictor agents are sometimes used for patients who are hypotensive because of a compensatory peripheral vasoconstriction that is inadequate to compensate for the low cardiac output; in this case inadequate tissue perfusion may be improved by the cautious administration of the sympathomimetic amines norepinephrine or dopamine which increase myocardial contractility and elevate peripheral resistance. In addition, in the patient with myocardial infarction the coronary vessels distal to the occlusion will be maximally dilated because of the local accumulation of vasodilator metabolites. Therefore coronary artery perfusion is largely dependent on aortic perfusion pressure, which may be improved by adrenergic agents. However, some studies fail to show improvement in survival with the use of these agents, and in addition they may promote arrhythmias and tachycardia. They also increase heart afterload by elevation of systemic blood pressure; this may worsen the already elevated left ventricular diastolic pressure by increasing the resistance to systolic ejection. It is important to recall that an increase in ventricular dilation increases the wall tension and elevates myocardial oxygen requirements, which may promote extension of infarct size.

Myocardial function may be improved in the acute heart failure of myocardial infarction by the intravenous administration of vasodilators such as phentolamine, sodium nitroprusside, or nitroglycerine, which reduce cardiac work by decreasing vasoconstriction and hence the afterload, the resistance against which the heart must pump blood. Reduction of afterload may lead to decreased diastolic pressure, lowered pulmonary capillary pressure and decreased pulmonary congestion, and will tend to promote increased cardiac output. It has been reported that in patients with congestive heart failure complicating acute myocardial infarction, sublingual and oral isosorbide dinitrate produces a significant decline in pulmonary artery end-diastolic pressure which may last over 3 hours, and may be associated with improvement in pulmonary rales, dyspnea, and in some patients, increased urinary output. Vasodilators should not be used, however, in the presence of too low an arterial pressure, because the vasodilation they produce would further lower the pressure, and decrease coronary artery perfusion.

Intraaortic balloon counterpulsation may be used to provide assistance to the failing circulation in acute heart failure and cardiogenic shock. The three-chambered balloon is inserted through the femoral artery and is positioned to lie in the descending aorta above the renal and below the subclavian arteries. The center chamber inflates first followed immediately by inflation of the outer two chambers. The balloon is filled with helium or carbon dioxide. It is timed by the patient's own electrocardiogram; it rapidly inflates at the T wave early in diastole, producing increased intraarterial pressure to provide increased coronary blood flow and peripheral tissue perfusion. It rapidly deflates toward the end of the P wave in early systole, which decreases afterload, enhances ventricular systolic ejection, lowers resistance against which the left ventricle ejects blood, and therefore decreases its workload and oxygen requirement. Cardiac output increases, and this leads to a decline in left ventricular diastolic pressure (left ventricular diastolic volume) and decreases myocardial lactate production, indicating improved heart muscle oxygenation.

In spite of the initial favorable changes in the circulation with the balloon pump, reversal of cardiogenic shock does not often occur. Its use is generally reserved for patients who have been unresponsive to volume expansion, control of arrhythmias, oxygen administration and relief of pain, or administration of appropriate pharmacologic agents. Some studies show that perhaps one fifth of patients who receive IABA survive to leave the hospital; however, long-term survivors appear to be rare, probably because of the extensive myocardial damage which prompted its use in the first place and the severity of the underlying organic heart disease. It is not without significant complications, including iliofemoral vascular occlusion at the insertion site which may necessitate further surgery or amputation.

Another use of the balloon pump may be in providing circulatory support for the few carefully selected patients in whom angiographic and other evaluation for potentially operatively correctable cardiac abnormalities is indicated.

The difficulty of designing and conducting a suitably controlled randomized prospective study to evaluate possible long-term benefits of the balloon pump in severe AMI limits the possibility of objectively assessing its value.

Echocardiography, radioactive thallium imaging, and other noninvasive procedures provide means for assessing myocardial performance in AMI; abnormalities of left ventricular function and structure discerned by these methods appear to be well correlated with CI, LVEDP, and other values obtained by more invasive methods, and with clinical signs and symptoms of circulatory status.

PRESERVATION OF THE ZONE OF ISCHEMIC MYOCARDIUM SURROUNDING THE INFARCT

The preservation of the zone of ischemic myocardium surrounding the infarct has become an increasingly important consideration in the management of AMI. It is not only the short-term, in-hospital survival that is correlated with eventual infarct size; the long-term prognosis for the patient depends very significantly on the overall amount of normally functioning myocardium remaining after the acute phase of the process, and the subsequent healing and scar formation.

Studies of experimentally produced myocardial infarction in laboratory animals indicate that following coronary occlusion there is a central area of irreversibly necrotic tissue surrounded by a zone of ischemic myocardium the fate of which, in a sense, hangs in the balance determined by the ratio between myocardial oxygen supply and myocardial oxygen requirements. This area of abnormal but still potentially viable tissue may increase in size over a number of hours following the acute infarction. The area of infarction which it surrounds may expand into it, or remain relatively stable without extension, depending to some extent upon the presence of factors which, on the one hand, increase or decrease myocardial

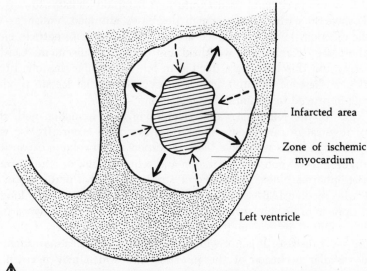

= Extension of infarct, by increased myocardial oxygen demand or decreased myocardial oxygen supply

= Confinement of infarct, and prevention of extension, by decreased myocardial oxygen demand or increased myocardial oxygen supply

Figure 5-5. Concept of preservation of the zone of ischemic myocardium surrounding the heart. Influences which tend to increase the extension of the infarct are those that increase myocardial oxygen requirements or reduce myocardial oxygen supply.

Factors increasing myocardial O_2 requirements:
tachycardia (arrhythmias, sympathomimetic drugs, catecholamines)
increased contractility (sympathomimetic drugs, catecholamines, digitalis)
increased wall tension from ventricular dilation
increased peripheral resistance to systolic ejection (elevated BP)
Factors decreasing myocardial O_2 supply:
poor coronary artery perfusion from
tachycardia (decreased diastolic filling time)
hypotension and hypovolemia (decreased diastolic filling pressure)
low cardiac output
arterial hypoxemia
anemia

oxygen supply; or, on the other hand, increase or decrease myocardial oxygen requirements. An increase in oxygen demand or a decrease in oxygen supply will tend to increase the encroachment of the infarcted area into the ischemic zone. A decrease in oxygen need or an increase in supply would be expected to prevent such extension and confine the eventual size of the necrotic area.

Factors Which Influence the Oxygen Requirements of the Myocardium

There are four major factors determining the rate of oxygen consumption by the heart: heart rate, inotropic state (degree of contractility), tension on the myocardial wall, and systolic arterial pressure. Wall tension, in turn, is determined by two factors: intraventricular volume and intraventricular pressure. Myocardial oxygen consumption is therefore increased by elevated heart rate, by increased contractility (or inotropic state), by increased ventricular volume (that is, increased LVEDV, which is also increased preload) and increased pressure in the arteries into which the ventricle ejects blood (that is, increased peripheral resistance which is also increased afterload). Therefore, in the clinical setting, factors which produce tachycardia, increased contractility, increased left ventricle dilation, and elevated arterial blood pressure, would be expected to increase myocardial oxygen requirements. If coronary artery oxygen supply remained the same, such factors would be predicted to increase the infarcted area, other things equal.

The catecholamines, which increase heart rate, increase myocardial contractility, and produce peripheral vasoconstriction, would increase myocardial oxygen consumption and extend infarct size. Conversely, β adrenergic blocking agents such as propranolol; and vasodilators, such as phentolamine and nitroglycerine in modest amounts (insufficient to produce hypotension and a too low cardiac output) would be predicted to inhibit infarct extension.

Factors Which Influence Oxygen Supply to the Myocardium

Coronary artery perfusion pressure and arterial O_2 content are the major determinants of myocardial oxygen supply. Therefore factors which improve coronary artery blood flow and oxygen content, such as adequate diastolic filling time and diastolic filling pressure, and oxygen inhalation, would be assumed to preserve the ischemic zone from infarction. Clinically such measures would be O_2 supplements, pharmacologic control of arrhythmias, and treatment of hypovolemia and hypotension (volume repletion and mild vasoconstrictors), and elevation of cardiac output through improved myocardial contractility (inotropic agents).

Be it noted that some of these measures are physiologically contradictory from the standpoint of the balance between myocardial oxygen consumption and coronary artery flow. Catecholamines, which elevate contractility and cardiac output (thereby improving coronary artery flow), also elevate oxygen consumption. A factor which increases venous return may cause excessive ventricle dilation. A vasoconstrictor which may improve coronary perfusion may also increase resistance to systolic ejection and worsen ventricular dilation. Thus a careful titration of drugs to obtain a desired effect without eliciting an undesired one may be possible: the combined use of a positive inotropic agent with a peripheral vasodilator is an example of such titration. Less conservative measures might include IABA or surgical coronary revascularization.

Factors which impair oxygen supply to the myocardium are a decline in coronary artery perfusion pressure from any cause: tachycardia, hypotension and hypovolemia and low cardiac output; arterial hypoxemia; and anemia.

Other measures which have been tested with the aim of reducing infarct size are increasing the availability of metabolic substrate to the myocardium by the infusion of glucose, insulin and potassium; and reduction of myocardial edema and inflammation by infusions of hypertonic mannitol, adrenal glucocorticoids, or hyaluronidase. These are experimental procedures which have been used in the management of human AMI with the aim of reducing infarct size. In experimental animals they have been shown by histologic and electron microscopic criteria, and by measurements of lactate production and cardiac enzymes, to limit infarct size as compared with controls. The mechanisms of action of these agents in limiting infarct size in experimental animals is uncertain; the assessment of their effects in human AMI awaits the development of reliable objective criteria. The rate of resolution of ST segment elevation and subsequent alterations in the QRS complex have been proposed as possible methods of evaluating their usefulness.

PREVENTION OF REINFARCTION AFTER ACUTE MYOCARDIAL INFARCTION

A recent study exploring the value of the antiplatelet agent sulfinpyrazone in the prevention of a second AMI reports that this drug in doses of 200 mg four times a day, as compared with placebo, results in an annual 48.5% reduction in cardiac deaths and a 57.2% reduction in rate of sudden cardiac death, over the first 8.4 months of the study. Aspirin, dipyridamole, and other antiplatelet agents are being evaluated for similar effects in other studies.

The precise mechanism of action of sulfinpyrazone and other antiplatelet agents in reducing embolic phenomena is uncertain. Platelets have a number of characteristics which promote thrombus formation and vascular spasm, including adherence, aggregation, stimulation of blood clotting, and secretion of vasoactive chemicals. Antiplatelet agents and in particular sulfinpyrazone, inhibit several of these platelet activities but in the doses used clinically appear not to increase bleeding time.

An important component of prevention of reinfarction is a program of cardiac exercise rehabilitation as described in Chapter 8.

REFERENCES

Beeson PB and McDermott, editors: *Textbook of Medicine*, 14th ed. Philadelphia, Pa.: Saunders, 1975.

Bourassa MG, et al: The anturane reinfarction trial research group. Sulfinpyrazone in the prevention of cardiac death after myocardial infarction. *N. Engl. J. Med.* 298:289–295, 1978.

Braunwald E: Salvage of ischemic myocardium. In: Lefer AM, et al, editors: *Pathophysiology and Therapeutics of Myocardial Ischemia*. New York: Spectrum Publications, 1977.

Cady LD, et al: Quantitation of severity of critical illness with special reference to blood lactate. *Crit. Care Med.* 1:75–80, 1973.

Flaherty JT and Weisfeldt ML: Myocardial infarction. In: Willerson JT and Sanders CA, editors: *Clinical Cardiology*. New York: Grune & Stratton, 1977.

Frohlich ED, editor: *Pathophysiology*. Philadelphia, Pa.: Lippincott, 1976.

Ganong WF: *Review of Medical Physiology*, 8th ed. Los Altos, Calif.: Lange Medical Publications, 1977.

Goldberger E and Wheat MR, Jr.: *Treatment of Cardiac Emergencies*, 2nd ed. St. Louis, Mo.: Mosby, 1977.

Guyton AC: *Textbook of Medical Physiology*, 5th ed. Philadelphia, Pa.: Saunders, 1976.

Jackson G, et al: Intra-aortic balloon assistance in cardiogenic shock after myocardial infarction or cardiac surgery. *Br. Heart J.* 39:598–604, 1977.

Olivia PB and Breckinridge JC: Arteriographic evidence of coronary artery spasm in acute myocardial infarction. *Circulation* 56:366–375, 1977.

Parmley WW and Tyberg JV: Determinants of myocardial oxygen demand. In: Klocke FJ, guest editor: *Symposium on Coronary Circulation*. Yu PN and Goodwin JF, editors: *Progress in Cardiology*. Philadelphia, Pa.: Lea & Febiger, 1976.

Romhilt DW and Fowler NO: Physical signs in acute myocardial infarction. *Heart Lung* 2:74–80, 1973.

Thorn GW, et al, editors: *Harrison's Principles of Internal Medicine*, 8th ed. New York, McGraw-Hill, 1977.

Vyden JK, et al: Hemodynamic alterations in acute myocardial infarction. In: Lefer AM, et al., editors: *Pathophysiology and Therapeutics of Myocardial Ischemia*. New York: Spectrum Publications, 1977.

CHAPTER SIX

Cardiac Arrhythmias

IMPULSE FORMATION, EXCITATION, AND CONDUCTION IN THE NORMAL HEART

Anatomic Divisions of the Specialized Conduction System

The Sinoatrial Node (Sinus Node, SA Node)

This structure is the normal primary pacemaker of the heart; it is located near the area where the superior vena cava enters the right atrium. Its blood supply comes from the right coronary artery in some individuals, and from the left circumflex coronary artery in others. It receives its nerve supply from both the sympathetic (adrenergic) and the parasympathetic (cholinergic) divisions of the autonomic nervous system. The adrenergic innervation comes from the cervical sympathetic ganglia via the cardiac nerves; the cholinergic innervation is mainly from the right vagus nerve (CN X). Impulses in the sympathetic nerves increase the rate of cardiac impulse formation in the SA node, and therefore the heart rate, while parasympathetic stimuli decrease it; if vagal stimulation is very strong, impulse formation may briefly cease altogether.

The Intraatrial Conduction System (Internodal Atrial Pathways)

There are specialized conducting fibers within the atria which convey the cardiac impulse from its origin in the SA node to the atrioventricular (AV node). Although impulse conduction through ordinary atrial myocardium no doubt also occurs simultaneously, it probably does so at a slower rate, and the impulse

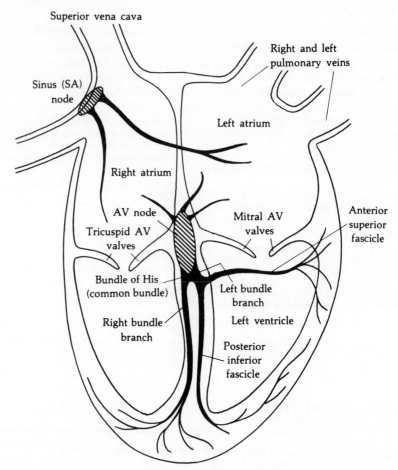

Figure 6-1. Anatomic divisions of the specialized impulse formation and conduction system of the heart: sinus node (SA node, sinoatrial node); intraatrial conduction system; atrioventricular node (AV node); bundle of His; right bundle branch; and left bundle branch and its superior and inferior divisions (fascicles).

there is weaker, so that transmission through the specialized atrial conduction fibers is the dominant process responsible for activating the AV node.

The Atrioventricular Node (AV Node)

This structure is located on the lower right side of the interatrial septum near the opening of the inferior vena cava. Its blood supply is derived mainly from the right coronary artery; therefore, AV node blood flow comes largely from the posterior surface of the heart. It is for this reason that a posterior (inferior) wall myocardial infarction often impairs conduction in AV junctional pathways. It receives a large nerve supply of both adrenergic and cholinergic fibers, the latter coming primarily from the left vagus. The node itself consists of large numbers of very small diameter fibers which form a complicated interconnecting network. Because of the structure of the node the velocity of conduction of the cardiac impulse through it is slow, and the strength of the impulse at this point is relatively weak.

The Bundle of His (AV Bundle, Common Bundle)

The His bundle is much larger than the AV node, and is a downward continuation of it. Both the rate and strength of the cardiac impulse are greater here than in the AV node. The common bundle is located at the lower portion of the intraatrial septum; its fibers travel in the subendocardial tissue toward the upper portion of the intraventricular septum. It then divides into the right and left bundle branches. The blood supply to the His bundle and its branches comes mainly from the anterior descending branch of the left coronary artery; therefore an anterior wall myocardial infarction often results in abnormalities of conduction in the His bundle, bundle branches, and the Purkinje system.

The Right Bundle Branch (RBB)

This is a thinner and more direct continuation of the His bundle than the left bundle branch. The right branch travels across the intraventricular septum and then courses down the right side of the septum. Along its first portion it is subendocardial, but then becomes more superficial as it approaches the apex. It branches into the Purkinje fibers supplying the anterior papillary muscle and the ventricular wall, and then ramifies throughout the myocardium.

The Left Bundle Branch (LBB) and Fascicles

The main left bundle branch is located beneath the endocardium on the upper portion of the intraventricular septum; it is usually larger in diameter than the RBB, but is considerably shorter. At the upper intraventricular septum it divides into two main groups of fibers: the anterior (superior) and the posterior (inferior) fascicles. These two divisions have a more rapid rate of conduction of the cardiac impulse than do any of the other specialized conduction tissues of the heart. They give off numerous branches—the Purkinje system—that has many interconnections throughout the myocardium, in addition to supplying the anterior and posterior papillary muscles.

The rapid conduction velocity and the strong impulse characteristic of both the right and left bundle branches result in a coordinated electrical stimulation to, and therefore mechanical contraction of, the myocardial fibers; this synchrony results in the optimal ejection of blood during systole.

Purkinje Fibers

These fibers are the ultimate portions of the specialized conduction system of the heart. They are the terminals of the right and left bundle branches and fascicles; they supply the papillary muscles and the entire myocardium.

The electrical excitation of the heart which precedes and is the stimulus for contraction, therefore, is initiated in the sinoatrial (SA) node and is propagated through specialized pathways in the atrium to the atrioventricular (AV) node. From there it enters the His bundle, bundle branches and fascicles, and ultimately traverses the Purkinje fibers. This sequential electrical activation leads to an orderly sequence of contraction of the four chambers, and therefore a coordinated movement of blood into, through, and then out of the heart. The coupling of electrical activation with mechanical contraction in the heart is discussed in Chapter 7.

Electrical Properties of the Specialized Conduction System: Automaticity, Excitability, and Conductivity

Automaticity refers to the ability of cells of the specialized conduction system of the heart spontaneously to depolarize and thus initiate a stimulus, or wave of excitation, which is conducted throughout the heart. *Excitability* denotes the capacity of a cell to respond to an electrical stimulus transmitted to it from another cell by depolarizing. *Conductivity* is the characteristic whereby the electrical impulse is spread from one excitable cell to the next so that the entire conduction system, and finally the entire myocardium, is electrically activated.

The Resting Transmembrane Potential

The cells of the various portions of the specialized conduction system of the heart, as well as the cells of the ordinary atrial and ventricular myocardium, have a difference in electrical charge across the resting (that is, nonactivated) membrane from the cell interior to the cell exterior. The inside of the cell is negative by about 90 mV with respect to the outside. This difference in charge is called the resting transmembrane potential, and is expressed as −90 mV.

In this resting steady-state condition, the electrical difference is based upon a difference in concentration of ions on the two sides of the cell membrane, especially of Na^+ and K^+. The extracellular concentration of Na^+ is over 10 times that of the cell interior. The intracellular concentration of K^+ is over 30 times greater than the extracellular concentration of that ion. The resting transmembrane electrical potential results largely from the difference in the concentration of K^+ between the cell interior and exterior. The difference in concentration of an ion on the two sides of a membrane is called the chemical gradient of that ion. Therefore, the resting transmembrane potential is mainly the result of the K^+ gradient. The potential, and the differential distribution of ions underlying it, are diagramed in Figure 6-2.

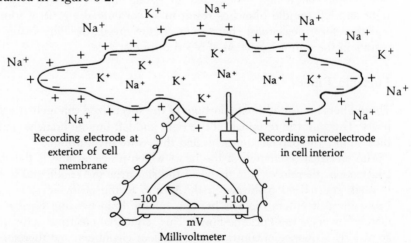

Figure 6-2. The resting transmembrane electrical potential, and differential ion distribution, between interior and exterior of a single heart muscle cell.

The difference in concentrations of ions on the two sides of the cell membrane is the result of an active transport process within the membrane itself, whereby Na^+ is continually pumped out of the cell, and K^+ pumped into and retained within it, so that the gradients remain stable within a normal range in the resting state. Ca^{2+} and Cl^- are other ions which are maintained in differential distribution between cell interior and exterior. The active transport processes responsible for ionic gradients result from oxygen- and energy-consuming metabolic activities within cell membranes; such ionic and electrical gradients are characteristic of essentially all living cells, not just myocardial cells. The natural tendency of ions to distribute themselves equally on the two sides of a membrane, according to their diffusion gradients, is thus countered by the active transport pumping processes within the membrane.

The Phases of the Action Potential

The events of depolarization, together with the recovery processes which restore the normal resting membrane potential, are collectively called the action potential.

The quality of automaticity in the specialized conducting tissues of the heart refers to their ability to depolarize spontaneously at regular intervals, thus initiating a series of action potentials which are then propagated throughout the heart. That portion of the specialized conducting tissues which regularly spontaneously depolarizes at the fastest rate is said to have the highest degree of automaticity, and it becomes the pacemaker. In the normal heart it is the SA node which possesses the most rapid inherent rate of impulse formation. The phases of the action potential in the cells of the specialized conduction system of the heart are diagramed in Figure 6-3.

Phase 0

The first event in the normal initiation of the cardiac impulse is a gradual decline in the resting membrane potential in the cells of the SA node from −90 mV to the threshold value of about −70 mV. This spontaneous drop in membrane potential occurs during the latter part of electrical diastole and is called phase 4 depolarization. As the potential declines (becomes less negative) to the threshold value, there is then a very rapid complete depolarization—that is, the potential difference across the membrane between inside and outside is rapidly abolished. In fact there is a temporary reversal, called the overshoot, in which the inside of the cell becomes briefly positive with respect to the outside. This wave of depolarization, or negativity, is very rapid, about 2 msec. It is called phase 0 of the action potential. The membrane is now stimulated; the wave of depolarization becomes self-sustaining, and is propagated in orderly fashion throughout the entire conduction system and thence through the whole myocardium. This constitutes the electrical impulse of the heart, and it initiates the contraction.

The rapid phase 0 depolarization of the membrane from −90 to about +20 mV which constitutes the inital portion of the action potential, results from a rapid increase in permeability of the membrane to Na^+. Specific so-called fast Na^+ channels in the membrane open up, permitting the rapid influx of Na^+ from the cell exterior to the inside. The overshoot is caused by entry of excess Na^+ above equilibrium levels. In addition, there is a loss of K^+ from the cell interior.

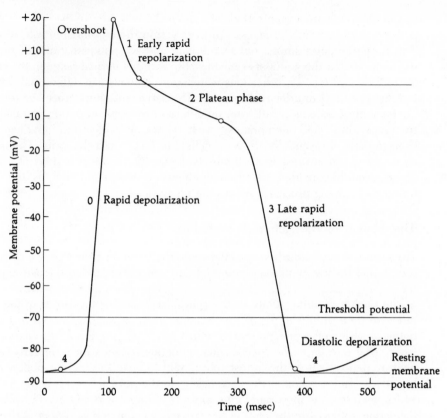

Figure 6-3. Diagram of the phases of the action potential in cells of the specialized conduction tissues of the heart.

The contractile response of the myocardium begins just after the onset of electrical depolarization and is not quite twice as long as the electrical events.

Phase 1

This is the initial rapid phase of repolarization of the membrane; it lasts only a few msec, and corresponds to a decreasing permeability of the membrane to Na^+, and extrusion of Na^+ out of the cell by the membrane pump; that is, the gates permitting Na^+ influx now close, and that which entered is transported back to the outside of the cell.

Phase 2

This is the stage of slower repolarization called the plateau phase; it lasts about 150 msec. The ionic movement characteristic of this phase is the opening of the so-called slow Ca^{2+} channels in the membrane and the influx of Ca^{2+} from the cell exterior to the inside. Ca^{2+} is the ion importantly responsible for excitation-contraction coupling, described in Chapter 7. The influx of Ca^{2+} and its resulting increased availability to replenish intracellular stores has a marked impact on actin-myosin interaction and therefore on contractility.

Phase 3

This stage of repolarization rapidly returns the membrane potential to close to its resting value. At this time there is an increased permeability of the membrane to K^+, and the intracellular content of K^+ increases as more K^+ is pumped into the cell from the outside. Repolarization is not complete until the heart muscle contraction is half over.

Phase 4

The transmembrane potential becomes restored to its normal resting value at the transition between phase 3 and phase 4. In cells of the specialized conduction tissue the resting membrane potential is maintained only briefly; in these cells having automaticity the transmembrane potential spontaneously declines to the threshold of about -70 mV at which point the next action potential is initiated. The spontaneous decline to threshold is called phase 4 diastolic depolarization. It occurs only in cells of the specialized conduction tissue. In contrast, in ordinary normal atrial and ventricular myocardium, there is no gradual depolarization in phase 4—that is, there is no slope. The membrane remains at resting values until it is depolarized by the action potential from the tissues possessing automaticity.

The Refractory Periods of the Heart

The absolute refractory period of the heart refers to that period during the action potential when no stimulus, no matter how strong, is capable of eliciting another action potential. It includes phase 0, 1, 2, and most of phase 3. The relative refractory period designates the relative inexcitability of the heart during the latter portions of the recovery process. During this period, lasting from the concluding section of phase 3 to just before phase 4, another action potential can be initiated by a stronger than ordinary stimulus. Briefly, at the end of the phase 3 to phase 4 transition, as the relative refractory period is ending there is a period called the vulnerable period, the coincides with the mid-portion of the T wave, when the heart is susceptible to developing fibrillation if stimulated. The relationships among these periods and the phases of the action potential are shown in Figure 6-4 for ordinary (nonpacemaker) myocardium.

Refractoriness is the state in which the myocardial cells in either the specialized conduction system or ordinary contracting atria or ventricles fail to respond to arriving stimuli; it results from the fact that repolarization is still incomplete. In this situation the transmembrane potential has not yet been restored to a degree sufficient to propagate the action potential. The cell is completely unresponsive when the transmembrane potential is below the threshold value. When the transmembrane potential is above threshold but below the resting value, a stronger stimulus is required to initiate an action potential.

The Hierarchy of Automaticity in the Specialized Conduction System

To recapitulate, pacemaker tissue possesses the ability spontaneously to depolarize without stimulation from outside itself. This capacity of self-excitation is

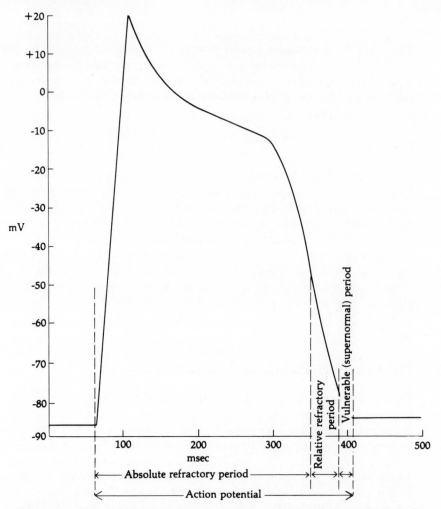

Figure 6-4. Diagram of the relation between the phases of the action potential; the absolute and relative refractory periods; and the vulnerable (supernormal) period in cells of the ordinary working (nonconduction) myocardium.

called automaticity, and it is characteristic of the tissue which makes up the specialized conducting system of the heart. These tissues spontaneously initiate repeated action potentials and this is what constitutes pacemaker activity. Unlike the ordinary normal myocardium of the atria and ventricles, the cell membranes of the conduction system have electrically unstable cell membranes so that in the resting (nonstimulated) state instead of maintaining a stable steady-state transmembrane potential as ordinary myocardium does, the membrane potential of pacemaker tissue declines steadily, without being stimulated, until the threshold value necessary to initiate another action potential is attained. This decline begins quite promptly following the recovery of the normal membrane potential after the prior wave of depolarizatization. The steady decline in membrane potential is called a prepotential or a pacemaker potential, and it results from ion movements across the membrane, in this case from a slow decline in permeability to K^+, which results in a gradual decrease in movement of potassium out of the cell, and therefore a drop of transmembrane potential. This occurs during diastole and is called phase 4 diastolic depolarization (Figure 6-3). Such pacemaker potentials do not occur in ordinary myocardial cells under normal conditions.

Under normal circumstances the SA node manifests the most rapid rate of spontaneous depolarization, and therefore has the highest degree of automaticity. Degrees of decline in automaticity in the various portions of the conduction system distal to the SA node, in decreasing order of pacemaker activity, are: AV junction, His bundle, bundle branches, fascicles, and Purkinje tissue. Therefore in the normal heart the SA node functions as the pacemaker for the whole heart. Because of its more rapid rate of spontaneous depolarization (=impulse formation) it discharges first, before the other pacemaker tissues lower in the system can attain their varying rates of spontaneous discharge to threshold. The impulse from the sinus node depolarizes them before they can depolarize themselves.

Under three sets of abnormal conditions, these subsidiary pacemakers (latent pacemakers) normally held in abeyance by the higher degree of automaticity from the SA node, can emerge and take over the pacemaker functions of the heart: (1) if the rate of impulse formation from the SA node is depressed; (2) if the transmission of the impulse from the SA node is delayed or blocked; and (3) if for some reason the rate of automaticity of subsidiary (latent) pacemaker tissue becomes enhanced above that of the SA node.

Under normal circumstances the various portions of the heart are electrically activated in an orderly sequence, which is followed by a coordinated wave of contraction. This coordinated appropriately sequenced function results in optimal heart diastolic filling and optimal systolic ejection. When the normal sequence of electrical activation is disturbed, then the normal sequence of mechanical contraction is altered, and myocardial performance declines.

Influences on Pacemaker Automaticity

When the sympathetic adrenergic nerve supply to the heart is stimulated via the cardiac nerves, the heart rate increases because of an increase in the rate of phase 4 diastolic depolarization. It is well known that sympathetic stimulation, as well as the administration of sympathomimetic pharmacologic agents, causes tachycardia and often leads to ectopic impulse formation and premature ventricular contractions. Conversely, during parasympathetic cholinergic nerve stimulation via the vagus, the heart rate slows because of a decrease in the rate of phase 4 depolarization. It is suggested that these effects are mediated by the action of norepinephrine and acetylcholine, respectively, on membrane permeability to K^+, and hence on the movement of K^+ across the cell membrane. Temperature changes and various pharmacologic agents also influence the rate of the phase 4 prepotentials and hence the automaticity. These influences also affect other phases of the action potential, and therefore the strength of the impulses, as well as the electrical stability of the resting membrane and the magnitude of the transmembrane potential. It is probable that, at the cellular level, the aforementioned factors exert their effects by influencing membrane permeability to ionic movement and membrane ion transport.

In addition to the neural influences on automaticity, abnormal states such as hypoxemia, hypercapnia, myocardial ischemia, electrolyte and acid–base abnormalities, cardiac dilation, and drugs, exert marked effects on resting membrane potentials and the various phases of the action potential.

Rate and Strength of Conduction Through the Specialized Conduction System

The Electrocardiogram (EKG)

The EKG is the graphic representation of the fluctuation in electrical potentials in the heart during the various phases of its electrical cycle. These electrical changes are transmitted from the surface of the heart to the surface of the body through the volume conduction of the ions in the body fluids, and are measured from the body surface. A lead II EKG, with the electrical events in the heart correlated with the various waves and intervals of the EKG, is shown in Figure 6-5.

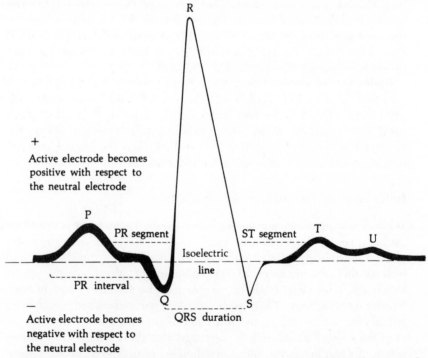

Figure 6-5. A lead II EKG showing the waves and intervals of the tracing and their correlation with the electrical events in the heart.

1. P wave—corresponds to atrial depolarization; the P wave occurs just prior to the beginning of contraction of the atria.

2. P-R interval—corresponds to atrial depolarization and conduction through the AV node; atrial repolarization is usually hidden by the QRS complex.

3. QRS complex—correlated with ventricular depolarization. The QRS complex occurs immediately before the onset of ventricular contraction.

4. QT interval—ventricular depolarization and onset of repolarization.

5. ST segment and T wave—ventricular repolarization.

6. U wave—coincides with the supernormal phase during ventricular recovery.

During the passage of the wave of depolarization across the ventricles, the heart is in an absolutely refractory state, meaning that it cannot be stimulated by a stimulus of any strength. The period of complete refractoriness is followed by the relative refractory period. In relative refractoriness a cardiac impulse can be initiated but only by a stimulus of extra strength. There is a short period during the relative refractory period where the heart is prone to develop ventricular fibrillation; this is called the vulnerable period. Under certain abnormal conditions, there is a period just at or after the close of the relatively refractory period when the heart may be excessively responsive to small stimuli; this is the supernormal period. These relationships with reference to the EKG are shown in Figure 6-6.

The procedure of His bundle electrograms has provided information concerning the speed of conduction to and through the SA node, the His bundle, and its major divisions. In this technique a balloon flow-directed catheter with a recording electrode tip is inserted through a vein in the arm to a location near the tricuspid valve in the right heart; from this point the electrical impulses passing through the conduction system can be recorded accurately. The responses of the electrode in the heart reveal the electrical changes within the conduction system during the P-R interval which are too small to show up on the surface EKG. The P-R interval is the time from the initiation of the P wave (atrial depolarization) to the beginning of the QRS complex (ventricular depolarization) of the surface EKG. The P-R interval can be divided into three subintervals on the basis of the His bundle electrogram. The electrogram records three deflections in individuals with an intact conduction system, and in normal sinus rhythm: (1) the A wave corresponds to depolarization of the right lower atrium; (2) the H wave is pro-

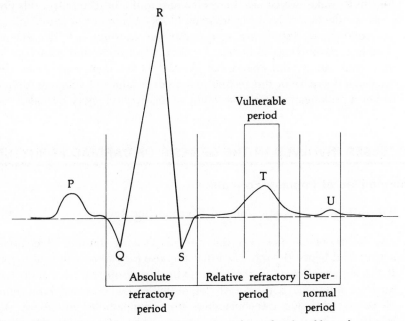

Figure 6-6. Absolute and relative refractory periods, and vulnerable and supernormal periods. Shown in relation to the EKG.

duced by depolarization of the His bundle; and (3) the V wave results from the wave of negativity spreading to adjacent portions of the ventricular myocardium.

The intervals are defined as follows: (1) the P-A interval represents the conduction time from the upper to the lower right atrium; (2) the A-H interval corresponds to the time required for conduction from the lower right atrium, through the AV node, to the depolarization of the His bundle (this interval therefore corresponds to AV nodal conduction time); and (3) the H-V interval records the conduction time through the His bundle and the bundle branch–Purkinje system to the ventricular myocardium. The normal A-H interval ranges between 90–140 msec and the H-V interval from approximately 35–55 msec.

Factors Influencing the Rate of Conduction

The markedly slow conduction through the AV node is correlated with a long absolute refractory period in nodal cells. This acts as a protective mechanism which prevents a too rapid rate of SA node or ectopic atrial impulses from penetrating to the ventricles and driving them at a high frequency. The importance of this adaptive device is evident when one recognizes that with excessively rapid ventricular rates, diastolic filling time is greatly reduced causing a drop in cardiac output and inadequate coronary artery perfusion.

In all cells of the conduction system, the speed of conduction is a function of the resting membrane potential at the time the action potential arrives; when the transmembrane potential is reduced then the speed of conduction is lowered. As the speed of conduction declines, the amplitude of the action potential is reduced, and eventually the wave of excitation may die out before the whole conduction system is activated. The term for this process of fading away of the action potential is *decremental conduction.* Since it leaves inadequately depolarized cells in its wake, which are then refractory to the next impulse, this process may cause conduction delay or conduction block. A number of pathologic changes in the conduction system are responsible for causing such decremental or incomplete conduction: ischemia, hypoxia, electrolyte and acid–base abnormalities, cold, drugs, and myocardial fibrosis. At the membrane level, the changes involve a decrease in the resting potential, a failure of adequate depolarization, and/or a prolongation in the absolute or relative refractory periods.

PROCESSES INVOLVED IN THE GENESIS OF CARDIAC ARRHYTHMIAS

Abnormalities of Impulse Formation

Alterations in the Specialized Conducting System

Any factor which increases the rate of phase 4 diastolic depolarization (see above), and hence the rate of cardiac impulse formation, will lead to tachycardia. If the increase occurs in the sinus node, the result will be a sinus tachycardia. Such an influence is produced, for example, by increased body temperature, elevated circulating catecholamines from sympathetic autonomic stimulation, and excess thyroid hormone.

If the increased rate of impulse formation occurs in some portion of the specialized conducting tissue beyond the sinus node, and the rate is faster than that from the node, then impulses formed at this site will take over as pacemaker of the heart, resulting in an ectopic tachycardia.

Conversely, any influences which depress the rate of impulse formation, such as parasympathomimetic drugs, hypothermia, or hypothyroidism, will lead to bradycardia. In addition to these systemic effects on impulse formation, localized influences such as hypoxia, ischemia, and electrolyte abnormalities, may produce alterations in the rate of phase 4 diastolic depolarization.

When marked slowing of impulse formation occurs, below the inherent rate of impulse formation of more distal tissues of the specialized conducting system, then sites farther along the system, such as the AV junctional area, may take over as pacemaker. This will occur because they are now no longer depolarized by the sinus node impulses before their own spontaneous depolarization could occur. Such emergence of a primary pacemaker leads to an *escape rhythm;* the contractions it produces are called postmature rather than premature, because they occur later than the next normal impulse from the primary pacemaker, rather than earlier.

Alterations in Atrial and Ventricular Myocardium

Ordinary myocardial fibers can, under abnormal conditions, develop spontaneous diastolic depolarization and therefore initiate abnormal impulse formation. This may result from some pathologic condition which produces a disturbance of the resting membrane potential, or a partial depolarization of the cell membrane; such membrane instability could result in automaticity and an *ectopic arrhythmia.* Ischemia, hypoxic cell damage, and local electrolyte imbalance have been proposed as mechanisms for such membrane alterations.

Abnormalities of Impulse Conduction

Factors Determining the Effectiveness of Impulse Conduction

There are two primary factors determining the effectiveness of transmission of the cardiac impulse through the specialized conduction tissues of the heart. One of these conditions is the strength in mV and speed of the impulse itself; a depolarization of large magnitude, traveling rapidly, is more effective in transmitting the excitation to fibers farther along in the sequence of activation. Some of the conditions known to affect strength and speed of the impulse are alteration in the content of K^+ in the serum, ischemia, hypoxia, and some drugs, including digitalis and quinidine.

A second factor affecting adequacy of impulse transmission is the excitability of the conducting fibers receiving the impulse from more proximal regions, in other words, a change in their threshold for excitation. If the diastolic threshold is increased, then a normal impulse is no longer capable of depolarizing it, and conduction block develops. One of the factors which standardly alters the capacity of a tissue to respond to a simulus is the absolute and relative refractory periods which accompany and follow a previous excitation. When fibers receiving a stimulus to contract are in the absolute refractory period, then no impulse can stimulate them; when they are relatively refractory, then a larger than normal stimulus is required, and the response that results is weak and slow. Therefore, the refractory period is an important determinant of the ability of tissues in the heart to respond to an impulse. Many influences are able to alter the refractory period of conduction tissues in the heart: adequacy of myocardial oxygenation, electrolyte balance, hormonal and neural influences, pharmacologic agents, and in fact the heart rate itself.

Examples of Types of Abnormal Impulse Conduction

Decremental Conduction

This term refers to a decline in both the speed and strength of the cardiac impulse, accompanied by a decrease in degree of response, as the wave of excitation proceeds along the conduction pathways. This decrementing is most likely to occur in tissues such as the AV node in which there is already under normal conditions a slowing in rate and decline in amplitude of the impulse.

Nonuniform (Irregular) Conduction

This term refers to a breakup or fragmentation of the wave of negativity because of a change in the structural or functional properties of a portion of the conduction pathway which the stimulus has entered. When the individual fibers of a portion of the conduction path are straight, regular and compact, as in the bundle branch system, the wave of negativity remains well integrated, fast and strong. However, in a portion of the conduction system with small, irregular, more dispersed individual fibers, such as the AV node, the impulse tends to disperse, slow, and weaken even under normal conditions. Local ischemia, hypoxia, or patchy arteriosclerotic changes, or local alteration in ionic balance, can disseminate and weaken the impulse still more until it is blocked.

Both decremental and nonuniform conduction are suggested by some workers to be responsible for conduction delay, conduction blocks, reciprocal beats, and the development of certain paroxysmal tachycardias.

Undirectional Block

This is a situation in which an area having depressed conduction permits the wave of depolarization to proceed in one direction, but inhibits its propagation in the opposite direction. Put another way, the impulse may be unable to proceed in the direction of the normal forward pathway (anterograde conduction) but may be able to pass in the opposite direction (retrograde conduction). This process is suggested to be responsible for the mechanism of reentry. A diagram of one form of unidirectional block and its relationship to the genesis of reentry is shown in Figure 6-7.

MECHANISMS FOR ARRHYTHMIAS RESULTING FROM COMBINED ABNORMALITIES OF IMPULSE FORMATION AND IMPULSE CONDUCTION

It should be emphasized that the electrophysiologic processes involved in the genesis of arrhythmias seen in the clinical situation are not known, and that the

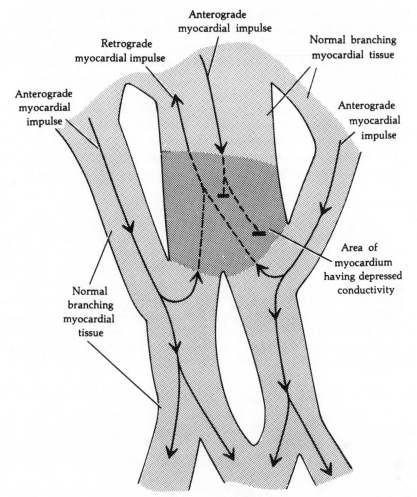

Figure 6-7. A proposed mechanism involved in the development of unidirectional block. The diagram shows a typical segment of branching myocardial conduction tissue. Normal direction (anterograde) of conduction of the impulse is downward. A portion of the wave of activation encounters an area of depressed conduction. When the tissue divides, the wave is weakened and dies out in the forward (downward) direction in the area of impaired conduction. In the normal areas of myocardium to either side the wave of activation continues, bypassing the depressed segment. Beyond it, the two normal anterograde portions of the impulse converge when the tissue reanastomoses; this strengthens the wave of activation which now is able to penetrate the block retrogradely, producing a reentry effect, as well as continuing anterogradely in the remainder of the myocardium.

following represents speculations of workers in the area, rather than demonstrated facts.

Premature Contraction of Atria or Ventricles

There are two theories of possible mechanisms responsible for this common arrhythmia. Some investigators suggest that the type of ectopic beat which follows a previous normal impulse and contraction by a constant interval (coupled beat) arises as a result of oscillations in the membrane potential of cells in the ectopic focus. The oscillations in membrane potential are an abnormal response to the previous action potential, and are proposed to involve the slow Ca^{2+} membrane channels active during the recovery process (phase 2 repolarization).

The second theory proposes a process of reentry caused by an area of conducting tissue or myocardium which has a prolonged refractory period or in which conductivity is depressed because of some abnormality such as local ischemia or hypoxia. The impulse fails to stimulate the area and goes around it. Then by the time the impulse has attained the other side of the obstacle, the latter has regained its excitability or conductivity and the impulse retrogradely reenters the formerly depressed area, resulting in an ectopic beat time-coupled to the prior contraction (Figure 6-7).

Parasystole

Unlike the above, this arrhythmia is suggested to result from a regular depolarization of, and therefore automaticity in, an ectopic focus independent of the normal rhythm. Therefore, it acts as an independent impulse-generating center which competes with the normal center generating the basic rhythm. It is speculated to be protected from the normal impulses by a ring of myocardial tissues with depressed conduction, which sets up a unidirectional block, called a protection block, which prevents impulses coming from the basic pacemaker from depolarizing and thus controlling the parasystolic focus. This process is shown diagramatically in Figure 6-8.

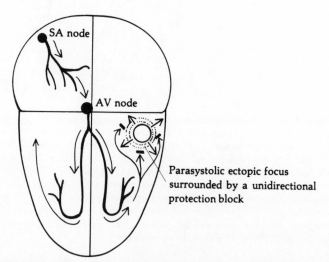

Figure 6-8. Proposed mechanism for arrhythmias caused by parasystole. The parasystolic ectopic focus of impulse generation is surrounded by a ring of myocardial tissue with abnormal conduction and a unidirectional protection block. The normal impulses generated from the SA and AV nodes are unable to penetrate the ring of tissue surrounding the parasystolic focus, depolarize it, and therefore suppress it. However, since the block in the ring of tissue is unidirectional, impulses generated from the parasystolic focus can spread to the remainder of the myocardium, generate impulses and contractions and therefore compete with the normal pacemaker. In short, the block around the focus is unidirectional so that normal impulses cannot get in but the abnormal parasystolic ones can get out, resulting in a parasystolic arrhythmia.

Ectopic Tachycardias

These common arrhythmias may result from an increased rate of phase 4 diastolic depolarization in some portion of the conduction system, or automaticity may develop even in regular atrial or ventricular myocardium. If the increased excitability and rate of impulse formation in the ectopic focus exceeds that of the basic (usually sinus) rhythm, then it may take over as the pacemaker for the heart. This is considered by some workers to be the mechanism for nonparoxysmal tachycardia.

Another possible mechanism for ectopic tachycardia is a repeating reentry process such as that shown in Figure 6-9; the impulses alternate or reciprocate, one coming directly but intermittently through an area of unilaterally impaired conduction from the pacemaker of the basic rhythm, which is conducted anterogradely; alternating with a reentry impulse conducted retrogradely around a unidirectional intermittent block. This is thought by some authors to be a mechanism responsible for paroxysmal tachycardia. If conduction improves in the blocked area, then the paroxysmal ectopic tachycardia will disappear because the reentry mechanism is abolished. Similarly, if the block becomes bidirectional, the tachycardia will also disappear because now neither antegrade nor retrograde pathways will conduct and so the reentry process is halted.

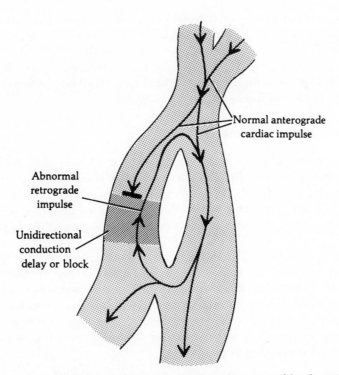

Normal anterograde cardiac impulse

Abnormal retrograde impulse

Unidirectional conduction delay or block

Figure 6-9. Proposed mechanism for an ectopic tachycardia generated by alternating or reciprocating impulses, one of which comes anterogradely and with intermittent unidirectional blocking through a region of impaired conduction; the other comes retrogradely from the impulses bypassing the block.

Flutter and Fibrillation

These common arrhythmias of older individuals are considered by some workers to result from a combination of electrical abnormalities, including multiple impulse formation in combination with multiple reentry sites. Therefore flutter and fibrillation could result from the processes illustrated in Figures 6-8 and 6-9 occurring at numerous sites throughout the myocardium.

CIRCULATORY CONSEQUENCES OF CARDIAC ARRHYTHMIAS

A cardiac arrhythmia may be asymptomatic or may produce symptoms and/or signs; the nature and magnitude of the consequences depend importantly upon the age of the patient and whether he has a basically healthy heart or one with organic disease.

Just as arrhythmias may be the consequence of either heart or systemic diseases, so such alterations of heart rate and rhythm may in turn be the cause of damage to the heart itself, especially if its function is already impaired, or to other body parts. These deleterious effects stem from the fact that irregularities of rate and rhythm alter cardiac function through several mechanisms.

Increased Myocardial O_2 Consumption

Tachycardia increases myocardial oxygen consumption; the need for increased oxygen to meet heart and peripheral tissue metabolic requirements rises with physical exertion, therefore a myocardium only marginally capable of meeting its own or systemic oxygen needs under basal conditions at a normal rate, may be unable to meet its oxygen need during a tachyarrythmia, and even less so with the added burden of increased physical activity.

Decreased Diastolic Filling Time

Another adverse effect of tachycardia is the shortening of diastolic filling time; as heart rate increases, the time during which venous return can adequately fill the ventricles is reduced. As ventricular filling declines, ventricular contractility similarly falls according to the Frank-Starling relationship which relates fiber length to force of contraction (Chapter 7) causing a further drop in cardiac output.

The bulk of blood flow through the coronary arteries occurs during diastole; in systole coronary resistance increases markedly because ventricle muscle is contracted. Tachycardia shortens diastolic filling time and thus decreases the period during which maximum coronary artery perfusion can occur. Decreased coronary perfusion, combined with ischemic heart disease and the elevated myocardial oxygen requirements of tachycardia, can lead to a worsening of myocardial ischemia or an actual infarction.

Decreased Cardiac Output

Bradycardia similarly results in a decline in cardiac output, particularly in those diseased hearts where compensatory increases in stroke volume cannot occur.

Since cardiac output is a function of stroke volume and heart rate, patients with a stroke volume restricted by heart disease are therefore dependent on increased heart rate to meet metabolic demand. Such patients, during bradycardia, may experience severe impairment of cardiac output, and therefore of exercise tolerance.

Alteration in the normal sequence of chamber contraction, because of abnormal patterns of electrical activation, may impair both the active atrial "booster pump" contribution to ventricular diastolic filling, and the normal synchronicity of ventricular contraction during systolic ejection. Asynchronous ventricular contraction leads to a slower rise in the rate of increase of ventricular pressure during systole, a lower systolic arterial pressure, and a less effective ventricular performance. A decline in cardiac output is the consequence. An orderly sequence of myocardial depolarization and hence of contraction in both ventricles is important for optimal effectiveness of cardiac action and maintenance of cardiac output.

Compensatory Vasoconstriction

These processes which cause a primary decrease in cardiac output in arrhythmias, also induce the secondary compensatory response of vasoconstriction. The reduced cardiac output causes a decline in perfusion to the aortic arch and carotid sinus baroreceptors, which in turn activate the brainstem vasomotor response mediated via the sympathetic adrenergic division of the autonomic nervous system. The renal and splanchnic vasculature receive reduced blood supply because of the lowered cardiac output; the perfusion to the organs is further reduced by differential vasoconstriction. The combined effects may be to reduce visceral blood flow by 25 to 50%. Progressive renal vasoconstriction may persist for long periods, even after correction of the arrhythmia, and may lead to oliguria, prerenal azotemia, proteinuria, and even acute tubular necrosis (Chapter 10). Mesenteric vasoconstriction may lead to vascular spasm and acute vascular insufficiency. The consequences may be adynamic ileus, abdominal pain and distention, acute ulceration or even bowel infarction.

Decreased Cerebral and Coronary Artery Blood Flow

Cerebral blood flow is also markedly impaired, to 25 to 50% of normal, depending upon the arrhythmia. A younger person with a normal cerebral vasculature may tolerate such reduction reasonably well, but in an older patient with atherosclerotic cerebrovascular insufficiency there may be marked symptoms of signs of cerebral ischemia: light-headedness or "dizziness," weakness, syncope, visual field defects, blurring or darkening of vision, paresthesias, mental confusion, seizures, or even cerebral infarction.

Cardiac arrhythmias may, and often do, feed back to cause further damage to the heart itself. Coronary artery perfusion may decline by half during certain arrhythmias. If this decline is coupled with underlying ischemic heart disease, as mentioned above, myocardial infarction may occur; or if it already has, it may extend, because of the discrepancy between myocardial oxygen requirements and coronary artery blood supply (Chapter 5).

SPECIFIC CARDIAC ARRHYTHMIAS

Disturbances of heart rate and rhythm may occur in individuals with apparently normal hearts as well as in patients with a wide variety of structural or physiologic cardiovascular abnormalities. They may be precipitated by metabolic disorders; fluid, electrolyte, or acid–base derangements; hormonal imbalances; arterial blood gas disturbances; vascular impairments; hypo- or hyperthermia; or secondary to drugs or toxins. Disorders of cardiac rate and rhythm may be a sign of some fundamental abnormality within the heart itself, or of a general systemic disorder. Therefore they constitute an alerting signal to evaluate the patient for such possible causative factors. Often cardiac arrhythmias are the manifestations of serious intrinsic heart disease, and frequently certain ones are characteristic of such specific diseases.

Alterations of Rate and Rhythm Arising in the Sinus Node

Sinus Arrhythmia

This is a normal phenomenon especially in young persons and consists of regular fluctuations in sinus rate correlated with the phases of the respiratory cycle. During inspiration, vagal cardioinhibitory impulses from stretch receptors in the lung inhibit the cardioinhibitory center in the lower brainstem and the heart rate accelerates. During expiration the rate again slows as normal vagal tone resumes. These changes are enhanced during slow deep breathing and are abolished with breath holding.

Sinus Bradycardia

Sinus bradycardia is defined as a heart rate less than 60 and is the expected finding in trained athletes. The usual rate is 45–59. It is sometimes found in elderly persons, especially during sleep and just after awakening, and may result from degenerative changes in the brainstem cardioregulatory centers, in the reflex pathways between the centers and the sinus node, or within the sinus node itself. It is not usually a matter of concern provided heart rate shows the normal increase with exercise. If the rate drops below the inherent rate of automaticity in subsidiary pacemakers below the sinus node, an escape rhythm generated in these latent pacemakers may emerge and control ventricular contractions. This may lead to AV dissociation or an AV junctional escape rhythm. Usually this condition is benign. Sinus bradycardia also is often caused by increased parasympathetic cholinergic stimuli from the vagus nerves in normal persons of all ages.

Sinus bradycardia is seen in certain systemic abnormalities such as hypothyroidism, elevated intracranial pressure, and hypothermia; and may be caused by pharmacologic agents: morphine, digitalis, propranolol, reserpine, and guanethidine. It may be an early sign of digitalis toxicity when it develops suddenly. It seldom causes symptoms in otherwise normal persons unless the rate drops below 35, when the person may experience lightheadedness. Syncope rarely occurs. If the patient has heart disease, such as congestive heart failure or a myocardial infarction, symptoms and signs may occur at a higher rate. If treatment is considered necessary, atropine (a cholinergic blocker) or a sympathomimetic amine such as isoproterenol or ephedrine may be used.

Sinus Tachycardia

Sinus tachycardia refers in adults to heart rates above 100 with a normal sinus rhythm and is a normal accompaniment to physical exertion, emotional arousal or exercise. It accompanies abnormal conditions such as fever by a direct, metabolic response of the heart to elevated temperature; and is an adrenergic (sympathetic autonomic) compensatory mechanism for the abnormally low cardiac output of dehydration, hypovolemia, hypotension and left ventricular failure. It is promoted by such parasympathetic blocking agents as atropine which interfere with the normal flow of tonic vagal impulses; and is caused by sympathetic adrenergic stimulation and the catecholamines norepinephrine and epinephrine.

Tachycardia is characteristic of certain systemic disorders such as thyrotoxicosis, pheochromocytoma, and pulmonary infections, especially if the latter are superimposed upon the hypoxemia of chronic obstructive pulmonary disease.

During tachycardia a functional systolic heart murmur may be present. In most persons tachycardia causes no symptoms, but in others it may lead to restlessness, apprehension and complaints of palpitations. Management consists of treating the underlying condition, whatever it may be, since the pathologic significance of sinus tachycardia depends on the causative factor.

Sick Sinus Syndrome (Bradycardia–Tachycardia Syndrome)

This arrhythmia takes a variety of forms and results from abnormal function of the sinus node; it may be manifested as sinus bradycardia which is often unresponsive to pharmacologic agents and which persists with exercise. It sometimes alternates with a supraventricular tachycardia. It is most frequently seen in patients who have underlying heart disease, hypertensive or arteriosclerotic, and is associated with a progressive fibrosis of the conduction system. Patients may complain of fatigue, dypsnea, or lightheadedness. A permanent pacemaker may be necessary in patients who are severely symptomatic, or who experience syncope and periodic sinus arrest.

Sinus Arrest

This is a failure of impulse formation in the SA node. It is caused by increased vagal tone or a hypersensitive carotid sinus reflex, or by quinidine or digitalis excess. Other causes are strong carotid sinus stimulation, hyperkalemia, a myocardial infarction, or myocarditis. When sinus arrest occurs, A-V junctional escape beats and rhythms may develop and control the ventricular contractions, but more often sinus rhythm is restored spontaneously before this occurs. If the pause is long the subject may faint. Death may result if the sinus rhythm does not resume and if no subsidiary pacemaker evolves.

Alterations of Rate and Rhythm Arising in the Atria

Premature Atrial Contractions (Ectopic Atrial Beats, Atrial Extrasystoles)

These are usually premature activations of the atria which originate in a spontaneous depolarization of some atrial area outside of the sinus node—that is, they arise in an ectopic atrial focus—usually (but not always) prior to the next normal impulse from the sinus node. Such an ectopic impulse will usually pass into the sinus node, depolarize it, and reset it. Therefore, there may be a pause in the next normal sinus impulse with respect to the previous normal one. This is called a postectopic pause. This arrhythmia is common and often occurs in normal persons as a consequence of excess alcohol, caffeine, or tobacco use, or in emotional stress.

In pathologic states, atrial arrhythmias tend to occur when pressures are increased in the atria from any cause. PACs are seen in patients with organic heart disease such as cor pulmonale secondary to chronic lung disease; rheumatic valvular disease, especially mitral stenosis; and occasionally in coronary artery disease. They may signal incipient atrial flutter, fibrillation, or ectopic atrial tachycardia; quinidine is usually effective in suppressing them. P waves of the EKG may appear abnormal because of the different sequence of atrial activation from that occurring in normal sinus stimulation.

Atrial Fibrillation

This disorder is 10 to 20 times more common than atrial flutter and is often associated with organic heart disease such as arteriosclerotic, hypertensive or rheumatic, and with the endocrine disorder thyrotoxicosis. The most common cause is rheumatic heart disease with mitral stenosis, because of enlargement of the left atrium. It is the most common atrial arrhythmia in older persons. It tends to last for hours or days rather than for a few minutes. It is sometimes precipitated by emotional upset, and is common in acute bronchitis superimposed on chronic obstructive pulmonary disease and cor pulmonale. It may originate anywhere in the atria outside the SA node.

It is thought to be caused by so-called circus movements low in the atria; a continuous ring of circling depolarizations give off series of separate wave fronts which then themselves initiate multiple smaller wave fronts of depolarization and non-coordinated contraction. There are no coordinated atrial contractions, only vermicular ("bag of worms") motion, so that the normal atrial contribution to ventricular filling is lost. This may result in impaired cardiac output especially in patients with the thickened ventricular wall of cardiac hypertrophy. Ventricular function is further impaired because of the chaotic nature of impulse conduction to the ventricles; some impulses are blocked because of the normal relatively long AV nodal conduction time, and some are conducted; the consequence for ventricular contraction is a rapid rate with an irregular irregularity of rhythm. Cardiac output then falls, and in the patient with impaired myocardial contractility, congestive heart failure may develop if the arrhythmia is protracted, because it increases ventricular rate above the level of dynamic efficiency. The EKG shows an absence of P waves and normal but irregular QRS complexes at a rate of 120 to 150 or more. However the ventricular rate may be normal, especially in elderly patients, because there may be an AV nodal conduction block of some of the impulses.

A serious consequence of the lack of coordinated blood flow and the turbulence in the atria is initiation of the clotting mechanism with the formation of thrombi and emboli. These may be released into the pulmonary circuit from the right atrium; or into the systemic circuit, including the cerebral circulation, from the left atrium.

The attacks may be paroxysmal and brief, or persistent for days. On occasion atrial fibrillation may become chronic and continue for years, particularly in rheumatic mitral valve disease. The patient may experience no symptoms, or may feel dyspnea, angina, or hypotension from the low cardiac output. Treatment includes pharmacologic slowing or conversion with digitalis, propranolol, or quinidine; or DC countershock conversion.

Atrial Flutter

This arrhythmia is characterized by rapid, very regular rates of atrial depolarization and contraction of about 220 to 320. It is often paroxysmal. Because of the AV node's refractory period, which inhibits it from conducting impulses to the ventricles at rates higher than about 200 to 250, AV block is usually present at a 2:1, 4:1, or 6:1 ratio, with ventricular rates of about 75 to 160 depending on the block ratio. Uneven number blocks are less frequent (3:1, 5:1). The usual ventricular response rate is 2:1. It may originate anywhere in the atria outside the SA node. Sometimes it is paroxysmal, but may persist chronically for extended periods. Although it is less common than atrial fibrillation, there may be changes back and forth between flutter and fibrillation; quinidine often changes fibrillation to flutter, and digitalis may do the reverse.

Atrial flutter is an arrhythmia of older persons and is often associated with organic heart disease: coronary atherosclerosis, valvular disease, or cor pulmonale. The degree to which the patient is symptomatic will depend not only on the underlying causative abnormalities but also importantly on the ventricular response rate. If this is low, the patient may be asymptomatic; but at high rates, angina, left ventricular failure, shortness of breath, and disturbing palpitations may occur. The atrioventricular conduction ratio is less predictable in flutter than in fibrillation; patients may have an abrupt transition from 4:1 to 2:1 precipitated by eating, emotional arousal, physical exertion, or even a change in posture. Thus the ventricular rate may go suddenly from 100 to 200 per minute on the basis of a changed ventricular response to the flutter. These rapid increases in ventricular response rate with minor activity may produce a rapid onset of increased pulmonary capillary pressure and dyspnea on the basis of sudden left ventricular overload.

The mechanism for atrial flutter is proposed to be similar to that of atrial fibrillation: circus movements with reentry, but in flutter the repeating circuit is suggested to be a larger portion of the atrium with more regular subsidiary waves of excitation and contraction, accounting for the regular rate of contraction.

A frequent treatment of flutter is digitalis which reduces the ventricular rate both by a direct inhibitory action on the myocardium and conduction system, and stimulation of vagal slowing of AV transmission. It increases the duration of refractoriness of the AV conduction pathway. Quinidine is then used for maintenance in an attempt to prevent recurrence. DC countershock may be successful in producing conversion to normal sinus rhythm where pharmacologic management has failed; digitalis may be withheld for several days prior to electrical conversion.

Supraventricular Paroxysmal Tachycardia

This is a perfectly regular very rapid rhythm with a rate of 140 to 250, having an abrupt onset and abrupt cessation, of which the patient is usually emphatically aware. Atrial to ventricular conduction ratio is almost always 1:1. There are two closely related types: paroxysmal atrial ectopic and AV junctional tachycardia, which are quite similar in their clinical signs and symptoms, causes and consequences. They are placed together by some authors because of the fact that electrocardiographic studies indicate the close electrophysiologic similarities between them and because it is often difficult to distinguish between them. They both occur in individuals of all ages including young apparently healthy persons (about 30% of cases) and may be seen in patients with a number of types of heart disease: arteriosclerotic, hypertensive and rheumatic. They also may occur in digitalis toxicity. In the otherwise well person the attacks sometimes seem to bear an association to gastrointestinal upsets, fatigue, use of coffee, alcohol or tobacco, and emotional arousal. It is thought to be caused in these cases by adrenergic stimulation mediated by the central nervous system.

Associated signs and symptoms may develop because of the reduced cardiac output (see above) including those of myocardial ischemia, diaphoresis, left ventricular failure, inadequate cerebral perfusion and even cardiogenic shock. If the patient has no heart disease palpitations may be the only symptom. The cardiac output declines significantly if the heart rate is over 180. Angina pectoris may develop with the onset of the tachycardia, even in patients with no known history of coronary artery disease, because of the high myocardial oxygen requirements caused by the tachycardia; S-T segment changes may accompany the anginal pain (Chapter 4).

The mechanism for the arrhythmia appears to be reentry (see above and Figure 6-9). When an ectopic beat encounters delay in the anterograde (forward) conduction system, because of refractoriness, the impulse may divert to an adjacent responsive pathway, bypassing the unresponsive area. It may then be conducted in a retrograde manner back to the atrium; if the anterograde normal pathway is now capable of being stimulated the impulse may traverse and activate it. The sequence can be repeated in a reciprocating manner, alternating between the two alternate pathways, one normal and the other abnormal, resulting in the very rapid regular pattern. It is the reentry process which appears to cause a high association of paroxysmal tachycardia with Wolff–Parkinson–White syndrome (see following).

Individuals susceptible to these attacks often learn to terminate them by self-stimulation of the parasympathetic cardioinhibitory reflexes mediated efferently by the vagus nerve: such procedures include inducing gagging, unilateral (usually right) carotid sinus stimulation by nonocclusive massage just below the angle of the jaw, or a Valsalva maneuver (straining against a closed glottis). These procedures increase vagal tone and cause cholinergic delay of AV junctional transmission by increasing the refractory period. Digitalis or propranolol produce similar effects pharmacologically, as do the cholinesterase inhibitors neostigmine or edrophonium. Edrophonium may be administered intravenously with simultaneous carotid sinus massage. Propranolol is the drug of choice for tachyarrhythmias secondary to Wolff–Parkinson–White syndrome. Where these arrhythmias are associated with emotional tension in a healthy young person without heart disease, giving phenobarbital or diazepam in a moderate dose may induce reversion to normal sinus rhythm. If these measures are not effective, an attempt may be made to induce reflex vagal stimulation with the use of a pressor agent such as phenylephrine or metaraminol. These agents raise blood pressure by causing vasoconstriction, and therefore elicit activation of the baroreceptor reflexes which in turn produces strong reflex vagal slowing of the heart. Prophylactic suppression of atrial extrasystoles by digitalis or quinidine may be required if attacks are frequent or severe, since premature atrial contractions are a common precipitating factor.

Alterations of Rate and Rhythm Arising in the AV Junction

There are two basic processes responsible for production of the various junctional arrhythmias: (1) so-called "active impulse formation," in which a subsidiary pacemaker may increase its rate of spontaneous depolarization above its normal inherently slower rate, so that it comes to exceed the rate of discharge of the more proximal pacemaker; and (2) "passive impulse formation," resulting from emergence of the natural rate of junctional impulse formation, either because of depression in the rate of the normal pacemaker, or a block in conduction of its impulses. Contractions resulting from "active" impulse generation are *premature* contractions, and cause AV junctional premature beats or an AV junctional tachycardia; the mechanism is abnormal acceleration of the rate of impulse formation in junctional tissue. Contractions resulting from "passive" impulse generation are called *postmature* contractions, because they arise after the normal sinus impulse should have arrived to initiate contraction. They result in AV junctional escape beats or rhythm.

Junctional Premature Contractions (Ectopic Junctional Beats)

This arrhythmia is the result of "active" impulse formation as described above. The impulses probably do not arise in the AV node itself, since His bundle electrograms have not demonstrated pacemaker activity in that area, but rather in areas proximal or distal to it. The impulses may show an abnormal P wave either preceding or following a normal or abnormal QRS, depending on whether the point of origin of the impulse is above or below the His bundle. The impulse generated in the AV junctional tissue is often conducted in two directions simultaneously: the retrograde impulse activates the atria (atrial capture) and the anterograde impulse activates the ventricles. Junctional premature contractions are much less common than either atrial or ventricular premature contractions; they often occur in normal hearts, do not usually cause signs or symptoms, and require no treatment. Digitalis, quinidine, or diphenylhydantoin suppress them.

Paroxysmal Junctional Tachycardia

See paroxysmal supraventricular tachycardia.

Nonparoxysmal AV Junctional Tachycardia

This arrhythmia results from enhanced automaticity of junctional tissue; its rate is 100 to 140, as compared with the usual inherent rate of 45–60 of AV junctional tissue. It has a regular rhythm, and lacks abrupt onset and termination. It almost always is seen in the presence of heart disease. The cause is thought to be an increase in the rate of phase 4 diastolic depolarization caused by altered membrane permeability resulting from ischemic or hypoxic cell damage, or the toxic effects of digitalis. It is seen in myocardial infarction, acute rheumatic fever and digitalis toxicity. In the latter cause it may presage ventricular tachycardia or fibrillation.

The atrial rhythm is often atrial fibrillation. When the sinus node or an ectopic atrial pacemaker controls the atria, and the junctional rhythm controls the ventricles, then these two centers fire independently, and complete dissociation of atrial and junction-initiated ventricular contractions occurs. This is called AV dissociation. Conversely, when the ventricular rate is higher than the atrial rate, and retrograde conduction of the impulse from the junction to the atria takes place, the junctional tachycardia acts as the pacemaker of the heart; the junctional beats are said to "capture" the atria. Alternatively, intermittent impulses from the atria may penetrate the junctional focus, periodically capturing the ventricles. Thus there may be complete AV dissociation, or combinations of AV dissociation alternating with atrial and/or ventricular capture.

Junctional tachycardia may occur in patients with myocardial infarction, myocarditis, or after heart surgery; the most common cause is digitalis toxicity. It may produce congestive heart failure, angina, weakness, lightheadedness, and apprehension. If digitalis is the cause, that drug should be stopped and diphenylhydantoin or other drugs (i.e., propranolol, potassium) may be used to suppress the arrhythmia.

AV Junctional Rhythm

This is an escape rhythm—an example of postmature beats or so-called "passive" impulse formation. It may arise when the rate of sinus impulse formation declines below the inherent rate of junctional tissue (that is, below about 45–60); or in a conduction block of the AV node. It is therefore a *normal protective mechanism* to activate the ventricles and maintain cardiac output in the event of failure of normal impulse formation or conduction. It may be seen in the presence of many different types of cardiac arrhythmia, including an ectopic atrial tachycardia, or atrial fibrillation or flutter, where the atrial impulses fail to be conducted to the AV junction because of an AV block. The AV junctional rhythm then arises as the escape pacemaker for the ventricles. AV junctional rhythm also occurs in conjunction with sinus arrest, sinus bradycardia and second or third degree AV block. The ventricular rate is about 45 to 60 and regular and the QRS is normal.

Most often AV junctional escape rhythms occur in conjunction with complete AV dissociation (see following). In complete AV dissociation the atria and ventricles beat independently, therefore the P waves and QRS complexes are unrelated to each other.

An AV junctional escape rhythm may occur as a consequence of digitalis toxicity, in ischemic disease of the myocardium, in congestive heart failure, in myocardial infarction, or in normal persons with sinus bradycardia. If the rate is so low as to cause impairment in the circulation, atropine or isoproterenol may be indicated. The management depends upon the cause and is therefore related to treatment of the underlying condition.

Alterations of Rate and Rhythm Arising in the Ventricles

Ventricular arrhythmias may develop on the basis of either "active" (premature) or "passive" (postmature) impulse formation. In the case of *premature* beats and rhythms, ventricular arrhythmias develop as a result of enhanced automaticity above that of the normal rate of impulse generation in the ventricles, which is always very slow. In the case of *postmature* beats and rhythms, they develop as a consequence of a delay or failure of conduction of a more proximal pacemaker impulse. Regardless of the mechanism, ventricular arrhythmias may originate from any region of the ventricles. The appearance of the QRS complex will depend upon the site of origin of the impulse. If the origin is high in the ventricles the QRS may be relatively normal. If the site is more distal, the pathway of conduction and activation of the ventricles is more aberrant and the complex will be distorted and wide.

Premature Ventricular Contractions (Ventricular Premature Beats, Ventricular Extrasystoles, Ectopic Ventricular Beats)

Ventricular premature contractions are the most common ectopic beats and probably are the most frequently occurring of all arrhythmias. PVCs occur in persons without heart disease, as a result of emotional arousal or anxiety, fatigue, and excessive use of alcohol, cigarets, or caffeine; in these circumstances they are often not of any significance. They sometimes occur after exercise in otherwise normal individuals after such activities as jogging, but tend to decrease or not occur once physical fitness improves.

The importance of the central and automatic nervous system in generating these ectopic beats has been emphasized by many authors. Fear, excitement, anxiety, and worry about the outcome of an important event all appear to be associated with increased incidence of PVCs. The mechanism for this observed relationship is probably an increase in sympathetic adrenergic impulses to the heart via the cardiac nerves; these stimuli then induce an increased rate of phase 4 diastolic depolarization, and therefore enhanced automaticity, in the fibers of the Purkinje system. PVCs are reported to decrease in frequency during sleep, especially slow-wave sleep. It is said that in patients without organic heart disease, PVCs tend to disappear with exercise; while in patients with heart disease, PVCs tend to appear or increase in frequency. In such patients, participation in an exercise rehabilitation program results in decrease or disappearance of PVCs as physical conditioning develops.

Ventricular premature beats increase with increasing age, and are common in older persons, even in the absence of any demonstrable heart disease. Often these contractions produce no symptoms, but sometimes patients may be aware of the forceful contraction which follows the compensatory pause. This pause results from the fact that the ectopic impulse, coming prior to the next normal impulse from the primary pacemaker (normally the sinus node), depolarizes the ventricular conduction pathways and working myocardium. Therefore, they are in their refractory period when the next normal stimulus arrives and cannot respond to the stimulus. This is often felt by the person as a "skipped beat." The compensatory pause in the series of ventricular contractions then occurs until the next normal sinus impulse arrives. Since this period has been longer than the usual time between ventricular contractions, the diastolic filling period is prolonged, the ventricle volume increases over the normal, and according to the Frank-Starling relation, the force of the next contraction is considerably greater than usual. This is felt as a "thump."

Frequently occurring PVCs, especially if they originate in different sites of the ventricular myocardium (multifocal PVCs) are very often indications of either organic heart disease, or digitalis intoxication, or both. In particular in ischemic heart disease from coronary artery atherosclerosis PVCs are associated with the development of ventricular tachycardia, ventricular fibrillation, and sudden death. Also, persons with asymptomatic coronary artery disease have been shown to have an increased incidence of this arrhythmia as compared with age-matched controls. Holter EKG monitoring of ambulatory patients over a 24-hour period, and graded treadmill or bicycle ergometer exercise stress testing during EKG monitoring, has shown considerably higher prevalence of PVCs than was formerly assumed. Some prospective studies of life expectancy and clinical course in patients who develop PVCs during exercise, as compared with those who do not, have indicated significantly greater incidence of sudden death or infarction in the former group. It has also been reported that in the months following recovery from a myocardial infarction the occurrence of many PVCs is correlated with a threefold higher incidence of sudden death. Thus prophylactic suppression of this ectopic activity constitutes a significant aspect of management in post-AMI rehabilitation regimens.

Among patients with established heart disease, PVCs are very common following myocardial infarction, especially in the early hours; they are of great significance in predicting ventricular tachycardia in the first few post-AMI days; and they often presage ventricular fibrillation. Criteria have been provided for evaluating the pathologic significance of PVC's, and their prognostic importance in heart disease. PVCs are said to be malignant if they show one or more of the following qualities: more than 6 or 7 per minute; originate in different sites (multiform and multifocal); occur in couplets or triplets; and appear early in the cardiac cycle, that is, if they encroach on the T wave. This latter situation is termed the R on T phenomenon. The vulnerable period of the ventricle coincides with the T wave; this is the time at the end of the relatively refractory period when a smaller than normal stimulus is capable of producing ventricular fibrillation, because the threshold for ventricular excitability is very low at this time.

Unifocal PVCs (those originating in a single ectopic site in the bundle branch, fascicle, or Purkinje system) usually have a constant coupling interval with the prior normal beat; the mechanism for initiation of the ectopic beat is dependent upon an abnormal response (such as incomplete repolarization or oscillation of membrane potential) to the prior action potential. The result of this coupling is ventricular bigeminy, in which a single ventricular extrasystole occurs at a regular interval following each normal beat. Or the PVC may occur regularly every third or fourth normal ventricular contraction. Conversely, when PVCs arise from two or more locales in the ventricular conduction system, the interval between the ectopic beat and the prior normal beat will vary. Characteristically the electrocardiographic appearance of a PVC is a wide and distorted QRS complex appearing without a preceding P wave and prematurely with respect to the QRS complexes of the basic rhythm.

Significant circulatory impairment is infrequent in occasional ventricular extrasystoles, but if the contractions are frequent, or occur in runs, then they result in a marked decline in cardiac output and may cause cerebral symptoms of faintness or lightheadedness, exercise intolerance and dyspnea, increased congestive heart failure, and weakness. Also the decline in cardiac output reduces coronary artery perfusion and impairs myocardial oxygenation, which may result in worsening of angina or even an infarction.

Frequency of PVCs increases in systemic abnormalities such as hypoxia, hypercapnia, electrolyte and acid–base disturbances, abnormally low or high body temperature, hypotension, and hypovolemia.

The management of this arrhythmia depends upon the causative or precipitating factors. The primary objective of treatment is to prevent ventricular tachycardia, fibrillation, and sudden death. When PVCs occur in otherwise healthy persons in association with emotional tension and injudicious lifestyle elements, a modification of these factors coupled with reassurance as to the benign nature of the arrhythmia is warranted.

Certain drugs are associated with an increased incidence of PVCs, especially the psychotropic drugs of the phenothiazine and tricyclic antidepressant groups. PVCs are also rarely a side effect of the cholesterol-lowering drug clofibrate. The association of digitalis toxicity with PVCs, especially in the presence of hypokalemia, is frequent; the incidence increases with the severity of the underlying heart disease.

Pharmacologic antiarrhythmic suppression of PVCs in ambulatory patients may be indicated if certain criteria are met: (1) if exercise induces runs of ventricular tachycardia, or if these appear with Holter 24-hour ambulatory monitoring; (2) if premature beats are frequent (more than 6/min); (3) if they are multifocal; and (4) if the R on T phenomenon occurs. Where digitalis toxicity is a cause, this necessitates temporary withdrawal, a check for a low serum potassium level, and possible use of diphenylhydantoin. In the case of myocardial ischemia from coronary artery disease, antiarrhythmic medication is given for the advent of "malignant" PVCs since studies seem to indicate that such intervention reduces the incidence of serious ventricular arrhythmias, although their effects in decreasing longer term morbidity and overall mortality have yet to be demonstrated in well-controlled clinical studies.

Antiarrhythmic pharmacologic agents used for suppressing malignant PVCs include: (1) quinidine, a widely used oral drug which decreases the rate of depolarization of the conduction system, and prolongs the refractory period; (2) procainamide, which is suitable for either oral or parenteral use and has actions similar to quinidine; (3) lidocaine, a parenterally administered agent which reduces depolarization rate as well as the refractory period; (4) propranolol, a β-adrenergic blocking agent; and (5) diphenylhydantoin, which has effects on the heart similar to lidocaine and is useful in PVCs caused by excessive digitalis. Disopyramide is a newer agent having an action like quinidine. All of these drugs have potential side effects; quinidine may cause rashes, light-headedness or dizziness, and thrombocytopenia; procainamide can lead to a lupus-like syndrome; and disopyramide may induce difficult micturition, constipation, abdominal discomfort, or syncope. Several other drugs are receiving clinical trials: verapamil, which slows depolarization; bretylium, an adrenergic blocker; oral agents with effect similar to parenteral lidocaine; and other β-adrenergic blocking agents related to propranolol.

Ventricular Tachycardia

This arrhythmia is defined as 6 or more consecutive premature ventricular contractions. The impulses may originate from any site within the ventricular conduction system, and on the EKG the QRS complexes are wide and distorted. The rate is usually 150–200/min and quite regular; it is frequently paroxysmal, that is, it is abrupt in onset and termination, and often triggered by one or more PVCs. In most cases the atrial and ventricular activation and contraction are completely independent, leading to complete AV dissociation. The atrial rhythm is usually sinus, and often sinus tachycardia, but often lower than the ventricular rate.

The abnormal pacemaker is located below the His bundle in the bundle branches, fascicles, or Purkinje system. Retrograde activation of the His bundle occurs and there may be atrial capture. The QRS complex is broad and abnormal because of the aberrant pathway of ventricular depolarization, and the P waves are usually independent of QRS complexes except when the ventricles may occasionally be captured by an atrial impulse.

For the most part this arrhythmia occurs in patients with organic heart disease, most commonly coronary artery disease with myocardial ischemia, but it also occurs in hypertensive and rheumatic heart disease. It is a frequent result of digitalis toxicity and hypokalemia; it occurs in hypoxemia and acid–base abnormalities; it is sometimes a response to quinidine, to adrenergic stimulation, and to mechanical stimulation of the heart such as cardiac catherization, surgery, and arteriography. It is occasionally seen in supposedly healthy persons. It may precede ventricular flutter or fibrillation and lead to death. It may occur in brief bursts or persist for hours.

Ventricular tachycardia very often leads to significant hemodynamic abnormalities (cardiac output may be reduced 50% or more), partly because of its frequent correlation with advanced organic heart disease. The rapid ventricular rate and lack of the appropriately timed atrial contribution to ventricular filling then leads to a further decline in ventricular performance, cardiac output, organ perfusion, and coronary artery blood flow. Signs and symptoms of the resulting abnormalities are dyspnea, pulmonary edema, angina, hypotension, mental confusion or syncope, and oliguria.

In conjunction with AMI, the most frequent cause of ventricular tachycardia, this configuration is more ominous and presages ventricular fibrillation; in the acute setting, intravenous lidocaine or procainamide is used promptly to terminate the attack. DC countershock may be used if the medication is not effective, but not in ventricular tachycardia from digitalis toxicity, since ventricular fibrillation may be the consequence. The patient's status relative to arterial oxygen and carbon dioxide tensions, electrolyte status, blood pressure, and acid–base balance should be evaluated promptly. Intravenous lidocaine is the most frequently used pharmacologic agent, since procainamide tends to lower blood pressure and cardiac output. Side effects from larger doses of lidocaine may be altered mental status, seizures, and decreased level of consciousness. Since lidocaine is metabolized in the liver, a patient with impaired liver function may show adverse reactions at a lower dose than usual. Other drugs that may be used are propranolol, quinidine, diphenylhydantoin, or disopyramide. These medications (except lidocaine) are also used in longer term antiarrhythmic maintenance. Some patients on long-term maintenance develop a reaction to procainamide which resembles systemic lupus erythematosus, but it is usually reversible after withdrawal of the drug.

Idioventricular Rhythm (Accelerated Idioventricular Tachycardia or Rhythm)

This is a slower ectopic ventricular arrhythmia than the preceding, with rates of 70 to about 100, intermediate between the very low rate of the usual idioventricular escape rhythm (40) and a ventricular tachycardia (120–200). It occurs as a result of enhancement of the escape rhythm which develops when there is a suppression of impulse transmission from the higher pacemaker. It most commonly occurs in patients with an acute myocardial infarction, or in digitalis toxicity, or severe hyperkalemia. It is regular, may produce slight adverse circulatory effects, and frequently needs no further treatment than digitalis withdrawal. It is sometimes referred to as a tachycardia, not because the rate is fast (it is within the normal range) but because it is fast for an idioventricular escape rhythm, which is otherwise very slow (40/min). The incidence of ventricular fibrillation is much lower than in a rapid ventricular tachycardia.

Ventricular Fibrillation

Ventricular fibrillation is hemodynamically equivalent to cardiac arrest. Although it may sometimes occur in brief episodes which subside spontaneously, usually it culminates in rapid death unless prompt measures are taken to reverse it. There is chaotic extremely rapid uncoordinated muscle movement stimulated by multifocal myocardial depolarizations. No effective pumping of blood occurs and the result is rapid loss of consciousness with a precipitous fall of blood pressure. It occurs often in coronary artery disease with myocardial ischemia and infarction, AV block, and digitalis and quinidine toxicity. It may also be precipitated by adrenergic agonists or sympathetic activation by any means. The goal in this disorder is prevention by attention to conditions likely to precipitate it: early recognition of arterial hypoxemia, hypokalemia, and developing congestive heart failure, and by alertness to premonitory ventricular ectopic beats. Effective treatment is prompt recognition, mechanical ventilation, and electrical defibrillation. If conversion fails, resuscitation must be started promptly. Establishing and maintaining the airway is of crucial importance; intubation with correction of hypoxemia and lactic acidemia should be accomplished without delay. Intravenous lidocaine may make a subsequent defibrillation attempt more effective.

Disorders Arising in the Conduction System: Conduction Delays or Blocks

Heart block is a term applied to the condition of impaired propagation of the wave of depolarization at any site along the conduction system of the heart. The impairment may consist of delayed or slowed transmission; a decrement in strength of the wave of negativity along the conduction pathways; or (less often) an outright obstruction because of physiologic or structural alteration, so that transmission ceases altogether at a given point. Blocks may be acute or chronic, reversible or irreversible, and uni- or bidirectional. In general, those occurring at more proximal locations in the conduction pathways tend to be less serious, while those at more distal sites are of greater significance. Blocks to conduction may occur at any one or more of the following places: in the AN region (atrial myocardium proximal to the AV node); in the N region (the AV node itself); in the NH region (the region of the His bundle immediately distal to the AV node); in the His bundle itself; the right or left bundle branches; the anterior or posterior fascicles of the left bundle branch; or in the Purkinje fibers of either right or left bundle branches (Figure 6-1). There may be combinations; for example, a complete right bundle branch block may occur along with a partial or incomplete block in the left His–Purkinje system. Therefore when the term AV block is used to refer to heart block, its use in this case is actually as a more general term for impaired conduction; the site of impairment is not necessarily in the AV node itself.

The impaired conduction appears on the EKG as a P-R interval of 0.21 sec or more, alone or in conjunction with other abnormalities, depending on the location of the conduction delay and its degree. At each possible site of delayed conduction listed above, the block may be partial (first or second degree) or complete (third degree). In addition, the various possible locations of block may occur singly or in combination with others. First degree heart block is defined as a P-R interval which is longer than normal but all P waves are followed normally by QRS complexes; that is, all atrial impulses succeed in passing through the conduction system, but at a slower than normal rate, and therefore all atrial contractions are followed by ventricular contractions. Second degree heart block refers to a more advanced delay; at intervals the atrial impulses (P waves) are unable to pass through the conduction system to stimulate the ventricles and a dropped beat results. Third degree (complete) heart block refers to the condition in which no atrial impulses succeed in reaching the ventricles; in this case the atria and ventricles are stimulated via separate pacemakers and maintain independent rhythms, leading to complete AV dissociation.

The causes of acute abnormalities of conduction include pharmacologic agents such as digitalis or quinidine which promote AV block by slowing conduction through the AV node; acute myocarditis, including rheumatic fever; metabolic abnormalities such as K^+, Ca^{2+}, or Mg^{2+} deficiency or excess; and, commonly, acute myocardial infarction. Delays of conduction which develop during the course of AMI usually do not persist after the first few days.

In chronic partial or complete heart block the cause is most often degenerative disease of the specialized conduction tissue, and takes the form of sclerosis and fibrosis which may involve any portion of the conduction system. The lesions are often widely distributed in a spotty fashion, but seldom is the block complete, in the sense that the tract is anatomically disrupted; more often the process involves patchy defects which correlate with varying degrees of conduction delay rather than outright block. The cause of this degenerative process, which is most frequently seen in persons over 60, is not established. Other common causes of chronic conduction delay are ischemic heart disease from coronary atherosclerosis and hypertensive heart disease. In some few patients conduction defects are congenital, and not infrequently in acquired partial or complete heart block the cause remains unknown.

Acute Conduction Delays in Myocardial Infarction

Acute heart block of varying degrees (first, second, or third) and in different sites of the conduction system, occurs frequently in acute myocardial infarction. AV conduction delay in inferior or posterior infarctions is more frequent and is usually of short duration, reverting to normal after the acute phase has resolved. This is thought to be caused by ischemia and edema in the region of the AV junction proximal to the His bundle bifurcation as a result of obstruction to blood flow in a branch of the right coronary artery; the His bundle and bundle branches are reported to be rarely involved. Block in this situation is usually transient and commonly is first degree of Mobitz Type I (see following). When the block is complete the escape pacemaker below the node takes over control of the ventricles with a rate of above 50/m. Since the escape pacemaker is high in the AV conduction system, the pathway of the activation of the ventricles is close to normal and therefore the QRS complexes are normal in appearance.

In the case of anterior infarctions from left main or anterior descending artery obstruction, the damage is more extensive; since it involves the septum there is often widespread impairment of conduction in the His bundle and/or bundle branches or fascicles. This form is less common but more serious. There may be a rapid transition from a block in one or two of the fascicles to complete heart block from left main or anterior descending artery obstruction. This form of acute block usually occurs as a Mobitz Type II second degree, or third degree trifascicular block (see following), is more likely to be permanent and irreversible, and is promptly treated by a temporary pacemaker.

When the block is complete, the escape pacemaker is located below the damaged area, in the bundle branches or lower in the Purkinje system, and therefore its inherent automaticity is low and the ventricular rate is often below 40/min. Since the pacemaker is low in the system, the pathway of activation of the ventricles is aberrant and so the QRS is widened and deformed. Impairment of the circulation may be severe, leading to Stokes-Adams attacks (see following) and sudden death. Complete heart block from major septal damage in an anterior AMI is associated with a high incidence of acute heart failure, cardiogenic shock, and a high mortality rate.

First Degree Heart Block

This common form of conduction defect is usually the result of impaired transmission of the impulse in the region of the AV junction. Usually there are no symptoms or signs beyond the EKG abnormality of a prolonged P-R interval, and it requires no treatment. It sometimes occurs transiently as a result of vagal stimulation. It also is caused by digitalis, and commonly results from acute rheumatic heart disease and less commonly from arteriosclerotic heart disease or systemic disorders which may affect the heart. In the acute care setting it may progress to a more advanced form of block.

Second Degree Heart Block

There are two types: Mobitz Type I (Wenckebach) and Mobitz Type II block.

Mobitz Type I Block

In this form of second degree block the P-R interval increases progressively (Wenckebach phenomenon) over several beats until finally one of the impulses from the atrium fails to be conducted to the ventricles, and the corresponding ventricular contraction fails to occur. That is, a P wave is blocked, and the corresponding QRS complex drops out. This usually results from a conduction delay in the AV junction; the conducted QRS complexes are usually normal in appearance.

The ratio of atrial to ventricular contraction is expressed according to the number of P waves per number of QRS complexes, so if one of four atrial impulses is blocked, that is a 4:3 ratio AV block. The P-R intervals of all conducted beats are usually constant, and the rhythm can be 2:1, 4:3, 5:4, and so on, although 3:2 or 4:3 are the most common AV conduction ratios. The ventricular rate is usually above 50/min. When it occurs acutely it is usually in association with an inferior infarction; but it also may result from any factor which increases vagal tone, such as carotid sinus stimulation or vomiting, and mild digitalis and quinidine toxicity. It also occurs in systemic infections and metabolic disorders such as electrolyte imbalance and uremia. It is usually transitory and requires no treatment aside from that of the underlying disorder, if present.

Mobitz Type II Block

This is less common and more serious than the above because, although it may be reversible, it is often associated with advanced organic heart disease and in that context may represent a stage on the way to third degree (complete) heart block and the occurrence of Stokes-Adams attacks (see following). It results in most cases from a conduction delay within the His bundle, or a trifascicular block, but is almost always distal to the AV node. The P-R interval may be either normal or increased, but it is fixed in length rather than variable as in the Wenckebach phenomenon of Mobitz I partial block. The dropped beats may occur in a regular AV conduction ratio of 2:1, 3:1, 4:1, or in irregular and fluctuating ratios. The pulse rate is slower than in Mobitz I. The conducted QRS complexes are usually wide because of the abnormal pathway of excitation in the ventricles. The conduction delay may be in the bundle itself, both bundle branches, or all three fascicles of the conducting system.

Mobitz II block is seen acutely in myocarditis or in myocardial infarction; in these situations it may be transient or may progress to complete block. The most common causes of *chronic* Mobitz II block are progressive fibrosis and sclerosis of the conduction system, and atherosclerotic coronary artery disease. This form of block often causes marked circulatory abnormalities because of the slow ventricular rate, the diffuse nature of the conduction defects such as bilateral bundle branch block, and the associated organic heart disease such as congestive heart failure. Patients often complain of palpitations, skipped beats, weakness, lightheadedness, or "blackouts."

Stokes-Adams attacks often occur in Mobitz II block because of inadequate cerebral perfusion from the low cardiac output, which causes ischemia of the brain. Neurologic symptoms from low brain blood flow may vary from a momentary lightheadedness to abrupt loss of consciousness. The syncope comes on in any position, including lying down; if the patient is standing, he falls down abruptly. There are no premonitory symptoms, and the attacks may vary from many per day to only occasional ones. The duration of unconsciousness is usually brief. The patient regains consciousness rapidly without any weakness, mental confusion, or drowsiness. The skin often shows an obvious postischemic flush resulting from vasodilation caused by the vasodilator metabolites which accumulated during the period of circulatory arrest. EKG monitoring during an attack of complete unconsciousness may show a brief period of ventricular asystole or fibrillation.

When the patient is symptomatic, especially if there are symptoms and signs of cerebral ischemia, shown by 24 hr Holter monitoring to be associated with periods of very low ventricular rates, or ventricular tachycardia or fibrillation, then a permanent artificial pacemaker is indicated.

It is important to point out that there are exceptions to the above differentiations between the two types of Mobitz block. Some EKG tracings show periods of both, alternating, demonstrating that shifts between them can occur in an individual patient.

Third Degree (Complete) Heart Block

This condition is characterized by atrial and ventricular excitation and contraction which are independent of each other. That is, there is complete AV dissociation. The atrial impulses fail to be conducted to the ventricles because of marked conduction delay, and a subsidiary pacemaker with the highest inherent rate just distal to the location of the block acts as the stimulus for ventricular activation. In third degree block (without treatment) the survival of the patient is completely dependent upon the emergence of this escape pacemaker distal to the block. If the block is low in the His bundle the escape pacemaker may be in the His bundle just below it and then the escape rate will be faster than if the block is in the bundle branches or fascicles, since the inherent rate of phase 4 diastolic depolarization decreases as one proceeds distally in the conduction system. These distal bundle or fascicle pacemakers are not only slower, but are less reliable and may fail, leading to Stokes-Adams attacks and sudden death.

Also, the farther distal in the conduction system the escape pacemaker originates, the wider and more distorted the QRS complexes will appear because of the slow and aberrant conduction of the impulse through the ventricles. In very slow rates of 40/min or below the patient will often be in congestive heart failure, and may be dyspneic, weak, and mentally impaired.

The rhythms originating below the bifurcation of the His bundle are called idioventricular and have rates of 30–40/min. Additional ventricular arrhythmias occur quite commonly in an idioventricular rhythm, for example, premature ventricular contractions, fibrillation, and ventricular ectopic tachycardia. The irritability of the myocardium tends to increase during a slow and unstable idioventricular rhythm, leading to spontaneous repetitive depolarization and ectopic beats.

Most instances of persisting complete heart block result from protracted conduction delay within the His bundle, from bilateral bundle branch block, or trifascicular block. The ventricular rate is usually low: 45/min or less, and the rhythm is regular. It is characteristic of a block in the His bundle or below that the ventricular rate does not increase with exercise, with vagal block by atropine, or from administration of sympathomimetic drugs or the catecholamines themselves, indicating that the effect of these agents is on the AV node.

The cause of complete heart block in the elderly is often a chronic progressive degenerative process in the conduction tissues; complete block is often preceded by EKG manifestations of incomplete bilateral bundle branch block. The management is surgical placement of a permanent pacemaker.

Bundle Branch Block

The EKG correlate of bundle branch block is a lengthened QRS complex; although lesions may be widely distributed in the conduction system, the EKG manifestation is often either right or left bundle branch block (BBB). The lesions are often slowly progressive degenerative changes. As is the case with the other conduction abnormalities, the physiologic change is more often a delayed conduction rather than an outright block, and the block therefore may be minor or partial in degree.

Right bundle branch block, especially partial, may occur in persons without organic heart disease. It is correlated with delayed activation of the right ventricle, which is not stimulated until after left ventricle activation has occurred, and the route of right ventricle stimulation is therefore abnormal and from the left ventricle. It may be associated with right heart failure (cor pulmonale) developing from severe lung disease. Left bundle branch block more often occurs in elderly persons with heart disease, often fibrosis of the conduction system or coronary artery or hypertensive heart disease. Left ventricular activation is delayed relative to the right, resulting in asynchronous ventricular contraction. Periodic 24-hr Holter monitoring of patients with either right or left bundle branch block often reveals brief intervals of more complete AV block, indicating the gradual progression of a disease process in a bundle branch to complete heart block, with time.

Hemiblocks

In hemiblocks one of the two fascicles (anterior superior and posterior inferior) of the left bundle branch has a delayed conduction, and the impulse to the papillary muscles and remainder of the ventricle is conveyed over the unblocked subdivision, instead of both papillary muscles and the ventricle being activated concomitantly, as normally occurs. Hemiblocks lead to left or right axis deviation on the EKG, indicating the aberrant route taken by the impulse in the case of either left or right hemiblock. (There are other causes of axis deviation in addition to hemiblocks.) Left anterior hemiblock is more common than right, and hemiblock in general is very common, occurring acutely in myocardial infarction, and chronically in ischemic, hypertensive, or degenerative heart disease.

Uni-, Bi-, and Trifascicular Blocks

A unifascicular block refers to a conduction delay in one of the three fascicles: the right bundle branch, or one of the two fascicles of the left bundle branch (in the latter case it is also a hemiblock, as indicated above).

A bifascicular block is a form of incomplete bilateral bundle branch block, the most common combination of which is right bundle branch block and left anterior hemiblock. Bifascicular block is most common in males 60 years of age or over. In bifascicular block with right bundle branch and left (either anterior or posterior) hemiblock, the ventricles presumably are activated via the third fascicle. In this disorder often major portions of the conduction system are involved in the disease process, although the patient may be quite asymptomatic. Periodic Holter monitoring and follow-up of patients to note the onset of possible symptoms of inadequate cerebral perfusion is appropriate.

A trifascicular block involves conduction delay in all of the three fascicles: the right bundle branch and the anterior and posterior divisions of the left bundle branch; therefore it is one form of bilateral bundle branch block, and hence is a type of complete, or third degree, heart block.

All of these variations are caused by the conditions which result in conduction system impairments alluded to previously, and represent EKG abnormalities which generally are correlated with extensive degeneration throughout the specialized conduction tissues. Often they are but way stations along the road to complete heart block.

Wolff–Parkinson–White Syndrome (Ventricular Preexcitation Syndrome, Anomalous AV Excitation, Accessory AV Conduction)

This is a disorder of the conduction system which may be either congenital or acquired. One common form is characterized on the EKG by normal P waves, a short P-R interval, an increased QRS complex duration, and a slurring on the initial portion of the QRS complex called a delta wave. In addition to the normal route of ventricular excitation from the atrium through the AV node, early activation of the ventricles along one or more of a group of accessory pathways may occur. These accessory pathways bypass all or a portion of the AV node and His bundle and therefore comprise strands of tissue which connect various portions of the atria and ventricles directly, in parallel with the normal conduction pathway. Epicardial mapping is a special diagnostic procedure which records the time and location of arrival of an excitation wave from the atria to the ventricles and thus localizes the precise site of the accessory connections. There are subtypes of WPW syndrome depending upon the location of the accessory conduction tracts.

WPW syndrome by itself is a benign condition. There are no symptoms and no circulatory or other signs. The syndrome is found in about 1% of the population; in about half of affected persons paroxysmal atrial arrhythmias occur, and this is the reason for the clinical significance of what would otherwise be merely an EKG anomaly. Most such atrial tachyarrhythmias occur in individuals who have no signs or symptoms of organic heart disease.

In a common form of WPW syndrome, the atrial impulse from the S A node is conducted simultaneously down the normal conduction system and down the accessory bypass tract—in other words, the impulse divides and travels in parallel fashion along the two routes. There are a number of theories to account for the high incidence of paroxysmal atrial tachyarrhythmias in WPW, as there may also be a number of mechanisms involved in its genesis. One theory suggests that atrial tachycardia occurs because of a difference in the refractory periods of the normal and accessory conduction pathways. Although the rate of conduction through the accessory pathway may be faster, its refractory period may be longer. When a premature atrial contraction occurs, the anomalous pathway is still refractory from the last SA impulse but the normal pathway is not; so in this case, instead of the impulse splitting as usual, it travels the normal pathway. By the time the impulse reaches the AV node, the accessory pathway is now excitable and the impulse splits, one portion continuing on anterogradely (forward) to stimulate the ventricles while the other enters the anomalous tract and is conducted retrogradely (backward) to restimulate the atria. Following this, the impulse then reenters the normal pathway again and is retransmitted forward again to the ventricles. This reciprocation then persists, resulting in a self-perpetuating circuit and producing a paroxysmal supraventricular tachycardia.

Management of the tachycardia of WPW consists in increasing the refractory period of the accessory conduction tracts sufficient to terminate the reentry process. Propranolol, procainamide, and quinidine are agents which accomplish this goal in many patients, with propranolol being preferred, especially when fibrillation is the atrial rhythm.

ANTIARRHYTHMIC PHARMACOLOGIC AGENTS

The goal in the pharmacologic management of abnormalities of impulse formation and conduction would ideally be to use a drug whose major action is directed against the specific disturbance causing the arrhythmia. Unfortunately the specific mechanisms involved in the genesis of abnormalities in rate and rhythm are seldom known. Moreover, the precise pharmacologic action of a given drug, as it relates to the control of an arrhythmia, is often not clear. Thus, to a large extent drug treatment of cardiac arrhythmias rests on an empiric basis.

Antiarrhythmic agents can be classified in broad terms according to their actions on the various phases of impulse formation and conduction in the different parts of the specialized conduction system, and in ordinary atrial and ventricular myocardium outside the system. Some of the aspects of impulse formation and conduction affected by antiarrhythmic drugs are: (1) the magnitude and stability of the resting membrane potential ; (2) the automaticity (impulse formation or rate of phase 4 diastolic depolarization); (3) the excitability (ability to respond to a stimulus); (4) the rate of conduction; and (5) the duration of the refractory period.

Digitalis

Digitalis is an important inotropic agent (it increases myocardial contractility) for the management of congestive heart failure, but in addition is of value in the control of supraventricular tachycardias. This effect is mediated in two ways: through an increase in cardioinhibitory stimuli from the vagus, and through a direct action on the conduction system and on ordinary myocardial cells. The indirect neural effect from the vagus (parasympathetic cholingergic influence) consists of decreasing the rate of impulse formation (that is, phase 4 diastolic depolarization) in the cells of the SA node. It also slows the rate of conduction through the AV node and the His bundle, and prolongs the refractory period of the AV node. The effect on AV nodal conduction appears to be mediated in part by vagal inhibitory action, and in part by direct effects on the cell membranes of conduction tissue. The result is a decrease in heart rate and a depressed rate and strength of transmission of the impulse through the conduction system. Direct membrane effects of digitalis on the conduction system are reported to be a decrease in strength and speed of the action potential in AV node and His bundle fibers. Therefore, the indirect effect, mediated by the parasympathetic nerve supply to the SA and AV nodes, and the direct effect, mediated via the action of digitalis upon cell membranes of the conduction system, appear to reinforce each other.

Other actions of digitalis which are directly on the myocardial cells occur at higher doses: an increased automaticity (that is, increased impulse formation) in AV junctional, His–Purkinje, and ventricular myocardium; and more responsiveness (that is, greater rate and strength of the action potential) of the distal Purkinje conduction system. It is these actions at higher dose levels that predispose to ectopic impulse formation and ventricular arrhythmias in digitalis toxicity.

The effects of excess digitalis on rhythm are sinus bradycardia and prolongation of the P-R interval; AV conduction block and AV dissociation; and ventricular premature contractions, tachycardia, and fibrillation. Clinically digitalis excess first causes anorexia, nausea, vomiting, mild diarrhea, and headache and visual disturbances.

Treatment of digitalis toxicity consists of withholding the drug. Potassium and antiarrhythmic agents such as propranolol or diphenylhydantoin are used only if necessary. Checking the serum K^+ is important in patients receiving diuretics who may be predisposed to digitalis intoxication by K^+ depletion.

Quinidine

Quinidine is a derivative of the antimalarial drug quinine; its antiarrhythmic action is related to four basic effects: (1) it decreases automaticity (slows the rate of diastolic phase 4 depolarization) and therefore depresses the rate of impulse formation, in both the normal AV node pacemaker, and any abnormal ectopic pacemakers which may be present; (2) it decreases the responsiveness (the degree of excitability) of conduction tissues to stimuli (that is, it prolongs conduction time which decreases conduction speed), thereby lowering the rate and strength of the impulse; (3) it prolongs the refractory period of the conduction pathways; and (4) it increases the duration of the action potential.

It has a cholinergic blocking action which shortens the refractory period of the AV node by decreasing vagal inhibition in this structure; note that this vagal blocking action may serve to counteract its action in depressing the rate of impulse formation—that is, its negative chronotropic action. So the direct and neurally mediated effects of quinidine are to some extent contradictory. This is the reason for the fact that when quinidine is used in the treatment of atrial flutter, the patient is often first digitalized to prevent a too-rapid ventricular response rate.

Toxic effects of quinidine include ventricular arrhythmias and asystole from depression of the SA node pacemaker. Side effects may be nausea, vomiting and diarrhea; tinnitus and vertigo; and skin rashes sometimes related to thrombocytopenia.

Disopyramide Phosphate

This is a newer antiarrhythmic agent with quinidine-like action which has proven effective in the management of a number of cardiac arrhythmias, including atrial fibrillation, paroxysmal supraventricular tachycardia, premature ventricular contractions, and ventricular tachycardia. Its membrane actions are in many respects similar to quinidine and procainamide: it decreases automaticity and velocity of impulse conduction, and increases the duration of the action potential and the refractory period.

Its side effects are those of its anticholinergic actions: difficulty emptying the bladder, dry mouth, and decreased gastrointestinal motility.

Procainamide

This drug is related to the local anesthetic procaine. Its pharmacologic actions are similar to those of quinidine: it decreases automaticity and excitability, slows the rate of conduction, and prolongs the refractory period. It has a number of side effects. Side effects are more common than with quinidine but are usually dose-related. There may be nausea, vomiting, and diarrhea; with long-term administration a lupus-like syndrome may develop including a positive antinuclear antibody test that usually clears when the drug is stopped.

Propranolol

Propranolol is a β-adrenergic blocking agent and acts by antagonizing the effects of the adrenergic mediators (catecholamines) epinephrine and norepinephrine and sympathetic nerve stimulation on the heart, thus prolonging the AV nodal refractory period and slowing AV nodal conduction rate. It also has direct effects on conduction tissues and on the ordinary myocardium which are not neurally mediated; like quinidine and procainamide, it decreases both automaticity and conduction velocity, prolongs the effective refractory period, and increases the duration of the action potential. Therefore, it is useful in suppressing all forms of tachyarrhythmias, and is used not only in treating acute arrhythmias but for prevention of chronically recurring ones.

Propranolol has a number of adverse side effects, including easy fatiguability, lethargy and weakness. More importantly, it is contraindicated in patients with heart failure since it markedly decreases myocardial contractility; and in patients with second or third degree heart block, where it may cause severe bradycardia or arrest. It is also not used for patients with asthma or chronic obstructive pulmonary disease, since its β blocking action increases bronchoconstriction and elevates airway resistance (chapter 9).

Lidocaine

Lidocaine is another local anesthetic with antiarrhythmic action; it has a brief duration of action which necessitates intravenous administration. It diminishes the automaticity of both the normal and ectopic pacemakers, especially in the His bundle–Purkinje system, and suppresses ventricular fibrillation. However, unlike the action of quinidine and procainamide, it does not prolong the refractory period or decrease conduction velocity. By shortening the refractory period and increasing conduction velocity it tends to counteract the decremental conduction which is thought to be responsible for many reentry mechanisms. That is, it enhances conduction in the terminal Purkinje fibers, and this appears to abolish the abnormally depressed conduction in these areas which makes reentry possible. Thus it is particularly effective in suppressing ventricular tacharrhythmias. It is less effective in atrial tachycardias. It has an advantage over quinidine and procainamide because it can be given rapidly in the acute situation without depressing cardiac output or blood pressure.

Toxic effects of lidocaine include central nervous system disturbances, including motor (muscle twitches or even seizures); sensory (paresthesios, numbness, tinnitus, dizziness); and level of consciousness and/or mental status alterations: drowsiness, disorientation, mental confusion, and euphoria.

Diphenylhydantoin (Phenytoin, DPH)

This anticonvulsant agent has been used for many years in the mangement of seizure disorders (epilepsy). DPH suppresses spontaneous depolarization (automaticity), especially in the Purkinje fibers of ventricular myocardium, and suppresses fibrillation in both the atria and ventricles. In this respect it is like quinidine, but unlike quinidine it speeds conduction velocity, decreases the refractory period, and shortens the action potential duration. Therefore in these latter three respects it resembles lidocaine. It is particularly useful in the control of cardiac arrhythmias resulting from digitalis toxicity. There is some evidence that the action of DPH in suppressing spontaneous neural firing in the central nervous system, especially the brainstem sympathetic centers, contributes to its antiarrhythmic actions.

Side effects of long-term administration are several: gingival hypertrophy; gastrointestinal symptoms; skin rashes; and neurologic symptoms and signs: dysarthria, ataxia, nystagmus. If it is given intravenously this must be done slowly and with EKG monitoring because since it increases AV block, asystole may occur with too rapid administration.

Atropine

Atropine is an anticholinergic agent which inhibits vagal influences on the heart and is therefore used in bradycardias. It increases the rate of spontaneous depolarization in pacemaker cells and increases conduction velocity through the AV node. Sometimes ventricular irritability may appear as the rate increases. The parasympatholytic effects are widespread and therefore numerous side effects occur: diminished secretion of exocrine glands, sinus tachycardia, micturition impairment, depressed gastronintestinal motility and secretion, and central nervous sytem stimulation. It is useful in digitalis toxicity, and contraindicated in glaucoma.

REFERENCES

Beeson PB and McDermott W, editors: *Textbook of Medicine,* 14th ed. Philadelphia, Pa.: Saunders, 1975.

Chung EK: *Principles of Cardiac Arrhythmias*, 2nd ed. Baltimore, Md.: Williams and Wilkins, 1977.

Fowler NO, editor: *Cardiac Arrhythmias, Diagnosis and Treatment*, 2nd ed. Hagerstown, Md.: Harper & Row 1977.

Froelich ED, editor: *Pathophysiology*. Philadelphia, Pa.: Lippincott, 1976.

Ganong WF: *Review of Medical Physiology*, 8th ed. Los Altos, Calif.: Lange Medical Publications, 1977.

Guyton AC: *Textbook of Medical Physiology*, 5th ed. Philadelphia, Pa.: Saunders, 1976.

Lynch JJ et al.: Psychological aspects of cardiac arrhythmia. *Am. Heart J.* 93:645–657, 1977.

Pollack GH: Cardiac pacemaking: An obligatory role of catecholamines? *Science* 196:731–738, 1977.

Sokolow M and McIlroy MB: *Clinical Cardiology*. Los Altos, Calif.: Lange Medical Publications, 1977.

Thorn GW et al, editors: *Harrison's Principles of Internal Medicine*, 8th ed. New York: McGraw-Hill, 1977.

Watanabe Y and Dreifus LS: *Cardiac Arrhythmias. Electrophysiologic Basis for Clinical Interpretation*. New York: Grune & Stratton, 1977.

CHAPTER SEVEN

Heart Failure

THE CONTRACTILE PROCESS OF HEART MUSCLE

The Myocardial Cell

Heart muscle is comprised of a specialized branching and reanastomosing lattice-work of individual striated muscle cells, called myocardial fibers, each of which has its own cell membrane. Each myocardial fiber, in turn, is comprised of many individual strands—the myofibrils—each of which extend the full length of the myocardial fiber. Cytoplasm surrounds the myofibrils; it contains (1) the cell nucleus; (2) an intracellular set of membrane systems called the sarcoplasmic reticulum, which closely invests the myofibrils; and (3) large numbers of elongated mitochondria, which are also in close contact with the myofibrils and generate the energy for all cellular activities including contraction.

The myofibrils are made up of a longitudinal series of repeating units called sarcomeres; the sarcomere is both the structural and the functional unit of contraction. The boundary of each sarcomere is the vertical Z line; attached to the Z line is a series of longitudinal thin filaments—the actin filaments—which extend from the boundary Z line toward the center of the sarcomere and comprise the light I bands. At the center of the sarcomere between the two I bands is a dark broad band, the A band. The center of the A band is made up only of horizontal myosin (thick) filaments; on either side of this central region are two areas comprised of overlapping myosin (thick) and actin (thin) filaments. These relationships are diagramed in Figure 7-1a and b.

The distance between the Z lines, which mark the boundaries of the sarcomere, is variable depending upon whether the heart muscle is in a contracted state, in which case the Z lines are closer together, or in a relaxed or stretched state, in which case the Z lines are farther apart. The A band, made up primarily of myosin fibrils, in the center of the sarcomere, is of constant width regardless of the state of relaxation or contraction of the heart muscle. The I bands on either side of the A band differ in width, depending on whether the muscle is contracted or relaxed. It is the change in width of the I bands which is responsible for the changes in distance between the Z lines (Figure 7-1c).

To sum up: the *myocardium* is made up of *myocardial fibers*—the individual cells of the heart muscle. Each myocardial fiber is made up of *myofibrils*. The myofibrils are comprised of a linked series of *sarcomeres*. Each sarcomere is made up of two different kinds of myofilaments: actin and myosin: (1) the thin actin filaments comprise the sarcomere light I bands; and (2) the thick myosin filaments lie at the center of the sarcomere A bands. The two outer edges of the A bands are comprised of interdigitating, or overlapping, actin and myosin filaments. The thick myosin filaments lie entirely within the sides of the Z line, extend throughout the I band, and then into the outer portions of the A band. In the areas of the central A band of the sarcomere in which action and myosin filaments overlap, there are cross-bridges which extend between and connect the myosin and actin filaments during contraction.

Although the preceding and following discussion of muscle structure and function is presented with reference to cardiac muscle, the basic situation is the same for all muscle tissue.

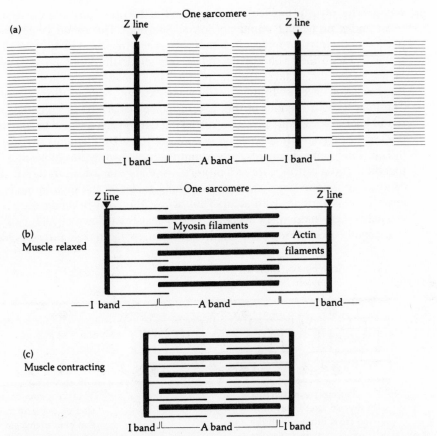

Figure 7-1. (*a*) Diagramatic representation of a portion of a myofibril made up of repeating units, sarcomeres, which are separated by the Z lines, and comprised of A bands and I bands. (*b*) Diagram of a single sarcomere showing the boundary Z lines, the I bands (thin actin filaments) and the A bands (overlapping actin and myosin filaments, with central thick myosin filaments alone). Muscle relaxed. (*c*) Same as (*b*), muscle contracted.

The Contractile Process

In considering the mechanism of muscle contraction, it is important to keep in mind that both the thick myosin and the thin actin filaments are always constant in length, both when the muscle is relaxed and when it is fully contracted. Thus muscle shortening is not produced by shortening of either the actin or myosin filaments, but rather by a sliding of the actin filaments farther into the myosin filaments; that is, during contraction the degree of interdigitation between actin and myosin filaments in the A band increases. This increased overlapping during contraction comes about as a result of a series of rapid breaking and reforming of the cross-bridges between the two sets of filaments, at successively overlapping levels, as they slide farther onto each other in a ratchet-like effect. The result for the sarcomeres and, therefore, for the myocardial fibers as a whole, is a net shortening in length: the contraction (Figure 7-1c).

We now descend a step further down into the subcellular interior of the sarcomere and examine the structure of the myosin and the actin filaments themselves. The myosin molecule is comprised of two portions: a long straight segment and a projecting round portion at one end. The round projection is the portion of the myosin molecule which acts as an enzyme (ATP-ase) for the breakdown of adenosine triphosphate (ATP); this yields the large amounts of energy necessary for the sliding of actin and myosin filaments over each other, and for the formation of cross-bridges as they increasingly overlap during contraction. The long straight sections of the myosin molecules are bound together with the round knoblike enzymic projections sticking out in such a way that they can form the cross-bridges with specialized portions of the actin filaments (Figure 7-2a).

The thin actin filaments are comprised of two actin molecules twisted together, and a central core of a protein, tropomyosin, which in the resting noncontracting muscle fiber covers the enzymic knobs on the myosin molecule that form the cross-bridges with actin. Thus at rest the cross-bridging sites of myosin are masked, or hidden, by tropomyosin so that breakdown of ATP and contraction cannot occur. Troponin, another protein, is located at intervals along the

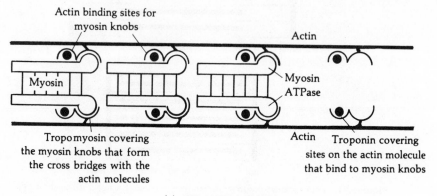

(a) RELAXED MUSCLE

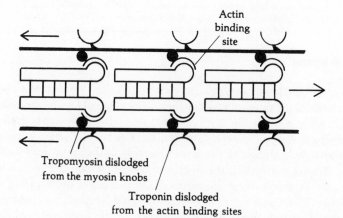

(b) CONTRACTING MUSCLE

Figure 7-2. Diagram illustrating mysoin and myosin knobs; actin and actin binding sites; troponin covering the actin binding sites; and tropomyosin masking the myosin knobs. (*a*) Relaxed muscle. (*b*) Contracting muscle. (*c*) Enlarged view of one set of interacting sites, in both the relaxed and the contracting configurations.

twisted actin filaments, and masks or hides the sites on the actin fibril which form cross-bridges with the myosin knobs during their overlapping. It is troponin which is the receptor for the influx of Ca^{2+}, binding to it and activating the contractile process. Thus the two proteins tropomyosin and troponin, which are in close approximation to the actin and myosin filaments, serve an inhibitory function which prevents the inappropriate interaction between actin and myosin while the muscle is in a resting noncontractile state (Figure 7-2d,e).

The Coupling of Cardiac Excitation and Contraction (Electrical-Mechanical Coupling)

The processes by which the wave of depolarization sweeping over the heart from the SA node and the conduction system initiates the mechanical shortening of the muscle fibril—the contraction process—is termed excitation-contraction coupling. The processes involved in impulse formation and conduction are discussed in Chapter 6.

The T-Tubule System

The wave of depolarization, which originates in the SA node and travels over the heart in a systematic and orderly fashion along the conduction pathways, is conveyed to each myofibril in the myocardial fiber along a system of transverse tubules wich are continuous with the cell membrane of the muscle fiber itself. This is the T-tubule system, and it extends down into the myocardial fibers along the ends of the sarcomeres at the Z lines (Figure 7-3).

When Ca^{2+} enters the area of the actin filament prior to the onset of contraction it binds to troponin, weakens its hold over the actin binding sites, and thus they become exposed to interact with the myosin knobs.

The dislodging of troponin from actin, in turn, dislodges tropomyosin from where it is covering the myosin knobs. The myosin ATPase therefore becomes unmasked, it hydrolyzes ATP and ADP (adenosine diphosphate) with the release of phosphate bond energy, which then supplies the energy to permit the formation of successive series of actin and myosin cross-linkages. Thr cross-bridging permits interdigitation of their filaments, and results in fibril shortening: the contraction (Figure 7-2b,c).

The phosphate bond energy for muscle shortening stored in ATP is generated in the large mitochondria from the oxidative phosphorylation of glucose and free fatty acids in the blood. Contraction requires large amounts of energy since each formation and breaking of cross linkages degrades molecules of the high energy ATP to lower energy compounds which must then be restored to ATP by further oxidative phosphorylation.

The Sarcoplasmic Reticulum

At the subcellular level, surrounding each myofibril and lying between the transverse (T) tubule system, is a complex network of weblike intracellular membranous channels called the sarcoplasmic reticulum. The channels form an interconnecting longitudinal tubular system which invests the myofibrils and also comes close to the surface of the individial sarcomeres, but does not open di-

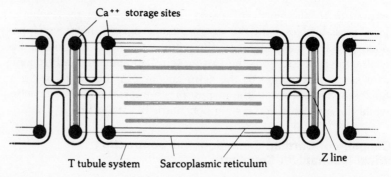

Figure 7-3. Diagram of one sacromere showing T tubule system, sarcoplasmic reticulum, and Ca^{2+} storage sacs. The Ca^{2+} is contained within these sites when the muscle is at rest (noncontracting). When the muscle is stimulated to contract, the action potential activates first the T-tubule system and then the sarcoplasmic reticulum, liberating Ca^{2+} from the storage sacs. Ca^{2+} then flows along the longitudinal sarcoplasmic tubules into the area of the actin and myosin filaments, activating the actual contraction process.

rectly to the muscle cell membrane. This reticulum contains numerous saclike structures which lie near the tubules and which serve as storage sites for Ca^{2+} during the periods when the muscle fibers are not contracting (Figure 7-3).

The action potential traveling across the heart along the muscle fiber cell membranes also activates the T-tubule system; this activation then spreads to the membranes of the sarcoplasmic reticulum, reaches the Ca^{2+} storage sacs in it, and promotes the movement of Ca^{2+} from these sacs, along the longitudinal sarcoplasmic tubules, and into close association with the actin and myosin filaments where it binds to troponin as described above. It is this binding which actually activates the contractile process itself, and therefore it is the movement of Ca^{2+} which, at the molecular level, acts as the transducer between the electrical energy of the action potential, the chemical energy of ATP, and the mechanical energy of the muscle contraction.

Heart Muscle Relaxation

Since phosphate bond energy is required for the withdrawal of Ca^{2+} from the vicinity of the actin and myosin filaments back into the sarcoplasmic reticulum, and thence to the storage sacs, relaxation is an active rather than a purely passive process. As this process of reaccumulation of Ca^{2+} by the sarcoplasmic reticulum proceeds, and the concentration of Ca^{2+} in the filaments declines, chemical bonding between actin and myosin decreases; the filaments slide back to their initial resting position relative to each other and muscle fiber relaxation occurs.

Cellular Basis of the Frank–Starling Relation

The Frank–Starling relation states that (within limits) the force of contraction depends on the initial fiber length. The basis for this relation is that when there is stretch on the myocardial fiber this tension pulls the actin and myosin filaments farther apart so that their amount of overlap at the edges of the A bands is very slight. Therefore, there are many potential cross-bridging sites available to produce a large amount of interdigitation and therefore an increased contraction.

Conversely, when they are already interdigitated to a large extent (low tension on the fiber) the contraction is minimal. However, if the fiber is stretched so much that the actin and myosin filaments are pulled apart altogether, no overlapping and therefore no shortening can occur. This may partially account for the very poor contractility of the greatly dilated heart in severe congestive heart failure.

HEART WORK

The function of the heart is to pump blood. Its ability to do so depends upon a number of factors. Some of these factors are inherent within heart muscle tissue itself, while others are extrinsic to it and constitute influences upon it from external forces: neural impulses from the autonomic nervous system, status of the blood vessels conveying blood into and out of it, and quantity and physical and chemical properties of the blood which it pumps, among others.

Contractile Properties of Heart Muscle

Load Size and Rate of Contraction (Force–Velocity Relation)

The greater the load a strip of heart muscle is called upon to move, the slower will be the rate of contraction. The reverse is true as well: the less the load the strip of heart muscle is required to move, the more rapid the rate of contraction will be. There are two factors which influence the force–velocity relation of

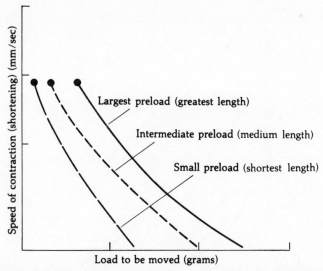

Figure 7-4. Force–velocity curves at three different initial fiber lengths (= three different degrees of stretch or tension, or three different preloads). In myocardial tissue the terms: preload, initial fiber length, and degrees of stretch or tension, all have essentially the same functional meaning. The three curves indicate that (1) an increased preload (or initial stretch or fiber length) enables the muscle to move a larger load, but there is no change in rate of contraction as a function of initial fiber length; and (2) the larger the load to be moved, at all initial fiber lengths, the slower the rate of contraction.

myocardium: (1) the length of the muscle fibers at the onset of contraction; this value is termed the preload; and (2) the contractility of the muscle fibers; this value is called the inotropic state. Figure 7-4 is a set of force velocity curves at three different initial fiber lengths; this figure illustrates three important qualities of myocardial tissue: (1) a longer fiber length at the onset of contraction enables the heart muscle to move a larger load than does a shorter fiber length; (2) initial fiber length has no effect on the *rate* at which the contraction occurs; and (3) the larger the load to be moved, the slower the rate of contraction at all fiber lengths. These characteristics of myocardium are directly relevant to heart failure; in failure the ventricles become distended with blood because the poor contractility causes decreased ventricular emptying. Therefore the ventricles dilate, which puts more stretch on the fibers, improving to some extent their contractile force, but causing them to contract more slowly.

Inotropic (Contractility) State and Rate and Force of Contraction

Figure 7-5 shows a set of force–velocity curves for myocardium in which the initial length of three strips of muscle is held constant, but the three strips are in different conditions of contractility (different inotropic states). This figure illustrates that the relative amount of a positive inotropic agent such as norepinephrine—one which increases myocardial contractility—not only increases the size of a load which the muscle is capable of moving, but also increases the *velocity* of the contraction. In the case of increased myocardial norepinephrine content, the heart muscle contracts more strongly and more rapidly; where the myocardium is depleted of norepinephrine, as occurs in heart failure, the muscle

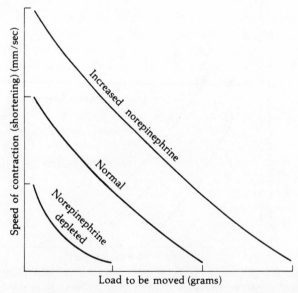

Figure 7-5. Force-velocity curves for three strips of myocardial tissue of the same initial fiber length (the same preload) but at three different inotropic (contractile) states: increased contractility, from norepinephrine; normal, without added norepinephrine; and the norephinephrine-depleted myocardium of heart failure. The curves indicate that an increased inotropic state increases both the rate and force of the contraction.

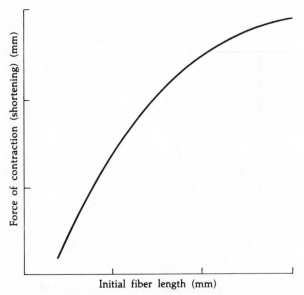

Figure 7-6. The Frank-Starling relationship between initial fiber length and force of contraction of heart muscle (see text).

contracts more slowly and less forcefully and so is not capable of moving as great a load.

Fiber Length and Force of Contraction (Length–Tension Relation; the Frank–Starling Relation)

The Frank–Starling law of the heart states that the force of contraction of heart muscle (other factors equal) is proportional to the initial length of the cardiac muscle fiber. This relation is illustrated in Figure 7-6, the Starling length–tension curve, which indicates that the degree of shortening is a function of the length of (or tension on) the heart muscle at the onset of contraction.

Ventricular End-Diastolic Volume (VEDV) and Stroke Volume (SV)

Translated into the function of the intact heart, what the Frank–Starling relationship states is that the amount of blood in the ventricle at the end of diastolic filling, and therefore at the onset of contraction (the preload), determines the amount of tension the ventricle is capable of developing, the strength and degree of the contraction which will occur, and therefore the amount of blood it will expel, at the next heart beat. This is true because in the heart the length of the muscle fibers at the onset of contraction, which equals the preload, is a function of the ventricular end-diastolic volume. The volume of blood in the ventricle at the end of the diastolic filling period determines the size of the ventricle, and hence the length of, and amount of stretch on, the muscle fibers in the ventricle.

The end-diastolic volume, in turn, is influenced by a number of factors such as the amount of venous return and the effectiveness of the atrial expulsion of blood into the ventricle, as well as the amount of blood remaining in the ventricle after its previous contraction (ventricular end-systolic volume). Other factors equal, it

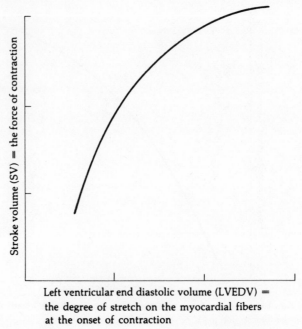

Left ventricular end diastolic volume (LVEDV) =
the degree of stretch on the myocardial fibers
at the onset of contraction

Figure 7-7. The relationship between the left-ventricular end-diastolic volume (i.e., preload), which in the intact heart is the factor determining stretch on the heart muscle at the onset of contraction; and the stroke volume, which is the consequence of the force of contraction. Note that this curve is identical with Figure 7-4. Figure 7-4 illustrates the Frank-Starling relationship as it applies to a strip of heart muscle; Figure 7-5 illustrates this relationship as it is seen in the intact working heart.

is the strength of ventricular myocardial contraction which determines the stroke volume. Therefore, another way of stating the Frank–Starling law of the heart is that, other factors (such as the afterload) held constant, stroke volume is a function of ventricular end-diastolic volume. This relationship between VEDV and SV is illustrated in Figure 7-7.

The Ventricular Function Curve

The ventricular function curve incorporates into the Starling or length–tension curve the factor of resistance against which the ventricle is required to pump blood; this *resistance* is essentially the mean aortic pressure (which is a major factor determining the afterload). Therefore in the equation for a ventricular function curve, stroke work (defined as stroke volume × mean aortic pressure) is substituted for the value: stroke volume (or force of contraction) on the ordinate. A similar curve to that of the Frank–Starling relation results if the mean aortic pressure is held within a steady normal range. Figure 7-8 is a group of ventricular function curves, showing the relation between myocardial performance (defined as stroke work) and ventricular end-diastolic pressure (which is taken as an equivalent of VEDV) over a range of inotropic (contractile) states.

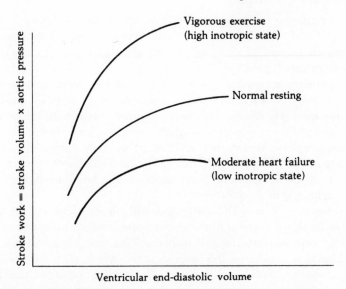

Figure 7-8. Ventricular function curves at several inotropic states of myocardium. Ventricular performance is equated with stroke work, which is defined as stroke volume times mean aortic pressure $(SW = SV \times \bar{X}AP)$. If the aortic pressure is held constant then the ventricular function curve resembles the Starling length–tension curve. With increasing myocardial contractility (increased inotropic state) myocardial performance is increased at each value of the LVEDP.

REGULATION OF THE CARDIAC OUTPUT

The cardiac output comprises the mechanical work of the heart; it is a product of the heart rate (beats per minute) and the stroke volume (volume per beat). So: CO = HR × SV. If either component increases while the other remains constant, cardiac output will increase; if either decreases while the other stays the same, cardiac output declines. Cardiac output in the normal adult is about 5 L-min, the cardiac index is the cardiac output per minute per body surface in square meters and averages a little over 3 liters.

Heart Rate Regulation

Heart rate is determined primarily by neural impulses to the heart originating in the cardiac control centers in the lower brainstem; these centers participate in a number of reflexes which mediate the responses of the heart to a wide variety of internal and external influences, including changing levels of physical activity, emotional responses, and the altered metabolic states of, for example, body temperature or thyroid hormone fluctuations.

Cholinergic (parasympathetic) neural influences on heart rate originate in the dorsal motor nucleus of the vagus nerve in the brainstem. This area is termed the cardioinhibitory center. Impulses traveling via the vagus to the heart decrease the heart rate (negative chronotropic effect) and the force of contraction (negative inotropic effect). The brainstem vagal nuclei maintain a continuous low flow of inhibitory impulses to the heart; this is called vagal tone. If the vagus nerves supplying the heart were severed, the tonic inhibitory flow would be interrupted and resting heart rate would increase. Administration of a parasympathetic cholinergic blocking agent such as atropine causes a marked elevation of basal heart rate.

Sympathetic adrenergic nerve impulses to the heart increase the heart rate (positive chronotropic effect) and increase the force of heart muscle contraction (positive inotropic effect). Although there are sympathetic centers in the brainstem, just as there are parasympathetic ones, evidence indicates that there is no cardioacceleration center, per se. Rather, neurally mediated elevation of heart rate appears to occur via inhibition of the cardioinhibitory center, and increased impulses in the sympathetic nerve supply to the heart originating at lower levels in the sympathetic nervous system.

The baroreceptors of the aortic arch and carotid sinus are the sensors for the afferent impulses to the cardioinhibitory center which influence its activity; thus, a fall in systemic arterial pressure resulting from hypovolemia or peripheral vasodilation is sensed by the baroreceptors, which alter their sensory (afferent) input to the cardioinhibitory centers. The result is both a decrease in vagal inhibitory tone and an increased firing in the sympathetic supply to the heart, resulting in increased heart rate.

Regulation of Stroke Volume

Stroke volume from each ventricle is around 80 ml; this is over half of the diastolic ventricular blood volume. Stroke volume, like heart rate, is also under dual neural regulation; sympathetic stimulation increases contractility and parasympathetic impulses have a negative inotropic (decreased contractility) action. When there is increased contractility, more of the blood present in the ventricle at the onset of contraction is ejected; therefore, less remains in the ventricles, resulting in a decreased end-systolic volume and an increased systolic ejection fraction. When there is decreased contractility, systolic ejection fraction declines and end systolic volume increases.

Stroke volume is determined by three factors: (1) the preload: the degree of stretch on the myocardial fibers at the onset of contraction; (2) the inotropic state (degree of contractility) of the myocardium; and (3) the afterload: the tension which the myocardium is required to develop during contraction; or, stated another way, the resistance which the heart muscle must overcome in order to eject the blood which it contains into the arteries.

Preload

Stroke volume is importantly influenced by the length, or degree of stretch, of the myocardial fiber at the onset of contraction, as discussed previously. The fiber length–contractility relationship is such that as the muscle fibers are stretched, the contractile tension which they are capable of developing during shortening is increased. This is the Frank-Starling relationship. This relationship has an upper limit; if myocardial fibers are stretched beyond a certain optimal limit then the strength of the resulting contraction may decline. In short, up to a point, the strength of contraction is directly proportional to the initial length of the muscle fiber at the onset of contraction. In the intact organism, the length of the heart muscle fiber is proportional to, or is a function of, the amount of blood in the ventricle at the conclusion of diastole: the end-diastolic volume. Put another way one can say that, other influences equal, stroke volume is a function of end-diastolic volume, since the degree of contractility (or force of contraction) determines each stroke volume. The term preload applies to the degree to which heart muscle is stretched at the onset of systole and therefore corresponds to end-diastolic volume.

End-diastolic volume, in turn, is determined by (1) venous return to the right heart; (2) strength of atrial contraction during ventricular diastolic filling; and (3) the amount of blood pumped out of the ventricle during the prior contraction, relative to the end-diastolic volume (systolic ejection fraction). It is important to emphasize, however, that in the intact healthy individual, the amount of venous return (as increased for example in muscular exercise or decreased in hypovolemia); the neural and hormonally mediated changes in myocardial contractility and heart rate; and the peripheral vascular resistance; may all be more important in determining cardiac output than changes in ventricular end-diastolic volume and the Frank-Starling relationship. In the normal exercising individual, ventricular diastolic volumes and filling pressures remain about the same (less than 12 mmHg) but cardiac output increases greatly. This increase in cardiac output without an increase in ventricular end-diastolic volume is attained largely via an increase in inotropic state (increased contractility) from sympathetic adrenergic stimulation.

Inotropic State

The degree of myocardial contractility is the major factor determining the level of ventricular performance at any given ventricular end-diastolic volume. That is to say that the position of the ventricular function curve (which relates stroke work to end-diastolic volume) is determined mainly by the inotropic state of the myocardium. This is illustrated in Figure 7-8 in which ventricular function curves are drawn for a number of different myocardial contractile states.

The most important factor determining myocardial contractility is the content and concentration of catecholamines in the heart muscle. The sympathetic adrenergic nerve terminals within the heart release norepinephrine directly into the myocardium itself to stimulate the myocardial β adrenergic receptors. In addition, the adrenal medulla produces both norepinephrine and epinephrine, and adrenergic terminals elsewhere release norepinephrine. These catecholamines enter the circulation and are carried to the heart via its blood supply. The action of these substances is to increase the heart muscle force of contraction, and therefore increase stroke volume, at any level of initial fiber length (end-diastolic volume). In addition, they increase the velocity of contraction. Thus, for a given end-diastolic volume (preload) and a given systolic pressure (afterload) a more rapid, forceful and complete contraction will occur if adrenergic neurotransmitters are present in adequate concentration. The greater the rate and force of contraction, given equal fiber length (preload) and given equal resistance to systolic ejection (afterload), the greater the stroke volume. Thus catecholamines elevate stroke volume and move the heart to a higher ventricular function curve; the higher curve is an expression of increased ventricular performance.

The inotropic effect of catecholamines on the myocardium is mediated via β

adrenergic receptors, the stimulation of which activates cell membrane adenyl cylase resulting in increased production of cyclic AMP; it is increased intracellular cyclic AMP which mediates the positive inotropic effects of the catecholamines.

Such myocardial depressant factors as hypoxemia, hypercapnia, acidemia (including lactic acidemia) and the myocardial depressant factors released from the viscera during shock, will produce a negative inotropic effect, and decrease ventricular contractility and output at any given ventricular end-diastolic volume (preload) and arterial impedance (afterload). Therefore, myocardial depressant factors shift the heart to a lower ventricular function curve; the lowered curve is an expression of decreased ventricular performance.

In chronic heart failure the content of norepinephrine in the myocardium is abnormally low and thus the heart performs on a depressed function curve. That is to say that the failing heart produces a lesser force of contraction (a lower stroke volume) for the same degree of stretch on the heart muscle fibers (i.e., the same end-diastolic volume) than the normal heart. The reason for this depressed inotropic state is a lower than normal content of norepinephrine in the myocardium, coupled with an inability to increase this amount during increased metabolic demand, for example, at the onset of exercise.

Afterload

The forces which impose resistance to the ejection of blood from the ventricle comprise the afterload on the ventricle. There are two factors opposing systolic emptying: (1) the impedance to blood flow through the aortic valves and the blood pressure in the aorta; and (2) the size, or degree of dilation, of the heart. Together, the resistance in the aorta and the degree of distention of the ventricle, determine the tension or stress developed in the wall of the ventricle during systolic ejection. If diastolic fiber length and myocardial inotropic state are held constant, then the speed and degree of myocardial contraction, and therefore the stroke volume, will decrease as the afterload increases. Figure 7-9 illustrates the relationship between stroke volume in ml and afterload expressed as systemic arterial pressure. As the afterload increases above normal levels, the resistance to systolic ejection increases and the consequence is a depressed stroke volume.

The elevated wall tension in a dilated heart combines with pressure in the aorta to effectively increase the resistance to systolic ejection, and hence the afterload. So, given the same mean aortic pressure, the enlarged heart has to cope with a larger afterload than one of normal size, and its produces a smaller stroke volume. Since, as we shall see, myocardial contractility is relatively fixed and impaired in heart failure, an increase in afterload such as would be produced by an elevated arterial blood pressure (for example, stopping antihypertensive medication), and excessive heart dilation as a result of ECF volume overload (such as would be caused by stopping maintenance diuretics) can rapidly produce a severe worsening of the heart failure. Since the pressure is relatively low in the pulmonary artery, because the pulmonary circuit is a highly distensible low-pressure circuit, pulmonary artery pressure is less of a factor in right ventricular output than aortic pressure is in left ventricular output. The systemic circuit is a high impedance circuit and thus peripheral (arterial) resistance is an important

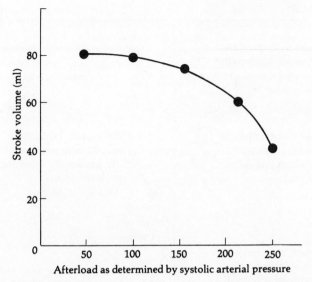

Figure 7-9. Relationship between stroke volume and myocardial afterload (resistance to systolic ejection). As the resistance to ejection increases, as occurs in increased systolic arterial pressure, then the stroke volume declines.

influence on stroke volume and on myocardial, especially left-ventricular, work load.

In the failing heart there exists a *depressed rate of contraction* for a given load to be moved; a *decreased force of contraction* for a given initial fiber length; and in the case of an hypertrophied and/or dilated heart, especially in the presence of elevated arterial blood pressure and volume, a greatly *increased resistance to systolic emptying* of blood from the ventricle. Thus in heart failure there is a depressed rate and force of contraction; an increased preload because of impaired systolic ejection; and an increased afterload, because of the dilated ventricle and peripheral vasoconstriction (see following). The increased force of contraction which would occur in the normal subject as a result of an increased preload, is largely nullified in the patient with heart failure by the depressed inotropic state and the fact that the ventricle is already overdilated.

The relationship between stroke volume and its major determinants is shown for the normal and the failing heart in Figure 7-10.

Interaction Between Preload and Afterload in the Regulation of Cardiac Output

If the afterload is increased (elevated systemic arterial pressure) the amount of blood which the left ventricle is capable of ejecting at a given fiber length is decreased—that is, stroke volume declines. The immediate consequence is an increased end-systolic volume and pressure. This produces an elevated end-diastolic volume, and an increased stretch on myocardial fibers prior to the onset of the next contraction. The increased stretch causes enhanced contractility and produces a more forceful systolic ejection, which is able to overcome the elevated arterial resistance. So stroke volume tends to return to normal, but at the metabolic cost of an increased workload on the myocardium. The reverse situa-

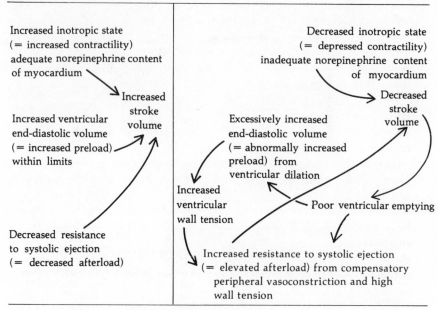

NORMAL   HEART FAILURE

Figure 7-10. Diagram of the three major determinants of stroke volume: inotropic state, preload, and afterload; and their interrelationships, (a) in the normal, and (b) in the failing heart.

tion would also apply. If aortic impedance falls (= decreased afterload), systolic ejection increases, ventricular emptying is more complete, end-diastolic volume and pressure drop, contractility declines, and stroke volume returns to the normal baseline level. Therefore, under normal conditions, and to some extent even in heart failure, there is a smooth integration of the effects of preload and afterload in the regulation of cardiac output.

THE FAILING HEART

Introduction

Definition

Heart failure is a condition in which the myocardium is unable to produce a cardiac output adequate to meet the metabolic needs of the tissues, especially for oxygen. The inability may occur as a result of either an excessive hemodynamic workload on the myocardium, such as hypertension; or a defect in the heart muscle itself which renders it unable to meet a normal workload, such as atherosclerotic cardiomyopathy. In either case the manifestations of heart failure are the consequence of a discrepancy between metabolic and hemodynamic requirements, and the capacity of the myocardium to meet the requirements. Decreased myocardial contractility (depressed inotropic state) is the common denominator of heart failure.

Types of Heart Failure

Left heart failure usually occurs before right heart failure, and is a more common abnormality; in fact, left heart failure is probably the most frequent cause of failure of the right ventricle, because of the high frequency of two common circulatory disorders which affect the left ventricle more than the right: coronary artery disease and hypertension.

When ventricular failure is marked and chronic, especially if both right and left sides of the heart are involved, the condition is then known as chronic congestive heart failure (CHF). This is the disorder with which we will be primarily concerned in this chapter.

Congestive heart failure is characterized by two categories of manifestations: (1) inadequate tissue and organ perfusion; and (2) systemic and pulmonary vascular congestion. These two categories have been referred to as "forward" and "backward" failure respectively; however, the manifestations are but two sides of the one coin: inadequate heart pumping. Decreased myocardial contractility, with low cardiac output, produces inadequate blood flow ahead of the ventricle which has failed, at the same time that it permits an increased volume and pressure of blood behind it. Nevertheless, the signs and symptoms of forward failure (inadequate tissue perfusion) may occur, for a time at least, independently of the signs and symptoms of backward failure (passive pulmonary and systemic, capillary and venous congestion).

Heart failure may occur acutely, as following a myocardial infarction; or may develop chronically and insidiously, in which case the patient may gradually become aware of a decreased tolerance of and capacity for physical exertion over a period of years; a more noticeable swelling of the ankles toward the end of a work week which resolves over the weekend; or the slow worsening over time of occasional substernal chest pain or shortness of breath while climbing stairs. This section will emphasize chronically developing heart failure. However gradually it may develop, the course of chronic congestive heart failure is often marked by episodes of worsening which may be precipitated by anxiety or physical overexertion, or an intercurrent infection, trauma, or surgery. These exacerbations constitute episodes of acute heart failure superimposed upon the underlying chronic failure.

Causes of Heart Failure

Underlying Causes

These may be divided into those which impose an excessive hemodynamic load on the myocardium such as arterial hypertension or heart valve stenosis or insufficiency; and those which directly impair the ability of heart muscle to cope with a normal workload, such as coronary atherosclerosis and myocardial ischemia, or toxic infections and inflammatory diseases of the myocardium.

Certain abnormalities which constitute the underlying causes of heart disease tend to affect one ventricle sooner than the other, and, although eventually congestive heart failure is likely to develop, early in the course of the disorder symptoms referable to right- or left-sided heart overload may occur. Usually the first symptom of left ventricular failure is shortness of breath with exertion, resulting from pulmonary vascular congestion. The usual causes are arterial hypertension and myocardial ischemia from coronary artery disease, and less frequently aortic or mitral valve disease. Often the first sign of right ventricle overload is pretibial and pedal edema; the more frequent causes are chronic obstructive pulmonary disease and mitral or pulmonic valve stenosis.

Precipitating Causes

Precipitating causes often operate by imposing an increased workload upon a myocardium already impaired by one of the abnormalities classed as underlying causes. Such precipitating causes, which may initiate an episode of acute heart failure in a patient with impaired but compensated myocardinal function, include an infarction; an acute exacerbation of arterial hypertension; an infection, especially one involving the lungs; distrubances of heart rate or rhythm; or lapses in the management regimen for chronic heart disease such as weight gain (usually caused by excess salt intake), stopping digitalis or diuretic, physical overexertion, or emotional upset.

Heart Cell Changes in Heart Failure

At the tissue level, the biochemical correlate of the functional abnormality in heart failure—decreased contractility of the myocardium—is a decreased overall content and concentration of norepinephrine, the adrenergic neurotransmitter of the sympathetic nerve endings in the heart, responsible for maintaining normal contractility at rest and increasing contractility during increased activity. Myocardial content of the catecholamine is reduced to one third of the normal value in patients with heart failure. Probably this depletion of myocardial norepinephrine results from a reduction in its release from adrenergic terminals in the heart muscle. The abnormal processes responsible for this depletion are not known, but a deficiency in the enzyme tyrosine hydroxylase, which catalyzes one of the steps in the biosynthesis of norepinephrine from its precursors is suspected, since there is a deficit in the activity of this enzyme in the failing heart.

The relationship between nonrepinephrine depletion and the subcellular processes of contraction responsible for the decreased contractility are not certain. Evidence indicates that there are subcellular β adrenergic elements in close conjunction with the contractile proteins, which act in some way, possibly involving the release or increased mobility or accessibility of Ca^{2+}, to enhance contractility when activated. Although a dearth of norepinephrine in heart failure results in lack of inotropic stimulation at rest and in exercise, evidence indicates that the more fundamental cellular deficits of heart failure have to do with decreased activity of the enzyme ATPase which releases the energy from ATP required for contraction; and a defect in the delivery of Ca^{2+} to the active sites of the contractile proteins.

Consequences of Decreased Myocardial Contractility

Impaired myocardial contractility is the basic defect in heart failure, and a decline in cardiac output is its first manifestation. Further physiologic consequences of the decreased cardiac output appear to take the form of compensatory adjustments which operate to increase cardiac output and maintain tissue perfusion near normal for extended periods of time.

Augmentation of Sympathetic Automatic Activation

The decreased cardiac output causes a reflex activation of the sympathetic nervous system which results in tachycardia and a peripheral arterial and venous vasoconstriction which is differential: blood is directed away from skin, viscera, kidneys and muscle, and to brain and heart—more vital organs. The venoconstriction aids venous return to the heart which improves diastolic filling. And the increased total peripheral resistance helps maintain the blood pressure within normal limits in spite of the decline in cardiac output. The elevated heart rate caused by adrenergic activation combines with vasoconstriction to sustain blood pressure and tissue perfusion. The receptors for the sympathetic autonomic activation are probably the baroreceptors in the aortic arch and carotid sinus which sense the decline in arterial pressure resulting from the low cardiac output, and respond by sending afferent impulses to the cardioaccelerator system and the brainstem vasopressor area. In addition, the increase in circulating catecholamines derived from adrenergic terminals outside the heart, and from the adrenal medullae, provide important extrinsic inotropic support for a myocardium which is deficient in its own intrinsic neural catecholamine supply. The concentration of norepinephrine in the plasma and urine of patients with heart failure has been studied at rest and during exercise and has been found to be markedly elevated above the levels in normal control subjects under both conditions.

Expansion of the Extracellular Fluid Volume (ECF)

The decline in cardiac output, combined with some degree of vasoconstriction in the renal arterial supply, and redistribution of blood flow within the kidney, results in inadequate renal perfusion. These changes have at least two consequences which probably contribute to an isosmotic hypervolemia: (1) low renal perfusion reduces glomerular filtration rate (GFR), decreases the amount of Na^+ filtered at the glomerulus, and causes a resulting decline in the Na^+ load passing the macula densa of the nephron; and (2) low renal blood flow reduces perfusion pressure to the juxtaglomerular cells of the afferent arteriole. These stimuli, plus the compensatory adrenergic activation occuring in heart failure (cited above) produce an increased secretion of renin by the juxtaglomerular cells; the resulting activation of the renin–angiotension–aldosterone system (described in Chapter 1) produces increased avidity for, and resorption of, Na^+ at the distal renal tubule. As Na^+ is retained, water is retained with it and ECF volume expansion results. In addition, low pressure receptors in the atria and central large veins send afferent impulses to the nuclei in the hypothalamus which produce ADH, so increased ADH secretion probably contributes to the ECF overload by stimulating increased resorption of water from the tubular filtrate in the distal tubule and collecting ducts of the kidney nephron.

The patient with congestive heart failure has an increased level of total body Na^+, an increased total body water content which may be proportionately greater than the Na^+ excess—that is, he may be hyponatremic—and a markedly increased interstitial and intravascular ECF volume. The amount of interstitial ECF is *proportionately* greater than that in the vasculature; in a patient with CHF and an increase of one-fifth in circulating blood volume, interstitial fluid content may be twice normal. Appearance of overt edema in heart failure has been reported to correlate with increased plasma levels of renin, angiotension and aldosterone, although other studies indicate that only renin levels are reliably elevated, aldosterone remaining often within normal limits. The metabolism of aldosterone is slowed in heart failure, probably as a result of impaired liver function because of inadequate liver perfusion. Thus aldosterone levels may be elevated even though secretion rate is normal.

The expanded ECF volume has both helpful and adverse consequences. (1) On the one hand, the expanded ECF increases venous return, left ventricular end-diastolic pressure, and myocardial fiber length, thus acting to elevate stroke volume according to the Frank-Starling relation, and to improve organ perfusion. Elevated end-diastolic volume caused by increased venous return (veno-constriction and an expanded ECF) and incomplete systolic emptying, increases myocardial fiber lengths and enables the heart to operate on a higher segment of the Frank-Starling curve which relates end-diastolic volume to stroke volume. The consequence is the maintenance of the cardiac output at levels nearer normal than could occur without the increased LVEDV. (2) On the other hand, the hypervolemia and increased venous return increases the workload on the myocardium (because of the increased volume to be pumped), elevates myocardial oxygen requirements, causes ventricular dilation, and eventually produces many of the disabling signs and symptoms characteristic of congestive heart failure: elevated pulmonary capillary pressure and pulmonary edema; and increased systemic venous pressure with peripheral capillary engorgement and edema. This is the typical patient in uncompensated, poorly managed heart failure.

Tachycardia

Tachycardia resulting from increased sympathetic activation helps sustain cardiac output in the face of decreased stroke volume (cardiac output = heart rate × stroke volume). The depressed contractility restricts stroke volume to a relatively constant quantity, which makes cardiac output in heart failure largely dependent on heart rate.

For a long time these compensatory mechanisms may interact to main cardiac output within normal levels, even at modest exertion, but at the cost of an increased end-diastolic volume and often an elevated resting heart rate. But as myocardial contractility continues to decline and ventricular end-diastolic volume increases, the onset of exercise, with its associated venous return, further dilates the ventricle without a corresponding increase in cardiac output. Pulmonary capillary pressure then becomes elevated and the patient experiences exertional dyspnea.

Hypertrophy of Heart Muscle

Hypertrophy of heart muscle is a compensatory mechanism which develops over a long period of time and occurs as a result of increased protein synthesis, as an adaptive response to chronic myocardial overload. In the course of hypertrophy increased muscle mass and increased capillary blood supply probably develop together, so that the myocardium may not "outgrow" its blood supply as is sometimes said to occur. Nevertheless in advanced hypertrophy the contractile properties of heart muscle decline, a development which appears to correlate with a decreased ability of the myocardial adrenergic terminals to synthesize norepinephrine. Hypertrophied myocardium appears to have a decreased rate of tension development and a slowed rate of contraction.

Dilation of the Heart

Dilation of the heart develops as the contractility declines, resulting in a progressively lower stroke volume; and as the ECF volume expands. Dilation also appears to act for a time as a compensatory mechanism, via further extension of the Frank-Starling relation, to sustain stroke output. But as dilation becomes more extreme, abnormalities in the structural integrity of the contractile elements develop as a result of chronic excessive stretch. Because of distortion and rearrangement of myocardial fibers, their ability to produce effective contraction which will result in useful external work (i.e., pumping blood) declines. In addition, in the dilated ventricle the wall tension becomes greatly elevated, producing an increase in afterload as described above. The consequences are increased oxygen consumption, inefficient energy utilization, and decreased effective work.

Each compensatory mechanism in heart failure, when developed beyond a certain extent, appears to contain the potential for eventually worsening rather than ameliorating the physiologic abnormalities. Enchanced activity of the sympathetic nervous system produces peripheral vasoconstriction which increases afterload by elevating resistance to systolic ejection; this increases myocardial hemodynamic load and work, and increases oxygen consumption and energy expenditure. Tachycardia increases myocardial oxygen consumption and reduces diastolic filling time of the coronary arteries and hence their perfusion, contributing to myocardial ischemia and a further reduced contractility. ECF volume expansion increases the hemodynamic workload of the myocardium, reduces alveolar ventilation and impairs tissue perfusion and oxygenation. It contributes to the development of dilation and hypertrophy, which (as indicated above) elevate afterload, impair contractility, and are costly in terms of oxygen and energy consumption.

It is important to note that the hypertensive patient with left ventricular or congestive heart failure offers a more complex management problem. It is essential to control the hypertension because of its contribution to increasing myocardial work by elevating afterload and LVEDP; yet many antihypertensive agents such as guanethidine, reserpine and propranolol either further deplete the myocardium of catecholamines, or block their effect, thus contributing to a withdrawal of the much needed positive inotropic effect of extrinsic catecholamines and a worsening of the heart failure. An additional effect of some of these antiadrenergic medications may also be to increase Na^+ and water retention with an increase of hypervolemic myocardial overload.

Values Measured in the Quantification of Heart Performance

Systolic Ejection Fraction

This value is the ratio of the stroke volume to the end-diastolic volume. Put another way, it is the amount of blood expelled from the ventricle during systole, relative to the amount of blood contained in the ventricle at the conclusion of diastole. It can be estimated angiographically, by radioisotope scanning, and by echocardiography. The failing heart demonstrates a low ratio, indicating that although it is functioning at an increased fiber length, because of increased ventricle blood volume, it is unable to expel a normal fraction of that blood at systole because of depressed contractility.

Left Ventricular End-Diastolic Pressure, Cardiac Output, and Total Body Oxygen Consumption

The left ventricular end-diastolic pressure, cardiac output, and total body oxygen consumption under basal conditions can be contrasted with the same values obtained during physical exertion. In the normal individual the cardiac output and stroke volume will rise a standard large amount for a given elevation in rate of oxygen consumption with increasing exertion, and the left ventricular pressure typically does not change much from its normal about 10 mmHg value, or may even decline. In the case of the failing heart, however, left ventricular pressure increases above 12 mmHg, but stroke volume may actually decline, and cardiac output increases only slightly; the increase in output is on the basis of elevated heart rate. The pressure in the left ventricle increases because the elevated venous return induced by exercise leads to increased left ventricular volume. But because of the poor myocardial contractility the ventricle is unable to increase its stroke output.

Change in Pressure with Change in Time (dp/dt)

The value dp/dt is the rate of increase in pressure within the ventricle as a function of time from the onset of systole. In heart failure there is a slowing in the rates of tension development and fiber shortening during systole. In addition, the rate of actual expulsion of blood from the ventricle during systole is slowed below normal both under basal conditions and during physical exertion.

Echocardiography

Echocardiography is a noninvasive method of evaluation of heart function in which ultrasonic waves are directed at and then reflected from various portions of the heart, by aiming the ultrasound impulses at the heart from different directions. This procedure can measure wall thickness, right ventricle size, and the end-systolic and end-diastolic dimensions; the resulting values are used in an assessment of ventricular performance.

Systolic Time Intervals

These values are determined by a simultaneous measurement of the heart sounds, the electrocardiogram, and the pulse wave of the carotid artery. The phonocardiogram is a method for exact timing of the heart sounds. The times between: (1) the electrical activation of the ventricle, as indicated by the QRS complex; (2) the ejection of blood out of the ventricle, as indicated by the carotid pulse wave; and (3) the conclusion of systolic ejection, as indicated by the sound of closure of the aortic valve (S_2) are measured and recorded.

The time between the QRS complex and the carotid pulse wave is the period during which the ventricle is increasing its pressure to the point where blood will actually be ejected from the ventricle; this period is the preejection period (PEP). The time between the carotid pulse wave and the closure of the aortic valve (marking the end of systolic ejection) is called the left ventricular ejection time (LVET).

Systolic time intervals compare the length of the preejection period with the duration of the left ventricular ejection time. In heart failure, a slowing of the rate of ventricular pressure development is shown by a lengthened PEP. A decrease in stroke volume is indicated by a shortened LVET. These changes occur as a shift in the *ratios* of the two values PEP and LVET, not as a change in the *overall* duration of electrical and mechanical systole, as measured from the time of the QRS complex (the wave of ventricular depolarization) to S_2 (the second heart sound). The change in ratio is called an increased PEP/LVET ratio and indicates that it takes the myocardium of the failing heart *longer* than normal to attain an adequate force to eject the blood in the ventricle; and then the ventricle sustains the expulsion phase for a *shorter* than normal period of time. When the PEP/LVET ratio is compared with the systolic ejection fraction (above) it has been shown that a high PEP/LVET ratio is correlated with a low ejection fraction, thus documenting the slowed and weakened myocardial contractility of heart failure.

Abnormal Response of the Heart to Exercise in Heart Failure

It is the case that in early heart failure the stroke volume and end-diastolic volume and pressure may be normal or close to normal when the subject is at rest; the heart may demonstrate abnormal changes, or the failure of the normal ones, only at the onset of increased exertion. This fact is a portion of the rationale for exercise stress testing as an important component of the complete evaluation of myocardial performance.

The alterations which occur in the normal subject during physical exertion are discussed more fully in Chapter 8. Briefly, they include marked vasodilation in skeletal muscle tissue; elevated venous return to the right heart; adrenergic stimulation of the myocardium; increased rate and force of cardiac contraction; and a greater stroke volume. But there is usually no increase in left ventricular end-diastolic volume and pressure. Cardiac output is markedly augmented. An increase in cardiac output is well correlated in the normal subject with an increase in oxygen consumption as exercise progresses.

In the subject with heart failure, however, the predicted rise in cardiac output, per unit increase in oxygen consumption, fails to occur. The increase in venous return induced by exercise is not balanced by a corresponding increase in stroke volume for a given exercise level; the consequence of this failure to increase stroke volume as venous return increases is an elevation of left ventricular end-diastolic volume and pressure. Blood accumulates in the left atrium and pulmonary vasculature behind the failing ventricle, and the patient experiences exertional dyspnea.

These differences in response to exercise between the normal and failing heart can be demonstrated by measurements of total oxygen consumption, and cardiac output and left ventricular end-diastolic pressure during cardiac catheterization or with newer noninvasive (and therefore safer) procedures, at rest and during physical exertion.

CLINICAL MANIFESTATIONS OF CONGESTIVE HEART FAILURE AND THEIR PATHOPHYSIOLOGIC BASIS

Symptoms

Dyspnea

Dyspnea is the most common and often the first chief complaint of a patient in early congestive heart failure. When he first becomes aware of the symptom it usually occurs at or soon after the onset of increased physical activity; he describes the sensation as shortness of breath or being easily "winded." The receptors for the sensations are not known, but the vagus nerve is the sensory neural supply to the lungs. The basis for dyspnea is probably the elevated pulmonary capillary pressure (elevated hydrostatic pressure in the pulmonary circuit) in the lung vasculature resulting from an expanded ECF volume, and the fact that the often stronger right ventricle pumps more blood into the lungs than the failing left ventricle can pump out and deliver to the systemic circuit, resulting in pulmonary vascular engorgement. First the left atrium dilates, and then hydrostatic pressure increases in the pulmonary venous circuit supplying the left atrium.

As pulmonary capillary pressure increases, the forces tending to retain fluid within the capillaries (Chapter 1) are exceeded, and extravasation of fluid occurs, first into the interstitial spaces (interstitial pulmonary edema) and then into the alveoli (intraalveolar pulmonary edema). This fluid accumulation has a number of consequences. (1) The resulting decreased pulmonary compliance requires an increased effort on the part of the respiratory muscles to move air into and out of the lungs. The resulting increased oxygen requirements of the respiratory muscles is coupled with a decreased oxygen supply to them because of the depressed cardiac output. (2) Fluid in the airways stimulates bronchoconstriction and increased resistance to airflow. (3) Increased pulmonary ECF volume results in decreased lung air volume. (4) Fluid in the alveoli impairs gaseous exchange, leading to alveolar hypoventilation and ultimately to hypoxemia. (5) Elevated pulmonary fluid and the increased work of breathing promotes a decreased tidal volume and increased minute ventilation (tachypnea); more air per respiratory cycle traverses respiratory dead space (that is, the large and small airways, where no gaseous exchange occurs) contributing to hypoxemia and elevated respiratory muscle oxygen consumption. As congestive heart failure progresses, the level of activity required to elicit dyspnea decreases and shortness of breath may eventually be present even at rest.

Orthopnea

Orthopnea is dyspnea which comes on after the patient lies down, is relieved by sitting up, and eventually prompts the use of two or more pillows to elevate the head and thorax during sleep. The degree of the symptom and its progress can be quantified by ascertaining how many pillows the patient uses at night at the present time as compared with one or two years ago. Orthopnea results from the circulatory readjustments brought about by recumbency. In the upright or sitting position, the effect of gravity causes increased hydrostatic pressure and accumulation of fluid in the blood vessels and interstitial spaces of the legs and lower trunk. On reclining, two changes occur. First there is a rapid elevation of central venous pressure as intravascular fluid moves from the lower body into the thorax, increases venous return to the right heart, and elevates pulmonary capillary pressure. The second mechanism takes longer—a matter of hours. Decreased hydrostatic pressure in the vessels of the lower body during recumbency permits interstitial fluid, which left the capillaries under the effects of gravity while standing, to reenter the vasculature, causing a marked increase in intravascular ECF and a decline in dependent ISF (occult, or in more severe cases, overt edema). Orthopnea, if severe, may be accompanied by wheezing and cough productive of watery fluid from the airways based on the processes described above for dyspnea.

Paroxysmal Nocturnal Dyspnea

Paroxysmal nocturnal dyspnea represents a progression of the above abnormalities. The patient, once asleep, may awaken suddenly with severe respiratory distress, a sense of suffocation, and feelings of extreme apprehension. This may be accompanied by cough with expectoration of clear frothy or pink blood-tinged sputum. In this condition the pulmonary capillary pressure has increased to the point where the capillary membranes have stretched enough to permit large amounts of fluid, plasma proteins, and even red blood cells to enter the interstitial and intraalveolar spaces. Probably a contributory factor to PND is the central depression of the brainstem respiratory control centers which occurs during sleep. This is associated with a decreased activation of the reticular formation characteristic of the sleep state. It results in hypoventilation marked enough to cause the PaO_2 to drop; this decline acts as a strong chemoreceptor respiratory stimulus. Also during sleep, sympathetic adrenergic activity and plasma catecholamine levels decline; this removes adrenergic inotropic support from the failing myocardium whose intrinsic adrenergic supply is greatly reduced. PND may be accompanied by nocturnal angina because of the increased myocardial work load imposed by the expanded circulating ECF, and hypoxia from sleep-induced respiratory depression.

Acute Pulmonary Edema

Acute pulmonary edema is a culmination of the pathologic alterations described above and essentially represents severe increase in pulmonary capillary pressure causing transudation of ECF into interstitial and intraalveolar spaces as a consequence of left ventricular failure. Severe arterial hypoxemia may result, often accompanied by hypocapnia and respiratory alkalemia from hypoxemic hyperventilation (Chapters 2 and 9).

Cheyne–Stokes Respirations

There are a number of theories accounting for the alternating hyperpnea and apnea which may occur in congestive heart failure, as well as in a number of neurologic brainstem impairments. The cyclic alteration in respiratory rate and depth is correlated with cyclic fluctuations in arterial blood gas oxygen and carbon dioxide tensions. During the phase of increasing hyperpnea, arterial PaO_2 rises and $PaCO_2$ declines, causing decreasing stimulation to the respiratory center. Hypoventilation then gradually develops, often culminating in a brief apneic period. During this time PaO_2 falls and $PaCO_2$ rises, again stimulating the respiratory center to another phase of hyperpnea. Chronic hypoxia of the respiratory center, or abnormal sensitivity of the center because of cerebrovascular disease, have been advanced as causes for the respiratory oscillations. In addition, it has been proposed that a prolonged circulation time from lungs to brain, resulting in a delayed feedback loop conveying arterial blood gas information to the respiratory control center from the pulmonary vascular circuit, results in the oscillation of the respiratory control reflexes.

Nocturia

The new development of this complaint, especially when it is accompanied by shortness of breath on exertion and/or elevated blood pressure, may indicate a worsening of congestive heart failure. Daytime accumulation of occult or overt systemic edema, which is elevated interstitial fluid content, occurs and the fluid is then mobilized back into the vasculature during the night's recumbent posture, causing a diuresis.

Signs

The patient may appear dusky or ashen because of the combination of the hypoxemia, which causes an increased amount of desaturated hemoglobin in the blood, resulting in cyanosis; and peripheral vasoconstriction caused by adrenergic activation, which results in pallor. There may be central cyanosis: the tip of the nose, tongue, and lips. Heart rate may be elevated and pulse pressure decreased (diastolic pressure elevated), both caused by the compensatory sympathetic stimulation which results in tachycardia and peripheral vasoconstriction. Jugular vein pressure may be elevated indicating increased central venous pressure. Heart enlargement may be indicated by palpation of an enlarged apical impulse which is displaced down and to the left, and a palpable thrust. Gallop rhythms resulting from audible S3 and S4 may be heard. Bibasilar fine pulmonary rales, often more marked on inspiration, and basilar dullness to percussion may be evident, the former from fluid in the airways, the latter from pleural effusion. The more severe the left ventricular failure, the more widespread the rales will be.

Symmetrical dependent edema may be present and is most marked in the ankles in ambultory patients. The degree of pitting can be assessed by estimating the depth of depression in millimeters after gentle uniform pressure over the tibia for a standard length of time. Liver enlargement from passive venous engorgement may develop. This is evaluated by percussing the liver span and estimating in cm its extent below the right costal margin. Pressing on the liver may cause reflux of blood into the jugular vein: hepatojugular reflux. The liver may be tender. Ascites may result from transudation of fluid from engorged capillaries in the splanchnic and portal circulation into the peritoneal cavity (Chapter 1).

Laboratory Values

A widened arteriovenous oxygen difference results from increased extraction of O_2 during slow flow through the tissues. A slowed cirulation time causes sluggish flow of blood through the systemic capillaries; since the transit time of blood through the capillaries is increased, a larger than normal fraction of the oxygen carried by hemoglobin is extracted to meet the metabolic needs of peripheral tissues. Therefore, the mixed venous blood returning to the right heart has a lower than normal content of oxygen.

Once the blood is returned to the lungs for oxygenation, the degree of oxygenation occurring there may be depressed because of alveolar hypoventilation caused by pulmonary edema. Interstitial and intraalveolar collections of fluid impede gaseous exchange between alveoli and pulmonary capillaries, resulting in ventilation/perfusion $(\dot{V}/\dot{Q})$ mismatch (Chapter 9) and a resulting below normal Pao_2 (hypoxic respiratory alkalemia). Blood urea nitrogen and creatinine may be elevated because of poor renal perfusion and a decreased glomerular filtration rate. This is prerenal azotemia (Chapter 10).

MANAGEMENT OF CHRONIC HEART FAILURE

Prevention and Control

The goal of management in chronic congestive heart failure is to attempt to reduce the discrepancy between the contractile capacity of the heart, and the myocardial work necessary to meet the patient's metabolic requirements—in other words, to increase cardiac output and decrease load on the myocardium. Since heart failure appears to develop as a consequence of a long period of excessive workload relative to the functional capacity of the heart, prevention should be the first concern, and life style is of prime importance in prevention (after careful selection of one's parents, since hereditary factors appear to be important predisposing elements in the development of heart disease). Two key factors in prevention are the prevention or control of hypertension and atherosclerotic coronary artery disease. Hypertension increases the chronic workload on the myocardium, and ischemic heart disease impairs the ability of the myocardium adequately to meet systemic metabolic requirements. Once hypertension and/or myocardial ischemia have developed, their control and/or reversal become of prime importance. The elements of both prevention and control comprise a list of elements of life style health habits: (1) a regular, preferably daily, vigorous exercise program appropriate to the patient's functional capacity; (2) maintenance of lean body weight; (3) a diet low in saturated fats, sugar, and salt; and (4) no cigaret smoking.

Once the signs and symptoms of heart failure have developed, the aims of treatment are measures to elevate cardiac output and to reduce myocardial overload. These aims may be attained by improving myocardial contractility with inotropic agents, especially digitalis, and decreasing the workload of the myocardium through: (1) reducing systemic arterial blood pressure (if it is elevated) with antihypertensive agents; (2) decreasing ECF volume by the use of diuretics; (3) and decreasing the level of physical activity, to reduce metabolic requirements of tissues.

Increasing Myocardial Contractility

Digitalis increases myocardial contractility. It shifts the heart muscle force velocity and performance curves upward. This is a positive inotropic action which appears not to be mediated via the β adrenergic system of the heart. The mechanism of the positive inotropic effect appears to relate to both the membrane and the intracellular excitation–contraction coupling described above. Digitalis inhibits the movement of Na^+ and K^+ across the heart muscle cell membrane, by inhibiting the enzymes involved in their active transport system. This enzyme-catalyzed active transport system is called Na^+–K^+ dependent (or stimulated) ATP-ase; it is contained in the sarcolemma. The mechanism by which these transmembrane alterations in Na^+ and K^+ movement and concentration influence contractility is not completely worked out, but the inhibition of their movement appears to promote increased amount and availability of Ca^{2+} at the subcellular shortening sites—the filaments themselves; the Ca^{2+} facilitates the contractile processes.

Digitalis also produces an increase in the refractory period of the AV node via both a direct action and one mediated by enhanced parasympathetic tone: increased vagal inhibition. The consequence is a slowing of the ventricular rate. Digitalis also exerts a negative chronotropic action at the level of the sinus node pacemaker. Again this effect is partly direct and partly parasympathetically mediated. The inotropic effect of digitalis improves cardiac output by elevating stroke volume, and the resulting increase in peripheral perfusion decreases the compensatory sympathetic activation, and production of renin by the kidney.

The inotropic effects of digitalis are manifested in the patient by a decrease in heart size because of elevated cardiac output; a lowering of left ventricular end-diastolic pressure, which decreases pulmonary vascular congestion; a decrease in compensatory peripheral vasoconstriction; improved peripheral tissue and organ perfusion; and a reduction in passive venous congestion. Although it does increase myocardial oxygen consumption, this effect is ameliorated by the reduction in myocardial oxygen needs resulting from decreased heart size and reduced wall tension. In addition, since it slows heart rate, it improves coronary artery perfusion by lengthening diastolic filling time. Toxic effects of digitalis are manifested by alterations of heart rate and rhythm, especially premature ventricular contractions, and are made worse by hypokalemia. Anorexia and change in heart rate or rhythm may be early signs of digitalis levels in excess of the therapeutic range (Chapter 6).

Decreasing Myocardial Workload

Decreasing ECF volume is an important component in the reduction of workload on the myocardium. Control of hypertension with antihypertensive medication is also necessary. Both diuretics and antihypertensive agents reduce heart work by lowering the afterload on the heart—diuretics by decreasing heart dilation and therefore wall tension, and antihypertensives by reducing the resistance to systolic ejection. A reduction in afterload leads to an increased stroke volume and elevated cardiac output. Management of hypervolemia with diuretics is discussed in Chapter 1, and hypertension in Chapter 3. Dietary salt restriction is often indicated in the management of both hypervolemia and hypertension.

Administration of pharmacologic agents which reduce afterload by dilating arteries, and reduce preload back to more normal levels by dilating veins, is proposed by some workers to be a valuable adjunct in the management of CHF. Recent studies of patients with severe chronic congestive heart failure have indicated that the addition of systemic peripheral vasodilator drugs to the basic inotropic (digoxin) and diuretic management has beneficial effects, both as concerns the patients' symptoms (persistent dyspnea and fatigue) and objective measurements of ventricular performance as assessed by cardiac catheterization, treadmill exercise tests, echocardiography, and other methods. The rationale for vasodilator therapy is that increased arterial tone causes increased resistance to systolic ejection; and increased venous tone leads to increased venous return, elevated left ventricular end-diastolic volume and pressure, and hence increased wall tension. The increased arterial resistance and elevated wall tension together comprise a heightened ventricular afterload which increases myocardial oxygen consumption and increases the workload on the myocardium. This leads to additional myocardial ischemia, decreased myocardial contractility, reduced cardiac output, and further increase in compensatory vasoconstriction. This in turn further increases afterload on the myocardium and perpetuates a vicious cycle which peripheral vasodilation counteracts.

One disadvantage of vasodilator therapy alone can be a decline in blood pressure and, therefore of aortic diastolic pressure, below levels adequate to sustain optimal coronary artery perfusion. For this reason some investigators have combined systemic vasodilators with inotropic agents under the assumption that the increased stroke volume produced by the increased myocardial contractility would ameliorate the decline in arterial pressure, and the two together would result in a greater increase in cardiac output than the decline in afterload caused by the vasodilator alone.

Combined Inotropic and Vasodilator Agents

Combination of various inotropic agents and systemic vasodilators have been used in treatment of congestive heart failure (especially that caused by chronic coronary heart disease) in both the ambulatory and in-patient clinical setting. Dobutamine is a new drug with both α and β adrenergic stimulating actions, but the β effects predominate so that during infusions there is a marked increase in myocardial contractility with little effect on the peripheral vasculature. It can be given orally; its actions resemble those of dopamine. This drug has been used with nitroprusside, which is a strong vasodilator of both arterial and venous beds;

it produces a decrease in impedance to left ventricular ejection, and a reduced left ventricular end-diastolic pressure and volume. The combination may lead to a higher cardiac output, lower pulmonary capillary wedge pressure and greater reduction in systemic and pulmonary vascular resistance than either alone. Other systemic vasodilators used in such treatment are phentolamine, isosorbide dinitrate (both oral and topical), hydralazine, and trimethaphan.

Prazosin, an oral systemic vasodilator agent, has been reported to result in sustained dilation of both venous and arteriolar vascular beds, with a marked decline in total systemic vascular resistance. The effects of orally administered prazosin begin in thirty minutes and persist for five hours; heart rate is unchanged, left ventricular end-diastolic pressure declines, cardiac index increases, and myocardial oxygen requirements decline. Heart size decreases and effectiveness of contraction increases, as demonstrated echocardiographically, and there may be a significant increase in treadmill exercise capacity. Correlated with the improved hemodynamic status, patients may report a marked amelioration of dyspnea, orthopnea, and fatigue.

The pharmacologic actions of prazosin are α adrenergic receptor blockade, and inhibition of an enzyme in vascular smooth muscle involved in vasoconstriction. This dual action produces generalized vascular relaxation in both the resistance vessels (arterioles) and the capacitance vessels (veins and venules), and leads to a decline in venous return to the right heart, lowering left ventricular diastolic volume to more normal levels, and alleviating pulmonary venous congestion. The decline in arterial impedance improves ventricular emptying, which contributes to the normalization of ventricular diastolic volume; and elevates cardiac output, improving organ and tissue perfusion.

Follow-up evaluation of patients with congestive heart failure treated with oral prazosin for several months indicates that the improvement in heart function and amelioration of symptoms shown on short-term assessment, persist on longer-term ambulatory management.

REFERENCES

Akera T: Membrane adenosine triphosphatase: a digitalis receptor? *Science* 198:569–574, 1977.

Awan NA, et al: Efficacy of ambulatory systemic vasodilator therapy with oral prazosin in chronic refractory heart failure. *Circulation* 56:346–355, 1977.

Awan NA, et al: Comparison of effects of nitroprusside and prazosin on left ventricular function and the peripheral circulation in chronic refractory congestive heart failure. *Circulation* 57:152–159, 1978.

Beeson PB and McDermott W, editors: *Textbook of Medicine*, 14th ed. Philadelphia, Pa.: Saunders, 1975.

Braunwald E: Determinants and assessment of cardiac function. *N. Engl. J. Med.* 296:86–89, 1977.

Braunwald E, et al: *Mechanisms of Contraction of the Normal and Failing Heart*, 2nd ed. Boston, Mass.: Little, Brown, 1976.

Dodge HT: Angiographic evaluation of ventricular function. *N. Engl. J. Med.* 296:551–553, 1977.

Ganong WF: *Review of Medical Physiology*, 8th ed. Los Altos, Calif.: Lang Medical Publications, 1977.

Gorlin R: Practical cardiac hemodynamics. *N. Engl. J. Med.* 296:203–205, 1977.

Guiha NH, et al: Treatment of refractory heart failure with infusion of nitroprusside. *N. Engl. J. Med.* 291:587–592, 1974.

Guyton AC: *Textbook of Medical Physiology*, 5th ed. Philadelphia, Pa.: Saunders, 1976.

Frohlich ED, editor: *Pathophysiology*. Philadelphia, Pa.: Lippincott, 1976.

Mason DT, editor: *Advances in Heart Disease*. New York: Grune & Stratton, 1977.

Mikulic E, et al. Comparative hemodynamic effects of inotropic and vasodilator drugs in severe heart failure. *Circulation* 56:528–533, 1977.

Parmley WK and Chatterjee K: Combined vasodilator and intropic therapy: a new approach in the treatment of heart failure. In: Mason DT, editor: *Advances in Heart Disease*. New York: Grune & Stratton, 1977, Chap. 3, pp. 45–57.

Rackley CE, et al: Hemodynamic effects of sublingual and oral long-acting nitrates. In: Mason DT, editor: *Advances in Heart Disease*. New York: Grune & Stratton, 1977, Chap. 4, pp. 59–69.

Segel LD and Mason DT: Alcohol and the heart. In Mason DT, editor: *Advances in Heart Disease*. New York: Grune & Stratton, 1977, Chap. 30, pp. 481–488.

Thorn GW, et al, editors: *Harrison's Principles of Internal Medicine*, 8th ed. New York: McGraw-Hill, 1977.

Weissler AM: Systolic time intervals. *N. Engl. J. Med.* 296:321–324, 1977.

Wikman-Coffelt J and Mason DT: Mechanism of decreased contratility in chronic hemodynamic overlaod. In: Mason DT, editor: *Advances in Heart Disease*. New York: Grune & Stratton, 1977, Chap. 31, pp. 491–504.

CHAPTER EIGHT

Exercise and the Heart

PHYSIOLOGIC CHANGES DURING EXERCISE IN THE NORMAL SUBJECT

Local Changes in Muscle Tissue

Cholinergic Vasodilation

At rest, skeletal muscle tissue has a low blood flow and a low degree of extraction of available hemoglobin-bound oxygen from blood. An increase in blood flow to muscle tissue occurs even prior to the onset of exercise, apparently initiated by psychic processes associated with the intention to begin muscle activity; then immediately at the onset of exertion muscle blood flow increases even more. These preliminary blood flow increases appear to be neurally mediated via a special innervation to muscle blood vessels called the sympathetic vasodilator system. All blood vessels throughout the body are innervated by norepinephrine-secreting adrenergic vasoconstrictor fibers from the sympathetic division of the autonomic nervous system. These vasoconstrictor fibers are tonically active in the resting state, which produces a continuous low level of vascular smooth muscle tone. However, skeletal muscle arteries and arterioles have in addition to the sympathetic adrenergic supply, a specialized vasodilator innervation; these fibers are cholinergic and, unlike the adrenergic supply, have no tonic activity. However, when they receive appropriate reflex stimulation from higher brain centers, associated with the intention to increase physical activity, the consequence is vasodilation. At the same time there is reflex neural inhibition of the tonic vasoconstricting impulses in the adrenergic vasomotor innervation, which produces a further vasodilation.

Production of Metabolites

As actual muscle contraction occurs during exercise, local metabolic rate increases and this maintains a greatly enhanced vasodilation and elevated blood flow. Because of the increased cellular metabolism, there is a drop in local O_2 content, an increase in local CO_2 content, increased H^+ production, K^+ liberation from the intracellular space, and production of adenosine and lactate. These substances are called vasodilator metabolites. Release of potassium ions from muscle cells appears to occupy a position of prime importance in mediating the vasodilation which occurs during the rhythmic muscle contraction of exercise. In the presence of hypokalemia the degree of increase in muscle blood flow from vasodilation may be inadequate to sustain muscular effort. This may be the basis for the muscular weakness sometimes experienced by the hypokalemic patient. All of these metabolic influences combine to produce marked relaxation of the arterioles and precapillary sphincters.

Temperature and Hormonal Effects

Increased heat production by actively contracting muscle causes yet more vasodilation by a direct temperature effect. Epinephrine released from the adrenal medulla during exercise also increases muscle vasodilation. The consequence of these processes is that blood flow in actively exercising muscle tissue may increase 20 to 40 times over baseline values, and the total cross-sectional diameter of the arterial tree in an active muscle is greatly increased.

Arteriovenous Oxygen Difference (A–V O_2) in Muscle

The arterial to venous oxygen difference (A–V O_2)—that is, the concentration of oxygen in the precapillary arterioles as compared with the concentration of oxygen in the postcapillary venules—is greatly increased during exercise. This is simply another way of stating that during active exercise, muscle tissue extracts a greatly increased amount of the available oxygen, over that amount which it extracts during resting metabolism. Muscle blood A–V O_2 is about 84 ml/L at rest;

that is, the oxygen content of arterial blood entering muscle capillaries is 8.4 ml O_2/100 ml blood greater than that of the venous blood leaving the capillaries in the nonactive state.

The $A-V$ O_2 may increase two- to threefold during vigorous exertion to 16 or even 24 ml O_2/100 ml blood, indicating the extraction of larger amounts of oxygen from the blood by working, as opposed to resting, muscles. The mechanisms by which this increased oxygen extraction occurs in active muscle, especially in the physically trained subject, are several. At the subcellular level there are increases in the number and size of the mitochondria, increased stores of oxidative energy substrates (fuel: glycogen, triglycerides, and others) and an increased metabolic enzyme content and activity. The hemoglobin–oxygen dissociation curve is shifted to the right, meaning that the hemoglobin gives up its oxygen to the metabolizing tissues more readily, by lowered pH, increased temperature, and increased 2,3-DPG production (Chapter 2). And because of rapid oxygen use, the gradient for diffusion of oxygen from the blood to the metabolizing cells is greatly increased. These are but some of the processes accounting for the two- or threefold widening of the $A–V$ O_2 occurring in vigorous exercise.

Systemic Cardiovascular Responses to Exercise

The systemic responses to exercise differ depending on the type of exercise: isometric vs. isotonic. There are basically two patterns of muscle contraction in exercise: dynamic and static. Dynamic exercise is also called isotonic, meaning that the tension on muscle fibers remains the same, but the muscles alternately contract and relax, that is, their length changes. Static exercise is also called isometric, meaning the length of the muscle fibers remains the same, but the tension increases and remains steadily high. In dynamic exercise such as brisk walking, jogging, swimming, bicycling, or rowing, there is alternate rhythmic contraction and relaxation of antagonistic muscle groups; though muscle fiber length changes, producing external movement, there is relatively little alteration in muscle tension. In static exercise, such as weight lifting, hand grips and bar chinning, there is a great degree of increased tension produced, with relatively little change in length, and slight production of external movements.

When skeletal muscle contracts it compresses the vascular bed within it; the greater the intensity and length of maintained contraction, the greater the degree of compression and hence the less the blood flow, even to the point of almost complete cessation of flow at maximal tension development. During relaxation between contractions however, greatly increased flow occurs. The larger the relaxation–flow phase in exercising muscle relative to the contraction–compression phase, the greater the degree of blood flow. This is but a part of the reason that the systemic response to exercise, as well as its long-term effects physiologically, depends largely on the nature of the exertion: isotonic or isometric (see following).

Isotonic (Dynamic) Exercise

When the brain events occur which are associated with the decision promptly to initiate muscle exercise, the heart rate increases even before the onset of muscle contraction; this elevation of heart rate occurs therefore probably as a consequence of a reflex involving higher brain centers, the brainstem, and the sympathetic cardiac nerves; it is mediated both by an inhibition of vagal parasympathetic cardioinhibitory tone, and an increase in discharge of the cardiac sympathetic nerve supply. Then, promptly after the onset of rhythmic (dynamic) muscle contraction, there is a moderate increase in stroke volume of the heart accompanied by a fall in total peripheral vascular resistance because of marked vasodilation in the contracting muscles. The systolic blood pressure rises slightly and the diastolic changes little. The heart rate increases markedly; the increase may be over 80 beats/min. This elevation in heart rate accounts for a larger share in producing the elevated cardiac output than does the increased stroke volume (cardiac output = stroke volume × heart rate).

The decline in skeletal muscle vascular resistance because of vasodilation is accompanied by varying degrees of vasoconstriction in the visceral vascular beds, depending on the intensity of exercise, producing a redistribution of blood flow to enhance the supply to working muscles. Cerebral blood flow apparently undergoes only minor variations with exercise unless exercise is continued to extremes, when vascular collapse and syncope may occur. Therefore, during dynamic exercise the myocardium is subjected primarily to an elevated *volume*, rather than an elevated *pressure*, workload. The myocardium responds more favorably to volume work than it does to pressure work, because pressure work increases myocardial oxygen consumption more than volume work does. One reason for this is the elevated resistance to systolic ejection (increased afterload) caused by increased aortic pressure.

Isometric (Static) Exercise

Isometric (static) exercise leads to muscle hypertrophy, and thus weight training is used in muscle-building programs and for athletes training for certain kinds of competitive sports in which muscle mass is of importance. However, isometric exercise training has little or no place in physical reconditioning programs for patients with even mild cardiac impairment. An exception is training patients in methods for doing necessary lifting with minimal adverse effects; lifting while breathing with the mouth open helps avoid the increase in blood pressure and cardiovascular strain resulting from the Valsalva maneuver (see following).

Prior to and at the onset of long-maintained static exertion, heart rate increases as it does in isotonic muscle work, but very rapidly after the onset of contraction both systolic and diastolic blood pressures rise markedly. In isometric exercises increases of 50 mmHg have been reported for each value (i.e., from 120/80 to 195/125), but the heart rate may increase only 20 bpm. There is evidence that in the person with latent, early, or labile hypertension, isometric muscle exertion produces an elevation of blood pressure even higher than in the normal subject. Thus the afterload on the heart (that is, the resistance in the aorta and systemic circuit against which the left ventricle must eject blood) is greatly elevated, as is the myocardial oxygen requirement. The stroke volume changes very little or may actually decline, especially in a heart with poor contractility. And blood flow to the contracting muscles declines during static contraction as a result of the compression of their vasculature caused by the maintained high muscle tension.

The differences in physiologic response to isotonic·(dynamic) and isometric

Table 8-1
Cardiovascular Response to Exercise

	Isometric (static)	*Isotonic (dynamic)*
Stroke volume	Slight or no increase	Moderate increase
Heart rate	Slight increase	Large increase
Peripheral vascular resistance	Large increase	Decrease
Blood pressure	Large elevation	Slight elevation or no change

(static) exercise may be summed up in the following way: isotonic exercise results in a moderate increase in stroke volume, a very large increase in heart rate, a decline in peripheral vascular resistance, and a slight increase in blood pressure; conversely, isometric exercise produces a slight or no increase in stroke volume, a slight increase in heart rate, a large increase in peripheral vascular resistance, and a large elevation in blood pressure. These responses are shown in Table 8-1.

Because of the inadequacy of blood flow to the contracted muscles during isometric exertion, oxygen supply is inadequate to sutain aerobic metabolism; pyruvate, instead of entering the aerobic Krebs cycle, forms lactate as a result of the need to use anaerobic glycolysis as the energy source, hence lactic acid accumulates and an oxygen debt occurs. Thus static exertion produces greater pressure work (increased afterload) for the myocardium than does dynamic exertion, and results in markedly elevated myocardial oxygen consumption. It is important to avoid this kind of exercise in cardiac rehabilitation because the patient with ischemic heart disease, in which myocardial blood and hence oxygen supply is already compromised, is much more likely to develop angina and arrhythmias with static than with dynamic exercise. Hemodynamic studies also show elevated ventricular end-diastolic volume and pressure under such conditions, indicating that the increased peripheral resistance and elevated afterload is impairing the ability of the left ventricle to empty adequately during systole.

An additional difficulty with this type of work for the patient with heart disease is the tendency to perform the Valsalva maneuver at maximal exertion: the glottis is closed, chest muscles braced, air is retained in the lungs, and a greatly elevated intrathoracic pressure immediately develops with straining. This produces a rapid and marked decline in venous return to the right heart and a precipitous fall in cardiac output, which greatly impairs coronary artery perfusion and enhances myocardial ischemia in the face of the elevated myocardial oxygen requirements resulting from the pressure work.

The remainder of the discussion of systemic cardiovascular response in exercise will be confined to dynamic (isotonic) muscular activity rather than static (isometric).

Cardiac Output in Exercise

Cardiac output is a function of both heart rate and stroke volume: $CO = HR \times SV$; since both of these parameters increase during dynamic exercise, the cardiac output elevates greatly. The cardiac output in a subject at rest is about 5 L/min, whereas during vigorous exercise it may increase six- to sevenfold, to 35 L/min. Cardiac output varies in relation to body size; therefore, cardiac output is often expressed as cardiac index (CI), which is the cardiac output divided by the surface area of the body in square meters: $CI = CO/m^2$. It is expressed as liters per minute per square meter. The cardiac index of an average-sized normal individual at rest is about 3.5 L per min per m^2. In light to moderate muscle exercise it may increase to 4.5, and in maximal exercise may attain as much as 9–10.

Stroke volume is increased chiefly because of the enhanced myocardial contractility produced by adrenergic stimulation to the heart occurring during exercise. The heart muscle contracts more forcefully and completely; therefore, the systolic ejection fraction (the amount of blood expelled from the ventricle during systole) increases relative to the amount of blood left in the ventricle at the end of systole (end-systolic volume), which declines. But to an even larger extent the increased cardiac output of exercise depends on the increase in heart rate occurring during isotonic exercise. This elevated heart rate is caused by stimulation from the sympathetic adrenergic nerve supply to the heart, and by the stimulating effect of circulating catecholamines. Therefore both chronotropic (rate) and inotropic (contractility) changes are involved in the elevated cardiac output of exercise.

However, the large cardiac output of exercise could not be sustained without a corresponding elevation of venous return to the right heart. This increase is promoted by the pumping action of the contracting muscles and by the increased rate and depth of respiration; at inspiration, intrathoracic pressure declines, fostering entry of blood into the thoracic great veins to the heart; at expiration, intrathoracic pressure rises, fostering right atrial filling. In addition, the generalized adrenergic activation of exercise produces venoconstriction which decreases the amount of blood stored in the veins, and mobilizes it into the systemic arterial circuit.

Oxygen Consumption (Uptake) and Arteriovenous Oxygen Difference (Whole Body) in Exercise

In the normal subject at rest, overall whole body O_2 consumption is about 250 ml/min. During light to moderate isotonic exercise this value may double, increasing to 500 ml/min; and in heavy exercise the value may exceed 1000 ml/min. The increase is caused by an elevated metabolic rate in vigorously contracting muscle.

The A–V O_2 in ml/L in the normal subject at rest is about 50 ml/L; the normal PaO_2 is about 90 mmHg and the normal PaO_2 is about 40 mmHg. Light to moderate exercise may increase the difference in oxygen content between arterial and mixed venous blood to over 75 ml/L, and at maximal exertion the A–V O_2 may increase from resting values of about 50 to over 120 ml/L. This increase results from an increased extraction of oxygen from hemoglobin by actively metabolizing tissues.

The Fick Principle: The Relationship Among Cardiac Output, Oxygen Consumption, and Arteriovenous Oxygen Difference

The Fick principle states that the amount of oxygen taken up by the cells of the body per unit of time ($=O_2$ consumption in ml/min) is equal to the arterial content of oxygen minus the venous content of oxygen ($= A - V O_2$) in ml O_2/L blood, times the blood flow (=cardiac output) in L/min.

Therefore, O_2 consumption (ml/min) = A–V O_2 (ml/L) × CO (L/min). Normal values for a subject at rest would be about

$$250 \text{ ml/min} = 50 \text{ ml/L} \times 5\text{L/min}$$

The relation among these three variables, CO, O_2 consumption, and A–V O_2, forms the physiologic basis for the exercise test as an evaluation of the ability of the cardiovascular system of a given subject to meet the oxygen requirements of his peripheral tissues.

The increase in cardiac output which occurs in exercise is directly proportional to the increase in oxygen consumption occurring during exercise. Since most of the increase in cardiac output is accounted for by an elevation in heart rate, the increased heart rate in exercise is proportional to the increase in oxygen consumption. This relation between heart rate and oxygen consumption is the basis for the use of the heart rate attained during a specified level and duration of standardized exercise, as an assessment of circulatory function, both with respect to the adequacy of ventricular performance and the efficiency of extraction of oxygen by the peripheral tissues.

AEROBIC CAPACITY, OXYGEN COST, AND FUNCTIONAL AEROBIC CAPACITY: $VO_{2 \text{ (max)}}$

Definitions

Maximal oxygen uptake is the $VO_{2(\text{max})}$. This term refers to the largest amount of oxygen which a subject is capable of consuming (or taking up) during the highest level of dynamic exercise of large muscle groups he is capable of performing. $VO_{2(\text{max})}$ is expressed in milliliters of oxygen taken up per kilogram of body weight per minute of maximal exercise: ml/[kg·min]. Essentially it represents the subject's maximal physiologic capacity to transport oxygen from the lungs to the metabolically active cells via the heart, vessels, and blood. Functional aerobic capacity is another term for $VO_{2(\text{max})}$.

Maximal oxygen uptake ($VO_{2(\text{max})}$) is a function of the values for the maximal cardiac output and the maximal arteriovenous oxygen difference determined during the greatest physical exertion the subject is able to perform. Therefore: $VO_{2(\text{max})} = CO_{(\text{max})} \times A - V O_{2(\text{max})}$. Note that this is the Fick equation couched in the terms of values at the maximal exercise level of which the subject is capable. $VO_{2(\text{max})}$ is correlated with lean body weight, is higher (corrected for weight) for males than females, is higher in physically trained and active than in sedentary persons, and it declines with age, although the rate of the decline can be slowed by a regular program of vigorous physical exercise. $VO_{2(\text{max})}$ is the standard measure of cardiovascular performance and yields an objective evaluation of the functional capacity of the circulatory system from the standpoint of (1) the function of the heart as a pump; (2) the oxygen transport capacities of the blood and blood vessels; and (3) the oxygen-extracting capacity of the peripheral tissues. Average maximal O_2 uptakes ($VO_{2(\text{max})}$) for normal subjects are shown in Table 8-2.

Table 8-2
Average Maximal O$_2$ Uptake (VO$_{2\ (max)}$)
in ml/[kg·min] for Normal Subjects
Accustomed to Average Levels of Activity

Age	Males	Females
20–29	38	34
30–39	34	30
40–49	31	27
50–59	29	24
60–69	26	20

Methods of Determining VO$_{2(max)}$

Research Testing

Determinations of VO$_{2(max)}$ may be done either directly or indirectly. If it is done directly, the volume and composition of the subject's respiratory gases are measured in successive samples at 1-min intervals during the concluding few minutes of a multistage exercise test. When done in the research laboratory, the test consists of first a warmup period during which the subject makes the physiologic transition from basal conditions to exertion. Then there are two or three 3-min periods of increasing exercise according to a multistage exercise protocol chosen on the basis of the subject's age, sex, and physiologic status, both as concerns his accustomed level of physical activity, and his cardiovascular status (Table 8-3). Actual measurement of the subject's oxygen uptake during the maximal exertion of which he is capable provides the value for the oxygen consumption (Table 8-2). This maximal oxygen uptake is the consequence of both (1) the maximal delivery of oxygen to the cells by the circulation (cardiac output) and (2) the maximal degree of extraction of oxygen by the peripheral tissues (A-V O$_2$).

The criteria for determining the maximal level of exercise of which a healthy subject is capable is based on his own symptoms: fatigue, leg claudication, lightheadedness or faintness, shortness of breath, weakness, or chest pain. The VO$_{2(max)}$ is the oxygen uptake just prior to and during the onset of symptoms which dictate the termination of the test. The signs of such fatigue include a leveling off of the heart rate, an increase in blood pressure (if a drop in blood pressure occurs this may indicate impending syncope) and an endpoint of marked dyspnea and other evidences of fatigue. These mark the maximal exercise level of which the subject is capable.

Clinical Testing

The determination of VO$_{2(max)}$ as outlined above requires methods too expensive, time consuming and uncomfortable to be useful in routine testing in the clinical setting. However, the data derived from such research studies on healthy subjects provide the basis for calculation of normal values of the VO$_{2(max)}$ based on sex, age, and accustomed level of physical activity (Table 8-2). These values are used as yardsticks for evaluation of a subject's cardiovascular status, and the effects of various management regimens for patients with ischemic heart disease. These measurements of the VO$_{2(max)}$ in research studies of large numbers of healthy male and female subjects at various ages have provided data for establishing correlations between oxygen consumption and maximal exercise levels on the multistage treadmill test. The stages of exercise level at various treadmill speeds and grades, for varying periods of exercise time, are based on the MET (metabolic equivalent), which is an expression for the metabolic cost of exercise. One MET is the amount of oxygen consumed per kilogram of body weight per minute, seated, at rest; it is about 3.5 ml/[kg·min]. The stages in treadmill exercise protocols are categorized in multiples of one MET. An example is shown in Table 8-3.

The metabolic costs of both recreational and vocational physical exertion have been similarly calculated; examples are shown in Tables 8-4 and 8-5. These data from normal subjects have been used to define ideal normal limits to which the results of a maximal multistage exercise test in a given patient can be compared. The data from a test include the stage (number of METS) attained and the duration of elapsed time at a given maximal stage. A determined value in a patient, therefore, based on stage and duration, may be compared with the predicted value for a healthy person matched for age, sex, and activity level.

Table 8-3
Excerpt from a Table of METS for Various Treadmill Grades and Speeds

METS	2	4	6	8	10	12
1.6 mph grade	1.5	10				
2.5 mph grade		4.5	10.5	16.5	22.5	
3.4 mph grade		2	6	10	14	18
3.75 mph grade			4	8	12	16

Functional Class	Class IV	Class III	Class II	Class I
	May be symptomatic at rest and becomes so with any degree of physical activity	Asymptomatic at rest but symptoms with less than the normal range of activity leading to marked restrictions on exercise	Asymptomatic at rest, some symptoms with ordinary activity, and slight overall exercise limitations	No exercise limitations and asymptomatic with the full range of normal activity

Table 8-4
Excerpts from Tables of Metabolic Costs of Two Forms of Exercise

O_2 Consumption ml[kg·min]	METS	Walk			Bicycle		
		mph	miles	time (min)	mph	miles	time (min)
9	2½	2	¾	22			
16	4½	4	1	15	6	1½	15
20	5¾	4½	1½	20	9	3	19
35	10	6½	2	18	15	4	16

Table 8-5
Excerpts from Tables of Metabolic Costs of Various Forms of Activity

METS	Recreational	Vocational
2	Talk, play cards, hand sewing	Drive car, desk paper work, sweep floor
3–4	Golf with pull-cart, horseback ride (trot), level walk, slow bicycle ride	Mop floor, clean windows, machine repair, bricklaying
6	Tennis, ski (easy slope)	Cut grass, push mower shovel snow or spade garden
8	Jog–run squash	Move furniture

Correlation of VO$_{2(max)}$ with Heart Rate

Since the heart rate correlates very closely with the level of oxygen consumption occurring at a given level of activity, the heart rate may be used as an estimate of the exercise level attained during a period of exertion. Maximal heart rate attainable with exercise declines with age; this decline is correlated with the decline in VO$_{2(max)}$ with increased age, and is different for men and women. A formula for maximal heart rate in males is reported to be 220 − age in years, and in females 216 − (0.88 × age in years). It has been reported that for sedentary women the decline in treadmill exercise capacity with increasing age is not significant. This is apparently not the case for men. Percentages of maximal heart rates as a function of age in males are shown in Table 8-6.

Table 8-6
Various Percentages of Maximal Heart Rates as a Function of Age (Males)

Age	70%	90%	100%
25	140	180	200
30	136	175	194
35	132	169	188
40	128	164	182
45	124	159	176
50	119	154	171
55	115	149	165
60	111	143	159
65	107	138	153

Functional Aerobic Impairment

The percentage deviation of an observed VO$_{2(max)}$ value from predicted normal age and sex matched control value is termed by some workers the functional aerobic impairment. Even in normal subjects without cardiovascular disorders there will be an about 10% or more functional aerobic impairment on a maximal exercise test if they are sedentary or obese, as compared with values for physically active persons who swim, jog, or bicycle regularly. *The VO$_{2(max)}$ will show lower than normal values whenever either maximal cardiac output or maximal ar-*

teriovenous oxygen difference, or both, are reduced. In the patient with heart disease, a reduced cardiac output is the usual major cause of functional aerobic impairment. Examples of factors causing a decline in A-V O_2 are sedentary life style resulting in impaired efficiency of oxygen extraction by peripheral tissues; a low PaO_2 because of pulmonary disease; and disturbances in oxygen transport and delivery to tissues such as anemia and carbon monoxide poisoning.

Relative Oxygen Cost: % $VO_{2(max)}$

The cardiovascular alterations occurring during submaximal exercise can be expressed either in terms of the absolute workload, or in terms of the relative oxygen cost of the workload to a given individual. Relative oxygen cost of a given degree of physical exercise is expressed by the equation:

$$\frac{\text{uptake of oxygen at submaximal exercise}}{\text{maximal uptake of oxygen at maximal exercise}} \times 100,$$

or

$$\% \ VO_{2(max)} \ (\text{relative oxygen cost}) = \frac{VO_2}{VO_{2(max)}} \times 100.$$

This value increases as the oxygen uptake in L/min and the absolute work load increase. At maximal possible workloads, as limited by the subject's physical capacity to perform exercise work, then % VO_2 would equal $VO_{2(max)}$.

The fact that % $VO_{2(max)}$ and % maximum heart rate are linearly related provides the basis for the use of heart rate as an assessment of the functional capacity of a subject's cardiovascular system in exercise testing (Table 8-6). If a subject who is physically conditioned by regular exercise and has a $VO_{2(max)}$ of 50 ml/[kg·min], bicycling at 15 mph, with an oxygen cost of 30 ml/[kg·min]; is compared with a physically untrained subject with a VO_{max} of 25 ml/[kg·min], bicycling at 7 mph, at an oxygen cost of 15 ml/[kg·min], then both subjects, in spite of the difference in actual external amount of work produced, would show the same *percentage of maximal* heart rate, once they have undergone exercise warmup. The reason for this is that both are producing muscular work at the same *percentage of their maximal oxygen uptake level*—that is, they are both working at the same relative oxygen cost or % $VO_{2(max)}$, which in this case is about 60%.

(The example should not be misinterpreted to mean that $Vo_{2(max)}$ is simply related to bicycling speed. The difference is related to the degree of physical conditioning in the two subjects and the differences in efficiency of exercise in the conditioned and unconditioned subject. The conditioned subject will not have as much increase in heart rate at the onset of exercise as the unconditioned one because there is a larger stroke volume reserve in the former. That is, the metabolic need to elevate cardiac output during increased physical exertion is met in the physically fit person by a large capacity for increased stroke volume. Also the difference in uptake and utilization of O_2 by the peripheral tissues of the two subjects is a function of their differences in physical conditioning; the trained subject is able to perform more work at a lesser metabolic cost because of a greater efficiency of O_2 uptake and use by peripheral tissues).

The % $VO_{2(max)}$ (relative oxygen cost) of a submaximal exercise test shows considerably greater variability for a given subject than does his $VO_{2(max)}$ (functional aerobic capacity); therefore, the maximal exercise test is a more accurate method for revealing the degree of deviation from a normal $VO_{2(max)}$ in a patient with heart disease than the submaximal exercise test (see following). The percentage deviation in $VO_{2(max)}$ for a patient, relative to values for age and sex matched normal controls, are important in assessment of the cardiovascular status and functional capacity of such an individual.

MYOCARDIAL OXYGEN CONSUMPTION AND EXERCISE TRAINING IN ISCHEMIC HEART DISEASE

Myocardial Oxygen Consumption

Myocardial oxygen consumption is determined by a number of physiologic factors but for the purposes of this discussion the determinants of heart muscle oxygen requirements are the heart rate, the pressure and duration of systolic ejection, and the inotropic state (contractility) of the myocardium. Two terms which are used in expressing this requirement, and which incorporate the determinants listed above, are the *double product* and the *triple product*. The double product = heart rate × peak systolic pressure; the triple product = heart rate × peak systolic pressure × systolic ejection time. The patient with ischemic heart disease tends to experience anginal chest pain and develop ischemic S-T segment depression (or sometimes elevation) during exercise testing at about the same value of double and triple products from test to test. Thus it appears to be the case that for each individual there exists a critical "ischemic threshold" at which myocardial oxygen requirements exceed the ability of the coronary vasculature to supply that need, because of a reduced blood flow to and through them.

Effects of Exercise Conditioning on Myocardial Oxygen Requirement

It has been shown in the *normal* subject that exercise conditioning may increase the functional aerobic capacity by 10 to 15%; this increase is brought about mainly by an increase in maximal stroke volume and cardiac output; the maximal heart rate declines about 3%. In addition, in some normal subjects, the arteriovenous oxygen difference increases; this tendency appears to be greater in younger than older subjects.

In patients with *heart disease* also, numerous studies have shown that exercise conditioning increases functional aerobic capacity; in fact evidence indicates that the percentage increase is greater with training in these subjects than it is in healthy individuals, probably because the initial $VO_{2(max)}$ values are lower. This is particularly true of patients with angina, perhaps because of their self-directed limitation of activity in order to decrease the frequency and severity of chest pain. This improved functional aerobic capacity in cardiac patients appears to result primarily from intracellular alterations in the trained skeletal muscle tissue itself rather than in the heart.

Because of the elevated $VO_{2(max)}$ resulting from training, the *relative oxygen cost* (% $VO_{2(max)}$) of any submaximal degree of physical exercise decreases.

Therefore, because of the reduced aerobic requirement necessary to perform the same amount of work which was previously performed at a higher metabolic cost, *the circulatory responses* (heart rate and blood pressure) *are proportionately decreased relative to the same amount of work performed.* Since heart rate and blood pressure, crucial determinants of myocardial oxygen requirements, are reduced per amount of work performed, *therefore heart muscle oxygen demand declines.*

In addition, since A-V O_2 is increased, which means that more of the available oxygen in the blood is removed and utilized to meet tissue metabolic needs, *peripheral oxygen demand also decreases,* lessening the workload of the myocardium. Thus in a patient with coronary artery disease, the amount of blood which the narrowed coronary arteries are able to supply to the myocardium, as a result of the changes induced by exercise conditioning, *more closely approximates myocardial requirements because hemodynamic load on the myocardium is reduced.*

Because the effects of training have enabled the individual with cardiac impairment to perform the same amount of work at decreased metabolic and myocardial cost—that is, functional aerobic impairment has declined with exercise conditioning—this individual may then become able to perform at higher external work loads than previously before reaching the ischemic threshold.

Other Effects of Exercise Training

The question naturally arises as to the effect of exercise training (1) on the development of significantly increased collateral blood flow to previously ischemic areas (exercise revascularization); and (2) on improving myocardial function directly, as opposed to a secondary improvement in performance owing to lessened hemodynamic workload. Both questions are somewhat controversial at the present time. With respect to the first, the balance of evidence indicates that increased formation of collaterals with exercise training, determinable by angiography, has not been demonstrated in the human. Collateral formation does occur over the years as ischemic heart disease progresses, but this appears to result from the natural history of the occluding disease itself rather than from neovascularization developing as a result of exercise (Chapter 4). This may be the reason that the likelihood of a fatality with an acute myocardial infarction is less above 65 years of age. Increased flow developing in smaller vessels supplying ischemic myocardium, as a result of exercise training, would probably not be demonstrable by angiogram.

With respect to the second question, that of increased stroke volume or myocardial contractility developing as a result of exercise training, reports vary. In this respect it is relevant that with exercise training, and the decreased exertional as well as resting heart rates accruing from it, improved myocardial contractility could result from the improved myocardial perfusion during lengthened diastolic intervals. Also, the increased completeness of systolic emptying would lead to lowered end diastolic volume and decreased wall tension. However, while exercise work capacity can be improved by exercise training in patients with ischemic heart disease, it has not been demonstrated that ventricular performance itself improves with such training.

The last and perhaps most important questions with respect to exercise and the heart relates to the effect of a regular program of vigorous exercise in (1) retarding the rate of progression of coronary atherosclerotic disease and, perhaps just as important, (2) altogether preventing its development. Many studies have reported evidence that such effects exist, but at the time of this writing there have not been reported sufficiently long-term, prospective, well-controlled studies to supply definitive answers. However, enough evidence has accumulated concerning the beneficial effects of exercise physiologically and psychoemotionally to justify its inclusion in every management regimen, whether it be preventive or rehabilitative. Its benefits in conjunction with other treatment modalities are well established. Regular vigorous exercise has been reported to decrease the incidence of myocardial infarction among middle aged persons; lower the mortality and morbidity when infarction does occur; and exert a protective or ameliorative effect against the major risk factors for ischemic heart disease.

Exercise Conditioning Guidelines

Specific criteria have been recommended for a program of exercise training adequate to meet the goal of elevating functional aerobic capacity in both normal healthy adults and those with cardiovascular disorders, particularly atherosclerotic coronary artery disease. In the latter case it is probably appropriate that the patient be evaluated in a treadmill laboratory before undertaking an exercise program. Exercise prescriptions are then made on the basis of the history, physical examination, and results of the treadmill test.

Nature of the Exercise

It should be of a type which involves dynamic isotonic activity in the large flexor–extensor muscle groups in the legs and hips, the arms, shoulders, back, and chest. Such exercises include walking–jogging–running progressions; bicycling (either regular or stationary); rowing; and swimming. Exercises should include a variety of forms involving all major muscle groups, since it is only the specifically conditioned muscles that increase their functional aerobic capacity. That is to say that although a program of, for example, only jogging will increase *total* aerobic capacity and reduce the hemodynamic stress on the heart occurring with exertion, the biochemical and microstructural adaptive changes in muscle tissue, which augment maximal oxygen uptake and optimal energy utilization, occur only in those muscles actually involved in regular exercise. This is one of the reasons for the fact that of all the forms of exercise swimming is perhaps the optimal conditioner, since it involves simultaneous use of all of the large muscle groups.

The Exercise Schedule

Intensity, duration, and *frequency* are the three components of an exercise conditioning program. Of the three, adequate *intensity* of exertion appears to be the most important component in producing a significant improvement in functional aerobic capacity. Intensity is usually directly related to the speed with which a given activity (running, bicycling, swimming, or whatever) is carried out. In order to produce significant improvement of $VO_{2(max)}$, the intensity of exercise should be about 70% of the $VO_{2(max)}$, which will correspond to approximately 80% of the maximal heart rate for a given subject; it is approximately this level of performance which constitutes the threshold for onset of symptoms: shortness of breath, sensations of fatigue and weakness, or in the patient with ischemic heart disease, substernal distress. The range of exercise tolerance between individuals is very great, so that setting forth arbitrary levels of performance (heart rate, work intensity, speed, distance) for strenuous activities, especially in the subject with impaired myocardial performance, is not of much value and may be dangerous. However, a failure to attain work intensity levels of about 70% of the $VO_{2(max)}$ in a regular exercise program is probably an inadequate physiologic challenge to induce the adaptive changes in function which lead to increased $VO_{2(max)}$ and decreased exertional hemodynamic stress on the heart.

One of the important uses of multilevel maximal exercise testing is to establish the baselines for work output, oxygen consumption, and heart rate during workouts, based on a determination of the actual $VO_{2(max)}$ for each individual subject. Because of the well-established direct relation between heart rate and oxygen consumption during exercise, subjects can estimate their own level of work attained. A sixty-year-old male with a maximal heart rate of about 175, as determined by his multistage maximal exercise test, producing a heart rate of about 140 at the conclusion of peak exertion in his regular exercise period, is working at 71% of his $VO_{2(max)}$. The risk of exercise-induced cardiovascular complications (serious arrhythmia, cerebral hypoxia, myocardial infarction, ventricular fibrillation) is lessened if this person does not exercise beyond 85% of his maximal heart rate, which corresponds to about 75% of his $VO_{2(max)}$. In persons who are symptomatic with vigorous exercise a good rule is to not exercise beyond 85% of that heart rate at which symptoms and signs occur: chest pain, arrhythmias, and S-T segment changes. In practice this is usually close to the point at which a person cannot carry on a conversation during exercise without having to interrupt talking to gasp for air.

Tables are available giving heart rate guidelines (target heart rates) that a person should not exceed in a rehabilitation program. However, the postmyocardial infarction patients who are participating regularly and doing well should be able to do close to 100% of the predicted maximal heart rate for their age by six months following the AMI.

Frequency and Duration of Exercise Periods

Frequency and *duration* of exercise periods should minimally be about 30 min, 3 to 5 times per week. Since there is some evidence that a lowered intensity of workload in an exercise period can in part be compensated for by an increased frequency of workouts, the subjects who are unable or unwilling, because of symptom development, to sustain 75% of their maximal heart rate for 10–15 minutes may increase the $VO_{2(max)}$-elevating effects of the exercise regimen by working out, say, six times per week for shorter periods at almost peak heart rate, rather than three times per week for 30–40 min.

Rather than setting arbitrary limits for the duration of each exercise period, the subjects may be encouraged to note subjective criteria such as a sense of shortness of breath, mild but unmistakable diaphoresis, and a generalized sense of fatigue as well as specific muscle fatigue in the muscle group involved in the exercise. Although the development of these symptoms is closely related to intensity of exertion, longer workouts will result in improved training effects and will eventually yield the subjective symptoms at a higher exercise intensity as physical conditioning improves.

Each exercise period should be comprised of the three phases of (1) about 5 min of gradual warmup to target heart rate range; (2) at least 20 minutes of continuous activity in the target heart rate range and/or at the level of subjective sensations listed above (symptom-limited maximal exertion); and (3) 5–10 minutes of cooldown in which the subject walks around and engages in intermittent light exercise. The last is of importance in that during vigorous exercise muscle vasodilation is maximal; with sudden cessation of exercise, there is a decline in muscle pumping to promote venous return. Since large volumes of blood are in the muscles, and also in the skin to facilitate heat dissipation, the consequence is a sudden drop in venous return, cardiac output, and cerebral and coronary perfusion. Abrupt stopping of exercise therefore can result in fainting, and in the patient with ischemic heart disease, angina or arrhythmias may ensue. Thus the postexercise cooldown of gradually decreasing exertion facilitates the circulatory adjustments involved in transition from the hemodynamic changes of exercise to basal conditions. Since hot showers, hot tub baths, and saunas increase peripheral vasodilation, they should not be used until cooldown is complete; and should always be used with caution or, in the case of older persons and those with heart disorders, avoided altogether. When nitrates are used to increase exercise tolerance in patients with angina, since they also produce peripheral vasodilation, postexercise cooldown and avoidance of standing still after exercise are of particular importance to avoid orthostatic hypotension and syncope, and a decline in coronary artery perfusion.

An important aspect of planning an exercise program in persons with possible ischemic heart disease is the initial multistage maximal exercise test, and periodic subsequent tests to evaluate the effects of exercise and to check on the progression of the basic disease process. In many symptomatic patients a program of regular symptom-limited walking, initially supervised, with gradually increasing distances and briskness of pace, forms an invaluable preconditioning period prior to more vigorous training. Increases in functional aerobic capacity may be promoted by the practice of slightly increasing the exercise intensity for a minute or two, just to the *onset* of the limiting symptoms (dyspnea, claudication, substernal distress, lightheadedness) and then dropping back to a slower pace, for a total of two to four such "sprints" in each exercise period. The facilitating effects of these interval effort increases in elevating $VO_{2(max)}$ apply whether the exercise conditioning is in the preliminary walk phase or later in the more advanced maximal exertion phases.

Improvement in exercise tolerance with gradual increase in $VO_{2(max)}$ occurs slowly, particularly in the older individual with the functional aerobic impairments resulting from years of sedentary life. Although improved psychoemotional status may appear quite rapidly, measurable objective increases in exercise tolerance may develop only slowly over two months or more. With cessation of regular training the decline in functional capacity is rapid; if the program is reinitiated subsequently, the subject should go back to a previous level of attainment if the lapse was longer than about two weeks. Thus, to maintain increased exercise tolerance and to delay the age-dependent decline in functional aerobic capacity, lifelong maintenance of a regular exercise regimen is required.

Types of Exercise Stress Tests

The reasons for performing a test can be to determine the etiology of chest pain; to assess the functional performance of the heart; to detect latent arrhythmias and labile hypertension; to determine baseline values for following the progress or evaluating the response to treatment; and finally to prescribe a program of exercise reconditioning (cardiac rehabilitation). It offers an objective measure of the ability of the coronary vasculature to increase the blood supply, and hence the oxygen supply, to the myocardium in response to the elevated heart muscle work required to supply active tissues. The subject is asked to perform gradually increasing amounts of muscular exertion, usually on a treadmill but sometimes on a bicycle ergometer, while being monitored electrocardiographically and with blood pressure measurements during the actual test and for a short recovery period following it.

Multi-stage treadmill gives $VO_{2(max)}$ values 3–5% higher than the bicycle ergometer. Some studies have shown that arm exercises, such as moving the pedals of a specially equipped bicycle ergometer by hand and arm movements, are comparable with leg exercise in producing ischemic responses in exercise testing, but the responses occur at a reduced workload (about 40%) as compared with maximum workload to induce ischemic response by leg work. Thus a measurement of functional aerobic capacity cannot usually be based on armwork. But such tests are important in certain individuals such as those with occupational arm work, and in leg amputees. Arm exercise tends to produce higher systolic and especially diastolic blood pressure, and also a higher heart rate, than leg work for proportional work loads, corrected for muscle mass. This difference in response is of great significance for the patient with impaired cardiac function and especially ischemic heart disease, since elevated blood pressure and heart rate together result in a great increase in myocardial oxygen requirements and reduced coronary artery diastolic perfusion time.

On the treadmill test, the O_2 requirements in ml $O_2/[kg$ body wt·min] are determined by the rate in mph and the % grade (Table 8-3). These are adjusted by the examiner to yield different levels of whole-body oxygen consumption in ranges appropriate to the characteristics of the subject: age; sex; cardiovascular history, status and symptoms; and accustomed levels of physical activity.

Studies have shown a good correlation between a subject's response to exercise testing and the status of the coronary arteries as revealed by arteriogram. It is reported to be 60–70% sensitive and 70–80% specific. The likelihood of a true positive test is enhanced if the patient has triple vessel disease, and if the test is performed in conjunction with nuclear cardiologic dynamic measures of mycardial perfusion and stroke volume (Chapter 4). Exercise testing has the advantage of being non-invasive and safe with careful patient selection and a standardized protocol. The treadmill has the two advantages that walking is an activity familiar to everyone, and that the examiner determines the speed and rate of increase of the work load. The test is useful for patients with angina as a means of assessing their cardiovascular functional capacity, since the amount of physical exertion a patient can safely perform is evaluated objectively. In addition it is valuable for detecting an ischemic myocardial response to exercise of increasing intensity in patients who are asymptomatic at rest, or in ordinary tasks of daily life, but who wish to be evaluated as a baseline for a regular exercise program to increase physical fitness. It is also essential in planning, and evaluating the consequences of, exercise rehabilitation programs for postinfarction patients, for those who have undergone coronary artery bypass operations, and for those who elect conservative medical management of symptomatic coronary artery disease.

The test, whether treadmill or bicycle ergometer, may be either a *submaximal* or a *maximal* one. In the submaximal test, the patient exercises at gradually increasing levels to 85% of the predicted maximal heart rate (the "target" heart rate) based on tables which correlate heart rate with oxygen consumption as a function of age, sex, and physical fitness (Table 8-6). The heart rate attained during exercise bears a linear relationship to oxygen uptake by the body during a given level of exertion. The ability of the circulation to transport oxygen to the tissues to meet metabolic requirements accurately reflects the adequacy of cardiac function. Therefore, the adequacy of an exercise test may be estimated by the heart rate attained during the test. A subject who can attain maximal predicted heart rate, and therefore is able to meet maximal tissue oxygen requirements without demonstrating abnormal electrocardiographic changes or disabling symptoms, probably has a functionally adequate coronary circulation and myocardial performance. Some authors believe that the submaximal test is safer than the maximal, and is better accepted by patients because of less fatigue, fewer within-test symptoms, and less post-test fatigue. However, it is less sensitive and will result in greater numbers of false negatives than a maximal test.

The test can be terminated before attaining target heart rate for a number of subjective (patient complaint) end points: anginal chest pain (in the absence of ischemic EKG changes, the test is usually continued until diagnostic EKG changes occur or the pain becomes relatively severe); signs or symptoms indicating the patient may faint from inadequate cerebral perfusion (dizziness, lightheadedness, ataxia); severe leg claudication; extreme sense of fatigue; or marked shortness of breath. Terminating a test for these reasons, although necessary, poses difficulties with respect to estimating the adequacy of the test, since subjects have a wide range of tolerance of such feelings, some of which may be induced or enhanced by anxiety, emotional instability, or unfamiliarity with the test procedure. The objective end point in the test is attainment of an individual stable maximal heart rate and maintenance of it for one to two minutes. ST-segment abnormalities diagnostic of ischemia; three or more consecutive, or multifocal, premature ventricular contractions; ventricular tachycardia; conduction abnormalities; supraventricular arrhythmias; or excessive elevation or fall of blood pressure; suggest an abnormal cardiovascular response to exercise and the test is terminated. (Normally, blood pressure rises to 160–190 mmHg systolic during maximal exercise.)

In the *multistage maximal* exercise test the target heart rates are not used but the level of exercise (and hence oxygen consumption) is gradually increased by increments to a degree of effort physiologically limited by that individual subject's age, sex, cardiovascular status, and habitual level of physical activity (Table 8-3). Reasons for termination are similar to those given for the submaximal test. In cases where the volume and composition of the subject's respiratory gases are being monitored, a plateau in oxygen uptake occurs when the maximal exercise level is reached. (It has been said that sympathy for a person doing a maximal exercise test begins 2 minutes after it has been completed.)

The duration of exercise and the level of workload (stage, or MET equivalents) achieved are reliable guides to a subject's degree of exercise tolerance and hence, cardiovascular function. The functional aerobic impairment, mentioned previously, compares a subject's performance in minutes of elapsed exercise time at a given stage on a multistage maximal treadmill protocol, to a predicted maximum performance for that subject based on age, sex, physical condition, and cardiovascular status.

In all tests resuscitation equipment and persons trained to expertness in its use should be present. A physician should be present or in the immediate vicinity. Monitoring is continued for 5 min after the conclusion of exercise or until the heart rate falls to less than 100 bpm and both subjective symptoms and objective signs are absent. Prior to testing, a history and physical examination should be performed and fully informed consent obtained.

In exercise stress tests false negative or false positive results may occur. A false negative test is one in which no abnormal EKG changes develop during or after the test, yet significant coronary atherosclerosis is present as demonstrated by other means such as coronary arteriography or at autopsy. Nitroglycerine or propranolol, a baseline abnormal EKG resulting from aberrant repolarization patterns, a submaximal test, or a "protective" (pretest) warmup may be causes of false negatives. A false positive test—one showing abnormal EKG changes where atherosclerotic heart disease is not present—may occur with hypokalemia or hypocalcemia, digitalis, psychoactive drugs, or with certain nonischemic cardiovascular abnormalities. For this reason digitalis should be stopped prior to exercise testing, and if the patient is on diuretics, his serum K^+ should be determined. There is also evidence that reversible coronary artery spasm sufficient to produce ischemic repolarization patterns on the EKG and/or anginal chest pain, may occasionally occur with exercise.

The ST-T changes which appear to be associated with a less favorable prognosis and are often a forerunner of clinically evident ischemic heart diseases are horizontal or downsloping depressions of the ST segment. Other changes such as cardiac arrhythmias, T-wave changes and intraventricular conduction abnormalities are reported to be nonspecific occurrences which may or may not be associated with ischemic heart disease. Most observers report that a 1.0 mm (0.1 mV) ST horizontal or downsloping depression of duration greater than 0.08 sec during a maximal or near-maximal test is a reliable index of ischemic change. The depth of depression is reported to correlate with the extent of coronary artery disease. ST-segment elevation occasionally occurs and is often correlated with so-called Prinzmetal angina, which is associated with a decrease, not an increase, in blood pressure. Persistent elevation can occur with hyperacute myocardial infarction. A normal treadmill test, however, does not rule out significant ischemic heart disease.

Many workers have reported on correlations between the treadmill exercise test electrocardiographic responses and the results of coronary arteriography. The presence of arteriographically demonstrated coronary artery narrowing needs to be graded and does not necessarily imply the presence of functionally significant ischemic heart disease. Therefore, it should be emphasized that *exer-*

cise electrocardiography is a test to determine myocardial ischemia and not coronary artery narrowing. The term "false negative exercise EKG" therefore is a misleading term for negative tests in some patients who show arteriographic lesions. It is known that large obstructions (75% or more) can occur in asymptomatic patients who are able to perform submaximal (85% of age-adjusted heart rate) exercise tests.

The reverse is also true: functionally significant coronary obstruction, particularly that associated with coronary spasm (Prinzmetal angina), may be present in spite of a normal coronary angiogram. Moreover, the functional significance of lesions demonstrated angiographically is often unclear. Evidence is accumulating that the correlation between stress electrocardiography and angiographic findings depends to some extent on the differences in populations studied: patients with symptomatic known ischemic heart disease being evaluated for the coronary bypass operation show a high correlation between major angiogram obstructions and exercise EKG abnormalities.

In patients with documented ischemic heart disease, exercise stress testing is of great value in establishing functional exercise capacity. It is also helpful after coronary bypass surgery to assess graft patency. The exercise test defines cardiovascular performance in objective terms. Recent reports of the diagnostic and prognostic value of exercise tests on large numbers of patients, who subsequently underwent angiography, and were then followed for up to 48 months, indicate that the ST-segment response, the overall duration of exercise, and the maximal heart reate achieved, are significantly correlated with the severity of coronary artery disease and the long-term survival.

Perhaps the most significant contribution of the exercise stress test is in objectively defining the limits of cardiovascular performance: as a basis for designing exercise prescriptions for rehabilitation of persons with known ischemic heart disease, and for evaluating the progression of the disorder; and monitoring the results of exercise and other treatment regimens. There are detailed guidelines for exercise rehabilitation of patients with coronary artery disease.

REFERENCES

Beeson PB and McDermott W, editors: *Textbook of Medicine*, 14th ed. Philadelphia, Pa.: Saunders, 1975.

Berra K, et al: The role of physical exercise in the prevention and treatment of coronary heart disease. *Heart Lung J.* 6:288–292, 1977.

Brammell HL and Niccoli A: A physiologic approach to cardiac rehabilitation. *Nurs. Clin. N.A.* 11:223–235, 1976.

Bruce RA, et al: Differences in cardiac function with prolonged physical training for cardiac rehabilitation. *Am. J. Cardiol.* 40:597–603, 1977.

Bruce RA: Exercise testing for evaluation of ventricular function. *N. Engl. J. Med.* 296:671–674, 1977.

Bruce RA: Progress in exercise cardiology. *Progr. Cardiol.* 3:113–172, 1974.

Degre S, et al: Therapeutic effects of physical training in coronary heart disease. Cardiology 62:206–217, 1977.

Dehn MM and Mullins CB: Physiologic effects and importance of exercise in patients with coronary artery disease. *Cardiovasc. Med.* 2:365–85, 1977.

Detry J-M R, et al: Diagnostic value of history and maximal exercise electrocardiography in men and women suspected of coronary heart disease. *Circulation* 56:756–761, 1977.

Fortuin NJ and Weiss JL: Exercise stress testing. *Circulation* 56:699–712, 1977.

Frohlich ED, editor: Pathophysiology. Philadelphia, Pa.: Lippincott, 1976.

Ganong WF: *Review of Medical Physiology*, 8th ed. Los Altos, Calif.: Lange Medical Publications, 1977.

Guyton AC: *Textbook of Medical Physiology*, 5th ed. Philadelphia, Pa.: Saunders, 1976.

Harris R and Frankel LJ, editors: *Guide to Fitness after Fifty*. New York, London: Plenum Press, 1977.

Kellerman JJ, et al: Cardiocirculatory response to different types of training in patients with angina pectoris. *Cardiology* 62:218–231, 1977.

Letac B, et al: A study of left ventricular function in coronary patients before and after physical training. *Circulation* 56:375–378, 1977.

McNeer JF, et al: The role of the exercise test in the evaluation of patients for ischemic heart disease. *Circulation* 56:64–70, 1978.

Sheffield LT, et al: The exercise test in perspective. *Circulation* 55:681–683, 1977.

Sheffield LT, et al: Maximal heart rate and treadmill performance of healthy women in relation to age. *Circulation* 57:79–84, 1978.

Thorn GW, et al, editors: *Harrison's Principles of Internal Medicine*, 8th ed. New York: McGraw-Hill, 1977.

Udall JA and Ellestad MH: Predictive implications of ventricular premature contractions associated with treadmill stress testing. *Circulation* 56:985–989, 1977.

Wenger NK: Exercise for the coronary patient. *Cardiovasc. Med.* 2:69–72, 1977.

Zohman LR and Kattus AA: Exercise testing in the diagnosis of coronary heart disease: A perspective. *Am. J. Cardiol.* 40:243–250, 1977.

CHAPTER NINE

Disorders of Respiration

NORMAL RESPIRATION

Neural Regulation of Breathing

The Brainstem Respiratory Center

Automatic respiration is under the control of two groups of nerve cells located in the reticular formation of the medulla in the lower brainstem. The two groups comprise the respiratory center; they are termed (1) the dorsal respiratory group, which are primarily inspiratory; and (2) the ventral respiratory group, which contain both inspiratory and expiratory neurons. The dorsal neurons are responsible for rhythmic stimuli in the phrenic nerves, which are the motor innervation to the diaphragm. The ventral group of neurons has two divisions: an anterior group which innervates the accessory muscles of respiration; and a posterior group which controls both inspiratory and expiratory movements of the intercostal muscles. The respiratory control centers are also under voluntary respiratory influences from a system of neurons in the cerebral cortex which send afferent impulses to them. Integration between automatic regulation of respiration, occurring in the caudal (lower) brainstem, and the voluntary regulation of

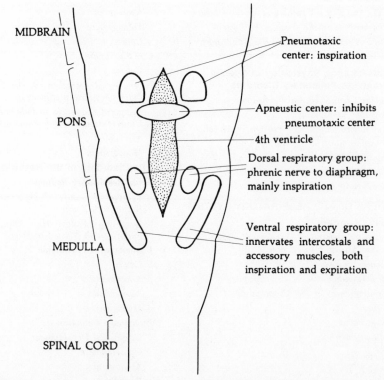

Figure 9-1. Brainstem respiratory control centers. Diagram of the lower brainstem, with the cerebellum removed, showing the pneumotaxic and apneustic centers of the pons and the dorsal and ventral respiratory group of the medulla. The apneustic center stimulates sustained inspiration. The pneumotaxic center produces intermittent inhibition of the apneustic center. The dorsal respiratory group activates the phrenic nerves to the diaphragm and is primarily inspiratory. The ventral group innervates the accessory respiratory muscles and the intercostal muscles and is both inspiratory and expiratory.

respiration, governed by the cerebral cortex, is accomplished within the spinal cord.

The rhythmic firing of the neurons in the respiratory center which cause inspiratory movements is automatic—that is, it demonstrates spontaneous discharge—but the strength, rate, and rhythmicity are influenced by nerve centers in the pons, a portion of the brainstem above the medulla, and by afferent impulses coming from the lungs via the vagus nerves, which are the sensory nerve supply to the lungs. The modulating center in the pons is divided into two sections, one which produces sustained inspiration, called the apneustic center, and one which periodically inhibits the apneustic center, called the pneumotaxic center. The neurons which control expiratory movements are not automatic and therefore do not discharge spontaneously but are subject to afferent impulses from several areas which stimulate them to fire, causing forcible expiration. They are not active in normal resting respiration.

Factors Influencing Activity of the Respiratory Center

CO_2, O_2, and pH Influences on Ventilation

Aortic and Carotid Chemoreceptors. There are specialized receptors in the aortic arch and in the carotid arteries near the bifurcation, called aortic and carotid chemoreceptors, which are sensitive to the tension of O_2 in the blood perfusing them, and which respond to a decline in Pao_2 by increasing the number of impulses in the afferent nerve fibers leaving them. Afferents from the aortic receptors travel to the medulla in the vagus nerves and those from the carotid receptors reach the medulla via the glossopharyngeal and carotid sinus nerves. These afferent impulses stimulate the respiratory center to increase the rate and depth of respiration. However, in the normal individual hypoxic drive to increase minute ventilation probably does not occur at a Pao_2 much above 60 mmHg. Therefore in the normal person increased CO_2 tension has a much greater effect as a stimulus to increased ventilatory response than does a decline in O_2 tension. The location of the receptors is shown in Figure 9-2.

Responses of the aortic and carotid receptors to stimuli differ in that the carotid ones respond to a decreased pH and increased $Paco_2$, in addition to a low Pao_2, while the aortic receptors respond to both low Pao_2 and high $Paco_2$, but apparently are not sensitive to changes in H^+ concentration. The degree of response of these chemoreceptors to hypoxia is potentiated by the simultaneous presence of hypercapnia and, in the case of the carotid receptors, by acidemia. (In man, hypoxic drive comes more from carotid than from aortic receptor stimulation.) The consequence of this potentiation is a greatly amplified stimulus to ventilation by combined abnormalities in arterial blood gas (ABG) composition, above that induced by an abnormality in a single value of Pao_2, $Paco_2$, or pH alone.

These chemoreceptors are also activated by a decline in blood pressure and an increase in sympathetic adrenergic stimulation.

Medullary Chemoreceptors. The brainstem receptors which produce increased rate and depth of breathing in response to elevated $Paco_2$ lie at the level of, but are different from, the neurons of the respiratory control center. They are

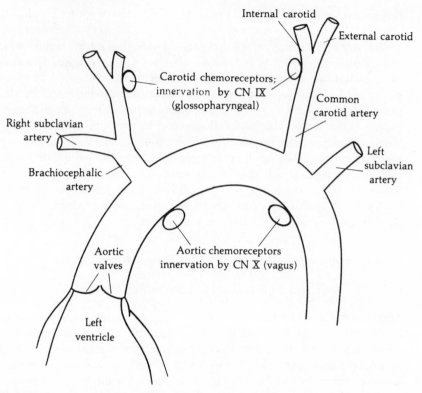

Figure 9-2. Aortic arch and carotid artery chemoreceptors for monitoring PaO_2 and $PaCO_2$; innervation is via the vagus and glossopharyngeal nerves, respectively.

on the ventral surface of the medulla and respond to changes in the H^+ concentration of either the brain interstitial fluid, or cerebrospinal fluid, or both. All membranes are very permeable to CO_2 but much less so to either H^+ or HCO_3^-. CO_2 in blood perfusing the brain readily enters the CSF and brain interstitial fluid and the following reaction occurs: $CO_2 + H_2O \rightarrow H_2CO_3 \rightarrow HCO_3^- + H^+$. That is, the CO_2 is hydrated and the carbonic acid then dissociates (ionizes), resulting in a local increase in H^+ concentration, which stimulates the H^+-sensitive chemoreceptors and leads to increased rate and depth of respiration. Acidemia interacts with elevated CO_2 tension to produce a greater respiratory stimulus than either exerts alone.

Sensors Within the Respiratory System

Airway Receptors. There are receptors in the nose which are sensitive to both mechanical and chemical stimuli; they are probably involved with the expiratory component of the sneeze reflex. They may mediate the reflex apnea and bradycardia occurring in response to such noxious stimuli as strong wind, cold air, and exposure of the nose and face to cold water.

Mechanical stimulation of the epipharynx activates neurons in the glossopharyngeal nerves, which produce rapid inspiration (aspiration or sniffing) and bronchodilation. This reflex clears the nose and brings material in it into the pharynx where it can be swallowed. Laryngeal and tracheal receptors are sensitive to noxious mechanical and chemical stimuli; activation of them has a number of possible reflex consequences: bronchoconstriction, coughing, apnea, and others, including elevation of blood pressure.

Lung Parenchyma Receptors. Pulmonary stretch receptors respond to distention of the lungs with air, and they induce reflex prolongation of expiration time, thus acting to inhibit respiratory rate and depth, as well as causing bronchodilation and circulatory changes: tachycardia and vasoconstriction. These are the Hering–Breuer reflexes, and they appear to exert a modulating influence on respiratory rate and depth. Elevation of Pa_{CO_2} inhibits this respiratory inhibition and this is probably of major importance in promoting the increased ventilation accompanying muscular exercise.

The lung parenchyma also possesses receptors for noxious stimuli of both mechanical and chemical types, such as ammonia and dust in inspired air. The reflex response is bronchoconstriction and hyperpnea. Response of these receptors may play a part in the respiratory abnormalities occurring during an attack of asthma, and may be mediated by release of histamine.

Some workers postulate the existence of a group of lung receptors located in close apposition to the pulmonary capillaries, or within their walls, called the juxtapulmonary capillary receptors (J receptors). It is suggested that these sensors respond to an elevation in pulmonary capillary pressure resulting from the pulmonary vascular congestion of, for example, left ventricular failure or a greatly expanded circulating blood volume. In experimental animals, activation of these receptors produces reflex hypotension, apnea, and bradycardia. Their role in normal respiratory regulation and their possible mediation of responses to pulmonary capillary engorgement remains to be established.

Other Factors Influencing the Respiratory Centers

The sensations of touch, temperature, pain, and proprioception from muscles, tendons, and joints appear to have marked influences on the respiratory regulation mechanisms, and operate via afferent impulses from these peripheral receptors traveling in the spinal cord to the brainstem. It has been suggested that impairment of spinal cord transmission of such impulses flowing from the periphery in the ascending spinal cord tracts to the respiratory center may result in abnormalities of respiratory function, such as obesity hypoventilation and sleep apnea (Chapter 15). The periodic apnea which occurs in some individuals during sleep, and which is reversed by arousal and awakening, is possibly an example of impaired peripheral influences on respiratory control, rather than an abnormality in either the respiratory centers themselves or of motor neuron stimulation to the respiratory muscles. It is proposed that a decrease of sensory imput to the brainstem reticular formation, resulting from defects in spinal ascending pathways, may lead to a decreased reticular formation activity and cause depressed levels of sensitivity and responsiveness in the respiratory center. Apnea and hypoventilation would be the consequence.

In addition, increased activation of the brainstem reticular activating mechanism from increased levels of arousal in the cerebral hemispheres appears to exert a stimulating effect on the respiratory control centers (nonspecific activation).

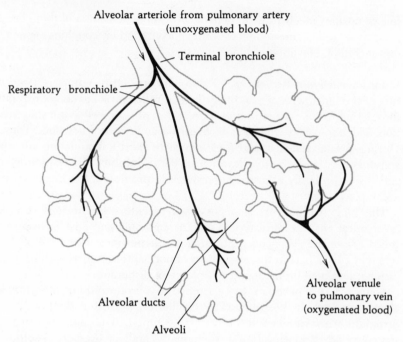

Alveolar arteriole from pulmonary artery
(unoxygenated blood)

Terminal bronchiole

Respiratory bronchiole

Alveolar venule
to pulmonary vein
(oxygenated blood)

Alveolar ducts

Alveoli

Figure 9-3. Alveolar–capillary units of the respiratory lobules.

Aspects of Lung Physiology of Special Relevance to Pulmonary Disorders

Alveolar Ventilation and Perfusion

The basic function of the lung is the exchange of the respiratory gases, oxygen and carbon dioxide, between venous blood in the pulmonary capillaries perfusing the alveoli and the gas mixture within the alveoli. The alveoli are comprised of a very thin membrane less than 1 mμ thick, have an average diameter of about 0.25 mm, and have a total surface area of 70 m^2. Within their walls is an extremely dense network of pulmonary capillaries. Thus the alveolar gas is in close proximity to the venous blood. An alveolar-capillary unit is shown in Figure 9-3.

Gaseous exchange between alveolar air and capillary blood occurs not by active transport but by simple diffusion along the two concentration gradients, for O_2 and CO_2, which exist between the partial pressures of these two gases in alveolar air, and the tensions of the two gases in the mixed venous blood of the pulmonary capillaries. The magnitude (steepness) of the diffusion gradients for O_2 and CO_2 between alveolar air and pulmonary capillary blood depends on the concentrations of the two gases in alveolar air and venous blood, respectively. In the capillary blood CO_2 leaves and O_2 enters. Between alveoli and blood, O_2 leaves the alveoli for the blood and CO_2 enters the alveoli from the blood. Between alveoli and respiratory passages, CO_2 leaves alveoli and O_2 enters them.

The partial pressures of O_2 and CO_2 in the alveoli (P_{AO_2} and P_{ACO_2}) depend upon a balance among a number of factors. The most important ones are (1) body tissue production of CO_2 and consumption of O_2, which adds CO_2 to alveolar gas and removes O_2 from it, and is determined by peripheral metabolic activity; and

(2) the effectiveness of alveolar ventilation in adding O_2 to and removing CO_2 from the alveolar gas. If the rate of removal of CO_2 and addition of O_2 to the alveoli by alveolar ventilation are low relative to metabolic O_2 consumption and CO_2 production, then the PaO_2 will fall and the $PaCO_2$ will rise. By definition, inadequacy of alveolar ventilation relative to metabolic activity is hypoventilation and the consequence is a decline in arterial O_2 tension and a rise in arterial CO_2 tension ($\downarrow PaO_2$ and $\uparrow PaCO_2$). Thus alveolar hypoventilation always results in both arterial hypoxemia ($\downarrow PaO_2$) and arterial hypercapnia ($\uparrow PaCO_2$). The common causes of alveolar hypoventilation are acute or chronic airway obstruction, depression of the brainstem respiratory control centers from trauma or drugs, and chest wall abnormalities. The reverse situation, excessive alveolar ventilation relative to metabolic need for O_2 and production of CO_2, is hyperventilation (discussed in Chapter 2). In all cases, the changes in arterial O_2 and CO_2 tensions then feed back to influence activity of the respiratory control centers as described above.

Alveolar Ventilation

The minute respiratory volume = tidal volume × respiratory rate (MRV = TV × RR) and is the total amount of air which flows into the respiratory airways each minute. Substituting average values in the equation above, average minute volume is about 7000 ml/min where tidal volume is 500 ml and respiratory rate is 14. These values are at rest. Exchange of O_2 and CO_2 between inspired air and pulmonary capillary blood occurs only in the alveoli; therefore the air in the conducting passages of the respiratory system—trachea, bronchi, and bronchioles—is not involved in respiratory exchange. These structures are called *anatomic* dead space. In a subject with a normal tidal volume of 500 ml, the first 350 ml of an inspired breath reaches the alveoli and intermingles with alveolar air; the remaining 150 ml stays in the airways. Then during expiration the first about 150 ml to be expired is this air from the anatomic dead space (and is therefore similar in composition to ambient air except for high water vapor). The following 350 ml is gas from the alveoli which participated in gaseous exchange with pulmonary capillary blood (and is therefore lower in O_2 and higher in CO_2 than ambient air). In patients with certain types of pulmonary disorders in which some alveoli are well ventilated but poorly perfused with blood (for example, pulmonary embolism) these alveoli are behaving like dead space—that is, they are not participating in gaseous exchange with pulmonary capillary blood, and the ventilation there is wasted ventilation. This is called *physiologic* deadspace.

The gas composition of alveolar air is markedly different from that of inspired air, as is indicated by the following comparisons:

	Inspired Air (mmHg)	*Alveolar Air* (mmHg)	*Mixed Expired Air* (mmHg)
O_2	159	104	120
CO_2	0.5	40	27
Water vapor	4.0	47	47

The reasons for these differences are (1) the increased amount of water vapor in alveolar air, which of necessity lowers the partial pressures of O_2 and CO_2; (2)

only part of the inspired air at each breath reaches the alveoli and equilibrates with air there; the remainder stays in the deadspace airways; and (3) gaseous exchange of O_2 and CO_2 between capillary blood and alveolar air proceeds continuously.

Pulmonary Capillary Perfusion of Alveoli

The cardiac output of the right ventricle is, like that of the left, about 5 L/min at rest. This is mixed venous blood entering the pulmonary vasculature for oxygenation and the elimination of CO_2. Since the amount of air entering the alveoli is also about 5 L/min, the ventilation–perfusion ratio, that is, the ratio of alveolar ventilation to pulmonary blood flow at rest ($\dot{V}/\dot{Q}$) in the lungs as a whole is close to 1.0. However, since the rate of flow of air per unit time through the respiratory passages and alveoli is very low, and the rate of flow of blood per unit time through the pulmonary vasculture is very rapid (less than 1 sec for a red cell to traverse the pulmonary capillaries at rest), the ratio of alveolar air volume to pulmonary capillary blood volume at any moment is quite high: about 2500 ml alveolar air to about 100 ml pulmonary capillary blood, that is, 25:1. (The total amount of blood in the pulmonary circuit at any given time is about 0.8–1.0 L.) Thus, with respect to air, the alveoli are a high volume and low pressure system; with respect to capillary blood they are a relatively low volume and low pressure system. Pulmonary artery pressure is about 25/10 mmHg, and pulmonary capillary pressure is about 8–10 mmHg.

Ventilation–Perfusion Ratios ($\dot{V}/\dot{Q}$)

In order for adequate oxygenation of, and removal of CO_2 from, blood in the pulmonary capillaries during its very brief transit time through the pulmonary circuit, the tensions of O_2 and CO_2 in this "venous" blood (P_{VO_2} and P_{VCO_2}) must equilibrate with the partial pressures of O_2 and CO_2 in the alveolar gas (P_{AO_2} and P_{ACO_2}). If the blood flow (perfusion) is reduced, but ventilation remains the same, less O_2 is removed from alveoli and less CO_2 is supplied to them, and the result is an alveolar oxygen tension (P_{AO_2}) and an alveolar carbon dioxide tension (P_{ACO_2}) equal to inspired air. Conversely, if alveolar ventilation declines but capillary perfusion of alveoli is unchanged, then more O_2 is removed from them relative to the declining supply, and more CO_2 is added than can be removed by ventilation; the result is a decreased P_{AO_2} and an increased P_{ACO_2}. These changes will lead to $\downarrow P_{aO_2}$ and $\uparrow P_{aCO_2}$. When ventilation to a perfused lung segment is altogether blocked, then $P_{AO_2} = P_{VO_2}$; and $P_{ACO_2} = P_{VCO_2}$. Thus, in the case of no ventilation of adequately perfused alveoli, the $\dot{V}/\dot{Q}$ is zero; in the situation of full ventilation of nonperfused alveoli the $\dot{V}/\dot{Q}$ is infinitely great.

Although the *overall* ratio between ventilation and perfusion in the lung is about 1.0, there are very marked *regional* differences in the degree of alveolar ventilation, relative to the amount of alveolar capillary perfusion, among the millions of alveolar capillary units that constitute the pulmonary parenchyma. These regional differences have a profound effect upon pulmonary gaseous exchange in the normal subject, and account for many of the abnormalities of arterial blood gas composition seen clinically (Chapter 2). There are many compensatory mechanisms which operate to offset such regional $\dot{V}/\dot{Q}$ abnormalities (see following).

Ventilation–perfusion mismatch is the commonest cause of abnormalities in arterial blood gases in individuals with lung disease. The alveoli which are underventilated relative to the degree of their capillary perfusion are primarily responsible for the arterial hypoxemia seen in many pulmonary disorders. These alveolar–capillary units have a low $\dot{V}/\dot{Q}$ ratio. Essentially, the flow of large amounts of underoxygenated blood, caused by inadequate alveolar ventilation, into the left heart and hence out into the systemic circulation, acts like an anatomic right-to-left shunt: it adds venous blood to oxygenated blood coming from alveolar capillary units with a normal $\dot{V}/\dot{Q}$ ratio. This is called venous admixture.

In contrast to units with a low $\dot{V}/\dot{Q}$ ratio, alveoli which are overventilated relative to their degree of capillary blood flow have a major impact on CO_2 elimination from the blood rather than O_2 addition to it; their action is to add abnormal *physiologic* deadspace (i.e., wasted ventilation) to the normal *anatomic* deadspace of trachea, bronchi and bronchioles. These alveolar–capillary units have a high $\dot{V}/\dot{Q}$ ratio.

$\dot{V}/\dot{Q}$ mismatch occurs to varying degrees and in various distributions throughout the lung in the broad spectrum of pulmonary disorders which will be described in the following sections. It is likely that very frequently, more in some disorders than others, increased venous admixture in some alveolar–capillary units and increased physiologic deadspace in others, work together to produce abnormalities of arterial blood gas composition, the complications which they induce, and the compensatory mechanisms which operate to counteract them. Nevertheless it is probably also true that very often inadequate alveolar ventilation and impaired capillary perfusion occur together in various portions of the lung; that is, lung parenchyma which is poorly perfused also often tends to be poorly ventilated. One reason for this is the very intimate structural relationships in the lung between the air-containing structures and the blood-containing ones

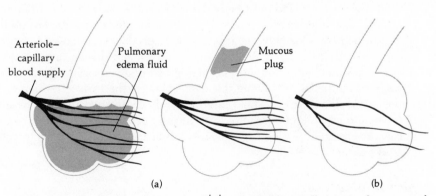

Figure 9-4. Ventilation–perfusion ratios $(\dot{V}/\dot{Q})$. (*a*) Alveolar–capillary units that are poorly ventilated, for example because of pulmonary edema fluid in the alveoli; or mucous plugging of the bronchioles; but are adequately perfused with capillary blood. This leads to venous admixture or pulmonary shunting. Such units have a *low* $\dot{V}/\dot{Q}$ ratio. (*b*) An alveolar capillary unit that is well ventilated but poorly perfused with capillary blood, for example because of small pulmonary emboli, or an obliterative or vasoconstrictive pulmonary vascular disease. This leads to increased physiologic deadspace. Such units have a *high* $\dot{V}/\dot{Q}$ ratio.

(Figure 9-3), so that disease processes, especially chronic ones, tend to affect ventilation and perfusion together.

There are compensatory mechanisms that operate to minimize $\dot{V}/\dot{Q}$ mismatch. Alveolar hypoxia has a direct local vasoconstrictive action on pulmonary arterioles; this tends to shunt blood flow away from poorly ventilated areas. In addition, in cases of impaired blood flow to a segment of lung, such as the obstruction of pulmonary embolism, it appears that there is a spastic contraction of the smooth muscle in the bronchioles and small bronchi, tending to close them off. This bronchoconstriction results from the local decline in CO_2 caused by decreased flow of high CO_2-content blood through the area. It reduces wasted ventilation. Thus these adaptive physiologic reactions function to ameliorate to some extent the effects of venous admixture and physiologic deadspace in pulmonary disorders.

Lung Compliance

Compliance of the lung refers to the change in lung volume produced by change in pressure in the airways (change in volume per unit of change in pressure or $\Delta V/\Delta P$) and in the normal subject is about 0.2 L/cm H_2O. It is a measure of the elastic recoil properties of the lung. Compliance is decreased—that is, a greater change in airway pressure is required to produce a given change in lung volume—in such conditions as pulmonary interstitial fibrosis and the increased pulmonary vascular congestion of left ventricular failure. Compliance is increased—that is, a lesser change in airway pressure is necessary in order to produce a given change in lung volume—in pulmonary emphysema.

Two factors which importantly influence lung compliance are the degree of flexibility versus rigidity of lung tissue (the more rigid the tissue, the less compliant); and the surface tension of the thin film of fluid which lines all alveoli. Surface tension is essentially an expression for the physical tendency of a liquid to round up into the smallest possible sphere; it is very low in such substances as oils but high in water and most body fluids. Thus the layer of interstitial fluid lining the alveoli would exert a physical effect tending to reduce the alveoli to their smallest diameter—namely, collapse (which produces atelectasis). This force would make alveoli very difficult to open and expand during inspiration. However, the presence of a protein phospholipid substance, surfactant, produced by specialized epithelial cells lining the alveoli, lowers the surface tension of the alveolar liquid film at the air–fluid interface and acts to keep them open and permits them to expand more readily, with a lesser expenditure of muscular energy, during inspiration. Inadequate amounts of surfactant in the lung greatly decreases pulmonary compliance.

Airway Resistance

Resistance of airways to airflow within them in the normal subject is relatively low but is nevertheless sufficient to cause the changes in lung volume to lag slightly behind the changes in intrapleural pressure during both inspiration and expiration. This frictional resistance occurs principally in the medium-sized bronchi and is greater at small lung volumes, and during expiration, because the airways are held less widely open during the elevated intrathoracic pressure occurring when the inspiratory muscles relax. Airway resistance is increased by several processes in various respiratory disorders. In chronic bronchitis, airways are narrowed because of edema, vascular congestion (hyperemia), and glandular hypertrophy of the mucosal lining, as well as the presence of large amounts of mucous secretions. In asthma there is a hyperreaction of bronchial smooth muscle, leading to reversible airway narrowing from bronchospasm and bronchoconstriction. Even in the normal nonasthmatic subject, inhaled toxic substances such as tobacco smoke, automobile exhaust, and industrial vapors cause bronchial constriction, airway narrowing, and increased resistance to air flow. In patients with emphysema and bronchitis the large airways become more collapsible—less resistant to compression by an elevation of intrathoracic pressure. Consequently, in the forced expirations required to empty the dilated alveoli characteristic of emphysema, the use of accessory muscles to produce forced exhalation elevates intrathoraic pressure to a degree sufficient to compress these weakened large airways. This airways collapse greatly increases resistance to expiratory air flow. The greater the effort, the greater the compression of large airways, and the higher the resistance.

The Work of Breathing

The work of breathing is accomplished by the respiratory muscles which produce the actual alterations in configuration of the thorax necessary to move air into and out of the lungs. This muscular work consumes O_2 and produces CO_2; in the normal subject the work of breathing is slight, but energy requirements of breathing in an individual with pulmonary disease may be very great because of abnormal lung compliance, increased airway resistance, disordered ventilation and perfusion relationships; or with chest wall defects (obesity, kyphoscoliosis, flail chest). The greater the energy expenditure required to move enough air into and out of the lungs to produce adequate alveolar ventilation, the larger is the percentage of the total bodily oxygen consumption that will be expended in the work of breathing. As the work of breathing increases in patients with lung disease, an adaptive response develops which tends to minimize the work: the patient breathes more shallowly and more rapidly. This has the compensatory advantage of decreasing the work of breathing, but it also carries a penalty. In tachypnea the percentage of the total minute volume which flows back and forth over anatomic deadspace is greatly increased. This acts to impair alveolar ventilation and alveolar–capillary gaseous exchange. Such patients with chronically increased work of breathing appear to make a compromise whereby decreased levels of alveolar ventilation, and hence increased blood gas abnormalities, are accepted for the decrease in O_2 consumption and CO_2 production that results from the reduced work of breathing of rapid shallow respirations.

This matter of the influence of rate and depth of respirations on overall alveolar ventilation and hence on arterial blood gas composition in pulmonary disorders, both chronic and acute, is a highly significant one, and it relates specifically to respiratory tree deadspace. Because of normal anatomic deadspace, the percentage of the air breathed in which actually reaches the alveoli is greater in deep and slow respirations than it is in rapid and shallow ones. Therefore the degree of alveolar ventilation, for a given respiratory minute volume, is less in rapid shallow breathing. For example:

	Tachypnea	*Normal*
respiratory rate/min.	28	14
total volume/breath	250 ml	650 ml
minute volume	7.0 L	9.1 L
alveolar ventilation	2.8 L/min	7.0 L/min
(= tidal volume minus deadspace volume times respiratory rate)		

DISORDERS OF THE RESPIRATORY SYSTEM

Chronic Disorders

The chronic abnormalities of the lungs which lead to respiratory insufficiency may be classified according to the characteristic dysfunctions which they produce in pulmonary function tests (PFTs). The results of these tests form the basis for a grouping of lung diseases based on the alterations in physiologic function characteristic of each disease. The two major categories of respiratory abnormality based on spirometry are *obstructive* lung disease and *restrictive* lung disease. These are not actual diagnostic terms for clear-cut clinical entities, but rather two types of change in lung function produced by a variety of pulmonary disorders. Two of the parameters measured in spirometry often used as the basis for division into the classes obstructive and restrictive are the vital capacity (VC) and the forced expiratory volume in 1 sec (FEV_1). The greatest amount of air that can be breathed out after a maximal inspiration is the vital capacity; it averages about 4.5 L in the normal subject. The fraction of this amount that can be breathed out with maximal effort in 1 sec is the forced expiration volume in 1 sec and is measured with a spirometer. In the healthy person the FEV_1 is about 75–80% of the VC.

In *obstructive* lung diseases (for example, emphysema, bronchitis, and asthma) which are characterized by a reduced rate of airflow, there is a diminished FEV_1, but the VC may be normal or only slightly changed. That is to say, the pulmonary system may or may not contain overall less movable air, but the air that does move does so too slowly because of airway narrowing. Therefore the ratio of the forced expiration volume to the vital capacity is subnormal: the FEV_1/VC is low. *Restrictive* lung diseases (for example, diffuse interstitial fibrosis and pleural scarring) are characterized by reduced lung volume (low vital capacity), because of limited lung, pleural, or chest wall expansion; but the resistance to airflow is often unchanged and so air moves readily; thus there are normal rates of air flow (normal FEV_1). In these diseases, then, the expiratory flow rates are high relative to the low vital capacity. In other words, in restrictive pulmonary diseases the ratio of timed forced expiratory volume to vital capacity is high: a high FEV_1/VC. In many patients these changes are mixed and the abnormalities revealed by pulmonary function tests are expressed as changes in the relationship or ratio between VC and FEV_1, as described above. In summary, obstructive lung diseases are characterized by a disproportionate reduction in expiratory flow relative to vital capacity (a low FEV_1 to VC ratio); and restrictive lung diseases typically reveal a reduced vital capacity relative to the expiratory flow rate (a high FEV_1 to VC ratio).

Chronic Obstructive Pulmonary Disease (COPD); Chronic Airway Obstruction (CAO)

The commonly used term COPD refers to the group of lung disorders in which there is increased resistance to airflow, especially on expiration, and which are comprised of the two distinct entities, bronchitis and emphysema, in varying proportions. In addition, many patients with COPD have an asthmatic (bronchospastic, reversible) component to their airway obstruction. The most characteristic manifestations are dyspnea and decreased exercise tolerance. Although these symptoms do not appear until the disease is well established, pulmonary function tests will often reveal decreased airflow rates much earlier. Exertional dyspnea generally occurs when the FEV_1 declines to about 50% of the expected value. The structural and functional abnormalities responsible for increased resistance to airflow are different in the three classes of abnormalities: bronchitis, emphysema, and asthma.

Causes

Cigaret smoking is the most common cause of emphysema and bronchitis. The incidence of COPD in pipe and cigar smokers is lower than in cigaret smokers but higher than in nonsmokers. Cigaret smoke inhibits the action of the cilia which line the respiratory tract and normally exert a continuous sweeping action to remove foreign materials from the lungs. Smoking causes inflammation of the respiratory mucosa and hypertrophy and excessive secretion of the mucous glands; and in addition it produces constriction of the smooth muscles of bronchial walls resulting in airway narrowing. Exposure to industrial fumes and dusts and air pollution are additional but much less significant etiologic factors.

Some patients with an early onset and severe progression of emphysema have a genetically determined deficiency of serum α_1-antitrypsin, a blood inhibitor of the action of proteolytic enzymes. Normal subjects have serum α_1-antitrypsin levels of around 250 mg/100 ml, whereas patients with this form of emphysema may have serum levels around 50 mg/100 ml serum. It is suggested that the mechanism of cause of emphysema and bronchitis in such individuals is that the protein-hydrolyzing enzymes (leukoproteases) which are released into lung parenchyma by leukocytes during respiratory infections also hydrolyze the proteins of lung tissue because inadequate antitrypsin levels are present to restrict their digestive action.

Abnormalities

In emphysema there is destruction of the walls of alveoli, dilation and loss of elasticity of air spaces distal to the terminal bronchioles, and overinflation of the lungs. The decrease of elastic recoil of the lung results in a decline in the radial traction on and support of the airways which tends to keep them open; in addition, the larger airways in emphysema are thinned and atrophic. These changes result in greater collapsibility of both large and small airways and lead to a marked increase in resistance to airflow.

Histologically there are two types of emphysema: proximal acinar (centriacinar) in which there are abnormal breaks in the walls of the respiratory bronchioles and alveolar ducts; and panacinar, in which there is a more uniform destruction of bronchioles, ducts, and the more distal alveolar spaces (Figure 9-3). The progressive destruction of alveolar compartments leads to distended empty-appearing spaces. The capillary circulation tends to be obliterated as the alveolar partitions and ducts are destroyed. This causes a great reduction in the alveolar–capillary surface available for gas exchange.

Chronic bronchitis is characterized by edema and hyperemia of bronchial mucosa, mucous gland hyperplasia and hypersecretion, and hypertrophy of smooth muscle, with mucous plugging of both the large cartilaginous and smaller noncartilaginous airways.

The asthmatic component in COPD refers to the reversible smooth-muscle bronchospasm which is often present in these patients in conjunction with emphysema and bronchitis.

Consequences of the Abnormalities

Usually chronic bronchitis and emphysema, along with some bronchospasm, are present together in varying degrees in COPD; and the airway narrowing and decreased airflow rates, especially expiratory, which they cause, result from a combination of decreased elastic recoil, reduced airway caliber, and increased airway compression. Because more change in pressure is required to produce a given amount of airflow into and out of the alveoli, the work of breathing is greatly increased. Airway resistance is defined as the ratio of airflow to the pressure change between alveolus and mouth; in COPD it is almost always greater during expiration, and is assessed by the amount of air that can be forcibly exhaled after a maximal inhalation in 1 sec: the FEV_1.

In addition to the mechanical difficulties of moving air through narrowed passageways, the unequal distribution of alveolar ventilation relative to capillary perfusion produces abnormalities of gaseous exchange in which some regions of the lung may be overventilated but underperfused (increased physiologic deadspace) while others may be underventilated but relatively overperfused (venous admixture). The result of the $\dot{V}/\dot{Q}$ mismatch is abnormalities in arterial blood gas tensions: elevated $Paco_2$, decreased pH, and decreased Pao_2. The chronic alveolar hypoventilation and resulting alveolar hypoxia causes pulmonary vascular constriction; this is a direct response of the blood vessels of the pulmonary circuit to low partial pressures of oxygen in the alveoli. The widespread pulmonary vasoconstriction causes elevated pulmonary vascular resistance and pulmonary hypertension. In the same way that chronic systemic arterial hypertension causes elevated left ventricular workload, so chronically increased pulmonary vascular pressure leads to strain on and eventually hypertrophy of the right ventricle: cor pulmonale.

Types

There is a spectrum of clinical types among patients with COPD. at one end of the spectrum is the patient with predominant bronchitis—called the blue bloater because he tends to be cyanotic and edematous. The blue bloater has a slightly or moderately elevated respiratory minute volume but markedly abnormal ABGs: ↑$Paco_2$ and ↓Pao_2. At the other end of the spectrum is the patient with predominant emphysema called pink puffer because, although his skin color tends to be normal, he is markedly dyspneic, often even at rest. The pink puffer is also tachypneic and may have a high respiratory minute volume which serves to maintain ABGs within relatively normal limits. Most patients with COPD occupy points along the continuum, with mixed characteristics of the two types, and also often manifest some degree of rapidly reversible (bronchospastic) airway narrowing.

For heuristic purposes it is useful to note the characteristics of the types at the extreme ends of the spectrum. It is thought that one of the major physiologic differences between the two extreme types is the nature and degree of responsiveness of their central brainstem and peripheral chemoreceptor mechanisms to the chronic alveolar hypoventilation caused by the lung disease. The bronchitic type manifests an abnormally low ventilatory response to hypoxia and hypercapnia, that is, he has a high tolerance for blood gas abnormalities; the emphysematous type shows a marked increase in ventilatory drive to hypoxia and hypercapnia (intolerance to $\uparrow PaCO_2$ and $\downarrow PaO_2$).

Another proposal which has been advanced to account for the different physiologic manifestations in the two forms of COPD is that in pure emphysema there is less ventilation–perfusion mismatch; that is, in lung regions where there is severe emphysematous lung destruction, the capillary supply is correspondingly obliterated, leading to less deadspace and venous admixture effects. In the pure bronchitic type it is suggested that there is marked and widespread $\dot{V}/\dot{Q}$ mismatch, with resulting major physiologic deadspace and venous admixture producing the severe ABG abnormalities: chronic hypoxemia, hypercapnia, and acidemia.

The bronchitic type of COPD patient is characterized by a persistent cough productive of mucopurulent sputum, a long history of cigaret smoking, frequent episodes of acute bronchitis, cyanosis and pedal edema, rhonchi, pulmonary hypertension, and right ventricular hypertrophy. $\dot{V}/\dot{Q}$ mismatch with hypoxemia and hypercapnia is present. The low PaO_2 stimulates the secretion of erythropoietin from the kidney which activates the bone marrow and leads to erythrocytosis (often mistakenly called polycythemia, which is an increase in all cellular elements of the blood, not just red cells), elevated hematocrit, and increased blood viscosity. Histologically the pulmonary tree shows the mucous membrane changes described above, with varying degrees of centriacinar emphysema. There may be mild to moderate response to bronchodilators depending on the amount of bronchospastic component in the airway obstruction.

The emphysematous type of COPD patient is markedly dyspneic, has markedly impaired lung elastic recoil, little cough or sputum, overinflated lungs and hyperresonant chest, is less hypoxic than the bronchitic, and may have a normal or even low $PaCO_2$ because of hypoxemic hyperventilation. These patients are less prone to acute episodes of bronchitis, but when they do have one it is very serious or fatal. Histologically their lungs show extensive panacinar emphysema, with variable airway mucous membrane changes. There is little response to bronchodilators.

Assessment

Subjective. The patient's complaints are shortness of breath, decreased exercise tolerance, cough, sputum production, wheezing, and frequent respiratory infections.

Objective. On physical examination there may be dyspnea at rest, cyanosis, and pedal edema. One may observe increased anteroposterior chest diameter, lung fields are hyperresonant to percussion and the hemidiaphragms are often low, both caused by lung hyperinflation, and there is minimal respiratory diaphragm excursion. There are rhonchi and wheezing on auscultation, especially with forced expiration; the rhonchi often clear briefly or change after coughing. Decreased breath sounds are characteristic. Maximal forced expiration requires more than 6 sec. The cardiac impulse may be displaced to just below the left costal margin near the epigastrium or midsternal line because of hyperinflation of the lungs. The patient with cor pulmonale may have an accentuated P_2 (the pulmonic component of the second heart sound) from forcible closing of the pulmonic valve, caused by pulmonary hypertension, and a heave at the lower left sternal border indicating right ventricular hypertrophy. There may be increased jugular venous pressure. In many patients the correlation between the symptoms, the physical signs, and the changes in the chest X-ray, are often not particularly good. The usual characteristics are hyperinflation and low flat hemidiaphragms.

Management

The most important consideration in COPD is prevention, which, in view of the significant role of smoking in etiology, means to encourage nonsmokers not to start and smokers to stop, a difficult task in either case, particularly the latter. Patients who are discovered to have an α_1-antitrypsin deficiency must take particular care in avoiding those factors which are known to hasten the onset of, and worsen the progression of, lung disease: smoking, air pollution, and frequent respiratory infections. Early recognition of reduced respiratory airflow is important because of the possibility of retarding the rate of progression in some cases by proper management. By and large, however, it is the case that by the time the patient seeks health care because of the symptoms and signs of COPD, the disease is already far advanced.

Unlike asthma, where resistance to airflow is to a large extent reversible, and sometimes precipitated by known and to some degree possibly avoidable factors, the progression of chronic bronchitis and emphysema is not altered to any major extent regardless of treatment. Thus, management is directed at identifying a reversible component which will respond to bronchodilators, improving pulmonary hygiene, reducing inflammation, and preventing and treating infection. Emphysema itself is irreversible. Improving the patient's exercise tolerance by a regular program of physical activity, and mental outlook by appropriate counseling where indicated, are important adjuncts. Thus the program of care is centered around rehabilitation and improvement of the quality of life. COPD represents one of our major health problems and appears to be on the increase; perhaps as many as one fifth of the persons in the United States have chronic pulmonary abnormalities, the majority of which are some form of COPD. Well-organized effective ambulatory care for these patients constitutes a major challenge to the health professions. Health care and instruction and assessment conducted by nurses trained in respiratory therapy, given in regularly scheduled visits to the patient at home, are a cornerstone in the successful ambulatory management of COPD. In this way the patient's health self-care becomes integrated into the pattern of the daily life style.

The initial workup consists of health history, physical examination, chest X-rays, EKG, the usual laboratory hematology and chemistry, including serum electrolytes, and pulmonary function tests. The latter are less routinely performed today since they are expensive (except for small office machines) and do not greatly influence the treatment program.

Education. Patient education in methods of self-assessment and self-care is perhaps more important in COPD than in any other chronic disease with the exception of diabetes mellitus. Patients may be offered individual or small group learning sessions given by pulmonary nurse clinicians or respiratory therapists on lung anatomy and physiology; the changes occurring in COPD; the methods of routine self-care involved in pulmonary hygiene; and prophylaxis: cessation of smoking, avoidance of air pollution (including all aerosol sprays), and prevention, early recognition, and prompt treatment of respiratory infections. Annual fall influenza vaccine is considered to be helpful by some authors, and pneumococcal pneumonia vaccine is often recommended.

Teaching patients to breathe properly is also helpful to them; most persons with COPD are tachypneic—rapid shallow respirations are wasteful as discussed previously. Slow abdominal-diaphragmatic breathing with exhalation against pursed lips has been shown to improve alveolar ventilation and decrease minute volume.

Pulmonary Hygiene. A daily program of bronchial hygiene consists of inhalation of isoproterenol, metaproterenol, or isoetharine (with or without phenylephrine) followed by inhalation of steam, and then expulsive coughing to clear mucus from the airways. β adrenergic bronchodilators have been shown to increase ciliary movement and to facilitate clearing of mucus in addition to dilating airways. Chest physiotherapy with chest wall percussion and vibration, with postural drainage, aids expulsion of secretions. Adequate hydration should be maintained at all times to thin respiratory secretions and aid in their removal—up to 3000 ml fluid intake in 24 hr.

Pharmacologic Agents. Oral bronchodilators such as theophylline, and sympathomimetic amines such as ephedrine, are effective; they are preferably used separately rather than in fixed dose combinations, since the fixed dosage does not permit flexibility in either medication.

For periods of increased dyspnea and hypoxemia oral adrenal steroids may be indicated for a few days to reduce inflammation and edema of the airways.

Respiratory Infections. Respiratory infections, signaled by increased coughing, fever, and purulent sputum production should be treated promptly with a broad-spectrum antibiotic such as ampicillin or tetracycline for a full 7–10 day course. A reliable, well-informed patient may appreciate having a course of antibiotics on hand at home to start self-treatment at the first sign of increased purulence of sputum, or systemic symptoms indicating a developing respiratory infection.

Physical Conditioning. As discussed in the section on exercise and the heart (Chapter 8) a program of graded physical training, although it may not measurably improve lung function, definitely does, in most patients, yield a sense of well-being and lead to increased performance ability. There is a decrease in oxygen requirement and consumption, and improved oxygen delivery to and utilization by peripheral tissues. Walking outdoors at a pace which just induces mild dyspnea is the best all-round conditioner for the COPD patient; in inclement weather home exercise devices such as a rowing machine or stationary bicycle, maintain exercise tolerance at improved levels.

Supplemental O_2.   For the patient with severe hypoxemia, ambulatory oxygen equipment is available. Continuous low-flow O_2 (1–3 L/m) relieves the alveolar hypoxia which induces pulmonary vasoconstriction and hypertension; it thus reduces the workload of the right ventricle which predisposes to cor pulmonale. Studies indicate that severely hypoxemic patients treated with low flow oxygen for 12–16 hr/day, as part of a complete management regimen, have improved survival rates over those not so treated. Indications for oxygen supplementation are erythrocytosis, right ventricular enlargement, severe dyspnea, and a PaO_2 below 50 mmHg.

Psychoemotional Aspects.   A study of psychologic and emotional factors in COPD has revealed that many of these people experience psychiatric impairment sufficient to interfere with quality of life and daily performance, including such symptoms as anxiety, paranoia, depression, and constant fears of suffocation and feelings of impending doom. One of the most significant findings is a marked fear of dyspnea which leads to avoidance of even minor physical activity. This, of course, results in physical deconditioning, decline in work performance and increased oxygen requirements. It constitutes a physical activity phobia which has been called respiratory panic and resembles the fear and avoidance of modest levels of exertion manifested by some patients with ischemic heart disease and angina. Granted some of the justification for such fears, and the depression which must result from having an inexorably progressive disease; nevertheless to the degree that such psychologic states interfere with enjoyment of the life a person does have left, and hasten his deterioration, its assessment and control is an important component of management. Perhaps one of the most successful aspects of such management is supervised monitoring of increasing activity levels, with reassurance that shortness of breath does not signal impending disaster. Repeated exercise in the presence of a health care practitioner constitutes a form of desensitization therapy which will help the patient break the dyspnea–anxiety cycle, learn self-monitoring of symptoms, and self-dependence.

Studies of the impact of a detailed, carefully specified, and monitored, maintenance and rehabilitation program encompassing the elements described above, have indicated that such a program may result in a slight delay in the inexorable rate of progression of COPD impairment. The baseline progression has been estimated to produce yearly decrements in FEV_1 of about 80 ml, which may be reduced to 50 ml/yr with a comprehensive management program.

Asthma

Asthma is a disease involving reversible bronchial and bronchiolar narrowing based upon increased bronchial smooth muscle tone, mucosal edema, and hypersecretion. The motor and secretory hyperactivity usually occurs acutely in recurrent episodes, but these acute attacks are superimposed on a more or less continuous hyperresponsiveness of the airways to a wide variety of internal and external stimuli. Hyperinflation of the lungs and increased resistance to airflow may be present even without the symptoms and signs of an acute attack. Therefore asthma is considered to be a chronic obstructive disease with periodic exacerbations, rather than a discontinuous series of discrete episodes. The attacks are characterized by dyspnea, wheezing, and cough.

Types

Extrinsic Atopic. This form of asthma is clearly immunologic and is seen in patients who tend to develop the Type I immediate form of hypersensitivity (Chapter 22) allergic responses (hay fever, hives) to a number of allergens present in the environment. Such persons are said to be atopic, and often have a family history positive for urticaria, respiratory allergies, and asthma; may have hay fever and other allergic manifestations themselves; and show positive skin test reactions to many antigens. The acute attacks can often be associated with exposure to such a known allergen which may be via inhalation, ingestion, or injection; emotional upsets, physical exercise, and respiratory infections may also trigger acute episodes. Patients having this form of asthma usually developed it during childhood or at least before about 30 years of age. Childhood asthma is easier to control, tends to occur in discrete attacks with complete absence of signs or symptoms in between, and has a good prognosis. Eosinophilia of blood and sputum is characteristic of this form.

Type I hypersensitivity responses, including extrinsic asthma, are mediated by an antibody, called reaginic antibody, which belongs to the IgE class of immunoglobulins. In patients with extrinsic (allergic) asthma blood immunoglobulin IgE levels are elevated. The processes involved in the various types of hypersensitivity responses are discussed in more detail in Chapter 22 and in the following section.

Extrinsic Nonatopic. This is considered by some workers, but not by others, as a separate category. This form is reported to occur more often in adults, there is a lesser association with other allergic manifestations, and it is suggested to occur as a Type III delayed hypersensitivity response which is mediated by circulating antibodies of the immunoglobulin classes IgG, IgA, and IgM (see Chapter 22). This type of reaction occurs not until several hours after exposure to an antigen; the subsequent antigen–antibody reaction leads to the formation of precipitins which then cause an inflammatory reaction. There is evidence that the Type III delayed asthmatic response is dependent on a Type I immediate sensitization having occurred as a result of exposure to an antigen at some previous time in the patient's history.

Intrinsic. This form is primarily a disorder of adults and is more serious, more difficult to control, and has a poorer prognosis. Onset is usually after the age of 30 or so; there is no elevated IgE; skin testing fails to reveal a hypersensitivity response, and there are seldom other allergic manifestations; genetic factors are less prominent; and protracted severe attacks are more often seen than in the extrinsic type. Factors tending to precipitate the attacks can seldom be identified, and the disorder may become progressively more severe with time. In these patients the increased airway resistance appears to be related more to internal factors and may result from reflex neural mechanisms, psychoemotional states, or pulmonary infections. There is a relatively high incidence of chronic mucopurulent bronchitis. Some authors define a subcategory of intrinsic asthma called asthmatic bronchitis, in which there is a positive clinical history of bronchitis; chronic physical findings of wheezing, diffuse rhonchi, and coarse breath sounds; and a more abnormal chest X-ray between acute exacerbations.

ASA Triad (Triad of Aspirin Sensitivity, Nasal Polyps, and Asthma).   This form of asthma occurs in patients who develop severe attacks of bronchospasm within an hour or two of ingesting aspirin; it occurs more often in older patients (35 to 70 years of age). The response to aspirin in these patients appears not to be a form of immunologic hypersentivity reaction. Nasal polyps and perennial rhinitis are common accompaniments; there is chronic nasal mucosal edema, probably based on increased capillary permeability, and mucosal protrusions occur which develop into the polyps. These patients appear to be unusually susceptible to environmental pollution.

Exercise-Induced.   In patients with this form of asthma there is a marked increase in airway resistance with a decreased airflow which develops a few minutes after exercise has ceased. During exercise in some persons there is a marked bronchodilation; it is suggested that exercise-induced asthma represents a reactive bronchoconstriction. The hyperventilation occurring during exercise may produce hypocapnia which triggers subsequent bronchoconstriction, and the catecholamines released by adrenergic nerve terminals and adrenal medulla during physical activity may cause bronchoconstriction in susceptible subjects by stimulating bronchial α receptors (see following).

Lung Abnormalities

Increased resistance to airflow, especially expiratory airflow, is caused by reversible airway narrowing from constriction of bronchial smooth muscle, hyperemia and edema of airway mucosa, and collections within the bronchial lumens of mucous secretions and cellular debris. In addition to the obstruction to airflow, these abnormalities cause alveolar hypoventilation which leads to a decline in arterial O_2 tension and O_2 desaturation of hemoglobin. The PaO_2 may be between 60 and 75 mmHg during an attack, and the $PaCO_2$ is often low. The hypoxemia stimulates hyperventilation which causes a decline in $PaCO_2$ (hypocapnia). There is hyperinflation of the lung in severe attacks, with trapping of air in the alveoli leading to areas of localized emphysema. Lung compliance is normal or increased. If the attack is very severe and protracted, then the alveolar hypoventilation may be marked enough to eventually lead to CO_2 retention and narcosis. This development indicates a life-threatening degree of airway obstruction.

Mucous plugging of bronchioles permits resorption of alveolar air distal to the obstruction, and these alveoli collapse, causing atelectasis. Continued pulmonary capillary perfusion of these collapsed alveoli leads to venous admixture—essentially the shunting of pulmonary blood, so that underoxygenated blood is returned to the left heart. This further lowers the PaO_2. The shunting is ameliorated to some degree by an adaptive vasoconstriction of pulmonary vessels supplying atelectatic areas; this response tends to minimize $\dot{V}/\dot{Q}$ mismatch.

Spirometry during severe exacerbations shows a decreased rate of expiratory airflow (FEV_1) and a decline in vital capacity (VC); residual volume is increased. There is a correlation between dyspnea and wheezing and objectively measured expiratory flow rates; when the patient is severely symptomatic, the FEV_1 may be less than half normal (below 1 L); during the recovery period airflow increases and is around 60–70% of normal when the wheezing and dyspnea clear.

Cellular Processes Underlying Bronchospasm and Hypersecretion

As is the case with most visceral functions, the motor and secretory responses of the bronchial smooth muscle and mucosa, as well as release of the mediators which cause capillary dilation and increased permeability, are under dual control. They are regulated by the major neural control mechanisms which have complementary or opposite effects. These two mechanisms are the parasympathetic (cholinergic) and the sympathetic (adrenergic) divisions of the autonomic nervous system.

Cholinergic. Branches of the vagus nerve (CN X) furnish both the afferent (sensory) and the efferent (motor and secretory) autonomic nerve supply to both the smooth muscle and the nucosa of the tracheobroncial tree. The vagus nerve is the pathway for neural reflexes which mediate motor and secretory responses of the lungs and airways to both local and systemic influences.

Pulmonary tissue has a rich parasympathetic innervation, much greater than the sympathetic autonomic nerve supply. The cholinergic division has as its neurotransmitter acetylcholine (ACh) which is released at cholinergic nerve terminals when parasympathetic nerves are stimulated. ACh then activates specific ACh receptors which are located on the membranes of both smooth muscle and mucosal secretory cells. Stimulation of these cholinergic cell membrane receptors results in activation of the enzyme guanyl cyclase which is bound to the surface of cell membranes. This enzyme catalyzes the synthesis of the cyclic nucleotide cyclic guanosine monophosphate (cGMP) from guanosine triphosphate (GTP). When cGMP levels increase in the cells which produce the mediators of hypersensitivity reactions, mediator release occurs. The mediators of hypersensitivity responses include a number of different substances which are released from tissue mast cells, circulating basophils, and some mucosal cells; in some cases as a result of antigen–antibody hypersensitivity reactions and in other cases perhaps as a result of cholinergic stimulation by ACh. These mediators include histamine, slow-reacting substance of anaphylaxis (SRS-A), eosinophil chemotactic factor of anaphylaxis (ECF-A), serotonin, bradykinin, and certain prostaglandins (Chapter 22). These mediators have a number of actions including the production of bronchical smooth muscle contraction, and vasodilation and increased capillary permeability. The former action causes airway narrowing by bronchoconstriction, and the latter actions cause airway narrowing by edema, hyperemia, and hypersecretion. Although the specific action of cGMP on bronchial smooth muscle to produce contraction has not yet been directly demonstrated, there is evidence that this occurs; cGMP is present in all cells and in

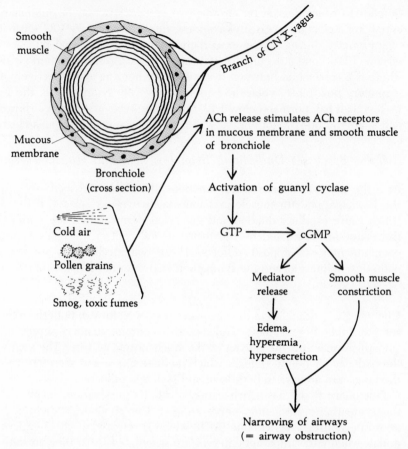

Figure 9-5. Diagram showing sequence of events in lung caused by stimulation of the cholinergic nerve supply, inhalation of allergens, cold air, or pollutants.

cholinergically activated ones ACh exerts many of its effects via this compound. Therefore, the consequences of cholinergic stimulation on the bronchi and bronchioles appear to be constriction and increased secretion.

The inhalation of respiratory irritants, whether physical, such as cold air; chemical, such as air pollutants or specific allergens; and respiratory infections; stimulate the sensory receptors in the bronchi, and elicit both bronchoconstriction and stimulation to the capillary supply of mucosal cells. This stimulation causes mucosal secretion by increasing capillary permeability and edema and also stimulates the release of the mediators of the hypersensitivity response as described above. In addition to the neurally mediated *reflex* response, respiratory irritants and antigens to which the subject has been sensitized, elicit *direct local* responses of bronchoconstriction, hypersecretion, and release of mediators. In addition to stimuli from the environment, these processes may be a portion of the mechanism by which a variety of internal influences, such as exercise, emotional tension, excitement, anxiety, and other neural effects precipitate the bronchoconstriction, edema, inflammation, and hypersecretion of an acute asthmatic attack.

Adrenergic. Autonomic sympathic (adrenergic) innervation to the lung exists but to a lesser degree than cholinergic innervation. Unlike the single type of ACh receptors of the cholinergic system, two types of adrenergic cell membrane receptors occur: alpha (α) and beta (β); the β receptors are further divided into two types, β_1 and β_2. β_1 receptors are mainly the cardiac adrenergic receptors, while most other β receptors are the β_2 type. The effects of β receptor stimulation are largely brought about by activation of membrane-bound adenyl cyclase, with a resulting increase in cyclic adenosine monophosphate (cAMP). Evidence indicates that at some sites, α receptors stimulation inhibits adenyl cyclase and thus antagonizes β receptor stimulation.

The catecholamines are adrenergic stimulators (agonists), and, depending on the specific compound, to varying degrees generally act on both α and β receptors. There are naturally produced (endogenous) catecholamines as well as an increasing variety of synthetic adrenergic or sympathomimetic amines, the latter showing a variety of mixed, or pure α or β, receptor stimulating effects. The principal endogenous adrenergic neurotransmitters are norepinephrine, synthesized and released by adrenergic nerve terminals and the adrenal medullae; and epinephrine, produced mainly by cells of the adrenal medullae. Both norepinephrine and epinephrine have both α and β receptor stimulating action, but epinephrine is primarily a β stimulator, while norepinephrine has much more α activity.

Stimulation of pulmonary β_2 adrenergic receptors antagonizes the cholinergic effects of bronchoconstriction, mucosal secretory activity, and mediator release. Thus, bronchial smooth muscle relaxation and decreased mucosal and mediator secretion results from sympathetic amines having β_2 agonist actions. These effects are mediated via stimulation of the cell membrane surface β_2 adrenergic receptors which increases membrane content of the enzyme adenyl cyclase. Adenyl cyclase then elevates intracellular synthesis of the cyclic nucleotide cyclic adenosine monophosphate (cAMP) from adenosine triphosphate (ATP). The consequence of increased intracellular cAMP content is bronchial smooth muscle relaxation and decreased mucous gland secretion and cellular release of mediators.

Evidence indicates that those effects of catecholamines and/or sympathomimetic amines which are mediated by α adrenergic receptors are brought about by a *decrease* in intracellular cAMP (and/or an increase in cGMP); α receptor stimulation results in decreased cAMP levels, increased mediator production and mucosal secretion and bronchoconstriction. Therefore in this situation α and β receptors have antagonistic actions. In the case of an adrenergic agent with both α and β actions, β overrides α effects so that the latter are counteracted, possibly because of the much larger number of β than α receptors in the tracheobronchial tree. For this reason ephedrine and epinephrine, which have both α and β stimulating actions, produce the overall effects of bronchodilation and decreased secretion and edema by increasing intracellular cAMP. (The β receptor blocking agent propranolol causes bronchoconstriction and mucosal secretion and mediator release).

In summary cGMP and the better-known cyclic nucleotide adenosine monophosphate (cAMP) often interact in a compensatory fashion, one producing inhibition and the other causing stimulation of a given process. This relationship appears to apply to the motor and secretory functions of the tracheobronchial tree as well. In addition, α adrenergic stimulation appears in some cases to have an

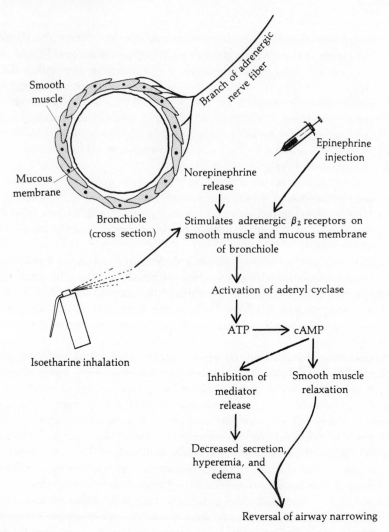

Figure 9-6. Diagram showing sequence of events in lung caused by stimulation of the adrenergic nerve supply, by injecting epinephrine, or inhaling isoetharine.

effect resembling cholinergic ACh stimulation, namely, both actions seem to promote increased bronchoconstriction and bronchial mucosal hypersecretion and edema, and occur by decreasing intracellular content of cAMP and/or increasing intracellular content of cGMP. So α adrenergic stimulation, β adrenergic blockade, and cholinergic stimulation, cause decreased intracellular cAMP and resulting bronchoconstriction and hypersecretion. β adrenergic stimulation increases cAMP and hence results in bronchodilation and reduced mucosal edema and secretions.

Pharmacologic Applications

Among the major pharmacologic agents used in the management of asthma, regardless of type, perhaps the two most important categories are the sympathomimetic amines (epinephrine, isoetharine, terbutaline) and the methylxanthines (such as theophylline and aminophylline). The bronchodilation and decreased edema and secretion effects of both of these types of drugs occurs as a result of their action in producing increased cAMP in the cells of the tracheo-bronchial tree. As discussed above, the β_2 adrenergic (sympathomimetic) agents accomplish this by increasing the action of the enzyme adenyl cyclase, which promotes increased cAMP synthesis. The methylxanthines, on the other hand, increase intracellular cAMP by inhibiting the action of the enzyme phosphodiesterase, which degrades cAMP to a less active compound. Since the two types of compounds increase cAMP by two different processes, they tend to complement and reinforce each other and to produce a better therapeutic response when used together than when either is used separately in the control of moderate to severe symptomatic asthma.

Assessment in an Acute Attack

The range of manifestations of asthma is broad; in mild or early forms the airway obstruction may be relatively slight and manifested by a persistent cough, often worse at night, but without wheezing or dyspnea. At one extreme, the patient may be asymptomatic and the airway narrowing manifested only by wheezing on examination of the chest or slight abnormalities on pulmonary function testing. (In some patients chronic bronchospasm, wheezing, and dyspnea of varying degrees may persist for long periods and be poorly responsive to treatment.)

At the other extreme the bronchospasm and hypoxemia, edema, and hyper-secretion may be so severe as to produce marked dyspnea and abnormalities of the arterial blood gases. Between attacks there may be no, or few, symptoms and signs. It is reported that the relation between the intensity of the bronchospasm and the severity of the attack is not consistent, so that some very severe attacks may be of short duration. Status asthmaticus refers to a very severe and prolonged attack which is resistant to treatment and which results in severe degree of hypoxemia as well as CO_2 retention and narcosis.

Factors which precipitate asthmatic attacks are similarly diverse and include contact with an antigen to which the patient has been sensitized, a viral respiratory infection, cold or polluted air, exercise, coughing, laughing, and emotional tension. Probably it is most often the case that the precipitating factor for a given attack is not known.

Evaluation of a patient with an acute attack of asthma should be prompt, and treatment should be started as soon as possible. It is said that the longer the dyspnea and wheezing have persisted, the slower the attack will be to resolve and the more intensive the treatment must be. Typically an attack reaches its maximum severity within a few minutes of the onset of symptoms; it may occasionally resolve spontaneously, often clears rapidly and completely with treatment, but if untreated may persist for hours.

If the attack is severe, the patient is in evident respiratory distress and prefers to sit up, often leaning forward with the arms on some supporting object. There is often anxiety and sometimes mental confusion. Coughing is frequent and may be dry or productive. Accessory muscles of respiration are active, with laryngeal and sternocleidomastoid muscle retraction on inspiration. There may be increased anterior–posterior chest dimension; decreased respiratory chest wall excursion; and because of overinflated lungs, cardiac and hepatic dullness to percussion are commonly decreased. The patient is often tachycardic and tachypneic and blood pressure may be elevated. Lung fields may be hyperresonant. Auscultation may demonstrate diminished breath sounds, a prolonged expiratory phase, and wheezing and rhonchi on both inspiration and expiration. The wheezes often increase on forced expiration. The attack may terminate with a paroxysm of coughing productive of viscous sputum. There may or may not be cyanosis depending upon the severity of the attack; its absence is never a reliable guide to adequate oxygenation of the arterial blood. If central cyanosis is present, it indicates severe hypoxemia.

Arterial blood gases show a low Pao_2 (60–80 mmHg) and O_2 saturation and if the attack is mild to moderate, a low $Paco_2$ and alkalemic pH. If the attack is severe and long, the hypoxemia will be more marked, perhaps below 60 mmHg, and there may be CO_2 retention and acidemia from the lactic acid produced by anaerobic metabolism and the elevated $Paco_2$.

The chest X-ray is often normal between attacks, but during an attack there may be overinflation of the lungs, low hemidiaphragms, and an increased retrosternal air space. If the attack is severe and protracted there may be evidence of atelectasis and infiltrates caused by mucus plugging. Spirometry during an attack reveals decreased vital capacity and decreased expiratory flow rate. In spite of the several abnormalities, death from asthma is rare.

Management

Management of asthma depends on the causes and the degree of severity.

Chronic Maintenance.   Since asthma is for the most part a chronic disease and not a series of acute episodes, many patients require some form of maintenance regimen. Perhaps the most important aspect of management is avoidance of known precipitating factors which may be revealed by a careful, detailed history. In extrinsic asthma attempts to eliminate environmental allergens to which the patient is sensitized is the primary goal and most effective treatment. Desensitization procedures tend not to be effective, besides having the disadvantages mentioned in Chapter 22.

Decreasing the patient's exposure to emotionally stressful circumstances, to general environmental pollutants, and to upper respiratory infections is important in decreasing frequency and severity of attacks. In intrinsic asthma there may also be identifiable from a careful history factors which appear to bring on attacks for the individual patient: physical or chemical tracheobroncial irritants such as cold air or fumes, muscular exercise, emotional tension, or others. It is important that these factors be avoided where possible.

Although asthma is considered by many workers to be a "psychosomatic" disorder (what chronic disease is *not* psychosomatic?), emotional problems are probably not a basic cause. Studies have failed to show that psychologic disturbances are greater in asthmatics than in control populations; where emotional disorders are present they may represent a response to the disease and the disabilities which it imposes, rather than the cause. Nevertheless, emotional upsets may act as a trigger for an attack in some patients and psychiatric intervention may be appropriate and helpful in a few.

Patients with reagin-induced asthma occurring during pollen season often respond well to around the clock administration of a bronchodilator such as oral aminophylline. If additional treatment is necessary, inhaled sympathomimetic bronchodilators may be effective, or ephedrine or a β_2 agonist such as oral ter-butaline may be added. Xanthine-type pharmacologic agents produce an increase in cAMP levels, and hence bronchodilation, by a mechanism different from but synergistic with β adrenergic receptor stimulation, namely, by inhibiting its in-tracellular degradation. Aminophylline, one of the most effective and frequently used bronchodilator agents, is a compound of theophylline and ethylenediamine; it is degraded to theophylline which is the active form. It has the specific action of producing bronchiolar smooth muscle relaxation. This drug is used in combi-nation with a β_2 agonist which increases intracellular synthesis of cAMP and therefore bronchodilation and decreased mediator release. The combination pro-duces very effective increases in the cross-sectional diameter of airways, and hence improved airflow and alveolar ventilation, with decreased tachypnea and work of breathing.

Other adrenergic agonists with predominantly β_2 action used for inhalation are isoetharine and isoproterenol. Terbutaline, salbutamol, and metaproterenol are oral β_2 agents. Patients should be encouraged to avoid overuse of sym-pathomimetic agents because of their cardiovascular side effects: tachycardia, cardiac arrhythmias, and palpitations.

In many patients the precipitating factors either cannot be eliminated or can-not be discovered. If the attacks are infrequent and the symptoms relatively mild then the above medications may be used only intermittently with the advent of symptoms. When symptoms are frequent and more severe, then the same com-binations of oral theophylline, oral β_2 sympathomimetic agents and inhaled bron-chodilators may be necessary on a regular basis. As mentioned earlier, abnormal-ities in pulmonary function tests between attacks indicate that increased resistance to airflow is often continuous in moderate to severe asthma and is as-sociated with an increased susceptibility to a variety of stimuli which lead to overt attacks; therefore, continuous bronchodilation treatment would seem ap-propriate. It is suggested by numerous authors that fixed dosage combinations of theophylline and a sympathomimetic be avoided; if the dosage of theophylline is adequate, the ephedrine may be excessive, and if the ephedrine dose is moder-ate, than the theophylline may be inadequate.

Disodium cromoglycate is a compound which inhibits the release of the medi-ators of anaphylaxis from mast cells and basophils. It is not a bronchodilator, and is of no value in the acute attack, but used in the maintenance of moderate to severe asthma it may reduce the frequency and severity of acute episodes. It is more effective in extrinsic than intrinsic, but is still very helpful to many patients in the latter category who experience exercise- or chemical or physical stimuli-induced attacks, as well as in patients in which the precipitating factors remain unidentified. Two or more weeks on a trial basis may be required to demonstrate its effectiveness. It is inhaled as a powder from a special device, and some pa-tients find this at first alarming or objectionable, so there is some resistance to be overcome in encouraging a trial. There is some evidence that it decreases the need for steroids in severe intractable asthma.

Adrenal corticosteroids may be necessary at intervals to control asthma in some patients. They are reported to be remarkably effective in the early weeks of use, but with continued administration the benefit wanes and eventually the adverse side effects come to outweigh the benefits. Systemic steroids appear to be useful primarily in the control of acute exacerbations, and then should be tapered and withdrawn as soon as possible. It has been suggested that the elevated blood eosinophil count which characterizes many adults with intrinsic asthma may be a useful guide for the management program, since there appears to be a correlation between eosinophilia and the activity of the disease as concerns signs and symptoms. Adrenal glucocorticoids, where necessary for control of exacerbations, produce a reduced eosinophil count which correlates with clinical improvement. Adrenal glucocorticoids probably act by stabilizing intracellular lysosomal membranes, thus inhibiting the release of intracellular enzymes which occurs in inflamed tissue. They also appear to increase cAMP levels by increasing the sensitivity of β adrenergic receptors to catecholamines. They also inhibit production of kinins and decrease the infiltration of inflammatory cells into the tracheobronchial tree. All of these actions reduce secretory and inflammatory reactions, decrease mediator release, and inhibit bronchoconstriction by direct β receptor activation.

Aerosolized dermatologic topical steroids have proven useful for inhalation and they have fewer systemic side effects because of their local action, and less pituitary ACTH suppression. Beclomethasone and triamcinolone are aerosol-administered steroids with minimal systemic absorption which exert antibronchoconstrictive and antiinflammatory actions. In severe asthma where steroids are necessary these agents which act locally on the tracheobronchial musoca may permit reduction in the use of oral steroids.

All pharmacologic agents used in the management of asthma have undesirable side effects. Since the results of the actions of β adrenergic agents and the methylxanthines are similar it follows that many of their side effects are also alike. The sympathomimetics may cause palpitations, tachycardia, hypertension, cardiac arrhythmias, restlessness, tremors, insomnia, and anxiety. The preferential β_2 agents have fewer cardiovascular side effects than the mixed β_1 and β_2. Aminophylline may promote nervous irritability, excitement, dizziness and vertigo, and even seizures; cardiac effects similar to the β adrenergic agents; and nausea, vomiting, and epigastric discomfort. Ephedrine (mixed α and β adrenergic) causes drying of mucosal surfaces and difficult micturition, especially in older patients. Cromoglycate generally is well tolerated but may induce hoarseness, cough, skin rash, and occasionally more serious lung reactions. Adrenal glucocorticoids cause osteoporosis, hypertension, fluid retention, peptic ulcers, cushingoid state and psychoemotional abnormalities. The inhaled nonabsorbed steroids sometimes produce cough and wheezing or may result in oropharyngeal yeast infections (candidiasis). Most of these agents also promote peptic ulcer disease.

A formal program of exercise rehabilitation as described in the preceding section of COPD is considered to be a very helpful addition to a maintenance regimen for asthma patients.

Acute Attacks. Epinephrine given subcutaneously continues to be the first choice in most cases for termination of an acute attack. Alternatively, a more preferential β_2 adrenergic agent such as terbutaline or salbutamol may be desirable in some instances since there are fewer cardiovascular side effects and the duration of action is longer. Depending on the severity of the attack, its duration, and the responsiveness to epinephrine injection, hospitalization and additional modes of treatment may be required. The adequacy of the patient's response to injected epinephrine is assessed by evaluating the relief of subjective distress, and auscultation of posterior lung fields for decrease or absence of wheezing. No further treatment may be required.

Adequate systemic hydration by oral and, if necessary, intravenous fluids is an extremely important aspect of management of the acute moderate to severe attack. Dehydration results in an increased viscosity of bronchial secretions and the sputum becomes thick, tenacious, and difficult for the patient to clear from the airways. If this material is not mobilized and removed by expulsive coughing it leads to mucus plugging of bronchioles, atelectasis, and physiologic shunting of pulmonary blood ($\dot{V}/\dot{Q}$ mismatch, venous admixture). Liquefaction and mobilization of pulmonary secretions may also be promoted by local hydration: inhalation of nebulized saline with a bronchodilator, and humidification of the inspired air–oxygen mixture. Chest physiotherapy is a useful measure in aiding removal of airway secretions.

Hypoxemia is an invariable accompaniment to an acute moderate or severe attack, so that in these patients arterial blood gas determinations are important in assessment and guiding treatment. Supplemental humidified O_2 via nasal prongs or face mask at controlled low flow rates is appropriate, particularly when bronchodilators are used. The reason for this is that bronchodilators produce vasodilation and increased blood flow in the pulmonary circuit; but there is poor alveolar ventilation because of plugging with bronchial secretions, and adaptive vasoconstriction of pulmonary vessels occurs in such hypoventilated areas. Therefore when a bronchodilator is given, although it produces increased cross-sectional diameter of airways with improved alveolar ventilation, nevertheless *perfusion may increase proportionately more than ventilation* until the secretions are removed. The temporary discrepancy in ventilation and perfusion ($\dot{V}/\dot{Q}$ mismatch) produced by bronchodilators may therefore contribute to a worsening hypoxemia; this should be countered by supplemental O_2.

O_2 administration in acute exacerbations of asthma does not in most cases pose the threat to continued spontaneous respiration that it does in the acute respiratory failure of COPD (see following). The asthmatic patient does not have chronic hypercapnia (and in fact has a low $PaCO_2$ during the attack) and therefore both the hypoxemia and hypercapneic drive to the respiratory centers are intact. So during the hypoxemia of an acute attack, supplemental O_2 is not as likely to lead to respiratory depression. An exception to this is the very severe and protracted asthmatic attack in which CO_2 retention and narcosis has developed. In this situation, as in COPD, hypercapneic respiratory drive may be blunted; hypoxemia remains the principal drive for respiration, and a too-marked elevation of the PaO_2 may lead to progressive worsening hypoventilation and/or respiratory arrest. An FIO_2 of about 30 is considered safe (2–3 L/min).

Oral or intravenous theophylline may be given depending on the severity of the attack. There is reported to be a wide range in variation of responsiveness of patients to theophylline; excessive blood levels may cause cardiovascular and central nervous system side effects: tachyarrhythmias, reflexely induced bradycardia, or seizures. Blood level determinations may be appropriate to guide rate of administration.

Adrenal corticosteroids may be required, orally or intravenously, in relatively high doses; this is particularly true if the patient is receiving maintenance oral steroids such as prednisone. It is important to recognize that there is a several hour delay between start of steroid administration and therapeutic effect.

Danger signals in acute severe asthma are reported to be a (spuriously) "normal" or increased $PaCO_2$ indicating marked inadequacy of alveolar ventilation from very severe acute airway obstruction; altered mental status (confusion, agitation) and/or decreased level of consciousness; and cyanosis, a PaO_2 of less than 55–60 mmHg, EKG abnormalities, and hyperinflated lungs revealed by the chest X-ray. Where CO_2 retention is occurring, where the hypoxemia is not adequately responsive to the above measures, and when hypercapnia and lactic acid accumulation from anaerobic metabolism are producing acidemia, then intubation and mechanical ventilation may be required.

Diffuse Interstitial (Infiltrative) Lung Disease

The group of lung disorders which lead to restrictive ventilatory defects are highly diverse as to cause (which is in fact very often not known); pathologic changes in the lung; rate of progression (acute or chronic); treatment methods and responsiveness to treatment; and eventual outcome (rapidly fatal, chronic slowly progressive, resolving). Nevertheless, they do have certain similarities: a diffuse generalized lung involvement with cellular proliferation and infiltrates of various kinds (cellular, noncellular, foreign naterial) which tend to occur outside the alveoli—that is, in the interstitial areas, but also commonly show intraalveolar components; comparable changes on pulmonary function testing; a uniform group of symptoms and signs; and similar longer term physiological consequences. In addition to the diversity of disorders included in the category of restrictive pulmonary diseases, there is a good bit of difference in terminology and classification of them used by various authors; a disease process may carry a number of different designations, which adds to the apparent confusion.

Causes

Some classifications of interstitial–infiltrative lung diseases are based on the nature of the histological process seen in lung biopsy and autopsy specimens, while others are grouped according to the etiology of the process. One classification of interstitial pulmonary disease based on the initiating factor includes those caused by: inhalation of toxic dusts and fumes; neoplasms; multiple thromboembolisms; ARDS (see following); systemic diseases such as rheumatoid arthritis, scleroderma, and lupus erythematosis; and a group of unknown or uncertain cause: idiopathic interstitial and intraalveolar diseases such as interstitial fibrosis, desquamative alveolitis, and interstitial pneumonitis.

In general terms, a sequence of changes within the lung appears to occur over time as a result of one of the initiating factors, and includes: an acute cellular infiltrate, the nature of which will depend on the causative agent; interstitial inflammation and edema; formation of fibrinous exudates and deposits of hyaline material; and eventually fibrous cell proliferation and fibrosis of broncheolar and alveolar membranes leading to scar formation and the destruction and distortion of lung parenchyma.

The type, and on occasion the cause, of the basic process can sometimes be established by lung biopsy. A careful history, physical examination, and special laboratory tests may be useful in establishing the cause, particularly in cases of lung disease from toxic substance in the occupational environment; from hypersensitivity reactions; and those associated with general systemic diseases, both acute such as viral infections, and chronic such as the rheumatic disorders.

Diffuse interstitial fibrosis, one form of diffuse infiltrative lung disease, is the term applied to the changes occurring in the lung as a result of a wide range of noxious agents and abnormal processes, some of the varieties of which are included in the etiologic classification, above. The processes in the lung, and their long-term consequences, have been compared to those of chronic kidney failure from chronic glomerulonephritis or pyelonephritis, and to chronic liver failure from biliary or alcoholic cirrhosis. That is, it is the nonspecific response of the organs to a number of destructive influences. Diffuse interstitial fibrosis may develop rapidly and terminate fatally as a result of a virus infection; more frequently the process is chronic and only gradually progressive over many years; occasionally it may remain stable over long periods, or sometimes resolve altogether.

Assessment

Subjective. The patient may complain of general systemic symptoms such as malaise, weight loss, shortness of breath made more severe by exercise, a generally decreased exercise tolerance, occasional arthralgias, and fatigue. There often is a cough, paroxysmal in nature, nonproductive or productive only of a small amount of mucoid sputum occasionally streaked with blood.

Objective. The physical examination may reveal no abnormalities. Often, however, if the disease process is well established, there will be tachypnea, and dyspnea on slight exertion or even at rest. Many patients have no physical findings on chest examination, or may have fine basilar rales. There may be clubbing of the fingers and, if the disease is advanced, cyanosis and evidence of right ventricular overload or failure (cor pulmonale, see following)

The chest X-ray may show cystic lesions and diffuse densities usually affecting both lungs and more marked at the bases. The lungs are often small and the hemidiaphragms elevated, which indicates reduced lung volume. The right ventricle may be enlarged and the pulmonary arteries dilated. These latter two changes indicate elevated vascular resistance in the pulmonary circuit because of progressive obliteration of the pulmonary capillary bed.

The lung abnormalities on pulmonary function tests are those of a restrictive lung disease, that is, a decreased vital capacity indicating low total lung volume, and an often normal airflow, indicating a lack of airway obstruction. If the fibrosis is severe then airflow rates may be reduced in the small terminal bronchioles, however. Lung compliance is often markedly reduced—that is, the lungs are "stiff," requiring an increased change in pressure required to produce a given change in volume. This increases the work of breathing and leads to tachypnea, as described previously.

Gas exchange at the alveoli is abnormally low, which produces a larger than normal difference in the Po_2 gradient between the alveolar and the arterial blood (increased $A-aO_2$ difference). At one time this poor gas diffusion between alveolar air and capillary blood was attributed to a thickening of the alveolar capillary membranes ("alveolar–capillary diffusion block"); however, it is now assumed to be the result of actual destruction of alveolar–capillary membranes and imbalances between alveolar ventilation and capillary perfusion; this results in venous admixture (physiologic shunting) and increased physiologic deadspace ventilation. Arterial blood gas determinations usually reveal an abnormally low PaO_2, with a low $PaCO_2$ because of the hypoxemia-induced hyperventilation. Elevated $PaCO_2$ occurs only in very advanced infiltrative disease.

Management

The management depends to a large degree upon the cause. In situations where inhalation of toxic dusts or fumes appear to be involved, avoidance would be indicated. In some types of infiltrative lung disease adrenal corticosteroids have proven beneficial in arresting the advancement; indications for a trial of prednisone are suggested to be the presence of respiratory symptoms, and/or evidence of significant progression of the disease. Results of treatment should be assessed on the basis of pulmonary function testing, chest X-ray, the patient's symptoms, and PaO_2. It is thought that if adrenal steroids are going to prove helpful they will have produced improvement in the patient's subjective and objective status by about a month of treatment. The dosage may then be slowly tapered, if possible, to avoid the well-known adverse effects of long-term administration (Chapter 13).

Course

Progression and outcome vary with the nature of the causative agent but also with unknown factors; in general there is great range of variation from remission to inexorable progression of lung destruction and hypoxemia. Often the lung changes are progressive and irreversible. Fatality results from pulmonary infections and pulmonary heart disease (cor pulmonale).

Cor Pulmonale

Cor pulmonale has a number of definitions; the term is used to refer to a group of interrelated abnormalities of the pulmonary vasculature, and of the right ventricle which pumps blood into these vessels. Cor pulmonale may be applied to conditions of (1) increased pulmonary vascular resistance; (2) elevated pulmonary artery pressure (PAP) resulting from an intrinsic disease of the lungs; (3) dilation or hypertrophy of the right ventricle occurring as a result of work overload from pumping blood into a high-resistance pulmonary circuit; or (4) congestive right ventricular failure secondary to the above abnormalities. In this discussion cor pulmonale is used in the sense of deranged structure or function of the right ventricle, primarily enlargement, caused by either vasomotor or anatomic increases in pulmonary vascular resistance, which have resulted in pulmonary hypertension.

Causes

The causes of the elevated pulmonary vascular resistance, in turn, may be several: (1) most commonly, intrinsic pulmonary diseases such as COPD or interstitial–infiltrative lung disease which have resulted in destruction or constriction of pulmonary vasculature; (2) lung blood vessel disease such as the rare primary pulmonary hypertension or the more common multiple pulmonary embolization; (3) depressed ventilatory drive by the brainstem respiratory control centers exemplified by idiopathic hypoventilation; or (4) abnormal musculoskeletal configuration of the thorax such as severe kyphoscoliosis. Moreover, cor pulmonale may develop acutely, as occurs in the case of extensive pulmonary embolization, and result primarily from dilation of the heart and therefore be largely reversible; or it may be a chronic and progressive disorder, as from severe bronchitic type COPD (blue bloater) in which case the enlargement may be mainly muscular hypertrophy. In the latter situation there may be acute exacerbations from superimposed acute bronchopulmonary infections, in which case dilation is superimposed upon the hypertrophied right ventricle, producing further enlargement.

In the normal individual the pulmonary vasculature is a low-pressure, low-resistance, remarkably distensible system. The blood pressure in the pulmonary circuit is only about one fourth that of the systemic circuit, yet it accommodates the same overall blood flow. With exercise, the cardiac output and therefore the total blood flow may increase two- or threefold without leading to a significant elevation of pulmonary artery pressure. The reason for this large accommodative capacity is that the pulmonary vasculature responds to an increase in blood flow by markedly decreasing its resistance. This is accomplished by a widespread pulmonary vasodilation in response to increased cardiac output from the right ventricle. This is a form of response called autoregulation.

Processes Involved in the Development of Pulmonary Artery Hypertension

In the disease processes enumerated above the pulmonary blood vessels lose their capacity to respond to an increased blood flow with the decreased resistance which normally serves to maintain pulmonary artery pressure within normal limits in the face of increased flow. Pulmonary vascular reserve capacity may decline either because of a reduction in the distensibility of pulmonary blood vessels, or because of a reduction in the actual number of open, functional blood vessels. The net result in either case is a reduction in the total cross-sectional diameter of the pulmonary vasculature. This reduction renders the pulmonary circuit increasingly less able to accommodate the elevated right ventricular output of exercise without an increase in pulmonary artery pressure.

When cross-sectional diameter has been reduced to about one third of normal, pulmonary arterial hypertension may be present even at rest. The elevated pulmonary artery pressure increases the overload on the right ventricle and requires greatly increased myocardial work and oxygen consumption to force blood through the vessels which are reduced in number or size by the disease process. Eventually the volume and pressure of the right ventricle increase, producing dilation. Ultimately, if the disease process continues and pulmonary artery pressure (PAP) remains chronically elevated, right ventricle hypertrophy develops.

In some patients with cor pulmonale left ventricular failure may evolve as a later complication; at that time combined failure or the right and left ventricles produces the characteristic signs and symptoms of overt congestive heart failure.

The processes leading to left ventricular involvement in cor pulmonale are several, and will be described shortly.

Returning to the underlying causes of the pulmonary hypertension which leads eventually to cor pulmonale, I stated that the changes accounting for the elevated pulmonary vascular resistance could be either functional (vasomotor) or structural (obliterative). As we shall see, there are interactions between these two processes.

Functional (Vasomotor) Changes. *Alveolar hypoxemia.* This category of cause of elevated pulmonary vascular resistance is the more common of the two, and is induced by the hypoxemia and acidemia characteristic of COPD at the more bronchitic end of the clinical spectrum described in a previous section. The abnormalities of the arterial blood gases and pH in this type of patient have a direct effect on the resistance to blood flow through the small arteries and arterioles of the lungs. A low content of oxygen in the alveoli (alveolar hypoxia) because of inadequate alveolar ventilation has the direct effect on pulmonary vessels of strong vasoconstriction. As these vessels constrict, pulmonary vascular resistance increases, and elevation of pressure in the pulmonary artery occurs. Hypoxic pulmonary vasoconstriction, if long continued, promotes actual hypertrophy of the smooth muscle layers of the pulmonary arterioles, so that functional vasomotor changes evolve into structural anatomic ones. This is well illustrated by the fact that a chronically hypoxemic patient with marked pulmonary artery hypertension and cor pulmonale, who is supplied with low flow oxygen (1–2 L/m), may show only a small decline in PAP over the short term, suggesting decreased pulmonary vasoconstriction in response to the increased alveolar oxygen content. However, when the oxygen supplementation is continued for several weeks to months, there may be a more marked decline in pulmonary artery hypertension, and corresponding further decrease in the signs and symptoms of cor pulmonale secondary to the decline, suggesting that some anatomic reversal of vessel smooth muscle hypertrophy has occurred.

An additional consequence of chronic hypoxemia is the stimulation of erythropoietin from the kidney which stimulates increased red blood cell production, erythrocytosis, elevated hematocrit, and increased blood viscosity; the latter increases the resistance to blood flow through all vascular beds, including the pulmonary circulation, elevating pulmonary artery pressure (PAP). Furthermore, hypoxemia itself, plus the lactic acidemia resulting from anaerobic metabolism, both cause depressed myocardial function and reduced cardiac output. The lowered performance of the heart then contributes to a worsening of chronic hypoxemia, and a vicious cycle is established.

Hypercapnia and acidemia. Inadequate alveolar ventilation causes hypercapnia as well as hypoxemia. The action of a high alveolar CO_2 concentration itself probably does not have the direct vasoconstrictive effect on pulmonary blood vessels that alveolar hypoxia does. Rather it appears that the elevated Pa_{CO_2} exerts its effects via other abnormalities secondary to it. (1) Severe chronic hypercapnia depresses the responsiveness of the respiratory control centers in the brainstem to the major physiologic stimulus to respiration, namely, an increase Pa_{CO_2}. (2) Chronically elevated Pa_{CO_2} stimulates the kidney to increased absorption of bicarbonate ions (renal–metabolic compensation for chronic respiratory acidosis,

Chapter 2); as serum HCO_3^- rises so does pH; there is some evidence that overcompensation (metabolic alkalemia) may occur which depresses ventilatory drive and worsens both hypoxemia and hypercapnia. (3) Chronic severe hypercapnia causes depression of both brainstem and higher centers in the central nervous system (CO_2 narcosis), cerebral vasodilation, and elevated intracranial pressure. Altered mental status and level of consciousness, occasionally with seizures, may occur. This is particularly true if there has been an acute increase in $Paco_2$ over the stable elevated level because of acute pulmonary infection. Central nervous system depression reduces the nonspecific activation component of respiratory drive. (4) Where the elevated $Paco_2$ has been acute and therefore renal metabolic compensation has not had time to return serum pH to more normal levels, the acidemia appears to potentiate the pulmonary vasoconstrictive effects of hypoxemia. These additive effects, particularly where there has been an *acute* further increase in $Paco_2$ and decline in pH and Pao_2, superimposed on the chronic abnormalities of bronchitic COPD, may overburden the right ventricle in cor pulmonale to the point where acute severe right heart failure develops.

In the pulmonary disorders characterized by marked hypoxemia and hypercapnia, cardiac output is often normal or high in spite of the increased resistance to flow of the pulmonary vasculature. Because of this combination of normal or high cardiac output and elevated flow resistance, pulmonary artery hypertension develops relatively early in the course of the disease, and increased PAP may be present even at rest, especially during acute infections which worsen the bronchial obstruction.

Structural (Anatomic) Changes. Obliteration of portions of the pulmonary vascular bed occurs in certain advanced stages of the pulmonary interstitial–infiltrative disorders which typify the restrictive lung diseases, in primary pulmonary hypertension, in multiple pulmonary embolization, and in the primarily emphysematous form of COPD. Again, the consequence is decreased cross-sectional diameter of the pulmonary circuit, from obstruction and narrowing of pulmonary arterioles, causing elevated pulmonary vascular resistance, and pulmonary artery hypertension. However, in many of these disorders alveolar–capillary gas exchange may not be sufficiently abnormal to produce marked blood gas alterations, so that the deleterious effects of hypoxemia, hypercapnia, and acidemia on the pulmonary vasculature are not marked during these early stages. In these patients cardiac output tends to be low. The decreased cardiac output operates to minimize the pulmonary hypertension, since arterial pressure in a circuit is the product of cardiac output and vascular resistance. Hypoxemia and elevated PAP may develop only at the onset of exercise, and be present at rest only later when the disease is far advanced.

Temporal Sequences in Pulmonary Hypertension and Cor Pulmonale

Acute. Dilation of the right ventricle occurs because of its inability to empty normally into an abnormal high-resistance, low-capacity pulmonary circuit. This may occur acutely as a consequence of pulmonary embolization, which will be discussed in a subsequent section.

Acute cor pulmonale more often refers to the increase in pulmonary hypertension, with distension of the right ventricle, occurring intermittently during acute exacerbations of bronchitic COPD from bronchopulmonary infection. The infection leads to increased airway obstruction, decreased alveolar ventilation, deterioration in ABG values ($\uparrow$PaCO_2, $\downarrow$PaO_2, $\downarrow$pH) and greatly elevated pulmonary vascular resistance. Although measures to control the infection and improve alveolar ventilation often result in amelioration of the elevated PAP and right ventricle dilation, some irreversible damage to pulmonary vasculature and parenchyma occurs with each attack, moving the patient along the continuum to chronic cor pulmonale.

Progressive.   Progressive pulmonary hypertension and cor pulmonale is usually the result of (1) an inexorably worsening pulmonary infiltrative–interstitial disease such as interstitial fibrosis; (2) a progressive pulmonary vascular disease (primary pulmonary hypertension or recurrent pulmonary embolizations); or (3) a COPD of such severity that blood gas abnormalities are extreme and continuous. It is in these interstitial and primary vascular diseases that progressive obliteration of the pulmonary vasculature occurs and leads to the greatest elevations in pulmonary artery pressure. Because COPD is a common disease, most cor pulmonale is seen in association with it, but more severe and protracted pulmonary artery hypertension occurs in the rarer vascular and interstitial lung diseases.

Just as chronically elevated systemic arterial pressure leads to elevated left ventricular end-diastolic pressure and volume, with dilation and eventual hypertrophy of the left ventricle; so chronically elevated pulmonary arterial pressure leads to similar changes in right ventricle structure and function. And just as the onset of left ventricular failure in chronic systemic hypertension is heralded by an inability to elevate systolic output at the onset of exercise, so the onset of right ventricular failure in chronic pulmonary hypertension is marked by a similar inability to empty normally. The result is an increase in pressure and volume of blood in the venous circuit supplying the failing ventricle, so that jugular venous pressure elevation, hepatomegaly from venous congestion, and pedal edema develop.

As we have seen in Chapter 7, left ventricular failure is the most common cause of right ventricular failure because of the increased load of pressure work imposed on the right ventricle by the inability of the failing left ventricle to pump blood out of the lungs. However, the deficits in left ventricular structure and function developing in cor pulmonale are on the basis of chronic arterial hypoxemia and systemic acidemia from the lung disease itself. Atherosclerotic coronary artery disease may also be present and, although unrelated to the lung disease, potentiates its effects. The two abnormalities may combine to produce chronic myocardial hypoxia and ischemic heart disease (Chapter 4).

Assessment

The history and physical examination may reveal the nature and severity of the pulmonary vascular or pulmonary parenchymal or interstitial disease which has led to elevated PAP and cor pulmonale. Symptoms are shortness of breath made worse by exercise, weakness and easy fatigability, and chronic cough (productive in COPD). Signs on physical examination may be cyanosis, elevated jugular venous pressure, enlarged tender liver with hepatojugular reflux, a cardiac thrust at the left sternal border, and a loud pulmonic component of the second heart sound. An S_3 indicates right ventricular failure. The chest X-ray may show evidences of the underlying pulmonary disorder, and distended pulmonary arteries. Comparison of the findings with those of previous films is useful. Right ventricular enlargement is not easy to detect. ABG determinations are valuable for assessing the patient's status at a given time as well as for following the progression of the disorder and evaluating the effects of a management regimen.

Management

Management of cor pulmonale depends largely on the control of the basic processes. Managements of COPD, heart failure, interstitial lung disease, and pulmonary embolism are discussed in other sections under the appropriate designations.

Acute Disorders of the Respiratory System

Acute Respiratory Failure

The term respiratory insufficiency refers to the inadequacy of gaseous exchange in the lungs to meet the metabolic requirements for O_2 necessary to maintain normal levels of physical activity. Respiratory failure, on the other hand, denotes a more severe degree of impairment of gaseous exchange, and implies inadequate oxygenation of pulmonary blood to meet metabolic requirements and maintain normal acid–base balance at rest.

Acute respiratory failure may be defined as rapidly developing, markedly abnormal arterial blood gas levels, because of inadequate pulmonary gas exchange, caused by intrinsic or extrinsic disorders of respiratory function. It may occur as a result of a wide range of physiologic abnormalities. It is said to exist when there is a sudden decline of the PaO_2 to 50–60 mmHg (depending on ambient barometric pressure) with or without an elevation of $PaCO_2$. When rapidly developing severe hypoxemia is accompanied by sudden increases of $PaCO_2$ to levels of 50 mmHg or more, some authors refer to the condition as ventilatory failure. This distinction between respiratory failure (hypoxemia alone) and ventilatory failure (hypoxemia in conjunction with hypercapnia) is often made because the causes, signs and symptoms, and management, may be quite different in the two cases. The definitive assessment of respiratory and ventilatory failure can be made *only* on the basis of arterial blood gas (ABG) analysis (by arterial puncture, if the patient does not have an arterial line) with laboratory determination of PaO_2, $PaCO_2$, HCO_3^-, pH, and O_2 saturation.

Ventilatory Failure (Hypercapneic Respiratory Failure)

Causes. This form of acute respiratory failure may occur in two different categories of patients: those with intrinsic lung diseases, and those with extrinsic respiratory abnormalities.

Intrinsic.   Examples of intrinsic pulmonary disorders which may lead to acute ventilatory failure are COPD, asthma, and interstitial fibrosis. In these chronic intrinsic lung diseases it is often the superimposition of an acute respiratory infection on the abnormalities of the underlying condition which precipitates acute ventilatory failure. (Pleural space defects such as pleural effusion, pneumothorax—especially tension pneumothorax—and pleural space fibrosis may also lead to ventilatory failure, especially when there is a prior intrinsic lung disease). In these pulmonary abnormalities there is either localized or generalized chronic alveolar hypoventilation which causes inadequate oxygenation of the blood, and permits the accumulation of carbon dioxide.

Extrinsic. Extrinsic respiratory disorders which may lead to acute ventilatory failure are categorized according to level of involvement: (a) abnormalities of the brainstem respiratory control center from depressive drug poisoning or brain trauma; (b) neuromuscular abnormalities such as myasthenia gravis, multiple sclerosis, or Guillain-Barré syndrome; and (c) chest wall disorders including multiple rib fractures with flail chest, and severe kyphoscoliosis. Any of these abnormalities may lead to alveolar hypoventilation with resulting hypoxemia and hypercapnia.

Chronic moderate levels of hypoxemia and hypercapnia, such as may occur in COPD, are well tolerated by most patients. One of the reasons that this is so is because of the several compensatory mechanisms elicited by the abnormal blood gases which operate to minimize their effects. In the case of chronic hypoxemia there is compensatory elevation of cardiac output, increased erythropoiesis, and a shift to the right in the oxygen–hemoglobin dissociation curve, all of which operate to increase delivery of oxygen to tissues in the face of a chronically depressed PaO_2. In the case of chronic hypercapnia, as discussed in detail in Chapter 2, increased renal resorption of bicarbonate ion returns the serum pH to a more normal level (renal–metabolic compensation for respiratory acidosis).

However, with rapidly developing hypoxemia and hypercapnia there is no time for these compensatory processes to evolve, so that a rapid decline in PaO_2 leads to a marked fall in tissue oxygenation; and a large rapid rise in $PaCO_2$ causes a severe fall in serum pH (acidemia). Hypoxemia causes impaired myocardial performance with declining cardiac output and further depression of tissue oxygenation; cardiac arrhythmias; pulmonary vascular constriction with pulmonary hypertension and right ventricular overload; and anaerobic cellular metabolism with developing lactic acidemia. Hypercapnia itself directly depresses levels of consciousness and alters mental status, adding to the effects of lactic acidemia caused by cellular hypoxia. A low serum pH and high $PaCO_2$ cause cerebral vasodilation, cerebral vascular congestion, and elevated intracranial pressure, which may be manifested as papilledema and reduced venous pulsation in disc vessels. Acidemia potentiates the adverse effects of hypoxemia.

Some of the above listed causes of acute ventilatory failure produce rapid, obvious, and dramatic changes in the patient's physiologic status. However, in patients with chronic ventilatory insufficiency (as from COPD) who develop acute respiratory failure from sedatives or superimposed acute respiratory infection, the transition from chronic compensated hypoxemia and hypercapnia to acute respiratory failure may be subtle and insidious.

Assessment. *Subjective.* If the patient's underlying condition permits awareness and expression of symptoms, there may be complaints of agitation, irritability or depression, drowsiness during the day, diplopia, muscle weakness and incoordination, insomnia and restlessness especially at night, headache, and tremulousness. These symptoms often indicate hypoxemia, with or without marked hypercapnia. Generally, however, especially if the patient is very ill, or if the abnormal blood gases have produced altered mental status and depressed level of consciousness, there will be no complaints. Thus close observation, combined with frequent monitoring of ABGs, are crucial to patient assessment.

Objective. ABG measurement of blood obtained by arterial puncture or from an arterial line is the only certain basis for an assessment of acute ventilatory failure; a $PaO_2 < 50$ mmHg and $PaCO_2 > 50$ mmHg is an arbitrary limit for definition of the state; serum pH below 7.0–7.2 is associated with increased mortality. Because of the fact that CO_2 is more soluble and diffusible than O_2, hypoxemia develops prior to hypercapnia. Clinical signs of hypoxemia and hypercapnia include mental confusion and bizarre behavior, restlessness, muscle twitchings or seizure, asterixis, cyanosis, delerium, lethargy and stupor, declining blood pressure, tachycardia and/or other cardiac arrhythmias, and papilledema. Early recognition and prompt intervention are essential in preventing complications and death, since the progressive decline in alveolar hypoventilation terminates in apnea and cardiopulmonary arrest.

Management. The first goal is reversal of the blood gas abnormalities. This involves securing and maintaining the airway through liquefaction and removal of mucous secretions, the use of an oropharyngeal or nasopharyngeal airway, or endotracheal intubation or tracheostomy where required. The use of enriched humidified oxygen inhalations is always necessary to combat hypoxermia. Nasal prongs are used to deliver oxygen at low flow rates; the key principle in use of O_2 is to administer the lowest possible fraction of inspired oxygen (FIO_2) which will return the patient's PaO_2 to an acceptable level, and maintain it there. Venturi masks are sometimes used; they deliver a fixed oxygen–air concentration (FIO_2) of various percentages, depending on the mask. However, they are not very comfortable, are expensive, and cannot be used during eating; removal of the mask even for brief periods may be dangerous to the COPD patient with acute ventilatory insufficiency and can result in a rapid decline in PaO_2, and increase in $PaCO_2$, because of an abrupt rise in alveolar CO_2 partial pressure ($PACO_2$). There is also evidence that the Venturi mask may not maintain an adequate PaO_2 in patients with hypoventilation and intrinsic lung disease. There are other types of masks available, but probably the two-pronged nasal cannula is best from the standpoint of patient comfort and convenience, as well as the maintenance of arterial oxygenation.

Regardless of the method of administration of oxygen (and simplest means are best, provided they attain the goal) a PaO_2 of 50–60 mmHg is acceptable. Referring to the Hb–O_2 dissociation curve (Chapter 2) it is evident that it is within this range that the curve plateaus. This means that when the arterial oxygen tension is below 50–60 mmHg, relatively *slight increase in PaO_2* will lead to a correspondingly *marked increase in Hb–O_2* saturation. However, above 50–60 mmHg, at the plateau, relatively major increases in PaO_2 result in only minor elevations in Hb–O_2 saturation. In addition, a high FIO_2, especially if long continued, causes oxygen toxicity and damage to alveolar–capillary membranes.

There is another well-established danger in uncontrolled high oxygen flow rates, particularly for the COPD patient in acute ventilatory failure; that danger is the threat of further respiratory depression, and poorer alveolar hypoventilation, caused by the enriched oxygen–air mixture. The solution to this problem resides in the administration of precisely measured, carefully controlled and monitored, low rates of oxygen flow. There are probably a number of mechanisms for the development of CO_2 narcosis and CO_2 retention in the patient with COPD who is given excessive oxygen for the hypoxemia of acute ventilatory failure.

In the normal subject, an elevation of $Paco_2$ provides a strong central brainstem and peripheral chemoreceptor drive to increased respiratory rate and depth, which will rapidly lower $Paco_2$ to normal levels. However, the COPD patient is *chronically* hypoxemic and hypercapneic. Renal metabolic compensation has returned the serum and CSF pH to close to normal levels by increasing serum and CSF bicarbonate concentration. Further acute increases in $Paco_2$ and decline of serum pH will not act as a strong respiratory stimulus, both because of pH buffering by high levels of bicarbonate in the ECF, and because the chronic hypercapnia has blunted the CO_2 ventilatory drive response of the respiratory center and peripheral chemoreceptors. Thus in these patients, the principal stimulus to respiration is hypoxia (plus the nonspecific cortical activation described in an earlier section).

When uncontrolled high flow rates of oxygen are administered, Pao_2 rises and this abruptly lowers the hypoxic drive to breathing and hence to alveolar ventilation, with resulting rapid elevations in both alveolar and arterial CO_2 content, causing central CO_2 narcosis. If the patient has received sedatives or tranquilizers for "restlessness" then the nonspecific cortical activation drive to respiration is also blunted, adding to depressed alveolar ventilation. Careful studies of precisely controlled low flow oxygen administration to COPD patients with acute ventilatory failure have demonstrated the safety and effectiveness of this mode of treatment in restoring Pao_2 to acceptable levels without adversely affecting alveolar ventilation or $Paco_2$ content. Since the degree of hypoxemia and the arterial blood gas response to oxygen supplementation in these patients is markedly variable, frequent ABG monitoring is essential.

Mechanical ventilation with a volume-cycled respirator may be required for patients whose ventilatory drive and alveolar ventilation are inadequate to return the Pao_2 to acceptable levels. Volume-cycled ventilators are preferable to pressure-cycled ones since they deliver a preset tidal volume in spite of alterations in pressure–volume relationships (from, for example, the decreased compliance of left ventricular failure) which require elevated pressure to maintain an adequate tidal volume. Intubation or tracheostomy is of course required for mechanical ventilation. There are four immediate benefits of mechanical ventilation to the patient with ventilatory failure: (1) it decreases work of breathing, thus conserving the patient's strength and lowering respiratory muscle CO_2 production; (2) it permits a decrease in FIO_2 because it produces a predetermined and stable tidal volume and respiratory rate, thus improving Pao_2 and $Paco_2$ levels without an increase in FIO_2; (3) it automatically compensates for altered responsiveness of the brainstem and peripheral respiratory control mechanisms by maintaining a stable predetermined respiratory rate and tidal volume; and (4) it improves ventilation–perfusion ratios throughout the lungs.

Once the ABG levels are corrected and stabilized, then attention may be directed to the primary cause of the acute ventilatory failure: respiratory infection, increased bronchospasm, increased bronchial secretions, drug overdose, or whatever.

Respiratory Failure (Hypoxemic Respiratory Failure, with Normal or Decreased Pa_{CO_2})

This form of acute respiratory insufficiency is characterized by a marked decline in Pa_{O_2} without carbon dioxide retention; it is caused by acute intrinsic abnormalities in pulmonary parenchyma which interfere with the ability of the alveoli to deliver sufficient amounts of oxygen to the pulmonary capillary blood; the result is sustained and substantial arterial oxygen desaturation. There are a number of causes: pneumonia, pulmonary thromboembolism, bronchiolitis and pneumonitis, atelectasis, and others. The impaired arterial oxygenation results from severe $\dot{V}/\dot{Q}$ mismatch, often as a consequence of the perfusion of inadequately or nonventilated alveoli which are filled with blood, edema fluid, exudates, and cellular accumulations. The fluid, unlike that resulting from the pulmonary edema of left ventricular failure, does not accumulate in interstitial and intraalveolar spaces because of elevated pulmonary capillary pressure; but rather does so because of abnormally increased pulmonary capillary permeability. The accumulated fluid leads to decreased lung compliance and increased work of breathing, which contributes to the hypoxemia. The accumulation of fluid leads to the appearance of diffuse infiltrates on chest X-ray, and the alveolar hypoxia (reduced $P_{A_{O_2}}$) induces increased pulmonary vascular resistance and pulmonary hypertension. Although there are a number of causes, the interesting syndrome of adult respiratory distress (ARDS) exemplifies the pathophysiologic abnormalities in perhaps their most extreme form.

The Adult Respiratory Distress Syndrome (ARDS, Shock Lung, Traumatic Wet Lung, Postperfusion Lung, Congestive Atelectasis). This complex of closely related pathophysiologic changes results from acute severe alveolar and capillary membrane injury from a wide variety of damaging and noxious factors, which may act directly on lung parenchyma itself, or indirectly by means of more widespread systemic abnormalities. In other words, although the initiating mechanisms may be remarkably diverse, it is as though the lung has but a limited repertory of responses to severe bodily harm. Thus the pathophysiologic abnormalities are much the same, and the management is similar in most cases, regardless of cause. The common denominator is an inability of the lungs adequately to oxygenate the arterial blood despite an adequate or high FIO_2, primarily because of increased lung fluid from abnormally increased alveolar capilliary permeability.

ARDS is characterized by a typical group of physiologic abnormalities: hypoxemia, decreased vital capacity and functional residual capacity, increased minute ventilation, decreased lung compliance, increased work of breathing, and elevated venous admixture and physiologic deadspace.

Several abnormalities that develop in the lungs in ARDS and result in decreased alveolar ventilation and impaired oxygenation of pulmonary capillary blood are caused by an excess of extracellular fluid in lung parenchyma. Basically, there are two quite different processes involved in the conditions which lead to an accumulation of fluid in the lungs.

The quantity of extracellular fluid in lung tissue depends on the balance of forces acting between the vascular and the interstitial fluid compartments of the lung. (These relationships are discussed more fully in Chapter 1 in the section on edema formation.) Under normal conditions there is a small net outward movement of ECF from the pulmonary capillaries into the interstitial spaces. This fluid is drained away by the pulmonary lymphatics so that it does not accumulate and interfere with pulmonary airflow and gas exchange at the alveolar capillary membranes. Fluid will accumulate in lung tissue whenever the net outward movement of ECF from pulmonary capillaries into pulmonary interstitium exceeds the capacity of the pulmonary lymphatics to drain it away.

The two different processes which may cause an extravasation of ECF in excess of the rate of removal by lymphatics are (1) increased pulmonary *capillary hydrostatic pressure* (that is, elevated pressure within the capillaries because of elevated intracapillary volume), which occurs in left ventricular failure (see Chapter 7, Heart Failure) and results in classical pulmonary edema; and (2) increased pulmonary *capillary permeability*, which permits extravasation of fluid from the capillaries into the interstitial spaces on the basis of loss of selective permeability, because of intrinsic damage to the capillary endothelium (rather than on the basis of elevated intracapillary pressure and volume). It is this latter process which is responsible for the increased lung parenchymal fluid content in ARDS. It is true that in some cases, especially in patients with prior organic heart disease, there may be impairment of myocardial performance in ARDS so that the elevated pulmonary capillary pressure of left ventricular failure may be superimposed upon the capillary membrane changes. The consequence would be a greater accumulation of lung fluid than would result from either process acting alone.

Causes. The diversity of etiology becomes evident on listing physiologic insults which have been reported to lead to ARDS: massive trauma and hemorrhagic shock, disseminated intravascular coagulation, aspiration of gastric contents, opiate drug poisoning, hemorrhagic pancreatitis, gram-negative sepsis, oxygen toxicity, fat emboli, severe viral pneumonia, and direct trauma to the chest and lungs. Thus in assessing patients for early ARDS, the underlying disorder and the immediate prior history are of prime importance.

The cause of ARDS in various forms of trauma is not known, but some authors suggest that a period of severe hypotension resulting from blood loss and third spacing (see Chapter 1) may be involved. The hypotension leads to underperfusion of the lungs, and it is proposed that continued ventilation of greatly underperfused lungs leads to vasoconstriction of the bronchial arterioles, possible intravascular coagulation in the lung microcirculation, and resulting ischemic damage to the distal bronchioles and alveolar–capillary membranes. Other workers believe that the lung is markedly resistant to ischemia from hypoperfusion, and suggest that a generalized intravascular coagulation in the systemic circulation develops during hypotensive shock; then when resuscitation occurs and the circulation returns to normal, these microthrombi are embolized into the pulmonary circulation, causing damage to and altered permeability of the alveolar capillary membranes. The increased circulating humoral agents in the blood during hemorrhagic or hypotensive shock (histamine, bradykinin, catecholamines, serotonin) are suggested by some authors to produce pulmonary vasoconstriction and alveolar capillary membrane damage which increases their permeability and permits extravasation of first ECF, and then plasma proteins, into the interstitial and then intraalveolar spaces.

In severe gram-negative sepsis from an infection outside the lungs, ARDS is a frequent and often fatal complication; it is reported to occur most often in conditions which cause peritonitis: gunshot wounds of the abdomen, ruptured gallbladder, intestinal perforation, and pancreatitis. Such patients have a positive blood culture, but the lungs are not infected, and it may be that the bacteria release some toxin which directly damages alveolar–capillary membranes.

ARDS occurring after aspiration of gastric contents is said not to be caused by the digestive enzymes, but possibly by some abnormality produced by the low pH of gastric fluid, which spreads rapidly through the lungs once aspiration has occurred. Severity of the reaction is correlated with the amount aspirated, and subsequent pulmonary infections are frequent if the patient survives the acute phase of the ARDS.

The processes involved in ARDS development following pulmonary thermal burns, and the inhalation of smoke and other toxic fumes, are readily explained on the basis of direct heat and chemical injury to and inflammatory reaction of the mucosa of the tracheobronchial tree, with resulting loss of selective permeability of the alveolar–capillary membranes.

In O_2 toxicity there is a quite clear relationship between the duration of exposure necessary to produce ARDS and the FIO_2; the higher the FIO_2 above 0.5 (50% O_2), the less time is required for development of pathologic changes in the lung. The sequence of such changes is reported to be accumulation of interstitial edema and fibrin; cellular infiltration with leukocytes, macrophages, and platelets; disruption of capillary endothelium; and finally in late stages, degeneration of alveolar epithelium.

Fat embolism to the lungs may occur as a result of release of marrow from long bones following fractures, but in addition is suggested to occur in trauma as a result of mobilization of body fat deposits into the blood by the high circulating levels of catecholamines, and alterations in the stability of blood lipids during shock. The pulmonary capillaries contain a fat-hydrolyzing enzyme, lipoprotein lipase, which hydrolyzes neutral fat into free fatty acids; these are suggested to be the destructive agent responsible for the increased pulmonary capillary permeability leading to ARDS.

Lung abnormalities. The common denominator for the lung abnormalities in ARDS appears to be the loss of selective permeability by the pulmonary capillaries, which permits first, excessive amounts of fluid and electrolytes to diffuse from them into the interstitial spaces; and later as their integrity is further disrupted, allows plasma proteins and formed elements of the blood to leak out into the lung.

In the normal subject there is always a net leakage of ECF from the pulmonary capillaries into the interstitial spaces (see Chapter 1) and this fluid is drained away by the lymphatic drainage system of the lung. However, when the capillary membranes are damaged, much larger amounts of fluid escape the vessels, including blood proteins and cells which normally are retained within them.

When the amount of fluid leaving the capillaries exceeds the capacity of the lymphatics to drain it away, then the fluid accumulates in the interstitial spaces and causes decreased lung compliance, increased work of breathing, and tachypnea.

Eventually as the amount of free fluid increases, it penetrates into the alveoli and respiratory bronchioles, and alveolar ventilation declines. Since the alveoli continue to be perfused, $\dot{V}/\dot{Q}$ mismatch (venous admixture) develops, and the PaO_2 falls. Since CO_2 is soluble and diffusible, and since the patient has a high minute respiratory volume (i.e., he is hyperventilating) the $PaCO_2$ is low and respiratory alkalemia develops.

Fluid and protein in the alveoli interfere with the production of surfactant, the phospholipoprotein which lowers the surface tension of the liquid film lining the alveoli to prevent their collapse. As surfactant production is impaired, alveolar surface tension becomes increased, alveoli are more difficult to inflate with air, and eventually they collapse, producing areas of atelectasis. As perfusion of unventilated alveoli increases, this increases the amount of unoxygenated blood returning to the left heart.

Disruption of capilliary blood flow occurs in other areas, caused by intravascular coagulation and microemboli, and in this case there is underperfusion of adequately ventilated alveoli which increases the physiologic deadspace; in other words, the amount of wasted ventilation increases. These two processes combined: increased venous admixture and increased physiologic deadspace, produce a worsening of the hypoxemia. Eventually pulmonary capillary membranes become so disrupted that there are areas of hemorrhage into lung tissue.

Formation of hyaline membranes lining the alveoli and terminal bronchioles frequently occurs. This layer of noncellular material is thought to be a coagulated protein exudate. It appears to add to the impairment of gaseous exchange in ARDS.

Assessment. Prevention, to the extent that it is possible, consists in early recognition and adequate treatment of shock, and appropriate management of the underlying abnormalities. A prime component of early recognition of ARDS is awareness of the circumstances under which it is likely to occur.

The time of onset of early signs, which may be restlessness, tachypnea, and cough, may be from two to more than 48 hr after the original trauma or damage, whatever it may have been. If the patient is receiving mechanical ventilation an early sign may be an increase in pressure required to deliver an adequate tidal volume, indicating decreasing lung compliance. At this stage chest X-ray and chest physical examination may reveal no abnormalities. Arterial blood gas determinations will show a gradual decline in the PaO_2; and, because of the tachypnea (if the patient is breathing on his own), an elevated pH, and a decrease in $PaCO_2$. These signs are at first generally ameliorated by oxygen administration at low flow rates; 4–6 L/m is probably approximately equivalent to an FIO_2 of about 0.35 to 0.46.

As fluid content in the lung increases, chest auscultation may reveal dispersed fine inspiratory rales. Chest X-ray is likely to be normal even in this stage, but by 12 hr after the onset of dyspnea there are likely to be diffuse, symmetrical bilateral pulmonary infiltrates; the appearance of the lung fields is called ground glass or whiteout; the reason is the relative airlessness of the lungs because of the accumulation of fluid. (Air is radiolucent and appears on the film as black; fluid and cellular debris are relatively radioopaque and appear in the film as white.) A greatly increased minute ventilation develops: 29–25 L/min; the normal value is less than half this. This increased minute ventilation has been referred to as high-output respiratory failure, by analogy with high-output cardiac failure (Chapter 7) and high-output renal failure (Chapter 10). The tachypnea contributes to increasingly severe hypoxemia by moving increased amounts of air over anatomic respiratory deadspace, as discussed previously. Tachycardia, diaphoresis, and decreased levels of consciousness may be observed.

With progression of the infiltrates, rapid deep respirations with obvious effort (dyspnea) develops, as well as cyanosis resulting from arterial O_2 desaturation of hemoglobin. At this stage the PaO_2 no longer is maintained by a low FIO_2 via nasal cannulae or mask, and in fact may even continue to decline in the face of greatly increased FIO_2 and mechanical ventilation. Rales and rhonchi become more prominent and widespread throughout the lung fields; the chest X-ray shows bilateral increasing alveolar infiltrates, less air, and further consolidations, caused by transudation of fluid from pulmonary capillaries into the alveoli.

Perfusion of alveoli which are not ventilated because they are filled with fluid leads to venous admixture—effectively, right to left shunting of unoxygenated blood. Mechanical ventilation becomes essential to sustain life, but is generally incapable of maintaining PaO_2 within tolerable levels unless a very high FIO_2 is used. It is also the case that high pressure is required to deliver an acceptable tidal volume, because of markedly decreased lung compliance. In the normal subject 10 cmH_2O pressure will deliver a 1 L tidal volume; in severe ARDS it may require 65–75 cmH_2O to deliver a tidal volume of 800 ml. Without mechanical ventilation the patient would be able to sustain only a very small and inadequate tidal volume, at the cost of a greatly increased, and exhausting, work of breathing.

Because of the large tidal volume and high respiratory rate required to sustain adequate minute ventilation in ARDS, marked respiratory alkalosis with alkalemia (pH > 7.5) develops because of abnormally low $PaCO_2$: to 20–30 mmHg or less. The hypocapnia may be corrected by adding mechanical deadspace in the form of an extra length of tubing between the ventilator and the patient (mechanical deadspace); this promotes the retention of CO_2 because the patient rebreathes the previous end-expiration high CO_2 air, but it has little effect on the inspired O_2 tension.

It should be reemphasized that the collection of fluid in the interstitial and alveolar spaces has additional significant deleterious action beyond producing venous admixture, increased deadspace ventilation, and reduced compliance. The sequence of changes can be summed up as follows. The alveolar transudates interfere first with the action of, and then with the production of, surfactant. Thus surface tension increases, tending to collapse those alveoli which are not already filled with fluid. This further lowers compliance, causes increased work of breathing, and results in an increase in pressure necessary to deliver an acceptable tidal volume. The collection of interstitial and intraalveolar fluid is not just ECF; there is a leak of plasma proteins and even cellular components of the blood, because of the severe disruption of alveolar capillary membranes. As plasma proteins accumulate in the interstitial and intraalveolar spaces, they raise the colloidal osmotic pressure of extravascular lung fluid and promote more extravasation of fluid from the capillaries.

Management.   Endotracheal intubation or tracheostomy and volume-cycled mechanical ventilation is usually essential. Tidal volume is adjusted to 15–20 ml/kg body weight, at a rate of 25–30 min, so that a minute ventilation over 20 L can be maintained. High concentrations of oxygen are often required to maintain an acceptable PaO_2, in spite of the fact that oxygen toxicity is itself a possible cause of ARDS. The minimum oxygen concentration possible to maintain the PaO_2 above 50 mmHg is used. One of the deleterious actions of high oxygen is that it impairs the action of lung macrophages, cells which are importantly involved with clearing particulate matter, cellular debris, and organisms, out of the lungs; this becomes an important issue in a disorder characterized by massive infiltrates.

The use of a ventilator equipped to maintain a larger functional residual lung volume has been a major advance in the management of ARDS. The use of a positive end-expiratory pressure (PEEP) of 5–10 cmH_2O maintains positive pressure throughout the tracheobronchial tree during the entire respiratory cycle. The resulting increased intrapulmonary pressure opens collapsed alveoli and prevents further atelectasis so that they can be ventilated, thus reducing $\dot{V}/\dot{Q}$ mismatch. It also increases the intraalveolar pressure so that there is less tendency for fluid to leave the capillaries and enter the interstitial and intraalveolar spaces. The response of an ARDS patient to PEEP may be dramatic, including clearing of mental status and improved level of consciousness; disappearance of cyanosis because of increased PaO_2 and hence improved tissue oxygenation; and an elevation of blood pressure, indicating that in most patients PEEP does not produce depression of cardiac output. An important action of PEEP is to steepen the gradient for the diffusion of oxygen from alveoli to pulmonary capillaries. The most significant benefit from PEEP is the maintenance of a satisfactory PaO_2 at a lower FIO_2. PEEP is indicated in the management of ARDS if the FIO_2 necessary to produce adequate arterial oxygenation is over 0.50. The response of the patient to mechanical ventilation, increased FIO_2 and PEEP is monitored by frequent ABG determinations.

The use of adrenal corticosteroids in the management of ARDS has been somewhat controversial. Few well-controlled studies have been reported. Their use appears to promote the production of surfactant; to maintain the integrity of capillary and alveolar membranes; to prevent platelet aggregation; to stabilize lysosomal membranes; to inhibit proteolytic enzymes, and the inflammatory response to them which would further destroy alveolar–capillary membranes; and to reduce leukocyte migration into the lungs which decreases the quantity of destructive leucoproteases released into lung tissue. On the other hand, one of the frequent serious complications of ARDS is the later development of sepsis; steroids predispose to it by depressing the immune response. Some workers suggest that, although prolonged steroid administration does increase the incidence of later infections, short-term, low-dose steroids given during the acute phase may be beneficial in some patients with ARDS. They are reported to be most useful in ARDS resulting from fat emboli, chemical airway damage, and aspiration of gastric contents.

Fluid restriction is a component of the management of ARDS. Because of the leakiness of the lung capillaries, and the excess interstitial and intraalveolar fluid in the lungs, the patients need to be kept on the dry side. This involves keeping crystalloid (saline) infusions to a minimum and substituting colloids such as salt-poor albumin that raise the colloidal osmotic pressure of the blood and help retain fluid in the capillaries, although this effect is reported to be of short duration. If necessary, renal function may need to be temporarily imperiled by withholding administered fluids to a degree which will maintain urinary output at or below 20–30 ml/hr; occasionally small doses of diuretics may be required, particularly if measurement of pulmonary capillary wedge pressure indicates hypervolemia and/or left ventricular failure. Many of the conditions which predispose to ARDS also promote SIADH, as described in Chapter 1, and thus tend to overhydrate the patient and cause hypoosmolarity of body fluids, making the pulmonary fluid content more difficult to control.

Prognosis and Outcome. The complications of ARDS are pneumonia, disseminated intravascular coagulation, lung abscesses, septicemia, pulmonary emboli, and heart failure. A complication of ventilator treatment, with or without PEEP, is tension pneumothorax, in which a break in the lung opens the pleural cavity to air from the pulmonary tree. Pressure from the ventilator may then fill the pleural space and collapse the lung. A portion of lung tissue at the break may exert a valvelike effect so that air can enter but then not leave the pleural space. The pleural space inflates, the lung on that side collapses, and a shift of mediastinal contents toward the other lung compresses it, as well as the heart, arteries, and especially the great veins. The result is a profound reduction in pulmonary oxygenation, impaired venous return, and greatly reduced cardiac output.

The early prognosis in ARDS can be assessed by the relation between the inspired oxygen partial pressures (PIO_2) and the resulting arterial oxygen tensions (PaO_2). Where the inspired-to-arterial pressure differences fail to narrow with time and treatment, and in fact widen, the prognosis is poor. Where an increasing PaO_2 results from gradually lowered PIO_2, the prognosis is improved. Thus a persistence of very low PaO_2 in the face of a high PIO_2 predicts a fatal outcome from consolidation and oxygen toxicity; while the reverse, correlated with radiographic and physiologic improvement, often leads to recovery. These relationships are illustrated in Figure 9-7a,b.

Patients who recover may show little or no functional respiratory impairments; others may go on to heal slowly with a greater or lesser loss of functional lung tissue, varying degrees of emphysema and interstitial fibrosis, and restriction of physical activity imposed by irreversible lung abnormalities.

Pneumococcal Pneumonia

Pneumonia is characterized by the sudden onset of a moderate to severe illness with a shaking chill, elevation in body temperature, increased respiratory rate, tachycardia, productive cough, a pleuritic type of chest pain, and dyspnea. Often the onset of illness has been preceded by several days of an upper respiratory infection. This picture is quite characteristics regardless of the organism causing the pneumonia.

Cause

Streptococcus (Diplococcus) pneumoniae, a gram-positive encapsulated coccus which usually occurs in pairs, is the cause of the great majority of bacterial pneumonias occurring both outside and within the hospital setting. *Staphylococcus* and *Klebsiella* (Friedländer's) pneumonia are reported to be second and third in

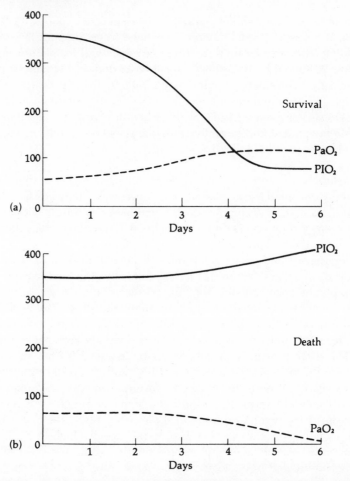

Figure 9-7. Diagram showing approximate relationship between the partial pressure of O_2 in the inspired air (PIO_2) and the arterial O_2 tension (PaO_2).

In (a) the fact that a gradually increasing PaO_2 is maintained during a gradual decline in PIO_2 predicts a favorable outcome for the patient. In other words the inspired-to-arterial O_2 pressure differences are narrowing with time and treatment, indicating improvement, since the patient is able to maintain an acceptable PaO_2 with lowered PIO_2.

In (b) the fact that a high and increasing PIO_2 not only fails to maintain an acceptable PaO_2 but the PaO_2 continues to decline, predicts an unfavorable outcome, death. That is, the inspired-to-arterial pressure differences are widening, indicating worsening alveolar ventilation and pulmonary gaseous exchange.

frequency in ambulatory populations. Bacterial pneumonia is a fairly common cause of death, and may be the commonest death caused by infection.

The upper respiratory tract of all normal persons is populated with large numbers of bacteria of various types, among them the organisms capable of causing pneumonia are present in perhaps half of normal individuals. The respiratory tract has a number of protective mechanisms which defend the lungs against infection, including the cough reflex, continuous expulsion of foreign material by cilia of the mucosal lining, phagocytic action of tissue macrophages, and possibly a bacteriostatic action of the mucus itself. Any abnormality which impairs the effectiveness of these defensive processes will predispose to the development of a bacterial pulmonary infection. Such abnormalities as a depressed cough reflex because of pharmacologic agents, decreased level of consciousness, or altered neural reflexes of the larynx and pharynx; anesthesia; irritation, edema, and inflammation of the tracheobronchial mucosa from toxic fumes or viral infections; heart failure and pulmonary edema; systemic illnesses and injuries; immunosuppression; localized obstruction; seizures; and alcohol intoxication; may lower tracheobronchial resistance and permit infection to develop. In many cases the passage of infected bronchial mucous secretions into more distal portions of the pulmonary tract, occurring in the course of a respiratory infection, appears to be the precipitating factor. It is reported that the presence of a specific infective organism in the oropharynx is an important determinant of the type of bacterial pneumonia which will occur.

In the normal subject, the lower respiratory tract below the level of the larynx is only sparsely populated with bacteria and there are usually none below the bifurcation of the trachea into the mainstem bronchi.

Abnormalities

The processes through which the bacteria produce damage to lung tissue in pneumonia are not known; although it has been suggested that bacteria elaborate toxins which are destructive to cells, these toxins have not been identified.

Lobar pneumonia is the usual form of bacterial pneumonia in adults. In this form there is a localized infection generally confined to a segment, or to a lobe: often the right lower or middle, or the left lower lobe. Bronchopneumonia, on the other hand, tends to be more a disease of the elderly, and is characterized by a patchy distribution which is not confined to anatomic lung divisions. The findings on physical examination may be different in the two types.

Once bacteria gain access to the lower respiratory tract they multiply rapidly in the warm, dark, and moist environment of the lung. Bacterial growth elicits the secretion of an edema fluid high in protein from infected alveoli and capillaries. This fluid acts as an ideal culture medium, and accumulates both in alveoli and interstitial spaces. As the quantity of the fluid and bacterial multiplication increase, the infection is carried to adjoining alveoli. The source of the proteinaceous edema fluid is probably the capillaries themselves, since the proteins are identical with plasma proteins; the bacteria appear to injure and disrupt the integrity of capillary membranes so that their selective permeability is lost.

The next stage in the sequence of pathological changes is the infiltration into the area of leukocytes, which engulf bacteria, and also of erythrocytes and platelets. Later, alveolar macrophages enter the region and, acting as scavengers, remove tissue debris, fibrin, dead cells, and bacteria. The changes in the lung occurring in pneumonia which are termed consolidation refer to the accumulation of edema fluid and cells of various kinds within the infected portions of lung, so that there is complete or almost complete airlessness of the involved lung segment. If the defense mechanisms fail to confine the infection to a localized area, then direct extension of the infection to adjoining lung areas may occur. If the infection reaches the pleura by contiguous extension, the result may be empyema; or if the inflammatory pleural response does not contain the infecting organisms, then a bacteria-free pleural effusion may develop.

Spread of the infection through the lymphatics of the lung may occur, with extension to the hilar lymph nodes, where an infection similar in most respects to the above may evolve. If the infection is not localized at this second stage, then bacteria may enter the major pulmonary lymphatic drainage, enter the thoracic duct, and then the systemic circulation. At this time bacteremia has occurred and blood cultures may be positive. This development carries a much higher mortality rate than the localized infection, and may lead to hematologic spread of the infection to other sites.

Antibody to the polysaccharide of the pneumococcus capsule probably develops locally in the lung, in the area of infection, between the leukocyte infiltration and the macrophage infiltration stages. The antibody greatly increases the phagocytosis of the bacterial invaders, and slows the spread of infection in the lung. As more antibody is synthesized it becomes detectable in the circulation; the appearance of antibody may correlate with a rapid decline in temperature to normal and it serves an important function in recovery from the infection by improving phagocytosis of bacteria and restricting their dispersion, both locally and systemically.

The recovery phase is characterized locally by a liquefaction of the consolidated material and removal of it from the lungs, both by expulsive coughing up of sputum and by drainage away through the lymphatic vessels.

There are a number of more systemic abnormalities which may accompany pneumonia if it is severe and/or inadequately treated. Hypoxemia is a frequent occurrence and may be accompanied by hypocapnia and alkalemia because of the hyperventilation induced by hypoxemia. The cause of the hypoxemia is a continued pulmonary capillary perfusion of non- or underventilated alveoli; this blood fails to be oxygenated and acts as a physiologic right to left shunt (venous admixture). Because of the increased fluid content in the affected region, and decreased air content, pulmonary compliance declines. There is also decreased surfactant production and this leads to atelectasis in the affected regions. These abnormalities combine to cause an increased work of breathing and tachypnea.

Assessment

The initial manifestations are the shaking chill, rapid elevation of temperature up to 40°C or more, general prostration, a persistent cough productive in a short while of pink or rust-colored purulent sputum, pleuritic chest pain which may be severe, tachypnea, and dyspnea. The patient appears prostrated and in acute distress. Although this is a characteristic picture in younger adults, older persons may have an atypical group of signs and symptoms often not readily referable to the respiratory system.

Characteristics of the illness which aid in differentiating viral from bacterial pneumonia are, in viral pneumonia: a history of exposure to persons with similar symptoms; a prodrome of flu-like symptoms (an upper respiratory infection, myalgias, anorexia, headache, malaise); gradual onset; hacking, nonproductive cough; absence of chest pain; negative sputum Gram stain; and a normal-range white blood cell count.

The findings in bacterial pneumonia on physical examination may be, depending on the stage and severity: restricted respiratory excursion of the chest wall and diaphragm on the affected side, dullness to percussion, increased tactile fremitus once consolidation has occurred (after a day or two following onset), bronchial breath sounds because of the increased transmission of sound from the central airways to the body wall caused by the consolidation, and fine high-pitched inspiratory rales over the affected area. There may be cyanosis, tachypnea, tachycardia, elevated temperature, and use of accessory muscles of respiration because of the increased work of breathing.

The chest X-ray may show no abnormalities early in the course but later infiltrates will appear in the affected area. The white cell count will show a leukocytosis over 12,000/mm^3. If the patient is encouraged in expulsive deep coughing by showing him how to splint the affected area of the chest with his arms, and explaining that saliva is of no use, it is often possible to obtain purulent sputum. This material should always be cultured. Properly prepared Gram stained smears of the sputum may reveal numerous polymorphonuclear leukocytes containing intracellular gram positive diplococci in pairs, indicating the likelihood of a *Streptococcus pneumoniae* infection. Blood cultures are reported to be positive early in the infection in perhaps a fifth or more of patients. Arterial blood gas determinations may be indicated.

Management

Penicillin is the agent of first choice in pneumococcal pneumonia unless the patient is sensitive to this drug in which case erythromycin is an appropriate second choice. If the patient is very ill with evidence of marked hypoxemia on ABG determination; if there is dehydration, signs of toxicity, hypotension, cardiac arrhythmias, or central nervous system depression, and if he is elderly or chronically ill with other disorders, hospitalization would be indicated. The temperature often returns to normal within 48 hr following start of treatment. Other aspects of management include chest physiotherapy, steam inhalations and expulsive coughing to clear secretions, supplemental O_2 and intravenous fluids if necessary. Smoking should be vigorously discouraged.

The most common complication of bacterial pneumonia is a delayed resolution, in other words, a protracted period required to remove the exudates from the affected regions of the lung. This period is reported to vary widely from two weeks to over four months, as indicated on the chest X-ray. The process is slower in older individuals, those with underlying systemic disorders, and/or chronic debilitation from alcoholism and heavy smoking.

Administration of the pneumococcal vaccine to debilitated and pneumonia-prone subjects is proving of great prophylactic value.

Pulmonary Embolism

Studies indicate that pulmonary embolism results in cardiovascular morbidity and mortality of a degree and severity exceeded only by coronary artery disease. Pulmonary embolism probably causes close to 200,000 deaths per year, of which approximately three fourths occur in acute care hospitals. The onset is characteristically sudden and without prodromal signs or symptoms. The great majority (over two thirds) are not recognized during life but are discovered only at postmortem examination. Thus recognition and diagnosis are difficult. Clinical manifestations of pulmonary embolism are relatively varied and nonspecific, and there are numerous acute pulmonary and cardiac disorders which may be confused with them: myocardial infarction, congestive heart failure, pulmonary infections, obstructive and infiltrative lung diseases, and many others.

Most pulmonary embolism occurs in persons of middle age or older and the incidence increases with age. Predisposing factors are surgery; acute myocardial infarction; congestive heart failure; chronic pulmonary disease, either obstructive or restrictive; prolonged immobilization in bed; long-distance travel; lower extremity fractures or other injuries; malignancy; oral contraceptive agents; obesity; diabetes, and others. Thrombophlebitis is a well-known risk factor for pulmonary embolism; yet in patients with documented pulmonary embolism, thrombophlebitis may be evident from history and physical examination in perhaps fewer than a quarter of these; even where venous thrombosis is known to exist on the basis of objective measures, physical examination of the lower extremities may be negative in half the patients.

Origin and Development

A clot which forms abnormally within a blood vessel is termed a thrombus, to distinguish it from normal extravascular clotting. Three general types of conditions predispose to this type of large clot formation within vessels. (1) Venous stasis, or slow stagnant flow of blood within veins, predisposes to clotting because small amounts of thrombin and other coagulating factors are being formed continuously in the blood; they are normally diluted and washed away by brisk blood flow in a vein and eventually are removed from the blood by elements of the reticuloendothelial system, mainly in the liver. In very slow flow, local concentration of these factors increases to levels where they may initiate clot formation. (2) Abnormalities in the endothelial lining of blood vessels such as the irregularities produced by atherosclerosis, local infectious processes, or slight trauma, may cause platelet aggregation and initiate the clotting sequence by release of thromboplastic substances, fatty acids, or adenosine disphosphate which results in activation of factor VII, initiating the intrinsic clotting sequence. (3) Changes in various components of the blood coagulation system itself; these are at present ill-defined and there is no good method of clinical testing for defining hypercoagulability states. Theoretically, thrombus formation can result from increased activation of the clotting processes, decreased inhibition of it, or inadequate fibrinolysis of clots.

Once a clot has formed in a vein, most commonly in the pelvis or lower extremity, blood flowing past it clots and increases its size by accretion at its various surfaces; it gradually tends to lengthen in the direction of blood flow and may become unstable at its point of original attachment to the vessel wall, in which case the whole thrombus may break loose and move along the vein toward the heart, becoming a massive embolus. Conversely small fragments may break off producing multiple emboli. In either event the embolus or emboli enter the vena cava and then travel through the right atrium, right ventricle, and into the pulmonary arteries. The clot is often broken into smaller fragments by the muscular contraction of the right ventricle as it pumps the blood. Depending on the numbers and size of the clot, one or more branches of the pulmonary artery become occluded; the embolus flows until its size causes it to become lodged in a vessel which it cannot pass through. Partial occlusion is more likely to occur than complete obstruction.

Consequences

The immediate result is an obstruction to the flow of blood in the affected artery to that portion of the lung which it supplies. This cessation or decrease in flow has a number of consequences, both respiratory and circulatory. Most patients who die from pulmonary embolism do so within the first hour, according to reports, and the majority of the remainder are said to do well with conservative management.

Respiratory. The segment of lung becomes physiologic dead space, that is, groups of alveoli are now ventilated but not perfused and therefore cannot participate in gaseous exchange with capillaries. Since there is no diffusion of CO_2 from capillaries to alveoli and terminal bronchioles in the affected lung tissue, the low alveolar CO_2 tension causes direct bronchiolar constriction, thus reducing ventilation in the physiologic deadspace. This is an adaptive response because by reducing the amount of wasted ventilation it decreases $\dot{V}/\dot{Q}$ mismatch. A subsequent respiratory consequence of the occluded blood supply is a decrease in synthesis of surfactant, the surface tension-lowering substance which maintains alveoli open. The result is elevation of surface tension in the liquid film lining the alveoli, and their collapse: atelectasis.

Circulatory. Because blood no longer flows in the segment of vessels blocked by the embolus, there is a reduction in the pulmonary vasculature available to carry blood and hence an elevation in pulmonary resistance. If the reduction in total cross-sectional diameter is large, then pulmonary hypertension, elevated right ventricular volume and pressure, and acute cor pulmonale may develop. Pulmonary artery pressure in excess of about 40 mmHg generally does not occur, however, because tricuspid valve regurgitation develops at pressures much above this unless hypertrophic cor pulmonale was preexistent. In patients who are debilitated from cardiac or pulmonary disease or by other disorders relatively small pulmonary emboli may cause death.

Probably more than 50% of the cross-sectional area of the pulmonary vascular bed must be obstructed before marked pulmonary hypertension develops in most patients, because of the large vascular reserve and distensibility of the system. Nevertheless lesser degrees of obstruction do, in some patients, produce marked elevations of pulmonary artery pressure. This fact has led some workers to postulate factors in addition to the mechanical obstruction alone to account for these elevations. Such factors could include reflex vasoconstriction from activation of neural impulses by the obstruction itself; or, indirectly, by the release of humoral agents such as histamine, the prostaglandins, bradykinin, or serotonin, by ischemic tissue or aggregates of platelets. There is in some cases evidence of vasoconstriction extending well beyond the boundaries of the actual obstructed area, which produces higher pulmonary artery pressure than the size of the obstruction itself would account for. These indicate the existence of humoral factors.

Infarction of the lung is one of the uncommon complications of a pulmonary embolism, and it has been estimated that actual necrosis of lung tissue as a result of the obstruction occurs in probably less than one fifth of patients. Lung parenchyma is well supplied by oxygen in the airways themselves, and by both bronchial arterial and pulmonary arterial circulations, accounting for the infrequent occurrence of infarction.

Assessment

Subjective. In spite of the fact that dyspnea, pleuritic chest pain, and hemoptysis are commonly considered to be the cardinal indications of pulmonary embolism, nevertheless the sudden onset of shortness of breath for which there is no explanation in the patient's underlying condition is reported to be *the most common*, and in fact may be the *only*, symptom. The mechanism for the symptom of shortness of breath and the sign of tachypnea are probably several. Studies indicate that in patients with massive pulmonary embolism there is a correlation between the degree of arterial hypoxemia and the percentage of occlusion of the vascular bed; however in the range of small to large emboli, studies have failed to correlate PaO_2 with degree of obstruction, and the PaO_2 is usually 55 mmHg or above. The $PaCO_2$ is usually decreased because of the hyperventilation. So hypoxic drive is probably an important factor in some patients. The hypoxemia results from the ventilation of nonperfused or markedly underperfused alveoli, resulting in increased physiologic deadspace. In addition, bronchiolar constriction occurs in response to low alveolar CO_2 tension (resulting from the embolus); therefore there is a decline in overall respiratory surface. Also, some workers postulate the presence of irritant receptors in the bronchiolar or alveolar membranes which may be stimulated by the release of the humoral or chemical agents alluded to above, or by increased pulmonary interstitial fluid content, and which may send afferent impulses to the brainstem respiratory centers causing reflex tachypnea.

Direct bronchospasm with elevated airway resistance may also occur as a consequence of the release of the humoral agents, and contribute to the dyspnea. It should be noted that dyspnea is present even in patients with small emboli and in whom there is minimal or no hypoxemia on ABG determinations. In such patients airway obstruction from reflex or direct bronchospasm, induced either by the released humoral vasoactive mediators or fluid in the airways, or both, may be the cause. Administration of large amounts of heparin rapidly ameliorates the dyspnea and tachypnea, and some investigators report that this amelioration results from the inhibition of platelet aggregation and release of serotonin, by the heparin.

Chest pain and hemotysis usually occur only when infarction of lung tissues occurs, and are therefore uncommon. When chest pain does occur it may be pleuritic (worsened by breathing movements); may mimic angina, taking the form of severe substernal distress; or may originate in the chest wall from spasm of the intercostal muscles, which may be tender to palpation. Complaints of upper abdominal pain also occur from involvement of the diaphragmatic pleura. Pulmonary embolism is reported to be most frequently mistaken for myocardial infarction.

Objective. The physical examination may be normal. There may be rales and/or localized wheezing from bronchoconstriction and intraairway fluid. Tachypnea is often present. Decreased breath sounds from pleural effusion, and a pleural friction rub, occur only as a consequence of infarction and are therefore rare. Rales and rhonchi occasionally are heard. Central nervous system accompaniments to embolism are very often anxiety and a sense of impending doom. Less often loss of consciousness occurs, and other neurologic changes such as hemiplegia and seizures have been reported. These phenomena may be secondary to decline in cardiac output caused by increased peripheral vascular resistance, or to cardiac arrhythmias, and occur more often in large embolization. Tachycardia is the most frequent cardiac finding; other cardiac abnormalities including cardiac arrest probably occur only in patients with massive embolism or prior organic heart disease. The second heart sound may be altered because of greatly increased pulmonary vascular resistance and elevated pulmonary pressure; P_2 (pulmonary valve closing sound) may be louder than A_2 (aortic valve closing sound) and there may be fixed or paradoxical splitting of S_2 caused by elevated right ventricular pressure and failure. Other signs of RV failure are elevated jugular venous pressure and hepatojugular reflux. Fever is usually present only with infarction or infection. Signs of venous thrombosis occur in less than half of patients with pulmonary embolism.

Laboratory. When pulmonary embolism is suspected, an EKG, chest X-ray, and ABG determination should be done promptly. Routine laboratory values may be normal, although erythrocyte sedimentation rate and white blood count may be elevated in the presence of infarction. The electrocardiogram is often normal, except for elevated heart rate, except in massive embolism. Chest X-ray also may be normal, but later parenchymal infiltrates, pleural effusion, and elevated hemidiaphragm may occur, especially if there has been an infarction. Other X-ray changes may be a difference in size of the two main pulmonary arteries, abrupt cutoff or tapering of smaller arteries, and areas of increased lucency, indicating absence or decrease of blood flow. Arterial blood gas abnormalities are most marked when the embolization is very large: low PaO_2 and $PaCO_2$, and elevated pH (respiratory alkalemia from hyperventilation). But arterial hypoxemia is not always present, and some studies have reported a PaO_2 of about 80 mmHg in a significant number of patients, although most are below this value. Microatalectasis causing an overall decrease in respiratory surface is thought to be one factor responsible for arterial hypoxemia when it does occur.

Special Tests. There are other more specific diagnostic tests used to determine the presence and degree of pulmonary embolism: ultrasound, pulmonary angiography, pulmonary perfusion radioisotope scan (perfusion scintigraphy) and pulmonary ventilation radioisotope scan (ventilation scintigraphy). To date, ultrasound has not been widely used, but is suggested to be useful in the diagnosis of pulmonary embolism. A pulmonary angiogram is the definitive method for evaluating the status of the pulmonary vasculature, and demonstrates filling defects (caused by partial occlusion), abrupt vessel cutoffs (caused by complete occlusion) and delayed or incomplete filling and emptying of vessels. Even this procedure yields equivocal results, and this fact combined with the expense, complicated nature of the procedure, and risks for the patient, may tend to moderate enthusiasm for performing it. Yet it does remain the "gold standard" for diagnosing pulmonary embolism.

The perfusion lung scan involves injecting albumin aggregates, labeled with radioactive iodine or technetium, intravenously. The minute albumin particles are trapped in the microvasculature of the pulmonary circulation and cause no damage. A gamma counter then receives the patterns of emission from the lungs, demonstrating the distribution of pulmonary blood flow; an area of absent or decreased radioactivity may suggest embolic obstruction while uniform distribution tends to rule it out. Other lung (and also cardiac) abnormalities also cause perfusion defects (especially COPD) but in the parenchymal disorders which do so, ventilation defects also tend to occur in the same area.

Therefore a ventilation scan may be performed to differentiate perfusion defects caused by other lung abnormalities (which are almost always accompanied by corresponding ventilation defects in the same area) from perfusion defects caused by pulmonary embolism (which are almost always accompanied by an intact ventilation scan of the affected area). The patient inhales a radioactive isotope such as xenon and the patterns of gamma emission are determined and recorded. The combination of these two procedures is called ventilation–perfusion scintigraphy. If a parenchymal disease of the lung is the cause of a perfusion abnormality, then a defect in the ventilation scan will show up in the same area. If a perfusion defect is the result of an abnormality of the blood vessels alone (such as pulmonary embolism) then the ventilation in that area is intact as demonstrated by penetration of the radioactive gas into that same segment of the lung.

It should be noted that since the bronchospasm which occurs in pulmonary embolism can alter the results of the ventilation scan, equal perfusion–ventilation defects even in the presence of pulmonary embolism demonstrated angiographically can sometimes occur. Studies have been performed which correlate the results of pulmonary angiogram and perfusion–ventilation scintigraphy, and show that perfusion abnormalities in the presence of preserved ventilation correlate well with angiographically demonstrated embolism.

Prevention

As is always the case in physiologic abnormalities, prevention should be the first concern. Over three quarters of pulmonary emboli are said to be derived from venous thrombosis of the lower extremities; therefore, all measures which counteract or prevent venous stasis in the area should be employed prophylactically, including elastic support stockings, elevation of the legs, avoiding propping the knees up with pillows, and particularly getting the patients up out of bed for ambulation as early and as often as possible.

The recognition of patients who are at especially high risk for the development of venous thrombosis, and therefore of pulmonary embolism, is important: patients with congestive heart failure and with myocardial infarction; patients of middle age and older whose treatment for other disorders, especially fractures of the lower extremities, necessitates periods of immobilization; and patients undergoing major surgery: pelvic, abdominal, or thoracic.

Reports of studies indicate that prophylactic treatment of high-risk patients with anticoagulants significantly lowers the occurrence of venous thrombosis and pulmonary embolism. Since full anticoagulation carries a high risk of complicating hemorrhage, especially in patients susceptible to the development of serious bleeding (peptic ulcer, esophageal varices, intracranial or visceral trauma and established severe hypertension) trials of low-dose heparin given subcutaneously, which may provide inhibition to clot-initiation without significantly altering clotting time or prothrombin time, appear useful. The heparin is given every 8 hours preoperatively and continued until the patient is ambulatory. Decline in the development of venous thrombosis appears to be the result of this regimen. Other forms of prophylactic anticoagulation which are being evaluated include aspirin, dipyridamole, sulfinpyrazone, and other antiplatelet agents.

Another component of prevention of pulmonary embolism is an improved, reliable noninvasive method for the early detection of venous thrombosis. Physical examination is not accurate, as mentioned previously, and the definitive method for detection, venography, is expensive, invasive, and carries significant risks. Newer noninvasive methods for detecting deep vein thrombosis include the Doppler ultrasonic flowmeter, which measures flow velocity within a given vessel; the plethysmograph, which measures flow volume; and radioisotope studies, which involve injecting radioisotope-labeled fibrinogen intravenously and then scanning the legs frequently for regions having a high concentration of emission, indicating the incorporation of the fibrinogen into developing thrombi. The latter method is sensitive to developing thrombi in the calf and lower thigh but not reliable in the case of upper thigh, groin, or pelvis. In the Doppler examination, increase in arterial blood flow produces a typical increase in flow in patent veins; absence of this surge indicates venous outflow obstruction, as from a thrombus. In plethysmography, arterial augmentation of blood flow is followed by reduced venous outflow in the case of thrombotic obstruction, resulting in increased volume of the part. The use of these two methods in combination may reduce the necessity for venograms.

Management

Prompt hospitalization, EKG, chest X-ray, ABG determination, and supplemental O_2 support, may be indicated in suspected pulmonary embolism; however, diagnostic studies may be performed on an outpatient basis if facilities are available and if the patient's condition warrants.

Most pulmonary emboli resolve spontaneously, and do so within a short period of time; dissolution begins within the first few hours following the obstruction and resolution is probably established by two weeks, gradually restoring blood flow through the affected vessels and resupplying the involved segment of lung. There is a fibrinolytic system in the blood which operates effectively to dissolve fibrin thrombi and emboli and to prevent further clot initiation. The active agent in this system is the enzyme plasmin, also called fibrinolysin, which breaks down fibrin and fibrinogen with the production of fibrinogen degradation products. These substances feed back to inhibit thrombin, which is the substance which initiates clotting by converting fibrinogen to fibrin in the first step of the clotting sequence. Thus not only are already formed clots lysed, but the compounds released by the lysis act to inhibit clot initiation and thus the formation of new thrombi. Clots which are not dissolved eventually undergo transformation to relatively inconspicuous fibrous scar tissue within the affected vessel.

Studies have been reported on the results of administering enzymes such as streptokinase or urokinase to patients with pulmonary embolism. These fibrinolytic agents enhance clot dissolution by converting plasminogen to plasmin which, as mentioned above, hydrolyzes fibrin. The expectations were that these agents would facilitate embolism dissolution in vivo and that this earlier resolution would have a favorable influence on subsequent morbidity and mortality. Accelerated resolution of the clots, improved cardiovascular status, and relief of clinical signs and symptoms such as dyspnea, have been reported; but arterial oxygen saturation was no different in treated patients as compared with a control population. There are a number of contraindications to their use, including early postoperative status, trauma, and cerebrovascular hemorrhage. While their use does appear to accelerate resolution as compared with heparin alone, eventual patient outcomes appear not to be significantly influenced by their use.

The standard treatment of pulmonary embolism, as for deep vein thrombosis, in addition to general supportive treatment, is heparin, preferably intravenously, since subcutaneous administration is reported not to yield reliable anticoagulation. Heparin prevents platelet aggregation, inhibits the coagulation sequence, and facilitates fibrinolysis of new thrombi. It also inhibits the release of the humoral substances which stimulate bronchospasm and vasoconstriction. It is usually continued until the patient has been ambulatory for several days. Oral anticoagulants are advocated by most authors for several weeks.

A number of more heroic methods of management have been advocated for patients who have large emboli which do not resolve well, for those who do not respond satisfactorily to more conventional treatment, or who appear to be having repeated emboli. Embolectomy, occlusion of the inferior vena cava, and insertion of a straining device ("umbrella") within the inferior vena cava to trap emboli on their way to the heart, are advocated and employed by some workers in certain cases.

REFERENCES

Agle DP and Baum GL: Psychological aspects of chronic obstructive pulmonary disease. *Med. Clin. N. Amer.* 61:749–758, 1977.

Beeson PB and McDermott W, editors: *Textbook of Medicine.* 14th ed. Philadelphia, Pa.: Saunders, 1975.

Berger AG, et al: Regulation of respiration. *N. Engl. J. Med.* 297:92–97, 138–143, 194–201, 1977.

Blaisdell FW and Lewis FR Jr: *Respiratory Distress Syndrome of Shock and Trauma. Post-traumatic Respiratory Failure.* Philadelphia, Pa.: Saunders, 1977.

Broughton JO: *Understanding Blood Gases. Reprint 456.* Ohio Medical Products medical article reprint library, August 1971.

Burrows B, et al: *Respiratory Insufficiency.* Chicago, Ill.: Year Book Medical Publishers, 1975.

Burton GG, et al, editors: *Respiratory Care. A Guide to Clinical Practice.* Philadelphia, Pa.: Lippincott, 1977.

Frohlich ED, editor: *Pathophysiology.* Philadelphia, Pa.: Lippincott, 1976.

Ganong WF: *Review of Medical Physiology.* 8th ed. Los Altos, Calif.: Lange Medical Publications, 1977.

Guenter CA and Welch MH, editors: *Pulmonary Medicine.* Philadelphia, Pa.: Lippincott, 1977.

Guyton AC. *Textbook of Medical Physiology.* 5th ed. Philadelphia, Pa.: Saunders, 1976.

Lieberman JS: Newer diagnostic methods in peripheral vascular disease. *Cardiovasc. Med.* 2:729–742, 1977.

MacDonnell KF: Adult respiratory distress syndrome. In: MacDonnell KF and Segal MS, editors: *Current Respiratory Care.* Boston, Mass.: Little, Brown, 1977.

Petty TL: *Intensive and Rehabilitative Respiratory Care.* 2nd ed. Philadelphia, Pa.: Lea and Febiger, 1974.

Rogers RM, editor: *Respiratory Intensive Care.* Springfield, Ill.: CC Thomas, 1977.

Rotman HH et al: Long-term physiologic consequences of the adult respiratory distress syndrome. *Chest* 72:190–192, 1977.

Segal MS and MacDonnell KF: Bronchial asthma: Nature and management. In: MacDonnell KF and Segal MS, editors: *Current Respiratory Care.* Boston, Mass.: Little, Brown, 1977.

Thorn GW, et al., editors: *Harrison's Principles of Internal Medicine.* 8th ed. New York: McGraw-Hill, 1977.

Takino M. *Pathogenesis and Therapy of Bronchial Asthma.* Baltimore, Md.: University Park Press, 1976; Tokyo: Igaku Shoin, 1976.

Tomashefski JF et al: Chronic obstructive pulmonary disease. *Postgrad. Med.* 62:87–136, 1977.

Vismara LA, et al: Pulmonary embolism update: Recent advances in detection and medical therapy. In: Mason DT, editor: *Advances in Heart Disease.* New York: Grune & Stratton, 1977.

West JB: *Pulmonary Pathophysiology—The Essentials.* Baltimore, Md.: Williams and Wilkins, 1977.

Wilson JE III and Ritter WS: Pulmonary embolism. In: Willerson JT and Sanders CA: *Clinical Cardiology.* New York: Grune & Stratton, 1977.

Renal Disorders

The primary functions of the kidney are the elimination from the blood of metabolic waste materials and the regulation of fluid and electrolyte balance. The nephron is the structural and functional unit of the kidney; there are approximately one million such units in each kidney. Each nephron is comprised of a glomerulus and a tubule. The glomerulus is the site of glomerular filtration; and the tubule, into which the glomerular filtrate flows, is the site of resorption from and secretion into the filtrate of various substances. Figure 10-1 shows a diagram of a cross section of the kidney indicating the relative positions of the two types of nephrons, cortical and juxtamedullary. Diagrams of representative nephrons and their blood supply, and the localization of several tubular functions, respectively, are shown in Figures 1-4 and 1-6. Kidney function is discussed in more detail in Chapter 1.

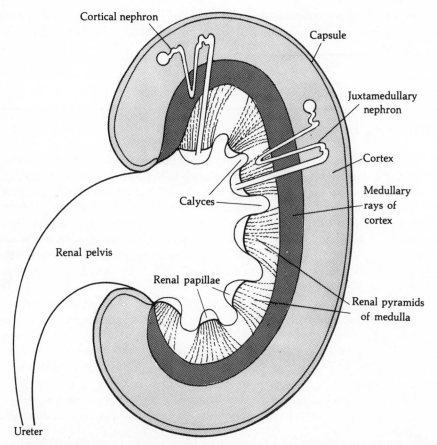

Figure 10-1. Cross-section of the kidney. The outer cortex contains the glomeruli, Bowman's capsules, and proximal and distal convoluted tubules. The inner cortex (medullary rays) contain loops of Henle and collecting ducts. The collecting ducts empty into the apices of the pyramids in the medulla; tubular filtrate, now actually urine, then flows into the papillary ducts, the calyces, and finally into the renal pelvis.

The two types of nephrons, cortical and juxtamedullary, are indicated in their relative positions within the kidney.

There are two types of nephrons in the kidney: cortical and juxtamedullary (Figure 10-1). Cortical nephrons have their glomeruli toward the outer portion of the kidney cortex and have short loops of Henle that do not penetrate very far into the medulla. Juxtamedullary nephrons have their glomeruli deeper within the cortex and have long Henle's loops which descend well into the medullary pyramids. The juxtamedullary nephrons resorb large amounts of water from the tubular filtrate, returning it to the ECF, and therefore are able to produce a concentrated urine. In the human there are more cortical than juxtamedullary nephrons.

The glomeruli filter over 150 L/24 hr of plasma; the tubules resorb most of the components of this filtrate, the greatest bulk of which is water and sodium, the latter as chloride and bicarbonate. The consequence of renal glomerular filtration and renal tubular resorption is the excretion of soluble end products of cellular metabolism, and regulation of the volume, ionic and molecular composition, and osmotic concentration of the extracellular fluid. Composition of the ECF is determined by not only what is taken into the body, but perhaps more importantly by what is selectively removed from it, or selectively resorbed and therefore retained.

NORMAL KIDNEY FUNCTION

The Glomerulus

The glomerulus consists of a group of several capillary loops with surrounding epithelial cells and a supporting material called mesangium. The capillaries are comprised of an inner layer of endothelial cells, an intermediate basement membrane composed of a glycoprotein, and an outer layer of epithelial cells which line the inner surface of Bowman's capsule. The latter receives the glomerular fluid which filters into it from the blood flowing into the glomerulus from the afferent arteriole. The filtrate entering Bowman's space from the glomerular capillaries then flows directly into the proximal tubule, which is continuous with Bowman's space. From about 1300 ml of whole blood flowing through the glomerular capillaries per minute, about 650 ml of which is plasma, roughly 120 ml of fluid—the glomerular filtrate—passes across the glomerular membranes and enters Bowman's space.

The rate of formation of this filtrate is called the glomerular filtration rate (GFR). The hydrostatic pressure necessary to push the filtrate from the glomerular capillaries into the space surrounding them is about 44 mmHg—about one half of the mean systemic arterial pressure—and is a direct consequence and extension of that pressure. Unfiltered plasma leaves the glomerulus through the efferent arteriole.

GFR will decline as a result of any factor that lowers hydrostatic pressure in the glomerular capillaries: systemic hypovolemia and hypotension, renal artery stenosis, or afferent arteriolar vasoconstriction. In addition, the colloidal osmotic pressure of the blood influences GFR; when it is low, as from hypoproteinemia, the effect of the low oncotic pressure is additive to the hydrostatic pressure, and GFR will increase. However, GFR tends to remain quite stable over a fairly wide range of systemic arterial pressures. There are several processes contributing to this stability; an important one of these is autoregulation by the afferent arterioles: their smooth muscle responds by direct changes in vascular resistance (constriction or dilation) in response to changes of perfusion pressure to them. With an elevation of pressure afferent arteriolar constriction occurs; in response to a decline in perfusion pressure there is arteriolar vasodilation. This response operates to maintain the stability of GFR in the face of fluctuations of blood pressure of 20 to 30 mmHg by directly regulating intracapillary hydrostatic pressure at the local level. Glomerular filtration declines to close to zero at around 60 mmHg systolic arterial pressure, and hence urine formation ceases.

The Proximal Tubule

The proximal tubule extends from Bowman's space to Henle's loop, and here the volume of glomerular filtrate is reduced to about 20% of the original amount filtered—that is, from roughly 165 L/d to about 35 L/d. The resorption occurring in the proximal tubule is isosmotic: H_2O and Na^+ are resorbed by active transport in quantities which maintain the Na^+ to H_2O ratio the same as that filtered, and therefore the same as that in the blood. Conversely, both Cl^- and H^+ concentrations increase in tubular fluid and HCO_3^- concentration decreases: HCO_3^- is resorbed into the blood, and H^+ is secreted from the blood into the filtrate. Most of the elimination of H^+ from the blood into the urine occurs here in the proximal tubule. Although Cl^- increases in concentration in the proximal tubule, much is still resorbed into the blood from the filtrate, along with HCO_3^- and Na^+. Water is returned from the filtrate into the blood along the osmotic gradient produced by Na^+ and Cl^- resorption.

The Loop of Henle

The loop of Henle is the area of the nephron between he end of the proximal tubule, as it turns downward to extend into the medulla of the kidney, and the point at which it reenters the cortex. Henle's loop has two structurally and physiologically distinct portions: the thin, descending segment is the first portion (from the proximal tubule to past the hairpin turn); the thick ascending segment continues from above the turn to the macula densa of the juxtaglomerular apparatus (Chapters 1 and 3). Since the renal medullary area is hypertonic with respect to the ECF, the loops of Henle of the juxtamedullary nephrons are exposed to a hypertonic interstitium. The hypertonicity is caused by high concentrations of sodium salts and urea. From the descending portion of Henle's loop, water moves along the osmotic gradient from filtrate into the high osmotic pressure interstitium and capillaries; thus the filtrate becomes highly concentrated. In the ascending limb the filtrate becomes more dilute because in this portion of the tubule Cl^- is actively pumped out of the filtrate back into the capillary blood, and Na^+ travels with it along the electrochemical gradient. The result of the loss of these ions is a decline in osmotic pressure of tubular fluid to the point where it may be somewhat hypotonic to body fluids as it enters the distal convoluted tubule.

The Distal Tubule

In the distal tubule section of the nephron Na^+ is resorbed from tubular filtrate in exchange for K^+ and H^+ secreted into it and hence out into the urine. It is sometimes referred to as the distal renal tubule cation-exchange site (DRT-CES) discussed in more detail in Chapter 1.

The Collecting Ducts

If the individual is well-hydrated, tubular fluid in the collecting ducts is hypotonic to body fluids and there may be little further resorption of water back into the blood. In the dehydrated subject, however, ADH from the hypothalamus renders the ducts more permeable to water. Water then is resorbed by osmosis from the ducts and conserved in the ECF as the fluid flows through the hypertonic interstitium of the papillary portion of the medulla (Chapter 1).

Urea Excretion

Urea that has filtered at the glomerulus gradually increases in concentration along the course of the renal tubule. Apparently active transport of urea out of tubular fluid does not occur in the human. The reason for the progressive increase in urea concentration is that much of the water and electrolytes that filtered with it at the glomerulus is progressively resorbed back into the ECF. As the tubular concentration of urea increases, so does its diffusion gradient, so that increasingly along the tubule it tends to move by passive diffusion from the filtrate back into the ECF.

The higher the glomerular filtration rate, and therefore the greater the rate of urine formation, the less urea is resorbed from tubular filtrate into the ECF. In normal to high rates of urine formation, over 50% of the urea filtered is removed in the urine; as GFR falls, 80–90% may be retained in the ECF. Therefore in kidney disorders in which there is depressed GFR there is a tendency for retention and an increased BUN.

However, in both normal subjects and those with a depressed GFR, the tendency for back-diffusion and therefore retention of urea to occur is countered by the fact that the concentration of urea in the renal interstitium of the medullary pyramids is very high, much higher than that of urea in the filtrate. Therefore at the part of the nephron which passes through the pyramids the diffusion gradient for urea is reversed and urea now diffuses from the interstitium back into the tubular filtrate and out in the urine.

GLOMERULAR DISEASE

In glomerular disease the glomeruli are injured and as a consequence their functions are impaired; with chronic destruction of glomeruli, subsequent abnormalities develop in the tubules, blood vessels, and interstitial tissue. Chronic renal failure of a degree severe enough to necessitate maintenance hemodialysis and eventual kidney transplantation is most commonly the result of chronic glomerulonephritis (GN); immune processes are involved in several types of glomerulonephritis. Some authors consider that the term GN should be applied only to those kidney disorders resulting from inflammatory and proliferative changes produced by immune processes, and that the other nonimmune kidney disorders, presently called forms of GN, should receive new names. According to present terminology, in some cases of GN patients may have an antibody in their blood which is directed against an antigen in their own glomerular basement membranes. This disorder is termed antiglomerular membrane GN. More commonly, antigen–antibody complexes (immune complexes) develop in the blood as a result of formation of antibodies to some exogenous factor, such as a virus or bacterium; or to some component of the patient's own tissue, such as the contents of cell nuclei as in lupus erythematosus. Antigen–antibody complexes then circulate to the kidney where they become trapped and deposit out in the glomeruli. Probably these complexes themselves are not directly responsible for glomerular damage, but rather initiate an inflammatory process involving activation of the complement system. Release of the mediators of inflammation, coagulation factors, in-migration of blood cells with release of proteolytic enzymes, fibrin deposition, and kinin formation occurs. The consequence is a destructive inflammatory process culminating in fibrosis and obliteration of glomeruli and Bowman's spaces. The sequences of events occurring with the formation of antigen–antibody complexes and activation of the complement cascade are discussed more fully in Chapter 22.

There are several basic glomerular changes occurring to varying degrees depending on the type of GN: (1) proliferation of all cell types of the glomerular capillaries: endothelial, mesangial, and epithelial; (2) infiltration by leukocytes and monocytes; (3) thickening of the basement membrane itself with additional deposition of amorphous material, possibly immune complexes; and (4) the deposition of a noncellular homogeneous material in the glomerulus—a process termed hyalinization or sclerosis.

The cause of much of glomerular disease is not known; since this is the case it is difficult to classify GN on the basis of etiology. Therefore, histologic characteristics may be used to categorize them.

Types of Glomerulonephritis

Antiglomerular Basement Membrane Disease

Goodpasture's syndrome, affecting mainly young men, is an example of antiglomerular basement membrane disease, in which renal insufficiency develops rapidly from necrotizing glomerulitis and is accompanied by pulmonary infiltrates and bleeding from the lungs. Since alveolar and glomerular basement membranes cross-react immunologically, the suggestion has been made that some antigen in these membranes has been altered by a chemical or infectious agent (virus, bacterium) in such a way that it becomes capable of stimulating autoantibody formation, which then fixes to the membranes and elicits humoral and cell-mediated immune responses. Progressive renal failure is the consequence.

Immune Complex Glomerular Disease

The type of glomerulonephritis known as immune complex glomerular disease is the most common of the forms caused by immune processes. In this case the antigen is derived from either (1) an exogenous source such as a streptococcus; or (2) as a result of some injury to the subject's own tissue which has either modified the native antigens so that they initiate an immune response, or has exposed antigens previously sequestered from recognition and attack by the immune system. A common example of an exogenously caused GN is acute poststreptococcal GN, which often affects children but may occur in persons of any age. The organisms responsible are certain types of Group A beta-hemolytic streptococci; the usual primary sites of infection are pharynx, tonsils, or skin. The organisms do not colonize the kidney.

The latent period between the primary infection and symptoms of GN may be longer than two weeks, indicating the time during which antistreptococcal antibodies are developing. Immunoglobulin and antigen complexes and complement components are deposited in the glomeruli, and serum complement titers are low, indicating consumption of complement in the deposition of antigen–antibody–complement complexes in the kidney. Glomerular lesions consist of inflammation, cellular proliferation, leukocyte infiltration and release of lysosomal enzymes, exudation, fibrin deposits, and thrombus formation.

The patient's symptoms may be bilateral flank pain, anorexia, and easy fatigability. Occasionally there are no symptoms. Males are affected more often than females. Signs may be edema, microscopic or gross hematuria, oliguria, often hypertension, and ECF volume overload, which in the older patient may predispose to signs and symptoms of left ventricular failure. The kidneys may be tender to palpation and palpable. Fluid retention results from a marked decline in GFR caused by obstruction of glomerular lumens by inflammation, edema, and cellular proliferation. The urinalysis will reveal red and white cells, casts, and protein. Elevated erythrocyte sedimentation rate and white blood cell count may be present. In severe cases the BUN and creatinine may be elevated. While the prognosis is good in children, many adults develop rapidly progressive GN or chronic GN with progressive renal failure. The management in the acute phase is bed rest, antihypertensive medication where indicated, and restriction of fluid intake. Resolution occurs with diuresis, lowering of blood pressure, and clearing of blood cells and protein from the urine, although proteinuria and hypoproteinemia may persist for many weeks and disappearance of all abnormalities may take longer than a year.

Proliferative GN, membranous GN, and rapidly progressive GN are three other disorders which are sometimes classified under the category of immune complex glomerulopathy. Often no evidence of a history of infection or toxin can be discovered, and there is usually no sign of a related systemic disease. Complement levels may be normal or decreased. *Proliferative GN* may lead to nephrotic syndrome, hypertension, and/or chronic renal failure. Conversely there may be no symptoms, and the only signs may be the finding of hematuria and proteinuria on routine urinalysis. There appears to be no effective treatment; a fairly long but progressive course is usual, but there is a wide range of variation. *Membranous GN* is typically manifested by the nephrotic syndrome; in adults it is the most common cause of this syndrome. Microscopically the glomerular capillary walls are thickened, there is no inflammatory process, and immunoglobulin and complement deposits occur in the basement membranes of the glomeruli. The onset is gradual and the progression of the disease is variable, sometimes with spontaneous remissions and a fairly high five-year survival. Hypertension and hematuria may or may not occur.

Rapidly progressive GN is a more severe disorder, with no satisfactory treatment, leading to renal failure, and characterized by hematuria, oliguria, and, histologically, by patchy distribution of glomerular thrombosis, necrosis, and cellular proliferation, and in some patients deposition of immune complexes or antiglomerular basement membrane substance. There is a proliferation of the epithelial cells which line the Bowman's spaces and deposition of fibrin, resulting in their occlusion and damage to the glomerular capillaries. The onset of this disorder tends to be more gradual than in other forms of GN, it occurs in males and females equally, and is most common in young adults. Early there may be hematuria, proteinuria, edema, and normal levels or mild elevation of BUN and creatinine. The development of oliguria and anuric renal failure is gradual but steady over several weeks or months, with severe proteinuria, edema, and increasing BUN. Treatment with immunosuppressive and anticoagulant agents is said occasionally to be associated with arrest or delay of the progression in a few patients.

The immune complex GN accompanying systemic and metabolic diseases such as systemic lupus erythematosus and diabetes mellitus are discussed briefly in Chapters 13 and 21.

Chronic Sclerosing Glomerulonephritis

Chronic sclerosing glomerulonephritis may represent the progressive, protracted consequence of glomerulonephritis originating from other causes, but usually seems to be unrelated to prior kidney disease. It is unusual following poststreptococcal GN, but may be a sequel in those who survive rapidly progressive GN and some other types of GN. Many patients with chronic sclerosing GN, however, have a history negative for a prior GN of any known variety. Chronic GN has a gradual, insidious onset and progresses slowly over many years to uremia and renal failure. It is accompanied by hematuria, proteinuria, and frequent sometimes severe hypertension and edema. It is considered by some authors to be caused by abnormal immune system response to unknown antigens. Most glomeruli are involved in a process of gradual destruction of the capillary tufts, cellular proliferation in the mesangium, and obliteration of Bowman's space. The tubules are also affected by dilation or atrophy and thickening of the basement membranes. Later, the intrarenal blood vessels undergo arteriolar sclerosis and fibrosis. There is also renal interstitial fibrosis. It is said to be the most common cause of chronic renal failure (see following). Hypertension contributes to the renal arteriolar sclerosis, intimal thickening, and worsening uremia.

Assessment

Patients with GN may manifest a wide range of signs and symptoms, from being entirely asymptomatic, with only laboratory findings of microscopic hematuria and proteinuria, through gross hematuria, edema, hypertension, and nephrotic syndrome, to the symptoms and signs of established chronic renal failure with uremia, ECF volume overload, and severe hypertension. Different histologic kidney lesions characterizing the several categories of GN may produce a similar set of signs and symptoms, indicating that a wide range of microscopic alterations lead to a similar constellation of physiologic abnormalities in renal function. In addition the causes, onset, course, and eventual outcomes may be quite different in the several categories, and a given set of even quite severe clinical manifestations may on the one hand lead to a favorable course, or on the other to a rapidly fatal progression. However, several manifestations are characteristic for GN regardless of underlying cause.

Changes in the urine in GN include hematuria, red blood cell casts, and proteinuria. When proteinuria becomes profuse edema and the other changes of the nephrotic syndrome develop. The term nephrotic syndrome does not itself imply a category of disease, but rather a group of abnormalities resulting from the loss of large amounts of protein in the urine because of alterations in the glomerular capillary filters which cause them to lose their selective permeability and permit the passage of plasma proteins into the tubular filtrate. Chronic renal failure is the expression of advanced glomerular disease and results in expanded ECF volume, hypertension, and the abnormalities characteristic of uremia (see following). Adrenal steroids and immunosuppressive agents are often used in the treatment of GN with varying degrees of success depending on the underlying process.

The Nephrotic Syndrome

The nephrotic syndrome is a complex of signs comprised of copious proteinuria, a decline in the plasma protein content, generalized edema, and elevated serum lipids. The loss of plasma proteins in the urine is the primary process; the other abnormalities develop as a consequence of this loss. Nephrotic syndrome may be defined on the basis of the amount of plasma protein lost from the blood into the urine; a stable proteinuria above about 3.5 gm/24 hr probably qualifies for that designation, although losses may be much greater, 10–15 gm/24 hr. The proteins lost in glomerular disease are the large plasma proteins, primarily albumin but also smaller globulins, which in the normal kidney are unable to penetrate the glomerular filter because of their size. But the abnormal alteration in the glomerular membranes appears to involve factors in addition to size restriction; evidence indicates that changed membrane electrical characteristics, of a still somewhat ill-defined nature, participate in the loss of selective permeability to protein in glomerular disease. Some studies suggest that a second reason for hyperproteinuria in nephrotic syndrome is increased protein breakdown. As a compensatory response to the decline in plasma proteins, the liver increases the synthesis of plasma proteins, so that the eventual plasma protein level is a balance between hepatic synthesis and urinary elimination.

Generalized edema (anasarca) develops when the serum albumin concentration declines to about 2.5 gm/100 ml of plasma or below. As has been discussed in detail in Chapter 1, the distribution of ECF between the intravascular and the interstitial fluid compartments depends on the relation between the hydrostatic and the colloid osmotic pressures on the two sides of the capillary membranes. Albumin is the smallest molecule of the plasma proteins, and therefore its contribution to plasma colloid osmotic pressure is the greatest. When its concentration in the intravascular fluid decreases, plasma colloid osmotic pressure falls, and the osmotic force tending to keep fluid within the capillary and out of the interstitium declines. Therefore, interstitial fluid volume increases because the intravascular hydrostatic pressure is increased *relative* to the intravascular colloid osmotic pressure. The result is an increased amount of fluid leaving capillaries and entering the interstitial compartment.

The loss of fluid from the intravascular into the interstitial compartment results in hypovolemia, hypotension, and a decreased effective perfusion pressure to the kidney. Then this decrease in renal blood flow activates the renin–angiotensin–aldosterone system, leading to increased distal tubular resorption of sodium and water, and an expanded ECF volume (secondary aldosteronism, Chapters 1 and 13). It is a vicious cycle, because as the ECF volume increases, the concentration of plasma proteins is relatively diminished because of hemodilution. This promotes fluid loss from capillaries into the interstitial spaces. The capillary hydrostatic pressure increases as the ECF expands, and more fluid is forced out of the capillaries, worsening the edema.

Hyperlipidemia occurs in nephrotic syndrome; there is elevation of triglycerides, cholesterol, and low- and high-density lipoproteins. The elevated blood lipids may occur as a consequence of accelerated protein synthesis by the liver, or because there is inadequate serum albumin, which is necessary for interconversion of the various plasma lipids. Whatever the processes involved, the result for patients with chronic nephrotic syndrome is accelerated atherosclerosis and both central and peripheral atherosclerotic cardiovascular disease.

The management of nephrotic syndrome is a high-protein diet (provided renal function permits), a low salt intake, and the administration of diuretics. Since the edema fluid is difficult to mobilize because of low plasma colloidal osmotic pressure, such patients are prone to hypovolemia and hypotension as a response to diuretics. This in turn decreases renal perfusion, reduces GFR, and may lead to prerenal azotemia or acute renal failure and uremia.

CHRONIC RENAL FAILURE

The kidney carries out a number of functions necessary for life: maintenance of volume, composition, and concentration of the ECF; acid–base homeostasis; elimination of metabolic wastes and toxins; regulation (with other mechanisms) of arterial blood pressure; and secretion of hormones essential to erythrocyte formation and calcium metabolism. As progressive destruction of renal parenchyma occurs in the course of chronic renal failure, regardless of the underlying cause or pathologic process, it is evident that these essential functions will be impaired.

All renal failure is associated with a decreased GFR. It may result from inadequate renal vascular perfusion (prerenal failure), from obstruction to the free flow of urine through the urinary tract to outside the body (postrenal failure); or, more often, from some intrinsic disease of the kidney (intrarenal failure).

In chronic renal failure the excretory functions of the kidney deteriorate over an extended period of time as a consequence of any one of a number of processes which progressively destroy nephrons. The basic cause of the damage may be glomerulonephritis, pyelonephritis, polycystic disease, or renal damage secondary to such systemic disorders as hypertension or diabetes mellitus.

The decline in the number of normal nephrons means that fewer nephrons are available to filter the blood; the result is an increase in GFR per nephron and an increase in solute load per nephron. The increased solute load per nephron induces an osmotic diuresis. The tubules hypertrophy as a result of the increased functional demands. Since each remaining functional nephron must filter a larger total volume (urea, creatinine, electrolytes, glucose, etc.), the solute osmotically obligates large volumes of water, and the kidney loses its capacity to excrete an osmotically concentrated urine (it loses its concentrating ability) and the ability to selectively resorb ions from tubular filtrate (it loses its diluting ability). So the early consequence of destruction of functional nephrons is polyuria of a urine approximately isosmotic to plasma.

In the normal subject less than 1.0% of the water that is filtered is excreted, and about 0.5% of the Na^+ that is filtered is excreted. In chronic renal failure, although the *overall* GFR is reduced, a larger than normal *fraction* of that which is filtered, is excreted. The normal GFR is about 100 ml/min. In early chronic renal failure it may decline to about 25 ml/min, and as failure becomes more advanced GFR may fall to 5 ml/min or below. In severe chronic renal failure, if the GFR is 1 ml/min the patient may excrete over half the filtered Na^+ and H_2O: as much as 1 L/24 hr of urine containing 100 meq/24 hr of Na^+. Thus, early in chronic renal failure there is a combination of (1) decline in overall glomerular filtration rate, and (2) a corresponding decline in the ability of the tubule selectively to resorb Na^+ and water. This is expressed as an increase in *fractional excretion ratios:* less overall is filtered, but more of what is filtered is eliminated. At this stage of osmotic diuresis the water loss necessitates a greatly increased water intake in order to eliminate the urinary solutes. Thus polyuria and polydipsia are among the first signs of developing renal failure, and nocturia may be an early complaint. The polyuria puts the patient at risk of dehydration and hypovolemia if fluid and solute intake is restricted in this early stage; salt restriction at this time may lead to hyponatremia because the patient is unable to eliminate free water while conserving Na^+ (i.e., the kidney has lost its diluting ability).

Renal failure is always characterized by azotemia, which is defined as the accumulation of nitrogenous waste products (mainly urea and creatinine). Azotemia develops when approximately 50% of renal function has been lost. Uremia refers to the group of abnormalities resulting from the accumulation of metabolic endproducts in the blood in renal failure. Blood urea nitrogen (BUN) level is determined primarily by the GFR (see above); as the number of functioning nephrons declines overall GFR falls and BUN increases. Early in renal insufficiency, when the GFR is still close to normal, the patient may have a BUN of 10 mg/100 ml. After several years of progressive nephron destruction the GFR may be 10 ml/min and the BUN may have risen to 100 mg/100 ml. But the rate of urea excretion is still equal to the rate of urea production. The fact that the elevated BUN has greatly increased the diffusion gradient for urea enables the urea excretion rate to equal the urea production rate.

Nitrogenous waste products such as urea and creatinine are relatively nontoxic, but other metabolic end-products which are not usually measured and may accumulate in the ECF are more so. It is generally not until the GFR has declined below 20 ml/min, the BUN has risen into the hundreds, and the creatinine is above 10 mg/100 ml, that signs and symptoms of uremia develop. It is in this later stage that normal dietary intake of water, salt, and protein produces more burden on the kidneys than they can remove. The patient becomes oliguric, ECF volume and total body sodium increase, and hypertension and edema ensue.

Uremia is accompanied by a group of systemic manifestations including anorexia, weight loss, weakness, lethargy, and altered mental function including depression, impaired ability to concentrate, and irritability. Hypertension and congestive heart failure are often complications of the uremic syndrome. Many of the abnormalities result not only from the accumulation of metabolic wastes, but also the hypervolemia, anemia, hypoproteinemia, and abnormal electrolyte status characteristic of severe chronic renal failure. The anemia is the result of reduced survival time of erythrocytes and depression of the bone marrow, partly caused by impaired production of erythropoietin. Pericarditis and cardiomyopathy as well as uremic pneumonitis and pulmonary edema may develop.

Inflammation and bleeding may occur at various sites in the gastrointestinal tract and in the pancreas. Skin abnormalities include poor wound healing, ecchymoses, pruritis, and rash.

Acidemia generally does not occur in chronic renal failure until the GFR falls below about one third of normal—that is, around 35 ml/min. In the failing kidney HCO_3^- retention and H^+ elimination are impaired. There is a reduction in the ability of the kidney to produce ammonia (NH_3). Chronic metabolic acidemia results and causes symptoms of shortness of breath with slight exertion, nausea, anorexia, and general malaise. Respiratory compensation with hyperventilation does not occur until later when the plasma pH has dropped further. Acidemia may be managed with oral alkali administration to maintain the serum bicarbonate over 18 mg/L.

Hyperkalemia may complicate chronic renal failure, especially when acidosis is present, according to the processes described in Chapter 2. Generally, hyperkalemia is not a problem until the GFR has declined to levels resulting in oliguria of around 800 ml/24 hr.

The ionized plasma calcium concentration may be low in renal failure, both because of the failure of the kidney to synthesize 1,25-dihydroxycholecalciferol resulting in impaired intestinal uptake of calcium from the diet; and because of the high serum phosphate content which depresses ionized Ca^{2+} levels (Chapter 13). Correction of acidemia may further depress ionized Ca^{2+} and lead to tetany and even seizures.

Stimulation of the parathyroid glands to secrete parathyroid hormone occurs in chronic renal failure largely on the basis of renal inability to eliminate phosphate ions. As renal failure progresses to a degree where GFR is reduced to about 20 ml/min, serum PO_4^{3-} increases. Ionized Ca^+ and PO_4^{3-} maintain an inverse relationship in plasma, and a combination of hypocalcemia and hyperphosphatemia stimulate parathyroid hormone release (secondary hyperparathyroidism) which causes demineralization of bone. This further increases serum PO_4^{3-} levels and perpetuates a vicious cycle. Aluminum hydroxide gels may be given to absorb PO_4^{3-} from the gut, and dietary PO_4^{3-} is restricted. The secondary hyperparathyroidism may lead to the development of autonomously secreting parathyroid adenomas. Consequences of hypoparathyroidism are bone pain, hypercalcemia, deposition of calcium in soft tissues, and osteitis fibrosa cystica—a characteristic bone lesion from parathyroid hypersecretion.

ACUTE RENAL FAILURE

Acute renal failure is a general term applied to a group of disorders of various causes in which there is a rapid decrease in urine formation. It is usually but not always associated with a marked acute decline in glomerular filtration rate and severe impairment of transport (both resorption and secretion) functions of the tubules. It is always associated with azotemia. There are three categories of cause of acute renal failure: (1) those resulting in urinary tract obstruction, called postrenal renal failure; (2) those caused by decreased renal perfusion, called prerenal renal failure; and (3) those resulting from damage to renal parenchyma either from intrinsic renal disease, such as acute glomerulonephritis; or extrinsic damage to renal parenchyma, as occurs in poisoning with nephrotoxins or ischemic renal injury. This is called intrarenal renal failure. Acute renal failure from either ischemic or toxic injury is called acute tubular necrosis (ATN).

Obstructive (Postrenal) Renal Failure (Obstructive Nephropathy)

In order to cause acute renal failure, the obstruction must be bilateral if it is above the bladder, or may be unilateral in a subject with a single kidney. Kidney stones, blood clots, malignancies, and retroperitoneal fibrosis are frequent causes of unilateral obstruction. Prostatic hypertrophy and neurogenic bladder are perhaps the most common causes of complete obstruction. When obstruction occurs, urine formation continues and the result is an elevation of hydrostatic pressure throughout the urinary outflow tract from Bowman's space to the site of obstruction, for example, the urethra as it passes through the prostate gland, in the case of prostatic hypertrophy. Tubules, calyces, the renal pelves, ureters, and bladder become distended with urine. Because of elevated hydrostatic pressure in Bowman's space, GFR declines. In addition, as the kidney expands in its inelastic capsule, the pressure becomes sufficient to compress the renal vessels; vascular resistance rises and renal blood flow declines. The combination of increased pressure and decreased blood flow reversibly damages the tubule cells. When the obstruction is relieved the temporary impairment of distal tubule capacity to resorb Na^+ and water results in a loss of those substances which may be great enough to cause hypovolemia.

Prerenal Acute Renal Failure (Prerenal Azotemia)

Prerenal acute renal failure is caused by decreased perfusion to the kidneys resulting from arterial hypotension of any cause: hemorrhagic shock, cardiogenic shock, or hypovolemia from dehydration or third spacing (Chapter 1). The kidneys receive a surprising one fifth to one fourth of the cardiac output—over 1 L/min. Any impairment of cardiac output decreases the effective renal perfusion pressure and leads to a decline in GFR.

Patients with congestive heart failure, even though they may be able to maintain a normal systemic arterial pressure, are especially prone to prerenal azotemia. Low renal perfusion is a characteristic accompaniment of heart failure because of the chronically reduced cardiac output. In addition reflex adrenergic activation occurs as a compensatory response to the low cardiac output, as described in Chapter 7. It induces a differential vasoconstriction that helps maintain blood flow to the brain and to the heart itself, but selectively deprives the kidneys and other viscera of adequate perfusion. The kidney responds to the low cardiac output and vasoconstriction by further constricting the efferent arteriole; this effectively increases hydrostatic pressure in the afferent arteriole and glomerulus. It improves GFR over what it would otherwise be, and helps maintain a more normal kidney function and urinary output. But these adaptive changes, coupled with the kidney's requirement for a large blood flow, lead to the fact that in the patient with chronic congestive failure, or impaired left ventricular function, any factor predisposing to cardiac decompensation (such as an increase in ECF volume, which will worsen left ventricular performance), a marked decrease in ECF volume (for example, from dehydration or an excess of strong diuretics), or hypotension from any cause, may lead to a further decline in renal perfusion sufficient to produce prerenal azotemia. GFR ceases when the pressure in the afferent arteriole declines to much below 65 mmHg and produces the oliguria or anuria of prerenal azotemia.

In patients having any of the precipitating conditions for prerenal failure listed above (whether or not they also have impaired cardiac performance), as perfusion pressure to the kidney declines the afferent arterioles dilate and the efferent arterioles constrict. This response elevates hydrostatic pressure in the glomerulus and helps to maintain GFR in the presence of an overall decreased renal blood flow.

BUN and plasma creatinine concentrations are useful indicators of renal function. In the normal subject, the usual range for the BUN is 10–20 mg/100 ml, and for the creatinine 0.6–1.2 mg/100 ml. Therefore the normal ratio of BUN to creatinine is not more than 20:1. When there is a decline in perfusion pressure to the kidney the GFR declines markedly, and the amount of urea and creatinine that is filtered falls with the GFR. As urine flow declines, the tendency for urea to diffuse out of the filtrate back into the peritubular blood increases (see above). However, creatinine tends to remain in the filtrate and be eliminated in the urine because the tubule membranes are less permeable to it. The result of this difference in response of the BUN and creatinine to a diminished flow of tubular filtrate is that the BUN will rise disproportionately faster than the creatinine, so that a BUN to creatinine ratio in excess of 20:1 is correlated with prerenal azotemia and is a sign of it.

Another characteristic finding in prerenal azotemia is a very low urine Na^+ concentration, below 20 meq/L and sometimes less than 5 meq/L. This low urinary Na^+ helps to distinguish prerenal azotemia from the other important oliguric state, acute tubular necrosis. In ATN the patient excretes a large percentage of filtered Na^+ and will likely have a urinary Na^+ of 40 to 90 meq/L; while in a patient with the hemodynamic alterations producing prerenal azotemia, such as volume depletion and hypotension, avid distal renal tubular resorption to promote conservation of Na^+ and expand ECF volume and renal perfusion results in very low urinary Na^+ content.

If the period of reduced renal perfusion has not been too long, or the degree too severe, then increase of cardiac output, elevation of blood pressure, and repletion of ECF volume will restore renal perfusion, GFR, and urine output. However, prerenal azotemia is perhaps the most prominent cause of the renal parenchymal damage which results in the form of acute renal failure called acute tubular necrosis. A failure to recognize or adequately treat prerenal azotemia may therefore result in ischemic acute renal failure, which is characterized by actual structural damage to renal parenchyma.

Acute Tubular Necrosis (Intrarenal Renal Failure)

The causes of acute tubular necrosis (ATN) are injury to the kidney from prolonged (longer than about half an hour) renal ischemia, or from nephrotoxic chemicals or drugs: some antimicrobial agents, some anesthetics, and specific kidney poisons such as mercuric chloride, ethylene glycol, and methyl alcohol. Common causes of severe renal ischemia are extensive hemorrhage, burns, shock, multiple trauma, hemolysis, heart and vessel surgery, sepsis, and heart failure. All of these may produce the profound hypotension that can cause structural kidney damage. Previous dehydration appears to increase the damaging effect of hypotension from any cause. In addition the hemolysis resulting from crushing muscle injuries or burns releases myoglobin or hemoglobin into the plasma, which then precipitates out in renal tubules, increasing the injury caused by the ischemia.

Mechanisms of Cause of ATN

Severe protracted hypotension causes intense renal vasoconstriction, with a more marked constriction in the outer cortex than in the medulla and inner cortex. There may be a strong afferent arteriolar constriction accompanying severe hypotension of long duration which could lead to the observed abrupt fall in GFR that accompanies ATN. Studies indicate that renal blood flow may remain reduced below one half of normal for several days after the onset of oligura, even when timely and adequate correction of the hypovolemia and hypotension has occurred. This cortical vasoconstriction, if in fact it occurs consistently and is the cause of the renal tubular abnormalities in ATN, would lead to a profound decline in glomerular blood flow and hence glomerular filtration pressure. The result could be a decrease in permeability of the glomerular membranes which would persist beyond the actual period of hypotension or hypovolemia.

Instead of, or in addition to, this possible mechanism of cause of renal parenchymal damage, some authors suggest that the damage may occur primarily to the renal tubules rather than to the glomeruli. Tubular edema caused by ischemic hypoxia, obstruction of the tubules by cellular debris, or abnormally increased permeability of tubular epithelial cells which permits backflow of filtrate into the interstitial fluid, have all been proposed as mechanisms of cause of the nephron damage and suppression of urine formation in ATN.

One theory of the pathogenesis of ATN involves the renin–angiotensin system (Chapter 3). Systemic hypotension causes profound renal vasoconstriction because of sympathetic adrenergic reflex response and a large outpouring of catecholamines. The renal vasoconstriction then leads to hypoxic ischemia of the tubular epithelium which causes impaired Na^+ resorption in the proximal tubule. Because of this there is increased concentration of Na^+ reaching the macula densa. The latter is stimulated to cause large amounts of renin to be released from the juxtaglomerular cells which could lead to intrarenal production of high concentrations of the powerful vasoconstrictor angiotensin II. The afferent arterioles would then respond by extreme vasoconstriction, and GFR would decline precipitously. The consequence would be a lack of tubular filtrate leading to structural damage of tubular epithelium.

The Kidney Lesions in ATN

All of these proposals have received support from the results of studies of acute tubular necrosis induced in experimental animals by a variety of methods; however, which of these mechanisms are involved in nephron damage in human ATN remains speculative. Whatever the mechanisms by which lesions are produced, two types of structural alterations have been described in human ATN. Where ATN has been precipitated by nephrotoxins, there is seen a diffuse necrosis of proximal tubular cells with the basement membrane largely intact. In the case of ATN caused by renal ischemia, the damage is distributed in an apparently random patchy fashion: small regions of necrosis of the renal tubular epithelium, frequently involving the basement membrane, occur throughout the entire tubular length of the nephron, with the glomeruli appearing relatively intact in most cases. (The fact that the glomeruli appear structurally intact does not rule out *functional* changes in glomerular circulation as the cause of the abnormalities, however.) The total disruption of small segments of tubule wall creates openings between tubular lumen and peritubular capillaries, accounting for the loss of tubular secreting and resorptive function characteristic of ATN. In addition, there is marked interstitial edema and inflammatory cell infiltration.

Where nephrotoxins have led to systemic effects such as vomiting, diarrhea, and gastrointestinal bleeding, then dehydration, hypovolemia, and hypotension may produce ATN on a renal ischemic basis. Thus the kidneys of such subjects could contain the lesions characteristic of the two categories of cause of ATN, both nephrotoxic and ischemic.

Physiologic Consequences of the Nephron Abnormalities

In the patient with normal renal function, only about 0.5% of the Na^+ and less than 1% of the water filtered at the glomerulus will be excreted in the urine. In the patient with ATN, however, up to 10% of the filtered Na^+ and 20% of the filtered water will be eliminated. As emphasized above, there is a marked decline in GFR. Therefore, this increased elimination of Na^+ and H_2O is the manifestation of a profound decrease in urine concentrating function; that is, there is a greatly decreased tubular capacity for resorption of Na^+ and H_2O. The correlate of this is an increase in *fractional excretion ratios* for both Na^+ and H_2O: though much less is filtered at the glomerulus to begin with, much less of that which is filtered is resorbed by the tubules, and therefore much more is excreted. In many patients with ATN the GFR drops to 1 ml/min and the urine output may be around 300 ml/24 hr, with a Na^+ content of about 15–18 meq/24 hr (greater than 50 meq/L).

About one fifth of patients with ATN demonstrate nonoliguric ATN—so-called high-output renal failure. In this situation there is the apparent paradox of increasing azotemia in the presence of a high urinary volume. The explanation is the mechanism described above: a low GFR—too low to filter adequate amounts of urea, creatinine, and other wastes—accompanied by a high fractional excretion ratio for Na^+ and water because of grossly inadequate tubular resorption. If the GFR is reduced to 9 L/24 hr and the damaged tubules are able to resorb only 7 L/24 hr, then urinary output will be entirely satisfactory: 2000 ml/24 hr. But the poor GFR produces a daily rise in BUN and creatinine which will cause uremia. The daily increase in BUN often averages 50 mg/100 ml/24 hr. In both oliguric and nonoliguric ATN the urine is approximately isosmotic to plasma; that is, the urine-to-plasma osmolarity ratio is approximately 1.0.

Because of the extreme decline in GFR, the plasma concentration of those substances normally eliminated in the urine will increase: urea, creatinine, uric acid, phosphate and sulfuric acids, organic acids, phenols, and potassium ions. A portion of the rapid increase in these substances in the blood is accounted for not only on the basis of decreased elimination of them by the failed kidneys, but their increased production resulting from the catabolic state caused by the severe systemic illness or injury which produced the ATN in the first place. In this situation the BUN may rise as much as 50–75 mg/100 ml/24 hr, and the uremic syndrome may develop rapidly.

Assessment and Course

Typically the patient's history will include one of the following conditions: hemorrhage from any cause, severe enough to produce marked and prolonged hypotension; sepsis; multiple trauma, especially with crushing muscle tissue damage; cardiogenic shock from a large myocardial infarction; rhabdomyolysis (breakdown of muscle cells) or hemolysis; or severe depletion of ECF volume from dehydration, vomiting and diarrhea, excessive strong diuretics, or third spacing. Where a nephrotoxic agent has been the cause, then ingestion of or exposure to one of the following will have occurred: antibiotics (gentamicin, kanamycin, streptomycin); an iodinated X-ray contrast medium; or specific nephrotoxins such as the inorganic salts of the heavy metals: Pb, Hg, Bi, or Ur; or organic compounds such as ethylene glycol.

The onset of ATN follows the causative agent by an interval of a few to 48 hours. Oliguria or anuria develops in most patients, with a rising BUN, creatinine, K^+, and salt and water retention. Complete anuria usually does not occur, but oliguria may consist of a urinary output of less than 200 ml/24 hr. The oliguria and uremia may last from 1 to 6 weeks or more, with an average being about 1–14 days. During the first several days the patient's condition is determined to a large extent by the nature and severity of the basic systemic injury or illness that precipitated the ATN. If the renal damage is not recognized, and especially if excess intravenous fluids are administered, hypervolemia leading to edema, dilutional hyponatremia, and left ventricular overload with pulmonary edema may develop. During the next phase of ATN, perhaps after a few days to a week of oliguria, central nervous system signs of uremia develop, and the results of overhydration become more apparent.

Weight gain is not always a reliable method for assessing fluid overload because tissue catabolism during severe injury or illness adds so-called water of tissue oxidation in amounts of perhaps 500 ml/24 hr. Insensible water losses amount to about 1000 ml/24 hr. An adult with a severe illness but kept adequately hydrated will lose about 0.5 kg/24 hr. If the patient is anuric, a fluid intake of under 500 m/24 hr will probably maintain normal fluid balance. Maintaining hydration adequate to keep body weight stable in such a situation will lead to hypervolemia and probably hyponatremia.

Central nervous system manifestations of the uremia of ATN may be asterixis (metabolic flap), altered mental status—irritability, restlessness, delirium, disorientation—and stupor or coma (Chapter 14). Gastrointestinal manifestations may include anorexia, hiccoughs, nausea and vomiting, thirst, and the more serious gastrointestinal bleeding. The mechanisms for this last complication are uncertain, but the uremia of ATN is often accompanied by mucosal sloughing and petechial hemorrhage of the digestive tract. The cardiovascular manifestations comprise the EKG changes of hyperkalemia; an elevated cardiac output caused by anemia, acidosis and often hypervolemia; hypertension in some patients; and left ventricular failure and pulmonary edema when hypervolemia is marked and left ventricular function is impaired. In a patient with severe tissue damage resulting in the release of intracellular contents (this includes hemolysis and gastrointestinal bleeding) the entry of large amounts of K^+ into the circulation from the disrupted cells will promote more rapid and higher serum K^+ elevations than would occur from the acute renal failure itself.

Regeneration of tubular epithelium generally occurs even after major damage to the tubules, as is demonstrated by the appearance of mitotic figures during recovery. Urinary output gradually increases, and the polyuria developing during the diuretic phase of recovery may be very great—up to 3000 ml/24 hr or more. During this phase the BUN and creatinine may continue to rise for several more days. This is explained by the fact that, although GFR is increasing, tubular epithelium has still not regained its resorptive functions, and the urine represents more an ultrafiltrate of plasma. That is, the GFR is still too low to filter enough urea and creatinine to lower the blood levels of these substances; and the large amount of urine output is a result of abnormally high fractional excretion ratios. Urinary Na^+ may be 50–75 meq/L and may cause hyponatremia and hypovolemia unless adequate Na^+ and H_2O replacement occurs. Careful monitoring of body weight and frequent urinary and serum Na^+ determinations are important during the diuretic phase to maintain proper water and electrolyte balance.

Management

Since in most cases ATN is self-limiting, provided the patient survives first the systemic illness or injury causing it, and then the consequences of the acute renal failure, the treatment is directed at these two components. Prompt recognition and reversal of prerenal azotemia is crucial, since it is the most frequent cause of ATN; thus maintenance of renal perfusion with adequate volume repletion, the avoidance of excess pharmacologic pressor agents (antihypotensives) which produce renal vasoconstriction, improvement of cardiac output, and restoration of blood pressure are the key elements. Management of shock is discussed in Chapter 1.

Early and frequent dialysis is recommended by many authorities, since it controls acidemia and hyperkalemia, permits daily protein intake of around 20–40 gm or more, and decreases the necessity for strict salt and fluid restriction. Indications for hemo- or peritoneal dialysis are considered to be a BUN over 100 mg/100 ml, acidemia, volume overload and oliguria which has failed to respond to trials of furosemide, hyperkalemia, and gastrointestinal bleeding.

Measures to reduce protein catabolism—breakdown of the patient's own tissues—are important in controlling azotemia. Glucose exerts a protein-sparing effect. Total caloric intake ideally should be in the range of 200/24 hr; so-called renal failure fluid comprised of essential L-amino acids and 30% glucose helps control BUN elevation and has been reported to facilitate recovery from ATN. The management of hyperkalemia is discussed in Chapter 1. Packed red cells may be given for a hematocrit below 20–30. Careful thought must be given to the route of elimination of pharmacologic agents which may be required in treatment; many antibiotics, digitalis, and others, are eliminated largely or entirely by the kidney and in renal failure may accumulate in the blood.

In ischemic ATN, where damage to the basement membranes has occurred, healing and recovery may be slower than with nephrotoxic injury in which the membrane, from which regeneration proceeds, is preserved. Thus in the former case there may be loss of nephrons with fibrosis and distortion of many renal tubules; a permanent decline in renal function may result. However, the kidneys have a very large functional reserve, and renal function is often restored to normal though it may require up to one year. The tubular resorptive functions, necessary to concentrate the urine, are the last to recover completely.

Mortality in acute intrarenal failure is high: over 50%. This is closely dependent on the severity of the underlying illnesses and injuries which caused the ATN to develop. A severe systematic disorder combined with delayed recognition and inadequate treatment increases the mortality and morbidity from ATN. The continued high mortality rate from ATN may also be a reflection of the fact that extremely ill and severely injured patients, who otherwise would have died from their underlying condition, are being kept alive by heroic life-sustaining measures only to succumb to acute intrarenal failure.

URINARY TRACT INFECTIONS and PYELONEPHRITIS

Lower Urinary Tract Infection: Cystitis

Normally the bladder urine is sterile, that is, there are no bacteria present in it. If bacteria are introduced into the bladder they are usually eliminated in a few days. There appear to be three mechanisms which operate to protect the bladder from infections in spite of the fact that urine itself permits bacterial growth. The first is a bacteriostatic action of urine itself which to some extent, because of high osmolarity and low pH, inhibits bacterial growth. This effect is more prominent in males than in females, and in urine formed during the night. The second is the elimination of bacteria from the bladder during voiding, if bladder-emptying is complete, and the bacterial-diluting effect of new urine entering the bladder from the ureters. The third factor is postulated to be a bladder mucosal substance or process which has an antibacterial action; the nature of this mechanism is not known but is suggested to be an immune process. There are two conditions which impair the ability of the bladder to maintain freedom from bacterial growth: an obstruction to the free flow of urine anywhere along the urinary outflow tract, including renal parenchyma; and a failure to completely empty the bladder of urine, which increases the population of bacteria and decreases the diluting effect of newly formed urine.

Asymptomatic bacteriuria results when the bladder urine contains bacteria which have not invaded tissue and therefore have not produced symptoms. The only sign would be the finding of bacteria on urine culture or Gram stain. However, once lower urinary tract tissue has been invaded symptoms of urethritis and cystitis occur—dysuria, burning on urination, frequency and urgency, and suprapubic pains—and the sign of suprapubic tenderness to palpation. Chills, fever, and other systemic signs of infection are generally absent. In female patients a thorough pelvic and genital speculum examination, with microscopic examination of the vaginal vault contents for *Trichomonas, Candida,* and gonococci, the external genitalia for herpes progenitalis, and in elderly women for atrophic vaginitis is advocated in complaints of dysuria. Studies have shown that a large percentage of women with these complaints do not have bacteriuria but rather one of the above disorders. Conversely, half of women with significant bacteriuria are asymptomatic.

There are a number of factors which predispose to cystitis. Any condition impeding free flow of urine and complete bladder emptying, such as benign prostatic hypertrophy or ureteral stricture, carries a considerably increased incidence of urinary tract infections. Sex is a factor; the incidence is about 10 times higher in females of reproductive age than in males. A number of factors are implicated in this difference: a shorter urethra, the local trauma of copulation, the greater degree of bacterial contamination of the external genitalia in females than males, and the lack of prostatic secretions which are bacteriostatic. Poor personal hygiene and wiping from back to front after bowel movement are often involved in the cause. Invasion of the urethra with catheters, cystoscope, dilating sounds or other instruments may increase proneness to infection by carrying in bacteria and damaging mucous membrane barriers to infection; the urethra has a considerable bacterial population along its outer one third. Autonomic nervous system abnormalities of bladder function such as spinal paraplegia, multiple sclerosis, and tabes dorsalis are predisposing factors because of overdistention and difficult emptying of the bladder and frequent catheterization.

Acute Pyelonephritis

Cause and Abnormalities

Since the mucous membrane of the urinary tract is continuous from urethra to kidney, once bladder urine and tissue have been infected, bacteria may ascend one or both ureters to the renal pelvis and cause infection and inflammation of the calyces and renal parenchyma itself. The usual organisms are the gram-negative inhabitants of the intestinal tract, usually *Escherichia coli* but also *Enterobacter, Pseudomonas,* and *Proteus.* Where there is associated chronic obstruction from stones, prostatic hypertrophy, or neurogenic bladder, and frequent catheterization or instrumentation, *Klebsiella* or *Pseudomonas* are frequently the pathogens. Hematogenous infection—that is, bacteria in the bloodstream from systemic infections or a focus of infection such as endocarditis—may occur, especially when there is some obstruction high in the tract from a kidney stone or ureteral stricture, and if the patient is debilitated or immunosuppressed. *Staphylococci* and *Streptococci* are gram-positive organisms that may be the cause in patients with chronic illnesses.

Some form of obstruction to the free flow of urine in various portions of the urinary tract is said to be present in about half of patients with acute pyelonephritis. The site of the obstruction may be in the urethra (stricture, prostatic hypertrophy); the bladder (tumor, neurogenic obstruction, calculus, chronic cystitis); the ureters (pregnancy, calculus, tumor, fibrosis, scarring); or within the kidneys themselves (calculi, crystals, polycystic disease, tumors, and other forms of chronic renal disease).

An important predisposing factor for pyelonephritis is vesicoureteral reflux. In the normal individual the ureters penetrate the bladder wall at an angle and their lower segment and point of attachment lies within the wall of the bladder itself. During urination the smooth muscle of the bladder contracts and exerts pressure on the intramural ureteral segments. Pressure within the bladder increases during micturition, but the compressed distal ureters tend to prevent the reflux of urine into the ureters and up toward the kidneys. In some individuals the ureters attach more directly and at a more obtuse angle, thus they are less readily compressed during urination and urine reflux occurs more readily. Cystitis promotes vesicoureteral reflux by causing inflammation and edema of the distal ureters making them less readily compressible. Chronic distention of the bladder also predisposes to reflux because of constant high intravesicular pressure which promotes backflow of urine into the ureters and kidneys.

Regardless of the predisposing factors, and often none can be found, bacteria colonize the renal pelvis in the case of ascending infection; where reflux has occurred, bacteria may be carried to the medulla or even the cortex. Bacteria then penetrate the mucosa and invade the interstitial areas of the medulla. The medullary portions of the kidney are particularly susceptible to infection. The osmotic pressure in this portion of the kidney is very high and the hypersomolarity impedes the leukocyte in-migration, phagocytosis, and the other tissue defense mechanisms which combat infection. The bacteria increase in numbers; inflammation, edema, exudation, and fibrin deposition occur. Necrosis of nearby renal tubules develops so that bacteria penetrate into the lumen and by this means the infection spreads from medulla into cortex, where small abscesses form. In most cases the glomeruli are not affected. The lesions in acute pyelonephritis tend to remain localized, and the result is a wedge-shaped area of affected tissue extending through from medulla to cortex; lateral spread does not usually occur.

Assessment

Pyelonephritis is common; in adults the incidence is highest in females during the reproductive years, and in elderly males as a correlate of prostatic hypertrophy. Symptoms are those of the dysuria of cystitis and sometimes aching pain in the flank or costovertebral angle. Systemic symptoms may include chills, fever, anorexia, nausea and vomiting, prostration, and malaise. In a surprisingly large number of patients the complaints may not be directly referrable to the urinary tract, for example, general fatigue and vague abdominal distress.

Signs may be costovertebral angle tenderness to percussion, hematuria, tenderness to palpation over the bladder and kidneys on the abdominal examination, more than 5 to 8 white blood cells per high-powered field if a centrifuged urine specimen is examined, white blood cell casts, many identical-appearing bacteria (rather than many different types of bacteria, which indicates vaginal or urethral contamination) in the Gram stain of a spun specimen, or any bacteria at all on the Gram stain of an unspun specimen. The definitive assessment of urinary tract infection is made by culture of a clean-catch voided urine specimen; more than 100,000 organisms/ml signifies infection.

Course and Management

The course of acute pyelonephritis generally runs well with a good response to appropriate antibiotics as determined by sensitivity studies of the bacteria. Frequently used antibiotic medications are sulfasoxazol and ampicillin. Fever, pain, dysuria, and other symptoms usually resolve within two days unless the pyelonephritis was very severe. It is desirable that patients return for a reculture after the course of antibiotics has been completed, even though they are asymptomatic. Asymptomatic urinary tract infections may persist for months or even years as demonstrated by positive urine cultures. Such chronic infections probably set the stage in many patients for chronic pyelonephritis. In a female patient with two or more severe urinary tract infections in one year, cystoscopy and an intravenous pyelogram may be indicated to rule out structural abnormalities. In men, a single episode may suggest the need for such a study, and in older men evaluation for prostatic hypertrophy is appropriate. Urethritis often produces dysuria in men and, although microscopic examination may reveal many white blood cells, the urine culture is often negative.

Chronic Pyelonephritis

Chronic pyelonephritis is a form of chronic interstitial nephritis that develops as a consequence of bacterial infection of the kidney. Often the infection has been of long duration, with recurrence of the same infection, or reinfections, over many years. It is frequently associated with vesicoureteral reflux or conditions that produce chronic obstruction at some level in the urinary tract. On the other hand, many patients with chronic pyelonephritis have negative urine cultures, a history negative for episodes of urinary tract infections, and no demonstrable obstructive lesions anywhere in the urinary tract. Thus in many cases the etiology of chronic pyelonephritis remains unknown.

Macroscopic changes in the kidney consist of patches of scarring, bilateral but asymmetric. The surface has coarse irregular pitting. The pelves and calyces may be dilated and deformed, especially where there has been obstruction, and there may be inflammation and scarring of these areas. Microscopically many glomeruli are often relatively intact; others are surrounded by fibrotic tissue. In some areas entire nephrons have been obliterated by fibrosis. In other areas there are patches of active interstitial inflammation and cellular infiltration involving both cortex and medulla. Some tubules are atrophic in certain areas, hypertrophied or dilated in others. In advanced disease the glomeruli may disappear or become hyalinized and the tubules filled with homogeneous deposits (colloid casts). As hypertension develops, the arteriolar abnormalities become more marked. These structural abnormalities are not specific for pyelonephritis but occur in many other renal interstitial diseases.

The patient may give a history of recurring urinary tract infections in adult life, or perhaps in childhood; the urine may contain white blood cell casts, and the urine culture may be positive. Intravenous pyelogram may show asymmetric patchy scarring of the kidneys bilaterally, areas of cortical atrophy, and deformed pelves and calyces. However, the culture and history may be negative for infection and the patient may come with pyuria, proteinuria, hematuria, established hypertension, and the complaints and laboratory and physical findings of azotemia or uremia.

There are a number of possible explanations for chronic pyelonephritis in the absence of a history of chronic urinary tract infection. Continued reflux of urine into the kidney can probably cause the tissue damage characteristic of chronic pyelonephritis without infection being present. Alternatively, given renal damage from early subclinical pyelonephritis in childhood or youth, the development of hypertension could continue a destructive process. Other proposed mechanisms are an immunologic process triggered by early infection and/or subclinical infections with atypical forms of bacteria.

The course of the chronic renal failure in chronic pyelonephritis tends to be prolonged if severe hypertension does not develop and is characterized by greater fluctuations in renal function than is typical of CRF from other causes, with periods of marked uremia developing from dehydration or recurrent illness or infection, interspersed with periods of semirecovery but at a lower level of function than previously. Severe azotemia is accompanied by a marked loss of concentrating ability, so that dehydration develops readily and, by decreasing GFR further, worsens the uremia. A favorable response in kidney function may be brought about by a careful control of urinary tract infections.

REFERENCES

Beeson PB and McDermott W, editors: *Textbook of Medicine.* 14th ed. Philadelphia, Pa.: Saunders, 1975.

Dans, PE and Klaus B: Dysuria in women. *Johns Hopkins Med J.* 138:13–18, 1976.

Flamenbaum, W: Pathophysiology of acute renal failure. *Arch. Intern. Med.* 131:91–928, 1973.

Frohlich ED, editor: *Pathophysiology.* Philadelphia, Pa.: Lippincott, 1976.

Ganong WF: *Review of Medical Physiology.* 8th ed. Los Altos, Calif.: Lange Medical Publications, 1977.

Golden A and Maher JF: *The Kidney.* 2nd ed. Baltimore, Md.: Williams & Wilkins, 1977.

Guyton AC: *Textbook of Medical Physiology.* 5th ed. Philadelphia, Pa.: Saunders, 1976.

Kurtzman NA and Martinez-Maldonado M, editors: *Pathophysiology of the Kidney.* Springfield, Ill.: CC Thomas, 1977.

Leaf A and Cotran RS: *Renal Pathophysiology.* Cambridge: Oxford University Press, 1976.

Massry SG, editor: The kidney in systemic diseases. *Contr. Nephrol.* v. 7, 1977.

Maude DL: *Kidney Physiology and Kidney Disease: An Introduction to Nephrology.* Philadelphia, Pa.: Lippincott, 1977.

Schrier RW, editor. *Pathophysiology of Renal and Electrolyte Disorders.* Boston, Mass.: Little, Brown, 1976.

Thorn GW, et al, editors: *Harrison's Principles of Internal Medicine.* 8th ed. New York: McGraw-Hill, 1977.

CHAPTER ELEVEN

Gastrointestinal Disorders

NORMAL FUNCTIONS OF THE GASTROINTESTINAL TRACT

The major contribution of the gastrointestinal tract to bodily homeostasis is the provision of nutrients, water, vitamins, and minerals. This function is accomplished by three types of processes: (1) motility—the orderly movement of alimentary contents through the canal and the mechanical breakdown of large particles into smaller ones; (2) secretion of digestive enzymes and the chemical substances facilitating their action, with the provision of an environment favorable to their actions, which is the hydrolysis (digestion) of complex substances to simpler ones; and (3) absorption of water, electrolytes, and the products of hydrolysis.

Gastrointestinal Motility

The several portions of the alimentary tract have a number of layers; from inside out they are the mucosal lining (which contains a layer of smooth muscle), the submucosa, a layer of circular muscle which by contraction narrows the lumen, a layer of longitudinal muscle which shortens and enlarges the lumen when it contracts, and the outer serosa which is continuous with the mesentery.

Smooth Muscle

As is the case with cardiac muscle, gut smooth muscle cells are in such intimate contact that the waves of electrical excitation which initiate muscle contraction pass directly—that is, they are propagated—from cell to cell, resulting in smooth coordinated waves of contraction. The smooth muscle cells of the gut undergo regular spontaneous waves of deplorization at rates differing in various portions of the tract (about 3 to more than 12/min), which result in the waves of contraction; these waves are called the gastrointestinal slow waves and they serve the function of a kind of basic pacemaker for gastrointestinal motor activity. Superimposed on them are other types of muscular contractions, the nature of which depends on the portion of the tract, the presence of food and fluid, and the influence of neural and humoral factors.

Innervation

Intrinsic Innervation

There are two major intrinsic networks of nerve fibers which extend throughout the gastrointestinal tract; together they are called the intramural nerve plexus. The *myenteric plexus* lies between the longitudinal and circular muscle layers and influences gut motility—that is, it is primarily a motor plexus. The *submucosal plexus* is primarily a group of nerve cells which have their origin in receptors—sensory cells—lying in the mucosa, and which respond to both chemical and mechanical stimuli from the inner layers of the gut wall. It is primarily a sensory plexus. Together these two intramural plexuses are involved in the local control of secretion, and the coordination of motility by means of local reflex arcs. When extrinsic innervation to the tract is interrupted, coordinated motor and secretory activity proceeds nevertheless because of the action of this intrinsic innervation.

Extrinsic Innervation

The source of the efferent nerve supply to the gut is from the autonomic nervous system. In general, parasympathetic cholinergic neural stimuli travel in the vagus nerve and enhance both motility and secretion in the tract. Sympathetic adrenergic stimulation generally inhibits both motor and secretory activity of the gut. The parasympathetic extrinsic innervation consists of preganglionic fibers which synapse extensively with neurons of the intramural plexus, but some innervate smooth muscle cells directly, and they also supply the blood vessels.

In addition there are extrinsic afferent nerve fibers traveling from receptors in the gastrointestinal tract to the central nervous system. Stimuli for activation of the afferent fibers are inflammation or chemical irritation of gut mucosa, and stretch on or distention of the gut wall. Some of these afferent impulses participate in local reflex control of motor and secretory activity via the intrinsic innervation. Others, including the pain afferents, enter the dorsal root ganglia of the spinal cord with the parasympathetic and sympathetic afferents and influence central nervous system effects on gut motility and secretion.

Motor Activity

There are two basic types of gut motility: peristaltic or propulsive movements, which act to propel ingested food and liquid along the tract; and mixing movements, which break solid material into smaller particles and churn gut contents to mingle them with enzymes and other compounds involved in digestion. Peristaltic movements are stimulated by distention and are an inherent response of smooth muscle tissue to stretch on its constituent fibers. However, in order for peristaltic contractions to function in a coordinated integrated manner that will promote orderly movement of gut contents through the lumen, normal structure and function of the myenteric plexus is essential. When it is absent or malfunctioning inherent smooth muscle contractility persists, but the contractions become incoordinated, feeble, and effectively nonpropulsive.

Gastrointestinal Secretion

Since the nature of secretions and their control and functions differ greatly in the various portions of the tract, this topic will be covered briefly for each anatomic division: stomach and intestine; and liver, gallbladder, and pancreas (Chapter 12).

Anatomic Divisions and Functions of the Gastrointestinal Tract

Esophagus

The esophagus propels food from mouth to stomach by waves of peristalsis initiated by swallowing. The sensory receptors for this reflex are located in the pharynx; mechanical stimulation of them initiates a brainstem reflex producing inhibition of breathing and coordinated pharyngeal muscle contractions, which not only prevent oral contents from entering the trachea but also move the bolus into the esophagus. At the junction between pharynx and esophagus there is a segment of esophageal muscle that has a high resting wall tension and thus acts as a sphincter; it is reflexly relaxed during deglutition. Then a ring of smooth muscle contraction forms behind the bolus and moves toward the stomach at about 4 cm/sec. The muscle above the junction between esophagus and stomach (esophagastric junction) is likewise specialized to remain tonically somewhat constricted and therefore also functions as a sphincter—that is, it has a high resting wall tension—which normally prevents reflux of gastric contents into the esophagus. This muscle ring is called the *lower esophageal sphincter*.

Stomach

The stomach has both motor and secretory functions.

Motor Activity

The motor functions of the stomach comprise (1) receptive relaxation, which permits it to receive and store dietary intake; (2) mixing of the food with the gastric secretions; (3) mechanical breakdown of food particles; and (4) release of gastric contents at a low controlled rate into the duodenum. Peristaltic contractions are coordinated by the gastric slow wave, which moves across the stomach from fundus to pylorus at about 3/min, and which is a major factor in the control of gastric emptying. These waves are the pacemakers for regular antral contractions that sweep over antrum, pylorus, and upper duodenum, and constitute the "antral pump." The pyloric sphincter exerts only minor control over the amount and rate of discharge of stomach contents. When the stomach has emptied there are more generalized waves of lesser intensity which gradually increase. These are the familiar hunger contractions.

The type of food eaten has a major effect on the rate at which food in the stomach is discharged into the duodenum. Carbohydrates leave the stomach most rapidly, proteins next, and fats more slowly. A number of other mechanisms influence the rate of emptying. The presence of a high hydrogen ion concentration, mechanical distention, and the products of protein digestion within the duodenum; initiate a reflexly mediated decrease in stomach secretion and rate of emptying which acts to prevent a too rapid inflow to the duodenum from the stomach; this response is called the enterogastric reflex. Any factor which inhibits vagal cholinergic nerve impulses, such as anticholinergic drugs (atropine, propantheline) delays gastric emptying. Vagotomy greatly delays gastric emptying and may lead to chronic loss of tone and to distention of the stomach.

Secretory Activity

In addition to the mucus glands present throughout the whole alimentary canal, the stomach contains two types of tubular glands: gastric glands in the body and fundus which put out digestive secretions; and pyloric and cardiac glands which release quantities of mucus, postulated by some authors to protect the pylorus against damage by strong acid-peptic secretions. The cells of the gastric glands release about 3000 ml/d of gastric juices comprised of water, electrolytes, mucus, hydrochloric acid (HCl), and digestive enzymes. The chief (peptic or zymogen) cells of the glands synthesize the enzymes, mainly pepsin; the parietal or oxyntic cells secrete strong (pH 0.8 or 150 meq/L) HCl against a large concentration gradient by active transport mechanisms which are still not completely understood.

Gastric gland secretion is regulated by both neural and humoral (hormonal) processes. Neural stimulation of both HCl and enzyme secretion originates in the brainstem in the dorsal motor nuclei of the vagus and acts via the myenteric plexus. The sympathetic nerve supply comes from the celiac plexus. The humoral stimulus to gastric gland secretion is the hormone gastrin, produced by G cells in the walls of certain glands in the antral portion of the gastric mucosa, as well as by cells in the mucosa of the duodenum. The main actions of gastrin are stimulation to HCl and pepsin secretion, and the growth of gastric mucosa. Release of gastrin is stimulated by vagal impulses, by distention of the stomach, and by the presence in the stomach of the products of protein digestion called secretagogues. The secretion of gastrin is inhibited by stomach acid, and the gastrointestinal hormones: secretin, gastroinhibitory peptide (GIP) (formed in the mucosa of the proximal small intestine when there is fat and glucose in the duodenum), and vasoactive intestinal peptide (VIP). All of these stimuli act via the intrinsic nerve supply of the myenteric plexus.

Gastrin does not act locally in the stomach as it is secreted. Rather, it is absorbed into the blood and then carried back to the gastric glands to produce its stimulating action. The secretion-stimulating effects of gastrin and vagal efferent impulses potentiate one another, in that when they are both operating the total amount of secretion is greater than the sum of each acting independently.

Histamine is a potent stimulus to gastric acid secretion and the histamine content of gastric mucosa is high. Some evidence suggests that those stimuli which increase HCl secretion do so by the release of histamine into the mucosa. There are two kinds of histamine receptors: H_1 and H_2. The histamine receptors which mediate hypersensitivity (allergic) reactions, and which are blocked by antihistamines such as diphenhydramine and chlorpheniramine, are the H_1 receptors; those antihistamines have slight if any effect on gastric acid secretion. It appears that it is the H_2 receptors which mediate the histamine stimulation of gastric HCl. Cimetidine is an H_2 blocker proving helpful in the control of acid release in many patients with peptic ulcer disease.

Small Intestine

In the small intestine partially digested food from the stomach is mixed with additional mucus, secretions of the intestinal mucosal cells, bile from the liver, and enzymes from the pancreas. The processes of digestion are completed here and the products are absorbed. In addition, the fluid and electrolytes which were secreted in more proximal portions of the alimentary canal are now resorbed into the circulation. The small intestine receives approximately 10 L/24 hr of fluid of which the greatest volume (8 L) is comprised of secretions into the tract from proximal structures, while about 2 L are of exogenous (dietary) origin. Of the total volume of all substances from both internal and external sources entering the small intestine, only about 1500 ml eventually enter the colon. The remainder is absorbed.

The motor activity of the small intestine consists of mixing contractions (rhythmic segmentation) and propulsive–peristaltic contractions. The small intestine slow wave rate is about 8–12/min depending on the level in the tract. The intact myenteric plexus is essential for these movements, and the extrinsic innervation influences them in a manner similar to its regulation of gastric motility.

Secretion of mucus and alkaline fluid similar in composition to the ECF occurs from glands of the small intestine, and bile and pancreatic secretions (Chapter 12) enter the duodenum at its proximal end. The digestive enzymes of the small intestine are almost entirely contained in granules in both intact and sloughed intestinal mucosa cells, rather than in the liquid secretions of the glands. Control of the secretion of mucus is largely mechanical distention and vagal impulses, both of which stimulate it. The presence of digesting food stimulates the secretion of intenstinal fluid and enzyme formation. Vasoactive intestinal peptide (VIP) is formed in the intestine, is carried in the blood back to the mucosa, stimulates intestinal secretion of isotonic water and electrolytes, and dilates peripheral blood vessels.

The absorptive surface of the small intestine is enormously increased by the many folds in the mucosa and the projections of multitudes of small villi from its surface. In addition, projecting from each mucosal cell is a brush border of microvilli which increase the absorptive surface still more. Absorption occurs both by diffusion and by a number of active transport processes. Fluid and the end products of digestion are taken in at this surface, and each villus contains a central lacteal for absorption of products of fat digestion into the lymphatics. These materials enter the portal circulation and are carried to the liver via the portal vein.

Colon

The principal functions of the colon are the removal by resorption of 90% of the water and many of the electrolytes from the contents entering it from the small intestine, and the storage of residual material until it can be eliminated during defecation. The proximal half of the colon primarily serves the absorptive functions, while the distal portions act as storage. As is the case with the small intestine, the colon has two types of motility: rhythmic segmental contractions called haustrations, and propulsive peristaltic movements. In addition it has a third type, seen only in the large intestine: a simultaneous contraction over a long area, which facilitates evacuating the distal colon during defecation. The colon also has the coordinating "pacemaker" slow wave present in the stomach and small intestine. The rate increases over the length of the colon from 2/min at the cecum to 6/min at the sigmoid.

There are no enzymes formed in the mucosa of the colon, and there are fewer villi than in the small intestine. Its princple secretion is mucus and the stimuli for mucus secretion are direct tactile stimulation of the mucus-secreting glands and a distention effect on the myenteric plexus, both produced by the contents of the colon. Both normal motility and normal secretion in the colon require the presence of adequate bulk in the lumen. Thus persons with refined processed food diets, low in natural fiber, often tend to have abnormal motor and secretory activity, resulting in dry hard stools and constipation, sometimes alternating with mucous diarrhea (functional bowel syndrome).

The ileocecal sphincter between the distal small intestine and proximal colon normally remains closed. Each time a peristaltic wave in the ileum reaches it, it opens briefly and a small amount of chyme enters the cecum. Also there is a gastroileal reflex, probably vagally mediated, in which emptying of the stomach induces relaxation of the ileocecal sphincter. When the cecum is distended the degree of constriction of the ileocecal sphincter increases, which delays entry of ileal contents into the cecum. In addition, sympathetic adrenergic impulses induced by irritation or damage in other viscera or originating in the central nervous system increase sphincter tone.

GASTROINTESTINAL DISORDERS

Esophagus

There are four symptoms which may occur as a result of disease of the esophagus. (1) *Dysphagia* is difficulty swallowing which may be felt as a sensation of something lodged in the deep substernal area. (2) *Pyrosis* (heartburn) is a burning sensation localized to beneath the lower sternum, tip of the xiphoid or upper epigastrium, which comes on in a wavelike fashion, and often ascends up the esophagus into the throat, at which moment there is sensed a bitter or acid taste in the mouth called water brash; patients may refer to this symptom as dyspepsia or (acid) indigestion. (3) *Pain* from the esophagus may or may not be associated with swallowing; if it is, it is called *odynophagia;* it is usually a deep substernal sensation which may radiate to the upper back, neck, or shoulder, and is of relatively long duration. Patients are often worried that the pain is associated with heart disease (angina pectoris). (4) *Regurgitation* is the passage back into the mouth of swallowed food or fluid which has failed to enter the stomach because of a mechanical disorder of the esophagus.

Diffuse Spasm of the Esophagus

Diffuse spasm is an abnormality of esophageal peristalisis causing dysphagia and substernal pain. It is caused by a number of disorders, including reflux esophagitis (see below) and abnormalities of the parasympathetic nerve supply of the esophagus, and is often precipitated by drinking cold liquids and by emotional tension and distress. It is a disorder of the middle-aged and elderly and the pain may be very severe, mimicking angina. The cause of the pain appears to be that the normal wave of peristalsis which is initiated by the voluntary act of swallowing becomes abnormal as it nears the distal third of the esophagus, and transforms into a diffuse nonpropulsive contraction which often includes a failure of the normal relaxation of the lower esophageal sphincter (LES). The disorder can be objectively demonstrated by esophageal manometry, a procedure in which pressure within the esophagus at various levels is measured by catheters which are open at the top, filled with fluid in order that they transmit luminal pressure, and connected with pressure transducers and a multichannel recording device. The patient is asked to swallow at intervals, and intraluminal pressures are recorded at various levels of the esophagus. These manometry studies show unproductive, noncoordinated smooth muscle contraction in the lower portions of the esophagus which usually correlate well with patient complaints of the characteristic pain.

Diffuse spasm is a benign and nonprogressive, though often distressing, disorder. Management consists of reassurance to the patient that the symptoms do not represent heart disease (if, in fact, this is the case). Since both angina and diffuse esophageal spasm may be brought on or made worse by psychoemotional tension, and relieved by nitroglycerine, it is important to differentiate chest pain that is brought on by physical exertion and relieved by physical rest (cardiac) from that which is not (esophageal spasm). If the spasm is associated with pyrosis, a reflux regimen (see below) may be helpful. Anticholinergic medication usually fails to bring relief. The smooth muscle relaxing agent nitroglycerine, taken sublingually, may be useful.

Achalasia

The principal symptom of achalasia is dysphagia, which is slowly progressive. It is a disorder of motility of the lower half or third of the esophagus and of the lower esophageal sphincter (LES); there is a failure of peristalsis of the distal esophagus, the resting pressure of the LES is elevated, it fails to relax in response to swallowing, and it is often structurally narrowed. The dysphagia occurs with both solid foods and liquids, and most patients also experience regurgitation—the spontaneous reentry of swallowed substances into the mouth without nausea or retching; this regurgitated material is not sour or bitter because it is being returned from the esophagus itself, not the stomach. About a third of patients also have wavelike substernal chest pain.

The cause is apparently an impaired parasympathetic (cholinergic) nerve supply to the lower esophagus and LES; the impairment appears to result from a degeneration of neural elements of the vagal nuclei in the brainstem, efferent fibers of the vagus nerve itself, and/or the intrinsic postganglionic cholinergic fibers comprising the myenteric plexus within the esophagus. In addition, over-responsiveness of the LES to the hormone gastrin appears to account for the elevated smooth muscle tension in that structure. Because of the lack of esophageal peristalsis and failure of LES relaxation, food and fluids are retained in the esophagus for hours, instead of entering the stomach; this leads to a gradual dilation and elongation of the esophagus which increases with time so that its eventual capacity may be over 1 L. When the patient lies down some of the contents may be regurgitated into the pharynx; if this material is not reswallowed it may be aspirated and cause aspiration pneumonitis, bronchiectasis, or pulmonary fibrosis. Eventually the patient becomes unable to eat and loses weight. A higher incidence of esophageal carcinoma in patients with long-standing achalasia than in age-matched controls has been reported.

The treatment of this disorder involves procedures to distend and disrupt the fibers of the LES. Simple passing of dilating sounds (bougienage) is not effective, and the procedure must be done surgically or more often with a special dilating balloon. When the LES is dilated by such a maneuver the ingested food and liquid is more readily able to enter the stomach under the influence of gravity. A complication of LES dilation is esophageal rupture. More conservative management with pharmacologic agents is not effective.

Gastroesophageal Reflux and Reflux Esophagitis

The LES is the mechanism for preventing gastroesophageal reflux. The sphincter marks the boundary between the esophagus and the stomach (the esophagastric junction) and normally lies at the level of the diaphragm. The pressure within the LES in the resting state is normally about 20 mmHg higher than pressure in either the esophagus above it or the stomach below it. Just after the voluntary act of swallowing, a coordinated wave of contraction exerting pressure upon the esophageal lumen of around 75 mmHg moves down the esophagus in orderly fashion. At this time pressure within the LES decreases, and it remains decreased until the propulsive peristaltic wave reaches it; as the wave passes, pressure within the sphincter again rises to its resting level. This wave initiated by a swallow is called primary peristalsis.

There are other stimuli for initiation of an esophageal peristaltic wave in addition to swallowing. Such stimuli as distention (as by a bolus of food) or an irritant (such as gastric juice) elicits a contraction at the point of stimulation, which then proceeds toward the stomach; this is a second protective mechanism for preventing esophageal damage by reflux of gastric contents, and is called secondary peristalsis (i.e., peristalsis which is not initiated by a swallow).

Although the mucosal lining of the stomach offers considerable resistance to the irritative and corrosive effects of gastric contents, the mucosa lining the esophagus does not, and therefore it is considerably more susceptible to the irritating action of HCl and pepsin, as well as to that of bile and pancreatic secretions (which often reflux into the stomach from the duodenum, gaining access to the esophagus).

Another reason for the importance of normal function of the LES in preventing reflux is that the pressure within the organs of the abdominal cavity, such as the stomach, is above atmospheric pressure, while pressure within organs of the thoracic cavity, including the esophagus, is below atmospheric pressure. Thus a positive pressure gradient exists between stomach and esophagus which favors reflux of gastric contents into the esophagus in the case of incompetence of the LES. Therefore, patients with decreased LES tonus tend to have gastroesophageal reflux.

Causes

Factors which lead to decreased LES tone appear to be decreased production of the stomach hormone gastrin, decreased gastric pH, increased production of the intestinal hormone secretin, and the increased secretion of cholecystokinin–pancreozymin, which occurs following a high-fat meal. Also any factors which tend to (1) elevate intraabdominal pressure such as obesity, large meals, pregnancy, straining, or tight clothing around the waist and abdomen; or (2) overcome the effects of gravity in preventing reflux, such as bending over or lying down, also tends to promote gastroesophageal reflux.

LES incompetence frequently occurs in conjunction with a hiatus hernia (below); however, although they often coexist, a structural abnormality at the diaphragmatic hiatus as a cause of LES incompetence and gastroesophageal reflux is another matter. Hiatus hernia is not always associated with low LES tone; gastroesophageal reflux occurs in many patients who have no hiatal abnormality; and in fact hiatus hernia may be present in perhaps one third of individuals, most of whom have no symptoms of reflux. It is also the case that there are marked individual differences in susceptibility of the esophageal mucosa to reflux of gastric contents. Some patients with a long history of symptoms of reflux may have no actual esophagitis, and others develop severe esophagitis shortly after experiencing symptoms of reflux. Effectiveness of secondary peristalsis in clearing the lower esophagus of refluxed gastric contents, differences in pH and enzyme content of refluxed material, and variations in mucosal resistance to such content, are probably all factors in explaining the different susceptibilities.

Consequences

The most frequent symptom of esophageal reflux is pyrosis and waterbrash. The "heartburn" is made worse by large meals, fatty meals, caffeine, alcohol intake, and lying down or bending over when food is in the stomach. It is relieved for a short time by drinking water and for a longer time by antacids. During sleep, reflux into the pharynx may occur and has been implicated as a precipitating factor in nocturnal asthma and as a cause of aspiration pneumonitis and pulmonary fibrosis. The patient may awaken from sleep choking on refluxed material.

Gastroesophageal reflux, if chronic and severe, may lead to reflux esophagitis. Although the former is common, the latter is not. In this situation there may be severe esophageal edema and inflammation, destruction of the epithelial lining in the distal esophagus, and marked odynophagia. Eventually erosions, an esophageal ulcer, or an inflammatory stricture, may develop, with bleeding, chest pain, and progressive dysphagia, especially for solids. In symptoms and signs of this nature, esophageal malignancy must be considered and may be ruled out by esophageal endoscopy and, if necessary, biopsy. Marked weight loss and severe odynophagia may occur in both esophageal malignancy and reflux esophagitis.

Assessment

Patient assessment consists of a careful history with attention to the symptoms and signs described above, together with special diagnostic procedures such as barium swallow, esophageal manometry, intraesophageal pH determination, and endoscopy.

Management

In management of gastroesophageal reflux and reflux esophagitis the main components are weight loss if obese; small (and if necessary, more frequent) meals; no constricting clothing; no fatty heavy food; no food after 2–3 hr before bedtime; sleep with the head of the bed elevated on blocks; and no lying down after meals. Antacids are a crucial aspect not only for the control of symptoms but for prevention of esophagitis. Depending on the severity and frequency of symptoms 15–30 ml of a commercial antacid such as Mylanta or Maalox every hour starting 1 hr after meals, and at bedtime, often controls the discomfort. As the symptoms are relieved the antacids can be tapered. Anticholinergic drugs should not be given for a number of reasons; although they do decrease acid–pepsin secretion, this helpful effect is overcome by the delay in gastric emptying, decrease in secondary peristalsis, lessening of alkaline salivary secretions, and lowering of tone in the LES, which they promote. If reflux esophagitis is severe and seems inadequately controlled by the above measures, the parasympathomimetic agonist bethanechol chloride may be tried. It stimulates gastric motility and emptying, and elevates LES tone. (It also stimulates bladder and bowel emptying.) Unlike acetylcholine it is not destroyed by cholinesterase and thus its effects are of longer duration. It should not be given if there is concurrent peptic ulcer, since it may promote perforation.

Hiatus Hernia

Hiatus hernia is simply defined as a protrusion of the stomach through the esophageal hiatus of the diaphragm into the chest cavity. There are two types. The direct, or sliding, type is the more common; here the esophagastric junction, LES, and proximal portion of the stomach pass through the hiatus and thus lie above the diaphragm. The indirect, or paraesophageal (also called rolling) type is characterized by the normal placement of junction and LES below the diaphragm, but the cardiac portion of the stomach slips through the hiatus and lies next to the lower portion of the esophagus above the diaphragm. This type is rare. Combined forms also occur. The cause is assumed to be a congenital abnormality in the diaphragmatic hiatus, although trauma, a loss of integrity of normal supporting structures in the area, or the elevated intraabdominal pressure of obesity or pregnancy may also be involved.

In the sliding type the LES and esophagastric junction may be seen on X-ray to move back and forth through the hiatus, and the assumption is that in patients who are symptomatic for gastroesophageal reflux, the junction and LES lie above the diaphragm most of the time. Most patients with this abnormality are asymptomatic, but early postprandial burning pain with feelings of fullness and eructation may also occur. When symptoms or complications develop in the sliding type, they are those of gastroesophageal reflux and esophagitis. In the paraesophageal (indirect or rolling) form there may be more serious consequences including obstruction to the esophagus, bleeding, and incarceration and strangulation, although these also are often devoid of signs or symptoms. The management of both types is usually control of the reflux as discussed above.

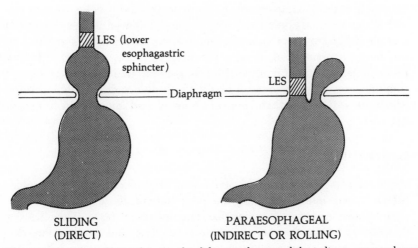

Figure 11-1. Types of hiatus hernias: the sliding, or direct; and the indirect, paraesophageal, or rolling. Various combinations of these abnormalities sometimes occur.

Peptic Ulcer Disease (Acid-Peptic Disease)

Peptic ulcers may be acute or chronic and may occur in any area exposed to gastric acid and pepsin. The most common sites are the lower esophagus, the stomach, and the duodenum.

Acute Ulcer (Stress Ulcer)

Acute ulcers are characterized by rapid development; they are superficial, being most often confined to the mucosal layer, and are more often multiple than single; and they usually occur in patients with serious systemic disorders: burns, multiple trauma, sepsis, brain lesions or trauma, treatment with cortisone, and other major abnormalities. They are called gastric erosions when they are superficial, but they can also invade submucosal and deeper layers. They are not typically accompanied by inflammation or fibrosis and do not often cause perforation or obstruction, but they frequently bleed. They ordinarily heal rapidly without tissue destruction or scarring upon resolution of the acute condition. The cause of these ulcerations is probably multiple: excess vagal cholinergic stimulation, causing hypersecretion of HC1 and pepsin; hypersecretion of adrenal glucocorticoid hormones; systemic hypotension leading to focal gastrointestinal ischemia in areas of high acid–pepsin content; and reflux of bile salts from the duodenum. Symptoms from the ulcer do not occur, and there may be severe bleeding or even occasional perforation with no warning. Acute ulcers also may develop from ingestion of alcohol, indomethacin, aspirin, phenylbutazone, ibuprofen, and other antiinflammatory agents including adrenal steroids.

Chronic Peptic Ulcer

Chronic peptic ulcers, whether gastric or duodenal, usually occur singly, typically last for many months, and often heal and recur over many years. A chronic ulcer at either site consists of a well-demarcated lesion with a base of necrotic tissue containing inflammatory material, surrounded by granulation tissue and deeper fibrosis. Characteristically there is a cyclic process of necrosis, erosion and ulceration, and edema and inflammation, followed by healing with the proliferation of fibrotic scar tissue. During erosion, blood vessels and the gut wall itself may be penetrated; during the healing phase scar tissue formation may produce deformities and obstruction. In general, peptic ulcers at any of the three common sites occur in areas of tissue which do not themselves secrete acid, but which are exposed to high concentrations of acid and pepsin from nearby sites that do.

Gastric Ulcer

Gastric ulcers comprise only about one fifth of chronic peptic ulcer disease (PUD), occur more commonly in older individuals (above 50 years), and are slightly more common in males than females (about 60%). They are sharp, well-demarcated lesions that penetrate the muscularis, and are therefore deeper than an erosion; they occur most often in the gastric antrum, especially in that area of central mucosa near the acid-secreting zone of the stomach, and on the lesser curvature. Most are smaller than 2 cm diameter. They leave a scar after healing. Gastritis is a frequent accompanying abnormality in gastric ulcer, which indicates that the ulcer is part of a more generalized disorder of the mucosa, another frequent manifestation of which is a generalized gastric hyposecretion. The basic abnormality is not known, but whatever it is it appears to predispose the mucosa to ulcer formation. Although incidence of duodenal ulcer is much higher than that of gastric, mortality rate from the latter is greater.

Causes. There are a number of theories as to the causes of gastric ulcer. It is proposed that in some patients the cause is an abnormality in motility of the pyloric antrum or duodenum, or both, which permits the contents of the duodenum to reflux into the stomach. The injurious substances may be HC1 and pepsin from the stomach itself, strong proteolytic enzymes from the pancreas, and constituents of bile. They injure the epithelial cells of the gastric mucosa and these cells then lose their capacity to resist ulceration and autodigestion by acid–pepsin. However, it appears that duodenal and bile reflux does not occur in many patients with gastric ulcer.

Another proposed cause is that some factor, such as local mucosal ischemia or the presence of irritating chemical agents (intrinsic to the body, or from an exogenous source), interferes with the normal mucous and mucosal cell protective barrier. This barrier is postulated to protect the mucosa from back-diffusion of H^+ from the lumen of the stomach. If it is disrupted, then back-diffusion can bring H^+ into contact with the mucosa, rendering the mucosal cells susceptible to damage by the strong chemicals. The acid injures both mucosal cells and blood vessels and results in inflammation, desquamation, and erosion. Another suggestion is that there is delayed gastric emptying because of pyloric malfunction, causing reflex hypersecretion of gastrin, with the stimulus being pyloric distention. Gastrin simulates excess HC1 release and mucosal erosion. Probably there are a number of causes, some of which are not yet known.

Some studies of populations with a high incidence of gastric ulcers have shown a correlation with habitual excessive use of aspirin (15 or more tablets a week) and with excess alcohol intake; both substances are thought to undermine the integrity of the mucosal barrier rendering it more susceptible to attack by the acid–pepsin secretions. Other dietary factors have also been implicated. There is said to be a familial tendency in gastric ulcers and they are reported to occur more often in persons of the type A blood group. Emotional factors such as chronic anxiety and depression may also play a role in cause, or at least they appear to be a correlate.

In addition to the back-diffusion of gastric acid, an abnormality of function of the gastric antrum and pylorus has been proposed as a causative factor in stomach ulcer formation. The pyloric sphincter in the normal subject functions to prevent reflux of duodenal contents into the stomach; in patients with gastric ulcer there is evidence that there is an impaired response of pyloric increased tonus to the stimuli of cholecystokinin–pancreozymin and secretin, and that this decreased pressure permits bile reflux from duodenum to stomach. Bile is found in excess amounts in the stomachs of many patients with gastric ulcer, and its effect in disrupting the protective mucous barrier is proposed by some workers to be a causative agent in ulcer development. The abnormalities of gastric motility reported for some gastric ulcer patients include impairment of the contractions of the antral area and delayed stomach emptying. Regardless of cause, it is known that both the total mass of parietal cells, as well as the amount of acid secretion, are low or (less often) within normal limits, in patients with gastric ulcer.

Assessment in Gastric Ulcer.   Gastric ulcers appear to produce more variable signs and symptoms than do ulcers of the duodenum, and it is not unknown for them to be altogether asymptomatic. Epigastric burning pain, nausea, anorexia, and upper abdominal distress, often to the left of the midline, may occur fairly soon after eating, and in fact some patients complain that eating brings the pain on or makes it worse. It is sometimes not relieved by eating, but is relieved by antacids or milk. Vomiting and weight loss may occur more often than in duodenal ulcers. Feelings of fullness and distention are quite common, as is a marked weight loss. Since the symptoms of gastric ulcer resemble those of gastric malignancy, the latter is an important ruleout which is accomplished by X-ray, endoscopy, gastric analysis and cytology, and biopsy; however, the vast majority are benign. If there is no acid secretion the lesion may be malignant, since in most gastric ulcer patients there is acid secretion; conversely, half of patients with carcinoma of the stomach have no acid production.

Management.   Gastric ulcers are less responsive to conservative treatment than are duodenal ones, and they tend to recur. Aspects of management are similar (see following). Hemorrhage from gastric ulcer is said to be more common, more copious, and more likely to recur than that from a duodenal ulcer. Studies have indicated that hospitalization for a period of two weeks or so facilitates healing, and use of the H_2 receptor blocking agent cimetidine appears to be helpful. Surgery may be indicated if conservative measures do not suffice to produce healing.

Duodenal Ulcer

Duodenal ulcer, the most common lesion of the gastrointestinal tract, is seen more often in males than females (although the incidence in females rises after the menopause), and is reported to develop most often between ages 30 through 55. The incidence seems to be on the decline in all groups. The ulcer is usually located immediately adjacent to the pylorus in the duodenal bulb, the first portion of the duodenum. It is usually deep and penetrates the muscle layer, and is generally less than 2 cm in diameter; about 15% of ulcer patients have more than one ulcer.

Causes.   Causes of duodenal ulcers are not known but are probably several; the two major categories of possible processes involved are increased secretion of gastric juice and lowered resistance of the mucosa to attack by gastric secretions. The mechanisms responsible for maintaining mucosal resistance to acid–pepsin are not known. Some patients who have duodenal ulcers secrete more acid in response to a standard meal than those who do not, and the mean pH in the duodenal bulb may be lower than in controls. However, large numbers of patients with ulcers have gastric secretory rates within the normal range.

The hormone gastrin is a potent stimulus to stomach acid secretion. Although serum gastrin levels are about the same in ulcer patients and controls during fasting, it has been reported that ulcer patients tend to have a postprandial rise in serum gastrin greater than that of controls. In addition, when ulcer patients are stimulated by histamine, another potent stimulus to gastric secretion, there appears to be a positive correlation between the number of parietal cells and the amount of gastric juice secreted. Parietal cell HCl secretion also correlates very well with the pepsin-secreting capacity of the chief cells, and the relative roles of HCl and pepsin secretion in the genesis of duodenal ulcer is still unsettled. Parasympathetic (cholinergic) stimulation via the vagus appears to be more of a stimulus to pepsin production than is gastrin, and gastrin and vagal stimulation together have a synergistic effect in promoting stomach hypersecretion. It is also probable that activation of the proteolytic enzyme pepsin by gastric acid plays a significant role in the development of duodenal ulcer.

The total number of parietal cells is a significant factor in determining the acid-secreting capacity of the mucosa; this is apparently under genetic control and is probably mediated via the trophic hormone gastrin. However, although some ulcer patients have a strong family history for PUD, others do not. A failure in the feedback process by which high acid content in the antrum inhibits gastrin production has been suggested as a contributory cause, as has failure of the normal hormonal secretin mechanism by which acid duodenal contents inhibit the release of gastrin. However, the role of such abnormalities in causing ulcer remains unclear. The participation of histamine, the other potent stimulus to acid secretion in addition to gastrin, in the genesis of duodenal ulcer is not known. Studies have shown that patients with duodenal ulcer have the greatest rate of gastrin secretion during the night (in fact, during their REM periods; Chapter 15) and that the low point in the 24-hr secretion is early in the morning. This is correlated with the fact that ulcer patients are frequently awakened around 2 A.M. from sleep by pain but rarely experience it in the early morning hours of 6 or 7 A.M.

Although psychoemotional factors have long been thought to be related not only to the original development of peptic ulcer but to exacerbations in its course, there is no clear evidence that either psychoemotional makeup of the patients or "stress"-inducing life circumstances are different in PUD from those in any other chronic disorder. Nevertheless it is known that emotional factors have a great influence on gastrointestinal functions, both motor and secretory, and perhaps no study has yet been devised which adequately tests the hypothesis.

Assessment. Peptic ulcer disease is one of the disorders with a highly characteristic history of present illness: typical periods of exacerbations with longer remissions, the sequence of epigastric pain with onset about 2 hr after meals, and relief by taking food or antacids. The pain is most severe when the stomach is empty, typically 11 A.M., 4 P.M., and 9 to 10 P.M., and is steady and burning in quality. It is localized to the epigastrium below or slightly to the right of the xiphoid process. It is brought on or made worse by alcohol, coffee, spicy foods, and acid fruit drinks and is relieved within a very few minutes, or immediately, by taking milk, food, or antacid. Although drinking water often relieves the burning pain of reflux esophagitis, it seldom does for duodenal ulcer. In the longer term the pain is characteristically intermittent and may be absent for long periods of weeks to months, or even years.

Duodenal ulcer is a chronic disorder marked by remissions and exacerbations which may bear little if any evident relationship to external life events or the nature of the management regimen. Exacerbations occur most commonly in spring and fall. A course which is reported to be quite common is an early stage of relatively mild, short, readily controlled episodes separated by long intervals. With the passage of years the frequency, duration, and severity of attacks may increase and the responsiveness to treatment decline. On the whole, however, most patients avoid severe progression and the various complications of duodenal ulcer.

Subjective.   Symptoms are characteristically a burning or gnawing steady pain in the upper epigastrium, which may radiate to the back, and which develops about 2 to 3 hr after a meal and often awakens the patient in the middle of the night but is not present on morning awakening or before breakfast. Distress on awakening may indicate the development of outlet obstruction from edema or fibrotic scarring. Ulcer pain may be relieved by taking milk or other food and by antacids. There are a number of theories as to the actual cause of the pain in PUD. Some suggest that it is stimulation of gastric or duodenal pain receptors by the strong acid to which the excoriated area is exposed, especially 2–4 hr after meals. Others suggest that it is altered motility and reflex smooth muscle spasm underlying and surrounding the injured tissue. More likely both mechanisms are involved. The relief of pain after eating results from dilution and neutralization of acid and pepsin, which elevates the intragastric pH for about 2 hr. Following this period there is a major increase in acid–pepsin secretion in response to the ingested food, and intragastric pH declines as the food leaves the stomach. Other symptoms in ulcer may be pyrosis and water brash from an incompetent LES and esophageal reflux.

Objective.   Signs of PUD are tenderness to deep palpation in the high midline epigastrium and a positive stool test for occult blood. Upper gastrointestinal X-ray with a barium contrast medium may reveal prominent mucosal folds, an ulcer crater often in the proximal portion of the duodenal bulb, and if the ulcer is of long standing, distortion of the bulb from fibrotic scarring. Perhaps a quarter of patients with PUD as demonstrated radiographically may have relatively few or no symptoms. Fiberoptic endoscopy reliably establishes the presence of an ulcer which may not have been visible on X-ray, but the procedure is not without risks and is not necessary in the majority of patients. The hematocrit is measured for evidence of blood loss, and, because of the occasional association of hypercalcemia with PUD, serum calcium level may be determined.

Management.   A tendency to spontaneous healing over a period of about 6 weeks, followed by a relatively long remission, and then recurrence, all relatively independent of management regimen, is characteristic in PUD. The objectives of the treatment program are the relief of symptoms, promotion of healing, prevention of recurrence, and avoidance of complications. Sometimes it is the only first objective which can be reliably attained. The basic aim underlying the other objectives is to reduce the concentration of acid in the stomach.

The systematic hourly use of non-absorbable antacids is directed at the aim of maintaining gastric pH at or above 4.5, which is purported to decrease or eliminate the enzymatic action of pepsin; relieve pain; and may reduce the destructive effect of acid on gastric mucosa, although there has been little objective evidence indicating that antacids alter the long-term course of the disease significantly, aside from alleviating symptoms. Few controlled studies show that antacids facilitate ulcer healing, reduce the incidence of complications, or increase the length of remissions. Antacids taken on an empty stomach elevate intragastric pH for only a short time because of rapid emptying of the antacid from the stomach when food is not present. On the other hand, adequate doses of an effective antacid taken one hour after meals are reported to reduce intragastric acidity by substantial amounts for about 3 hr after the meal in some patients. Antacids in liquid form are considerably more effective than tablets of the same compounds.

A recent controlled double-blind study of a large-dose antacid regimen for patients with duodenal ulcer which has been confirmed by endoscopy indicates that in 28 of 36 patients treated with a liquid aluminum-magnesium hydroxide antacid there was complete healing of the ulcer in about one month, as compared with 17 of 38 patients treated with placebo liquids. The dosage schedule was 30 ml of the liquid at 1 and 3 hr after meals and at bedtime. The relief of symptoms was not greater in the antacid group than in the placebo control subjects. During the last week of the study, symptoms were not well correlated with the degree of healing, but both antacid and placebo groups experienced a decline in symptoms over the month of the study period. Patients who continued to smoke cigarets healed less well than nonsmokers. Thus in this study improved healing but no improved control of symptoms occurred with antacid as compared with placebo management of duodenal ulcer.

The absorbable alkali sodium bicarbonate ($NaHCO_3$) should not be used in ulcer management, since it contributes a heavy sodium load to the ECF, produces metabolic alkalemia, and induces a large rebound gastric hypersecretion. While calcium carbonate is an effective antacid, it adds a considerable calcium load to the ECF which may cause a number of metabolic abnormalities: hypercalcemia, elevated serum bicarbonate with metabolic alkalemia, hyperphosphatemia, and renal damage with azotemia. Also, it is reported to have the net result of increasing gastric acid production both by stimulating gastrin secretion, and by a direct action on HCl production by parietal cells.

Some nonabsorbable commercial antacids in common use are Mylanta, Riopan, and Maalox in which the active alkali ingredients are a mixture of aluminum and magnesium hydroxides; Gelusil contains magnesium trisilicate and aluminum hydroxide; and Amphojel is a preparation of aluminum hydroxide. In terms of acid buffering potency Mylanta is reported in some studies to be most effective, with Maalox next. Another study reporting buffering capacity of common antacids cites Delcid (alumnium and magnesium hydroxides), Ducon (calcium carbonate and aluminum and magnesium hydroxides), and Mylanta II as the three most effective (in decreasing order). Those antacids containing magnesium tend to have a laxative action, while aluminum-containing ones tend to be constipating. Thus many patients find that they need to use a combination of antacids to avoid excess effects in either direction. Riopan is low in Na^+ and therefore is often recommended for use by patients with sodium-retaining states such as congestive heart failure. Antacids, 15–30 ml, should be taken every hour between meals, beginning one hour after each meal, at bedtime, and in the middle of the night if the patient awakens with pain. Most of these antacids also come in tablet form, which, although patients tend to prefer it because of convenience, is not very effective. The tablets do not exert their action until they are hydrated by gastrointestinal secretions; this requires so much time that by the time it has occurred the antacid may have largely left the stomach. In all cases the dosage should be gradually tapered, as symptoms decline, to 15 to 30 ml 90 min after meals and at bedtime.

Anticholinergic agents, such as tincture of belladonna and atropine, antagonize the stimulating effects of acetylcholine on structures innervated by the parasympathetic (cholinergic) division of the autonomic nervous system. They have been used for a long time in the treatment of duodenal ulcer on the basis of the known vagal cholinergic (parasympathetic) stimulating effects on gastric acid secretion, increase in gastric motility, and elevation of gastrin output. Anticholinergic agents reduce gastric secretion in fasting ulcer patients if given in doses large enough to induce the side effect of dry mouth; however, it is reported that in the patient receiving antacids and small, frequent bland feedings, the medications do not further lower the output of stomach HCl and pepsin. Some studies indicate decreased frequency and severity of exacerbations and reduced incidence of complications with prolonged use of anticholinergics, while others do not. Propantheline, an anticholinergic having the actions of decreased gastrointestinal motility and secretion, has been used, but there is no evidence that it promotes healing. Some workers believe that the delay in gastric emptying caused by all anticholinergics promotes gastric retention to a deleterious extent, and has an adverse effect on stomach content of acid and pepsin, thus doing more harm than good.

The H_2 *receptor antagonist cimetidine* appears to markedly inhibit the gastric acid secretory response to both gastrin and histamine stimulation. Histamine is considered by some workers to be the final common intracellular pathway by which increased HCl secretion is mediated via whatever stimulus pathway, be it hormonal (gastrin) or neural (cholinergic). Cell membranes have on their surfaces both H_1 and H_2 receptors and it is suggested that histamine stimulates parietal cell HCl production by binding to the H_2 receptors. When these receptors are blocked by a chemical antagonist, such binding and stimulation cannot occur, and HCl production declines. Studies show that cimetidine accelerates the healing of duodenal ulcer, relieves symptoms, decreases complications, and brings about remissions.

Dietary intake should be self-selected, with the patient choosing those foods which agree with him and eliminating those which he has found to increase his symptoms. Meals should be small, perhaps more frequent, appetizing, and selected on the basis of the patient's preference. Alcohol should be eliminated because it has been demonstrated to damage the gastric mucosal barrier and to increase gastrin and acid production. Caffeine stimulates gastric secretion, so tea, coffee, and cola beverages should be taken in moderation, with attention to the exacerbation of symptoms they may produce. PUD incidence is higher in smokers than nonsmokers; studies have shown that smoking inhibits the release of bicarbonate from the pancreas (thus lowering the buffering action of pancreatic secretions in the duodenum) and delays healing of stomach ulcers. Aspirin has an adverse effect on ulcer healing so should be avoided. There is apparently no evidence that diet has any effect on any of the management goals provided the patient avoids those substances which he has found by experience make him less comfortable. Sedatives, tranquilizers, and/or psychotherapy probably do not affect the course of PUD, but may make the patient more comfortable in the psychoemotional sense and therefore may be of value in some patients. A regular daily program of vigorous physical exercise in some sport, such as swimming, that the patient enjoys, promotes general feelings of mental and physical well-being, relieves frustrations, and improves health status.

Complications of PUD. These include hemorrhage (the most common complication), perforation or penetration, and obstruction. In addition, a failure to respond to conservative management with an amelioration of signs and symptoms may be considered a complication. Although the great majority of patients with PUD respond satisfactorily to conservative medical management, the occurrence of one of the serious complications may provide an indication for surgery.

Hemorrhage occurs somewhat more often in gastric than duodenal ulcers, and may occur in either without prior evidence of PUD. Signs of bleeding are commonly melena, a decline in hematocrit, and hematemesis. If blood loss is large, a liter or more, then signs and symptoms of hemorrhagic shock may develop. The management is blood replacement, nasogastric suction, ice-water gastric lavage, and other components of the management of blood loss. Most patients do not require operative intervention unless bleeding is persistent or recurrent.

Perforation into the peritoneal cavity often occurs suddenly with rapid increase in steady severe pain, and may be accompanied by bleeding. Escape of gastric or duodenal contents into the peritoneal cavity may result in free air under the diaphragm as seen on X-ray of the abdomen, and a chemical peritonitis which produces peritoneal signs of direct and rebound tenderness, abdominal muscle rigidity, and decreased bowel sounds (ileus). If large amounts of chemicals have entered the peritoneal cavity there may be extensive "third spacing": extravastion of ECF through capillaries of the peritoneum into the peritoneal cavity, leading to hypovolemia and hypotension. In this case surgery is often appropriate. With conservative management, the perforation site may become sealed off by the peritoneum, and after the acute episode the patient may show marked amelioration of signs and symptoms. Replacement of intravascular third space losses, continuous nasogastric suction, and antibiotics are important aspects of treatment.

Penetration of an ulcer into adjacent structures, as opposed to free perforation, may occur. In the case of a duodenal ulcer the penetration is often to the pancreas and less often into the biliary tract or colon. Symptoms of penetration are an increase in the severity and constancy of the pain, with radiation to the back, abdomen, or chest. Serum amylase may be elevated.

Gastric outlet obstruction occurs more often in duodenal ulcers that have been present for many years, and the symptoms and signs of obstruction are more likely to develop gradually than be of sudden onset. The intensity of symptoms and signs is related to the rapidity with which obstruction develops, and to its degree of completeness. The processes underlying the development of obstruction are two: edema, which is associated with a phase of active local tissue destruction in the ulcer; and the more gradual development of stenosis from fibrotic scar tissue formed during usually numerous phases of healing. The smooth muscle tissue of the antrum is capable of producing very strong contractions and therefore may be able to overcome marked outlet narrowing for a long time. In most cases the symptoms and signs of obstruction develop over weeks or months: anorexia, nausea and vomiting, progressive loss of weight, constipation, and epigastric distress and sensations of fullness during and after eating are the common ones. Dilation of the stomach usually occurs gradually as the obstruction becomes more severe.

The outcome of this complication depends on whether the obstruction is caused by edema, and is therefore reversible; or by stenotic scarring, where it is structural and therefore not reversible. The management is continuous nasogastric aspiration, maintenance of fluid and electrolyte balance, and assessment of the volume of residual gastric contents at intervals after the acute phase has passed (72 hr). Obstruction from edema often resolves spontaneously, while fibrotic stenosis does not. Surgery would be indicated in the latter case.

Disorders of the Small Intestine

Regional Enteritis (Crohn's Disease)

Crohn's disease is a chronic, usually relapsing, granulomatous inflammatory process involving all the layers of the gut wall and affecting persons of all ages. Although it may involve any portion of the gastrointestinal tract, it usually occurs in the small intestine, especially the terminal ileum. The age of onset is typically the mid-twenties, although it may begin at any age from childhood to old age.

Cause

The cause is not known but it is probably multifactorial, involving both hereditary and environmental factors. Although no bacterial, viral, or fungal agent has ever been demonstrated, its characteristic changes of inflammation and granuloma formation suggest some *infectious* cause, although there is no objective evidence for this. Many investigators have suggested an *immunologic* basis for the disease, including autoimmune responses or a hypersensitivity reaction. Abnormalities in both humoral and cell-mediated immunity have been cited in patients with Crohn's, but these may be merely an expression of immune system response to the disease, rather than part of the cause. Antinuclear antibodies are said to be present in perhaps one fifth of patients with the disease, and in more of their relatives than in control groups. Some families show a high incidence of both Crohn's and chronic ulcerative colitis, indicating some relation between the two disorders, and a genetic factor in both. The affected intestinal tissue in Crohn's is edematous and has a high concentration of lymphocytes, plasma cells, and eosinophils—all changes characteristic of immune-allergic responses. *Genetic* factors do appear to be contributory; it sometimes shows a familial incidence and has a higher incidence in Jews. *Social and economic factors* seem to be involved in that it is more a disease of white, urban, educated individuals than others. Some authors suggest that the absorption of some *irritant or otherwise noxious agent* in the small intestine, which is absorbed from the contents of the terminal ileum and causes blockage of the lacteals, may be involved in the cause. Both endogenous substances, such as a bile component, and exogenous ones, taken into the body from the environment in increasing amounts as widespread environmental pollution has developed over the last 10 to 20 years, have been suspected in the etiology. *Psychoemotional* precipitating factors have been cited as contributing to the onset and exacerbations of Crohn's; many persons with the disorder sometimes manifest psychiatric abnormalities, but whether this is more the case in Crohn's than in other debilitating chronic relapsing diseases is debatable. Primarily a disease of Western cultures, Crohn's was essentially unknown before the early 1930s but now appears to be greatly on the increase both in this country and abroad, having tripled in frequency in the past decade.

Abnormalities

The initial abnormality is presumed to be an obstructive process, initiated by an unknown factor, that occurs in the lacteals of the intestinal wall and leads to blockage of the lymphatics, nuclear infiltration, edema, and vascular congestion.

The process appears to be an inflammatory one that eventually involves all layers of the affected areas of the intestine, causing erythema, edema, and gross swelling as well as affecting lymph nodes and mesentery. The affected portions of bowel are edematous and hyperemic, with leukocyte infiltrations in the initial stage; this is succeeded by cellular infiltrates, a proliferative thickening and rigidity of the wall, and narrowing of the lumen by fibrosis. The stenotic narrowing may create an obstruction. The mucosa ulcerates, is destroyed, and is replaced with granulation tissue. The ulcerations may penetrate the full thickness of the wall leading to fistulas and abscesses and a matting together of adjacent segments of intestine. Lymph channels become dilated because of obstruction; the mesentery is thickened and mesenteric fat is drawn in irregular folds over the serosal layer. Characteristic of Crohn's is that segments of severely affected intestine may be interposed between normal-appearing ones.

Assessment

Symptoms and signs are extremely variable not only from patient to patient, but in a single individual at a given time and over the course of the disease. Remissions and relapses are characteristic.

Subjective. Early symptoms tend to be mild and rather nonspecific. The patient may describe right lower abdominal discomfort or a steady aching pain; a history of easy fatigability, weakness and malaise; weight loss; increasing diarrhea which does not contain gross blood, preceded by colicky pain; and anorexia, nausea, and vomiting. Diarrhea and abdominal distress are the first complaints in many patients, and in most they are usually mild for some time.

Objective. There may be mild iron-deficiency anemia, leukocytosis, elevated erythrocyte sedimentation rate, and a heme-positive stool test; there may be a tender palpable mass in the right lower quadrant. A continuous or intermittent low-grade fever is frequent. In a patient receiving regular health checkups, gradual documented weight loss may be the earliest manifestation. A polyarticular arthritis involving the large joints or spine occurs in a minority of patients. With the passage of time and progression of the disease the pain becomes more severe, the diarrhea more persistent, and weight loss and right lower quadrant tenderness and mass more marked. Abdominal and rectal fistulas or anal fissures may develop.

Contrast X-ray of the small intestine from first below and then above reveals segmental distribution of involvement; fissures, strictures with proximal dilation, fistulas, mucous membrane ulcerations, and a cobblestone appearance.

Complications

Intestinal obstruction from acute inflammatory proliferation and edema, and more chronic fibrosis and thickening, is a relatively frequent complication. Obstruction signs and symptoms may be intermittent because of fluctuations in the degree of edema and inflammation. Abdominal abscesses and fistulas are second in frequency; and perianal, anal, and rectal fistulas and abscesses next. Hemorrhage and perforation also occur. Malabsorption is relatively common because of impairment of the digestive and absorptive functions of the small intestine.

Crohn's disease is characterized by a number of systemic manifestations, but less so than chronic ulcerative colitis. Diseases of the skin, eye, and joints are not uncommon, including erythema nodosum, ankylosing spondylitis, asymmetric polyarticular arthritis, eczema, and uveitis. Some of these extraintestinal manifestations appear to correlate with the degree of activity of the intestinal disease. Liver disease is reported to occur eventually in the majority of Crohn's patients and takes a number of forms in which there is inflammation and injury of bile ducts both within and outside the liver. Gastrointestinal malignancy and the complications of treatment with adrenal glucocorticoids are said to contribute to the reduced life expectancy of patients with Crohn's.

Management

Care of patients with regional enteritis involves a large commitment of time and energy because of their psychoemotional responses to the disease and the necessity for educating them and involving their families. Adequate rest and a palatable nutritious diet is important, especially during exacerbations. Diphenoxylate is useful in controlling abdominal pain and diarrhea. Sulfasalazine may be useful in maintenance; its action is mainly antiinflammatory but also antibacterial. Adrenal glucocorticoids are useful in controlling acute worsenings when simpler measures have failed, and often relieve diarrhea, fever, and abdominal pain, but there is no evidence that they prevent complications or alter the long-term course. They are then gradually tapered to the dose that is just adequate to control the symptoms and signs. The major problem in Crohn's is maintenance of adequate nutrition. Many authors suggest that surgery be postponed as long as possible because of the almost inevitable recurrences following operations for obstruction, but it often becomes necessary when more conservative measures are inadequate to control intractable manifestations of the disease.

Disorders of the Colon

Irritable Colon (Functional Bowel Syndrome)

This disorder of motility of the large intestine is the most common of all the gastrointestinal disorders, accounting for perhaps half of the gastrointestinal complaints, and is probably equal to the common cold as a cause of minor illness. Patients experience periods of abdominal pain, alternating constipation and diarrhea, abdominal distention and flatulence, small diameter stools (regardless of consistency), and mucus in the stool.

Cause

The cause is not known, but the relation between this functional disorder and life "stress" and psychoemotional tension has been speculated about and explored in a variety of clinical studies for many years. Whatever the cause(s) may be, the signs and symptoms are the consequence of disordered motility in the large intestine. In addition, some studies suggest that motor activity of the small intestine is likewise abnormal. To state that abnormal intestinal motility is often observed in patients with psychoemotional disorders is a far different thing from stating that psychoemotional disorders are the *cause* of abnormalities of intestinal motility. It may be simply that they are but two manifestations of a more fundamental neural disorder involving the brainstem and limbic centers (both parasympathetic and sympathetic) which regulate both visceral function and emotional state. Thus to state that psychoemotional disorders are often *present in association with* the irritable colon syndrome would be more appropriate to the present level of knowledge concerning the relationship.

Some authors separate the irritable colon syndrome into two categories: the spastic colon type, in which the outstanding symptom is abdominal distress and pain, with predominant constipation; and the painless diarrhea type, in which pain is rare and diarrhea may be chronic or intermittent. Other authors are persuaded that most patients, perhaps three fourths, manifest a mixed type with alternating diarrhea and constipation with pain.

It is useful to recognize that intestinal hypermotility can be associated with either constipation or diarrhea, depending on whether the hypermotility is propulsive or not. If hypermotility is *propulsive* (peristaltic) then the intestinal contents are speeded along the lumen so rapidly that resorption of water and electrolytes does not occur to an adequate degree, and a copious watery diarrhea is the result. If the hypermotility is *nonpropulsive* (nonperistaltic) but is rather segmental and spastic, then pain and slowing of the passage of intestinal contents results, with reduction in mass, and a dry hard quality from too long retention in the colon, resulting in constipation.

Irritable bowel syndrome occurs very often in conjunction with the habit of aerophagia (air swallowing) which contributed markedly to the symptoms of distention, pressure sensations and flatulence of which these patients complain. Aerophagia contributes to the splenic flexure syndrome which may be seen in association with irritable bowel syndrome. It is characterized by left upper quadrant distress or, in the less frequent hepatic flexure syndrome, with right upper quadrant discomfort, which may be mistaken for gallbladder disease. Swallowed air and intestinal gas become trapped at the sharp turns in these areas of the colon. A strong propulsive peristaltic wave may push the gas (and feces, if present) against a strong spastic (nonpropulsive) segmentation beyond the lumen contents. This lack of motor coordination between adjacent segments of colon produces distressing abdominal symptoms.

It has been reported that different characteristic emotional states are correlated with, or accompany, the two phases of constipation and diarrhea. The emotional state accompanying the diarrhea is said to be an attitude of passive dependence and helplessness, guilt, and depression; the emotional state of the constipation phase has been described as confident, assertive, and independent. Both the somatic and the emotional state during diarrhea may be manifestations of activation of cholinergic (trophotropic) brainstem and limbic structures, while the somatic and emotional state correlating with the constipation phase may represent adrenergic sympathetic (ergotrophic) brainstem and limbic system activation.

Assessment

Symptoms are diffuse abdominal distress, often greatest in the left lower quadrant; periodic distention which patients call "bloating"; the pain may be relieved by defecation or expelling flatus; constipation alternating with diarrhea; and flatulence.

Signs are small hard pellet-like stools with much mucus in the constipated phase, long thin ribbonlike feces in the diarrhetic phase, palpable tender sigmoid, and enlarged areas of tympany over the ascending and transverse colon. Sigmoidoscopic examination may reveal hyperemia, mucus, and spasm at the rectosigmoid curve without other abnormalities. Laboratory and X-ray examinations are normal.

Management

A thorough workup may be performed if for no other reason than to be able confidently to assure these patients that there is no known dread disease present as the cause of their symptoms, to reassure them as to the benign (although annoying) course the illness will follow, and that it does not represent a prelude to inflammatory or malignant bowel disease. Examination and discussion of patients' life styles and their reaction to it is essential. Some patients will show a marked exacerbation of symptoms correlating with life stresses, while others will not. Patient teaching concerning the emotional correlates of the symptoms is helpful. The questions "How are things at home?" (or "at work?") and "Is there anything else you'd like to tell me?" are useful openers to such discussions, and patients should be given the time and receptive interest to encourage them to ventilate their feelings.

Management of the constipation is of central importance. The causes of constipation are almost always (1) inadequate dietary bulk; (2) ignoring the physical symptoms of the need to defecate so that feces become hard, dry, and difficult to expel (dyschezia), which may lead to painful anal fissures and hemorrhoids; (3) laxative and enema use; and (4) lack of exercise and adequate fluid intake. Painful anal lesions may be treated with Anusol-HC suppositories twice a day for 5 or 6 days, sitz baths, and stool softeners such as diocytl sodium succinate. Laxatives and enemas are to be *proscribed*. Dietary changes include whole grain cereals and bread, eliminating refined and processed foods, increased fresh and raw fruits and vegetable intake, with two teaspoons of unprocessed bran taken with each meal. Habit conditioning involves taking time after breakfast to heed and respond to the defecation reflex, and increased regular vigorous physical activity. Patients should be assured that a daily stool is not necessary, and that restoration of normal colon motility may take several weeks. While dietary habits are being changed daily psyllium preparation in water may be helpful, or suggested for patients who resist dietary change.

Diverticulosis

Diverticula are small herniations or outpouchings of the mucosal and submucosal layers of the colon through the muscular layers in areas where the latter are penetrated by small arteries. They are almost always multiple and in most patients occur in the distal colon and sigmoid, though occasionally they may occur throughout the colon. They are common and the incidence increases with age; perhaps half the people 65 or more have them, and apparently in most individuals they do not lead to symptoms.

Cause

Studies indicate that diverticula are probably caused by increased pressure within the lumen of the colon. In patients who have diverticulosis it appears that the mixing movements of the colon (rhythmic segmentation) are strong enough to close off adjacent segments of the colon completely; pressures within the closed segments increase as contraction occurs, and the pressure forces small outpocketings of gut lining through defects in the muscular layer where small arteries enter the muscularis. The cause of the increased strength of segmental motility appears to be the highly refined and excessively processed dietary intake of Western cultures, which fails to provide adequate roughage for normal fecal bulk. There is evidence that in order for the local coordinating reflexes of the myenteric plexus and appropriate intrinsic smooth muscle contractility to function in a normal and productive manner, adequate bulk to produce some degree of distention of the gut wall, and therefore to provide adequate stimuli for contraction, is required. Thus, with little colonic residue, increased force of contractions is necessary to move the small volume of colon contents along the lumen. Hypertrophy of the smooth muscle layers of the colon are reported to precede the development of diverticula. Diverticulosis apparently does not occur in countries where dietary habits provide adequate fiber from whole grains, and fresh and raw fruits and vegetables. Laboratory animals given a low residue diet develop diverticula. Unless complications occur, diverticulosis may be largely asymptomatic.

Complications

Complications of diverticula are inflammation within and around the outpouchings (diverticulitis) and bleeding. Bacteria and fecal material are probably constantly present within the herniations. The blood supply to the diverticulum may be compressed or occluded, which would predispose it to becoming ulcerated, inflamed, and infected; or partial obstruction of the neck of the protrusion may occur with the same result. The consequence may be formation of a small abscess and localized peritoneal infection and inflammation. Patchy necrosis and miniperforations may occur, leading to peridiverticular abscesses and bleeding. As the inflammations resolve and scar tissue forms, fibrosis and partial obstructions may develop. Degrees of severity in this sequence of events vary along a continuum from a low-grade inflammation and localized infection to a more widespread infection, larger perforation, extensive bleeding, and peritonitis.

Assessment

Subjective. Often patients relate a long history of constipation, or alternating constipation and diarrhea. There may be complaints of flatulence, periodic abdominal distention and distress, and/or lower left quadrant cramping abdominal pain, especially associated with meals and defecation. These symptoms often occur in patients with the irritable colon syndrome and in fact diverticulosis may be a sequel to that disorder. Acute diverticulitis is associated with more severe pain.

Objective. The sigmoid colon may be palpable as a firm tender mass during acute exacerbation of symptoms. Where microperforation and peridiverticular infection has occurred there may be rebound tenderness, guarding, elevated white blood count, and fever; rectal examination may elicit pain and show occult blood in the stool. When the acute phase has resolved barium enema and sigmoidoscopy is necessary to rule out malignancy of the colon, especially when there is a history of weight loss. Both diverticulosis and colon neoplasm occur in the same age group and give rise to similar symptoms. In diverticulosis sigmoidoscopy often does not show any abnormality, and the openings of the diverticula generally are not visible. X-ray shows a characteristic "sawtooth" appearance of the mucosa, deformities from fibrosis which developed as the acute inflammation resolves, and many small surface outpouchings, especially on the wall of the descending colon.

Management

Diverticulosis which is associated with the signs and symptoms of the irritable colon syndrome requires no treatment other than indicated for the syndrome (see above). In acute, mild diverticulitis antibiotics, dioctyl sodium succinate to soften the stool, bed rest, and oral liquids may be used. Long-term management of the chronic symptomatic disorder consists of a natural high-residue diet, supplemented with nonprocessed bran, adequate fluid intake, and regular exercise.

Chronic Ulcerative Colitis (CUC)

This is a chronic relapsing inflammatory disease of the colon, of unknown cause, characterized by uniform ulceration and hyperemia of the involved rectal and colon mucosa and submucosa, and manifesting abdominal pain and recurrent bloody diarrhea. There are usually a number of associated nonintestinal disorders. The incidence is greater in whites, highest in Jews, more prevalent in urban than rural areas, and more common in Western nations. It appears to be increasing in frequency, and often, with Crohn's disease of the colon (granulomatous colitis), has a familial occurrence. Both CUC and Crohn's of the colon have many aspects in common and they may represent differences in response to the same causative factors. CUC is several times more common than granulomatous colitis.

Cause

The cause is unknown, though many theories have been proposed, including immune responses, bacterial infection, allergic (hypersensitivity) reactions, and ingestion of toxic substances. Abnormalities of cell-mediated immune responses have been implicated in both CUC and Crohn's of the colon on the basis of association of these diseases with others of suspected autoimmune etiology (e.g., arthritis, erythema nodosum, uveitis), and because of the presence of lymphocytes with cytotoxic activity, antibody to colon epithelium, and other atypical cellular and humoral components in the patients' blood.

Psychoemotional factors have been implicated in the cause; some CUC patients seem to show traits of hostility, dependence, immaturity, and disturbed interpersonal relationships. On the other hand, about half of patients appear to have normal psychoemotional characteristics. It is understandable that patients with a disease such as CUC would experience adverse psychoemotional responses to the pain, debility, financial loss, and inconvenience which it causes.

Abnormalities

The mucosa and submucosa of the colon show intense hyperemia and vascular congestion, with edema, bleeding, infiltration of white blood cells, and ulcerations. In the early stages there is diffuse erythema and the granular-appearing mucosa bleeds readily with slight mechanical stimulation or even spontaneously. The degree of involvement of the colon varies from a short portion of the rectum to the entire colon; characteristically in an affected segment the abnormalities are uniform throughout its circumference. Later, or in more severe disease, pitting and ulcerations of the mucosa develop, the bowel wall becomes thinned, and the colon shortens apparently primarily because of spasm of the longitudinal muscle layer. Numerous small structures called pseudopolyps, or inflammatory polyps, develop in the mucosa as a result of deep erosions occurring in a circular area around patches of edematous inflamed mucosa; they are found uniformly distributed throughout affected areas of the colon. Multiple small abscesses containing infiltrates of white cells develop in the crypts of the colon and later may coalesce and eventually ulcerate. The submocosa and muscular layers become involved in more severe disease, and the haustra disappear.

Correlated with the structural changes are alterations in function. Absorption of fluid, electrolytes, and the products of digestion is impaired; the loss of the haustrations, which act as compartments to retard the progression of colon contents toward the rectum, combines with the failure of absorption, to produce frequent liquid stools. Motility is markedly decreased in CUC; there are very few smooth muscle contractions to retard the progression of the liquid contents. The diarrhea is promoted more by sheer volume of the intestinal contents, lack of retardation by haustral compartments, and the effects of gravity in the upright posture, than by the intestinal hypermotility which characterizes the diarrhea of many other forms of bowel disease.

Assessment

Diarrhetic stools contain pus, blood, and mucus; there is often fever; weight loss can be documented; abdominal pain is characteristic; and there is usually diffuse abdominal tenderness and sometimes distention. Tachycardia, pallor, anemia, elevated white blood count and erythrocyte sedimentation rate, dehydration, electrolyte imbalance, and hypoalbuminemia may all be present. In an acute severe onset, or exacerbation, some or all of these signs and symptoms may be present, but in most patients the symptoms are mild with only a few stools per day, no findings on physical examination, and normal laboratory values. Thus the range of manifestations is wide. The diagnosis is established by a proctosigmoidoscopic examination with biopsy and barium contrast colon X-ray.

Some authors consider there to be three clinical forms of CUC: ulcerative proctitis, ordinary ulcerative colitis, and fulminant ulcerative colitis. In ulcerative proctitis the characteristic lesions described above occur only in the rectum and subsequently extend to other areas of the colon in a third of patients; but in the majority of this group there are no manifestations of illness outside the rectum. Ordinary ulcerative colitis may have a gradual onset with slight bloody diarrhea or a much more severe initial attack with rapid spreading to involve major portions of the colon. In most patients the disease is first manifested in the rectum and spreads upward; the progression may be slow or rapid. The subsequent course for most patients is a chronic relapsing one with asymptomatic phases of months to years being interspersed with symptomatic periods of weeks. The frequency and severity of exacerbations and complications correlate with the extent of involvement of the colon.

The third form, acute fulminant ulcerative colitis, usually but not always occurs as an initial attack, and in it the acute inflammatory and destructive tissue process involves all of the layers of the colon. It is characterized by tachycardia, fever, dehydration, loss of electrolytes, moderate to small amounts of bloody diarrhea, abdominal pain, leukocytosis, hypoalbuminemia, and absence of bowel sounds. In the complication of toxic megacolon the colon becomes greatly dilated and distended with gas as a result of severe impairment of neuromuscular function in the transverse colon. Excessive use of intestinal motility depressants such as diphenoxylate or anticholinergics is said to sometimes precipitate this condition. Some writers consider emergency removal of the colon to be the definitive treatment for this form. Others consider that prompt appropriate conservative management with fluid and electrolyte replacements and ACTH or adrenal steroids, should be given a trial first. The mortality rate of toxic megacolon is quite high; cause of death is perforation, peritonitis, and septic shock. It is said occasionally to resolve spontaneously.

Management

During remissions the patient may take a low-residue or self-selected normal diet, depending on severity of the disease. Medications include maintenance sulfasalazine, which provides an antiinflammatory action from the aminosalicylic acid, and an antibacterial action from the sulfapyridine. Antispasmodics and anticholinergics (paregoric, diphenoxylate and atropine, tincture of belladonna) are often used. Some workers believe them to be helpful, while others suggest that they may not be, or may promote toxic megacolon. Rectal instillations of adrenal steroids appear to induce and maintain remissions when the disease is limited to the rectosigmoid. During a severe initial onset or when serious relapse occurs hospitalization is indicated; the patient is given intravenous ACTH or adrenal steroids, and intravenous alimentation sometimes is prescribed to permit complete "rest" of the colon. The adrenal steroids exert an antiinflammatory action by stabilizing cell and lysosomal membranes, reducing capillary permeability and edema, preventing in-migration of leukocytes, and inhibiting proliferation of fibroblasts. The response is a reduction in fever, abdominal pain, diarrhea, and anorexia. Following improvement steroids are given orally, and dietary intake and sulfasalazine are resumed. Eventually steroids are tapered and if possible finally withdrawn. The immunosuppressive agent azathioprine is used by some workers and may permit reduction of steroid dosage in those patients whose disease is severe enough to require maintenance steroids; it is not known whether azathioprine prolongs remissions.

Carcinoma of the colon is a complication of CUC; the risk is greater in those patients with severe disease involving large portions of the colon, especially if the onset was at a young age; the risk then increases with duration of the disease.

Colectomy may be necessary in the advent of toxic megacolon, as mentioned above; it is sometimes indicated also for patients who have severe disease unresponsive to medical management. Other indications are malignancy, hemorrhage, and obstruction from stricture.

Acute Intestinal Obstruction

Intestinal obstruction may result from a mechanical block to the passage of intestinal contents toward the anus; or from a failure of normal intestinal peristalsis, causing hypomotility. In either case distention of the intestinal lumen with fluid and gas proximal to the affected area is the result. Although the majority of all intestinal obstructions result from adynamic ileus, probably most severe obstruction is caused by mechanical factors.

Mechanisms of Obstruction

Mechanical Obstruction

Mechanical obstruction is of three types: (1) *Extramural (extrinsic)* obstruction is the most common type of mechanical obstruction. In this form, the whole circumference of the intestine, and hence the lumen, is constricted from some cause outside the intestine itself; examples are *herniation* of the intestine through a defect in the body wall (ventral, umbilical, femoral, inguinal), *adhesions* as a consequence of inflammation or prior abdominal operation, and *volvulus*, a twisting of the intestine upon itself. (2) *Mural (intrinsic)* obstruction is an occlusion of the intestinal lumen caused by some abnormality within the wall of the intestine itself: the inflammation and fibrosis of regional enteritis or diverticulitis, a tumor, and narrowing of a previous surgical anastomosis are examples of this type. (3) The least common type of mechanical obstruction is *intramural (intraluminal)* in which the lumen is occluded by some object within it, e.g., a

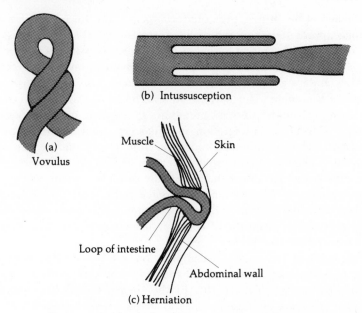

(b) Intussusception

(a) Vovulus

Muscle Skin

Loop of intestine

Abdominal wall

(c) Herniation

Figure 11-2. (a) Volvulus; (b) intussusception; (c) herniation.

foreign body, impacted feces, parasites, or intussusception (a telescoping of the intestine into itself).

In addition to this classification there are subtypes. Mechanical intestinal obstruction may be *complete* or *partial*, and it may develop rapidly (*acute*) or more gradually (*subacute*). Partial or incomplete obstructions sometimes resolve with conservative management. When there is compression or occlusion of the blood supply to a portion of the obstructed intestine, then *strangulation* is said to exist, as in a strangulated hernia, when a loop of intestine has slipped through an opening in the body wall, as opposed to a *simple* obstruction in which the vascular flow is intact initially and only becomes compromised later as pressure within the intestinal lumen increases, compressing vessels. In a strangulated obstruction, ischemia of the affected intestinal wall develops rapidly, leading to necrosis and infarction of the segment of intestine to which the blood flow is occluded. The consequence is often perforation of the wall and peritonitis from escape of intestinal contents into the peritoneum.

Another category of mechanical obstruction is the *closed loop* type; this is one in which there is a segment of unobstructed intestine interposed between two areas of occlusion; volvulus and incarcerated hernia are examples. In this situation the pressure of accumulating gases (from bacterial action) and fluid (secreted into the lumen by the isolated segment of gut) rises and is unable to equalize by movement in the proximal direction, as can occur in an ordinary obstruction. For this reason, intestinal decompression by means of a swallowed nasoduodenal tube, although it can lower pressure in the area proximal to the obstruction, cannot do so within the blind loop itself. As a result, the combination of increasing distention of the lumen and vascular compression at either end of the blind loop may lead quite rapidly to the sequence of ischemia, infarction, perforation, and peritonitis.

The most common causes of mechanical obstruction of the small intestine are hernias and adhesions, while in the large intestine carcinoma, volvulus, and diverticulitis are more frequent.

Adynamic (Paralytic) Ileus

Adynamic (paralytic) ileus is a failure of peristalsis because of decreased propulsive contractions of the intestinal smooth muscle, thus the normal progression of intestinal contents is slowed or stopped. It is a relatively common disorder which may occur secondary to a wide variety of injuries and systemic illnesses: physical or chemical peritoneal injury (as from blood in the peritoneum or digestive enzymes or bacterial contamination entering the peritoneal cavity from the gut lumen); surgery and other trauma; myocardial infarction; pneumonia; hypokalemia; gut ischemia from vascular insufficiency; sepsis; and others. Postoperative atony and peritonitis are the two most frequent causes.

The processes involved in the production of adynamic ileus from these various causative agents have not been clearly demonstrated. Possibilities include a direct suppression of inherent smooth muscle contractility; inhibition of the intrinsic (cholinergic) nerve supply of the smooth muscle; or a combination of decreased cholinergic (parasympathetic) and increased adrenergic (sympathetic) stimuli to the intestinal smooth muscle, via the extrinsic autonomic innervation. Yet another etiologic factor is suggested to be high levels of circulating catecholamines (norepinephrine and epinephrine), from both adrenergic nerve endings and adrenal medulla, occurring as a result of the prior injury or illness. Strong sympathetic autonomic inhibition of intestinal motility is well known to result from physiologic damage of various sorts.

Mechanical obstruction and adynamic ileus are related to each other in such a way that one may lead to the other. In the ileus of postoperative visceral atony, distention of a coil of intestine by secretions may cause it to bend or twist sharply upon itself, leading to mechanical obstruction; and an initial local mechanical obstruction leads to increased intraluminal pressure from accumulation of fluid and gas, then distention, and finally to a more generalized inhibition of neuromuscular tone resulting in adynamic ileus.

Consequences of Obstruction, Regardless of Cause

The intestine becomes distended with gas and fluid. The source of the gas is probably largely swallowed air but also is produced by the action of bacteria on the stagnating intestinal contents. The source of the fluid is not only the several thousand milliliters of gastrointestinal secretions normally entering the lumen from proximally in the tract (salivary, gastric, pancreatic, bile, and ingested fluids) but also an influx of water and electrolytes from the ECF into the lumen which occurs as a result of the obstruction itself. Thus not only cannot resorption of the normal gastrointestinal secretions occur farther on in the tract, as would occur under normal conditions, but even more electrolytes and water leave the ECF and fill the lumen because of the obstruction. Hypotension and hypovolemic shock often develop because of this "third spacing," and if ECF deficits are not replaced, prerenal azotemia may occur from inadequate renal perfusion as described in Chapters 1 and 10. In some forms of intestinal obstruction, persistent vomiting occurs, which further depletes ECF electrolytes and fluid.

The reasons for the influx of ECF from capillaries into gut lumen in acute obstruction are not well understood, but it appears to involve an impairment of transport of Na$^+$ from the intestinal lumen into the blood, perhaps because of abnormalities in mucosal capillaries induced by the obstruction. As Na$^+$ transport from gut to blood declines, water remains in the lumen with it. The consequence is dehydration, hypovolemia, and a sequestration of electrolytes and water within the gut lumen. The collecting gas and fluid produce increasing distention. As the lumen becomes more and more distended, pressure within it increases greatly, and blood flow within the wall becomes impaired. This causes a further decrease of electrolyte and water transport from gut lumen to ECF and the distention increases. Impaired blood flow to the intestine promotes local edema and loss of selective permeability, and the toxic products of bacterial decomposition not only enter the blood but diffuse into the peritoneum. As pressure rises in the lumen, venous outflow is compromised first, causing hyperemia, edema, and vascular congestion; later, further increases in pressure compromise arterial inflow with resulting ischemic hypoxia and necrosis. As distention increases, intraabdominal pressure does so as well, and respiratory excursions of the diaphragm are impaired, resulting in a decrease in alveolar ventilation, so that systemic hypoxemia may develop.

Assessment

The signs and symptoms of intestinal obstruction differ to some degree depending on whether it is adynamic ileus or mechanical obstruction, and whether the small or large intestine is affected.

Adynamic Ileus

There will generally be present an immediately predisposing condition, such as prior surgery, a severe systemic illness or injury, or some condition causing peritonitis, so that ileus comprises a complication of the underlying condition. The patient generally does not experience the colicky pain characteristic of mechanical obstruction, but there may be complaints of the discomfort of general abdominal distention. Vomiting of bile and gastric contents is common. There will probably not be passage of gas or feces. The abdomen will be distended and bowel sounds may be decreased or absent.

Small Intestine

The higher in the small intestine the obstruction, the less the abdominal distention and the more the vomiting. The patient may complain of epigastric and periumbilical colicky pain, and there may be the high-pitched pinging sounds characteristic of obstructive borborygmi which coincide with the pain. There may not be marked tenderness or rigidity early. Passage of loose stool and flatus may occur early in the course, but eventually obstipation develops.

With obstruction lower in the small intestine, vomiting may be less, and tympany to percussion and distention more, marked. The emesis may have a fecal character because of bacterial action on the upper stagnant intestinal contents. As time passes, the colicky pain gives way to more constant generalized pain, increasing distention occurs, bowel sounds diminish, and the peritoneal signs of direct and rebound tenderness and abdominal rigidity develop, along with signs of hypovolemia and hypotension. There may be a tender palpable abdominal mass.

Large Intestine

Abdominal distention and early obstipation are most marked here. Bowel sounds are lower pitched and less frequent and the pain may be lower in the abdomen. Vomiting occurs later and there may be a palpable mass, and blood on rectal examination.

X-ray may reveal proximally distended loops of intestine, the presence of air–fluid levels, and a decrease of gas in the colon distal to the obstruction.

Management

Management of mechanical obstruction consists of replacement of fluid and electrolyte losses, intestinal decompression with nasoduodenal suction, antibiotics, and operative correction of the obstruction, if it is complete. In adynamic ileus, treatment of the underlying disorders, fluid and electrolyte replacement, and intestinal decompression may suffice. In both cases oral intake is withheld. Where strangulation has occurred, mortality is higher than where it has not.

REFERENCES

References for Chapter 11 are included with those at the end of Chapter 12.

CHAPTER TWELVE

Disorders of the Liver, Gallbladder, and Exocrine Pancreas

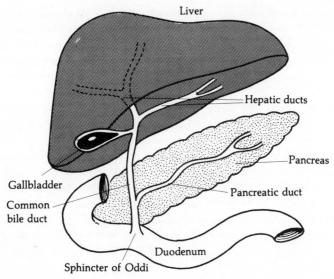

Liver

Hepatic ducts

Pancreas

Gallbladder

Pancreatic duct

Common
bile duct

Duodenum

Sphincter of Oddi

Figure 12-1. Anatomic relationship of liver, gall bladder, pancreas, ducts, and duodenum.

NORMAL FUNCTION OF LIVER, GALLBLADDER, AND EXOCRINE PANCREAS

Anatomic relations of liver, gallbladder, pancreas, and duodenum are shown in Figure 12-1.

Liver, Bile, and Gallbladder

The liver performs multiple complex functions in addition to the formation of bile; it regulates glucose levels in the blood by its glucostatic action of storing glycogen and releasing it as glucose as needed; it degrades hormones, drugs, and other substances; it forms the plasma proteins; it produces urea and ketones; it is involved in many aspects of fat metabolism.

Bile is secreted by cells of the liver at a volume of about 700 ml/24 hr, into small intrahepatic bile canaliculi which come together and exit from the liver as the right and left hepatic ducts. These fuse to form the common bile duct which drains into the duodenum either close to, or more frequently in conjunction with, the pancreatic duct. The sphincter of Oddi, which controls the exit of bile from the common duct into the duodenum, is usually closed when a person is not eating, and bile flows into the gallbladder and is stored. The capacity of the gallbladder is small—about 65 ml; it is able to store much of the bile secreted by the liver because it resorbs fluid and electrolytes from it. During a meal the sphincter relaxes and bile enters the duodenum from the common duct. Then when food begins entering the duodenum, cholecystokinin-pancreozymin (CCK-PZ) from the intestinal mucosa causes the gallbladder to contract and empty. Functions of the gallbladder are bile storage, bile acidification, and resorption of water and electrolytes.

Bile contains water, bile salts and pigments, cholesterol, fatty acids, and other substances. Bilirubin and biliverdin (derived from the breakdown of hemoglobin), conjugated with glucuronide, give the bile its characteristic color. The functions of bile in digestion and absorption are an emulsifying action on fat to facilitate its breakdown into minute particles, and the promotion of lipid absorption in the intestine by its formation with lipids of small complexes called micelles, which, unlike the lipids, are highly soluble and therefore more readily absorbable.

Bile pigments are formed from the heme of hemoglobin which is released when senescent erythrocytes break up. The hemoglobin is phagocytized by the reticuloendothelial system and then undergoes a structural change to form biliverdin, which is subsequently reduced to unconjugated bilirubin. Most of this is bound to albumin in the blood, is later taken up by liver cells as blood passes through the liver, and is bound to proteins which trap the free bilirubin inside the liver cells. Here it is conjugated with glucuronic acid to form conjugated bilirubin (bilirubin glucuronide). It is then actively transported into the bile canaliculi and thence into the hepatic ducts and finally into the duodenum. Some escapes into the blood, and part of this is excreted in the urine, but some remains in the plasma.

The intestinal mucosa is not very permeable to conjugated bilirubin, but is permeable to the unconjugated form and to urobilinogen, which is produced from bilirubin in the intestine by the action of bacteria. So these two soluble forms are absorbed by the small intestine into the portal circulation, transported to the liver, and the process is repeated. This recirculation of bilirubin is called the enterohepatic circulation. Some of the urobilinogen is also excreted in the urine. Total plasma bilirubin includes both free (called indirect-reacting) and conjugated (called direct-reacting) bilirubin. Bile pigment formation and circulation is shown in Figure 12-2.

Exocrine Pancreas

The exocrine (nonendocrine) glands of the pancreas secrete enzymes capable of hydrolyzing all of the major food categories: fats, carbohydrates, and proteins, and in addition secrete large quantities of bicarbonate ions (HCO_3^-). Total daily secretion is about 1200 ml. These enzymes are of major significance for the digestion which occurs in the small intestine. Pancreatic gland cells contain zymogen granules which are the stored enzymes; these are discharged into the minute pancreatic ducts which join to form the main duct of Wirsung. This duct enters the duodenum next to, or more often in conjunction with (since they join), the common bile duct at the ampulla of Vater. The pancreatic proteolytic (trypsin) and lipolytic (amylase) enzymes are very strong hydrolyzing agents, especially the former. It is important that the powerful enzyme trypsin not be released in active form into the pancreatic ducts where it could cause autodigestion. Therefore it is secreted in an inactive proenzyme form and converted into the active form, when it reaches the intestine, by the enzyme enterokinase. As an additional protective measure, trypsin inhibitor is secreted by the pancreas and is stored in cells surrounding the enzyme granules. Pancreatic lipase can also be damaging since it is capable of producing a substance which is toxic to cell membranes. In acute pancreatitis or trauma to the pancreas, the lipase may become activated within the gland leading to autodigestion of fat in it. Normally some amylase leaks out of the ducts into the plasma and does no harm.

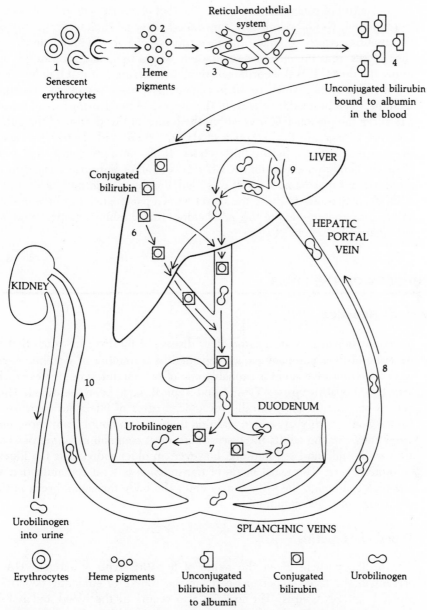

Reticuloendothelial system

Heme pigments

1
Senescent erythrocytes

2

3

4
Unconjugated bilirubin bound to albumin in the blood

5

LIVER

Conjugated bilirubin

6

9

HEPATIC PORTAL VEIN

KIDNEY

10

8

DUODENUM

Urobilinogen

7

Urobilinogen into urine

SPLANCHNIC VEINS

Erythrocytes | Heme pigments | Unconjugated bilirubin bound to albumin | Conjugated bilirubin | Urobilinogen

Figure 12-2. Diagram illustrating bile pigment formation and recirculation. (1 & 2) Senescent red cells break up, releasing heme pigments. (3) Heme is phagocytized by the tissues of the reticuloendothelial system and converted first to biliverdin and then unconjugated bilirubin. (4) Bilirubin (unconjugated) is carried bound to albumin in the blood. (5) Bilirubin is taken up by liver cells and conjugated with glucuronic acid to form conjugated bilirubin. (6) Conjugated bilirubin is secreted into the bile. (7) Much conjugated bilirubin is transformed to urobilinogen by the action of intestinal bacteria. (8) Most of the urobilinogen is absorbed into the vessels which join to form the hepatic portal vein and carried to the liver. (9) Urobilinogen is taken up by the liver and secreted in the bile. Steps (6) through (9) comprise the enterohepatic circulation. (10) Some urobilinogen is carried by the circulation to the kidney where it is excreted in the urine.

The control of pancreatic secretion, like that of gastric secretion, is both neural and humoral. Neural regulation is mediated via vagal cholinergic (parasympathetic) impulses which stimulate the formation of enzymes without much water or electrolytes; thus the enzymes stay largely within the gland acini rather than entering the ducts. It is the hormonal stimuli, occurring as a result of food entering the small intestine, which result in copious pancreatic secretions. The hormone secretin is synthesized by glands in the mucosa of the proximal small intestine as a result of the presence of acid within the lumen of this portion of the gut. Its actions are to increase the secretion of HCO_3^-, fluid, and electrolytes, mainly by the pancreas but also by the biliary tract. It also inhibits gastric acid secretion. Cholecystokinin-pancreozymin (CCK-PZ) is another hormone formed in cells of the duodenal mucosa as a result of stimulation by certain fatty acids and amino acids. Its actions are to cause the secretion of a pancreatic juice high in enzymes, and to cause contraction of the gallbladder. It also inhibits gastric emptying and potentiates the actions of secretin.

DISORDERS OF THE LIVER

Infectious Hepatitis

Infectious hepatitis is an inflammatory disease of the liver in which there is destruction of liver parenchyma accompanied by a number of systemic manifestations. The causative agent is probably one of several different viruses of which at least two, hepatitis viruses Type A and Type B, have been identified. There are said to be over 60,000 clinically recognized cases of infectious hepatitis in the United States each year, and in addition there are no doubt many more unrecognized ones. Among adults the diseases are most common in young persons, and are usually mild and self-limiting; however, in older individuals the illness may be quite severe. The usual mode of transmission is fecal contamination via the oral route, although the viruses may enter the body through a break in the skin or through mucous membranes.

Types of Hepatitis

A virus-like particle given the name of hepatitis type A antigen (HA Ag) is present in the feces of persons early in the course of epidemic hepatitis. It is probably an RNA virus. The antigen also occurs in the blood and is followed shortly thereafter by the appearance of an antibody to the antigen (anti-HA) which persists indefinitely and probably confers permanent immunity. Type A hepatitis is also called infectious or short-incubation hepatitis.

The hepatitis type B virus is a DNA virus; it is called the Dane particle, and has a core antigen (HbcAg) different from the viral coat or surface antigen: HBsAg. It is the latter, the coat or surface antigen, which is called the Australia antigen and is identified in laboratory diagnostic tests for the presence of the hepatitis B virus. The surface antigen may or may not itself be infectious. HBsAg is found in greatest frequency in patients with posttransfusion hepatitis and those who use illicit parenteral drugs. There are a number of separate strains or subtypes of hepatitis B virus characterized by minor differences in the viral coat antigens; these subtypes correspond to certain differences in both geographical distribution and clinical characteristics of the disease associated with them. Hepatitis B is also called serum hepatitis, or long-incubation hepatitis.

There is increasing evidence that additional viruses causing infectious hepatitis exist. Many persons who have had hepatitis following a blood transfusion are negative for both hepatitis A and HBsAg, and their antibodies. Thus there is probably at least one additional hepatitus virus, hepatitis C, and probably others. Other viruses, for example, cytomegalovirus (CMV) and herpes simplex virus (HSV), are probably also involved in causing hepatitis.

The routes of transmission of both hepatitis A and B can be both oral and parenteral as well as through contact with any mucosal surface including genital surfaces. Semen, saliva, and other body secretions and excretions are considered to be infective for both types. However, type A is more often transmitted by fecal–oral contamination, and type B more often by parenteral routes.

Some authors state that differences in incubation periods for the two types of hepatitis may depend more on the route of inoculation, the dilution or concentration of the virus in the inoculating substance, the relative freshness of the substance at the time of inoculation, and other factors associated with the actual process of transmission, than on any inherent quality of the viruses themselves or of the disease responses which they initiate. Thus the distinctions between type A and type B hepatitis based on routes of infection and length of incubation periods may be less clear than formerly thought. Usually the severity of illness in type B infection is greater than that in type A.

Hepatitis B virus is present in the serum of patients with acute hepatitis. It appears during the incubation period following effective exposure to the virus over variable periods of time from patient to patient. It may be present for as long as several weeks before the onset of the early symptoms in some individuals, and in others may be present only in undetectably low titers until several weeks following the clinical illness. In most uncomplicated hepatitis B the levels of coat antigen, HBsAg, decline and finally disappear before the peak of jaundice or AST (formerly SGOT) levels develop but in some patients it may persist for months or even years, both in apparently healthy subjects and in those patients with chronic active hepatitis (see following). Blood levels of HBsAg are highest before there are abormalities in biochemical liver function and HBsAg disappears altogether when the acute hepatitis has completely resolved. HBsAg is highest in symptomfree carriers; in mild chronic persistent hepatitis (see following) HBsAg levels are somewhat lower; and in chronic aggressive hepatitis and acute fulminant hepatitis, HBsAg levels are least. Therefore there seems to be an inverse relationship between the serum concentration of HBsAg and the amount of liver cell damage and severity of clinical illness. This inverse relationship may depend on the nature and degree of the immune system response to infection with the HB virus in various patients. A low level of cytotoxic T cell response may permit persistent antigenemia, but minimal liver damage and a mild clinical course; while excessive antigen–antibody, complement and cytotoxic T cell reactions may lead to activation of an immune complex disease resulting in widespread liver cell destruction and severe clinical illness.

Antibody to the hepatitis B virus core antigen (HBcAg) develops during the convalescent period in most patients but is found in only a small percentage of patients who have recovered from the disease; however, antibody to the hepatitis B virus surface antigen (HBsAg) occurs later and persists in most patients who have recovered from the infection. Immunity follows infection with both hepatitis A and B viruses. There is no cross-immunity between A and B, but cross-immunity between the various subtypes of hepatitis B probably occurs.

Liver Changes in Viral Hepatitis

Histologic changes in the liver appear to be similar in both type A and type B infections. The basic pathologic process consists of several phases: infiltration with mononuclear cells, necrosis of liver cells, inflammation, and foci of regeneration. For the most part, the extent of liver cell injury as indicated by biopsy is reasonably well correlated with the severity of the patient's signs and symptoms. Individual hepatocytes undergo degeneration and necrosis, and their normal arrangement is disrupted. Infiltration by inflammatory cells: lymphocytes, polymorphonuclear neutrophils and eosinophils, occurs. Normal bile flow is impaired, and bile thrombi appear in the ductules. The distribution of both the necrotic and inflammatory changes is diffuse and patchy. Kuppfer cells (mononuclear phagocytes) proliferate and engulf the necrotic debris. During convalescence, active regeneration occurs and the regeneration of hepatocytes and proliferation of newly formed ductules rapidly return the cellular relationships to normal, although minor abnormalities may persist for several months if the illness has been more severe.

Assessment

It is not possible to differentiate hepatitis types A and B on the basis of clinical manifestations alone. In type A the virus has usually gained access through oral intake and it remains in the gastrointestinal tract for variable periods before multiplying into the blood which introduces the stage of viremia. This stage, in turn, occurs prior to the localization of the virus within the liver. There are apparently three possible categories of response to the hepatitis virus: (1) restriction of the virus to a gastrointestinal tract infection, in which case there is virus in the alimentary canal and stool but no detectable change in liver function; (2) a mild liver inflammation without jaundice but with increased aminotransferase (formerly transaminase) values; and (3) jaundice, altered liver function, and clinically evident signs and symptoms. The first two forms are *anicteric hepatitis*.

During the *prodromal* phase, which may precede jaundice by a week or two, the patient, usually a young person, develops anorexia and nausea, malaise, easy fatigability, headache, tender cervical lymph nodes, and sometimes myalgia and arthralgias. There may be signs and symptoms of an upper respiratory infection. A few days later the gastrointestinal symptoms may become more marked, with nausea and vomiting, and diarrhea or constipation. Abdominal discomfort often is noted, and sensations of chilliness. Temperature is usually below 102°F, and a shaking chill seldom occurs. There may be an urticarial rash. The skin and joint manifestations are said to be the consequence of formation of antigen–antibody complexes between the virus and its antibody, which activate the complement cascade (Chapter 22). Patients with arthritic-type joint manifestations—which may be subjective only (pain and stiffness) or also objective (swelling, tenderness, warmth, redness)—are reported to have decreased levels of serum complement, indicating activation and consumption of the complement sequence; while those who do not have an arthritis phase have normal levels of serum complement. This preicteric phase may last a few days to over three weeks; in most patients clinical jaundice never develops, and the symptoms are interpreted as those of a different disorder. At this time laboratory values for liver function tests would be abnormal, and abdominal examination would probably reveal a tender palpable liver; but most patients with either hepatitis A or B probably do not seek health care, and if they do the hepatitis may go unrecognized.

The *icteric* or jaundice phase is usually introduced by dark urine and light-colored stools that precede jaundice by a few days. Jaundice is first visible in the scleras and mucous membranes of the mouth and occurs when the serum bilirubin rises above about 3.0 mg/100 ml. Many of the patient's symptoms except anorexia subside at this time and the temperature may return to normal, but often right upper quadrant pain and tenderness become more evident as the liver enlarges. Jaundice may increase for several days to two weeks, and this is correlated with increased serum bilirubin to about 20 mg/100 ml representing equal conjugated and unconjugated fractions. Absolute levels appear to correlate with the severity of the disease and the eventual clinical course. Persisting elevated serum bilirubin indicates a more severe disease and less favorable outcome. On occasion abdominal pain may be quite severe. When the icteric phase is prolonged over 14 to 21 days, subacute hepatic necrosis must be considered a possibility.

The *convalescent* or posticteric phase is accompanied by decreasing malaise, weakness, and anorexia. Liver enlargement and tenderness, with abnormal liver function, may last up to three months, but most patients are subjectively and objectively well within four months of the onset of jaundice.

Laboratory Values

Serum aminotransferase (formerly transaminase), either aspartate aminotransferase (AST) [formerly glutamic oxaloacetic transaminase (GOT)] or alanine aminotransferase (ALT) [formerly glutamic pyruvic transaminase (GPT)], is probably the most important. These values begin to rise above the normal 40 units before or during the prodromal symptoms and precede the rise in bilirubin. They reach a maximum, which may be over 1000 units, shortly after the onset of jaundice, and then drop fairly rapidly to normal within two to three weeks. Aminotransferase levels fail to correlate well with the severity of the disease. The serum bilirubin frequently rises just after the aminotransferase reaches a peak, rarely above 5–10 mg/100 ml, and usually returns to normal within two to three weeks. If the patient has a prolonged course, bilirubin may remain elevated for two or three months. Measurement of serum protein electrophoresis is an accurate index of liver function in hepatitis. Prolonged elevation of gamma globulin is an index of ongoing liver damage. Prothrombin time may occasionally be prolonged, but usually is not, provided the patient is following an uncomplicated course; when it does rise progressively this may be an index of severe disease.

HBsAg (see above) is the test that distinguishes hepatitis B from A and is detectable in the serum before symptoms develop and other tests become abnormal, perhaps for weeks. It may remain detectable during the jaundice phase and frequently returns to normal with the aminotransferase, but occasionally does so much earlier. As mentioned above, titer of HBsAg is not only unrelated to the severity of the disease but in fact may be inversely related to the degree of hepatic damage. In a few patients HBsAg persists for very long periods, or indefinitely. Some such carriers have chronic active liver disease, but others are entirely normal and asymptomatic. In considering the significance of HBsAg levels, it is important to recall that HBsAg is not itself the hepatitis virus, but only the antigen of the surface coat protein, and thus a lack of correlation of titers with severity of disease is not surprising.

Course and Complications

Most patients usually recover completely if they are healthy to begin with, and even those who have had a more severe illness generally do so. However, elderly persons and those with complicating or debilitating diseases, such as diabetes mellitus or congestive heart failure, tend to have a longer, more severe course. Serum bilirubin over 20 mg/100 ml, elevated prothrombin time, or hypoglycemia and/or hypoalbuminemia indicate a more serious disease.

Subacute Hepatic Necrosis

Subacute hepatic necrosis is a variant in which there is a more severe degree of liver damage, a longer, more serious illness, and poorer eventual prognosis. Protracted jaundice, depressed serum albumin, and elevated prothrombin time point to its development. Edema, ascites, and hepatic encephalopathy may develop. Laboratory abnormalities are more severe, and some of the patients who survive the acute illness may go on to chronic hepatitis or posthepatic cirrhosis.

Fulminant Hepatitis

Fulminant hepatitis (massive hepatic necrosis) occurs more often in type B hepatitis and is the most severe form of hepatitis, with extensive liver damage that may destroy so much of it that it becomes very small. Mortality rate is said to be well over 50%. Ascites and bleeding often occur. The indications of the liver failure may be rising bilirubin levels, prolonged prothrombin time, and the signs and symptoms of hepatic encephalopathy: decreased level of consciousness, altered mental status with confusion, agitation, and delerium; and neurologic signs: asterixis, seizures, abnormal reflexes, hyperventilation, and muscular rigidity. Ascites and edema may be present. Jaundice and hyperbilirubinemia may be severe and prothrombin time markedly increased. Cerebral edema and brainstem compression are often the cause of death. Surprisingly, if recovery does occur, the patient may regain a close to normal level of liver function.

Chronic Active Hepatitis

Chronic active hepatitis (autoimmune hepatitis, or chronic aggressive hepatitis) is a later complication of hepatitis B and is characterized by active hepatocellular necrosis, extensive chronic inflammation, and the development of liver fibrosis. It may lead to postnecrotic cirrhosis, with replacement of functional hepatic tissue by large nodules of fibrotic scar material. The patient experiences fatigue, weight loss, increasing weakness, and anorexia. Abdominal distress and diarrhea are common, and hepatomegaly may persist. Some patients also develop skin rash, joint symptoms, and other manifestations resembling a collagen-vascular disease or autoimmune disorder. This form of the disease has been called "lupoid" hepatitis. Some characteristics in the course of hepatitis B which may indicate a progression to chronic active hepatitis are persistence of symptoms for over three months, continued abnormal serum aminotransferase and bilirubin values, elevation of serum globulins above 2.5 gm/100 ml and protracted presence of HBsAg for several months following the acute phase.

The immunologic reactions in chronic active hepatitis appear to involve both humoral and cell-mediated immunity, and there is some evidence from histocompatibility typing studies that there is a genetic predisposition in some patients (Chapter 22). There is a wide range of signs and symptoms from a relatively long asymptomatic course to a more rapidly progressive cirrhosis and liver failure. Adrenal glucocorticoid administration for extended periods appears to induce remission and prolong survival; azathioprine is sometimes used with the steroids to permit a lower maintenance dose and therefore minimize the adverse effects of the latter. Immunosuppressive agents alone appear to be without benefit.

Chronic Persistent Hepatitis

Chronic persistent hepatitis is not a progressive disorder; it involves infiltration of inflammatory cells into the liver but little or no necrosis of hepatocytes, slight if any fibrosis, and it seldom or never leads to cirrhosis. The prognosis is good and generally the only aspect of management consists of reassurance to the patients that they do not have chronic active hepatitis.

Management

There is no specific treatment aside from the usual ones of adequate rest, nutrition, and fluids. Drugs and alcohol are usually proscribed. The pruritis caused by bile salts in the skin may be relieved by cholestyramine, a bile salt binding agent. Patients who are dehydrated, and having marked continued nausea and vomiting, a serum bilirubin above 15 mg/100 ml, prolonged prothrombin time, or are elderly and have other complicating conditions, are usually hospitalized. Patients should be instructed in careful personal hygiene measures including avoiding intimate contact with others, isolation of dishes, and most importantly frequent handwashing.

The period of maximum infectivity occurs during the preicteric phase, and in most patients there are no signs or symptoms which point to infectious hepatitis before this stage; therefore, all of the patient's close contacts have been exposed by this time. Stools are infective two to three weeks before the onset of jaundice, but those collected beyond the nineteenth day after the onset of jaundice probably are not. Gamma globulin (standard immune globulin) is effective in preventing overt hepatitis A in subjects with a known close exposure if given during the incubation period. The usual doses lead to development of an asymptomatic infection, but the histologic liver alterations probably occur. It is more effective if given soon after exposure and is of no value once symptoms have developed. For prevention of acute hepatitis B after a known exposure, high titer hepatitis B immune globulin appears to be protective. However, follow-up studies have been reported to show that after several months patients who received the high titer globulin have developed nearly as much hepatitis as those who received the standard globulin, and patients in the latter group are more likely to have developed both active and passive immunity. This may suggest that the high titer globulin may be protective against immune damage to liver cells from the virus only during the short period that the globulin is present, and that it impairs the development of active immunity. Nevertheless, in the short term, modification of the course of hepatitis B appears to be an appropriate goal.

Alcoholic Liver Disease

Excess alcohol intake is the most important drug problem of industrialized countries. The volume and duration of alcohol consumption is well correlated with liver pathology and mortality from cirrhosis in these countries. Liver cirrhosis, caused mainly by alcoholism, ranks as sixth in the causes of mortality in the United States.

Fatty Liver

Fatty liver is one of the most frequent disorders of the liver; the causes vary in different parts of the world, but in North America and in Europe at least three fourths of persons with fatty liver have a history of excess alcohol intake. The disorder develops in spite of an adequate diet, although malnutrition appears to have an additive effect in some patients. Genetic factors play an important role in determining individual differences (which are wide) in susceptibility to the sequence of pathologic changes which comprise alcoholic liver disease. Alcoholic fatty liver is an early stage in this sequence.

The normal liver does not have a large fat content—less than 5%, while in severe fatty liver the fat content may approach 50%. Fatty liver is readily induced in both humans and experimental animals by alcohol. The main constituent is triglycerides, which accumulate first within hepatocytes, distending and distorting them. Accompanying this fat accumulation, if it is severe, are varying degrees of inflammation and cellular necrosis. Whether these latter changes are due directly to the presence of fat, or whether the fat, inflammation, and necrosis are all the consequences of the hepatotoxic effects of alcohol is not fully established. However, alcohol has hepatotoxic actions which seem to increase liver fat content: it stimulates the liver to form triglycerides, and it mobilizes fat from peripheral stores and promotes its transport to and storage in the liver.

Alcohol is metabolized by oxidation in the liver in two stages: alcohol to acetaldehyde and acetaldehyde to acetate. Free acetate is the main end product; some is metabolized in the liver, but most leaves the liver and is metabolized elsewhere, mainly in muscle tissue. It is thought that alcohol induces fat deposition in the liver at least partially as a consequence of the high aldehyde and acetate content resulting from liver metabolism of alcohol. In addition, alcohol and its degradation products exert markedly abnormal effects on protein synthesis in the liver.

Symptoms and Signs of Fatty Liver

The manifestations of fatty liver may take one of two forms. The less serious appears to be asymptomatic chronic enlargement. The more serious is called acute fatty liver, in which there is right upper quadrant pain and tenderness, probably resulting from inflammation and destruction of liver parenchyma, cholestasis, and distention of the liver capsule. Jaundice is relatively frequent and may last for several weeks; it is suspected to be obstructive in nature and caused by the pressure of distended fat-containing hepatocytes on bile ductules and ducts. Ascites and edema may be present, and even bleeding from temporary esophageal varices may occur. Spider angiomas may be seen. The liver is palpable and tender. Liver function studies will demonstrate abnormalities in serum proteins (which may persist for many months), BSP retention, bilirubin, cholesterol, and prothrombin. Aminotransferase values are usually low and this helps distinguish the disorder from acute viral hepatitis. The only effective management is abstinence from alcohol. In patients whose livers are susceptible to the toxic effects of alcohol, probably on a genetic basis, continued alcohol intake causes fatty infiltration to be succeeded by alcoholic hepatitis and ultimately cirrhosis, portal hypertension, and their consequences.

Alcoholic Hepatitis

There is a large range in not only clinical manifestations but histopathologic changes in the liver, as revealed by liver biopsy, in the group of heterogeneous syndromes lying along the course of alcohol excess between fatty liver and alcoholic cirrhosis. The signs, symptoms, and laboratory abnormalities are similarly diverse. Some biopsy studies show remarkably slow progression of alcoholic hepatitis, even with continued drinking, during a three-year period in half of the study population. One third of the drinking group had developed cirrhosis within that period, as had some patients who had stopped drinking. This diversity of response probably correlates with individual differences in genetically determined susceptibility to the hepatotoxic effects of alcohol.

The most common symptoms of alcoholic hepatitis are anorexia, vomiting, abdominal pain, and abdominal distention. The liver may or may not be enlarged and tender, there may be jaundice, and weight loss and fever are frequent. Laboratory values are variably abnormal; the prothrombin time is reported to be of most accurate prognostic value, and if abnormal and unresponsive to vitamin K is predictive of nonsurvival. Liver biopsy is the only certain method of diagnosis and the histologic criteria are suggested by some authors to be active inflammation, polymorphonuclear infiltration, hepatocyte necrosis, and the presence of alcoholic hyaline (the so-called Mallory bodies) in liver cells, which are said to be accumulated necrotic cell organelles. The reported mortality rate varies widely in various study populations. Management consists of abstinence from alcohol and an adequate diet.

Laennec's Cirrhosis

Cirrhosis is a chronic process, probably eight times more common in alcoholics than nonalcoholics (although only about 1 in 10 chronic drinkers develops it),

which probably has a major genetic predisposing factor. Cirrhosis is characterized by the presence of regenerative nodules, made up of small masses of hepatocytes, blood vessels, lymphatics, and ductules; connective tissue septa; and
increased networks of fibrous tissue throughout.

The reported incidence of cirrhosis at autopsy among unselected populations
ranges from 1.0 to about 6.0%. The degree and duration of alcohol intake correlates with the severity of cirrhosis in most cases; excess use precedes the onset of
signs and symptoms by between 5 and 15 years.

Signs and Symptoms

Liver malfunction is signaled by easy fatigability, muscle weakness and wasting,
anorexia, ankle edema, jaundice, and abdominal distention from ascites. Right
upper quadrant pain, which is made worse by sitting up or leaning forward, is a
prominent symptom. Diarrhea is another frequent complaint, but whether this is
related to alcohol intake or the cirrhosis itself is uncertain.

Physical examination often reveals a palpable enlarged liver, jaundice, palmar
erythema, spider angiomas, sparse body hair; and gynecomastia, a small prostate, and testicular atrophy in males. With progression, liver size decreases
because of reduced cell mass and it becomes indurated and atrophied. Signs and
symptoms are exacerbated following alcohol intake. Acute and chronic pancreatitis and peptic ulcer are reported to have a high incidence in patients with
Laennec's cirrhosis. Fluid and electrolyte abnormalities develop as a result of the
hypoproteinemia (Chapter 1), and include secondary hyperaldosteronism and
sometimes dilutional hyponatremia because of further water retention in excess
of Na^+, perhaps because of ADH hypersecretion. Altered mental status and
decreased level of consciousness indicates hepatic encephalopathy. In some alcoholics with cirrhosis a massive gastrointestinal bleed from esophageal varices or
from a large peptic ulcer may be the first overt development.

Laboratory values show widespread abnormalities. Hematocrit and white cell
count are usually low because of hemolysis, bone marrow depression, and sple-
nomegaly. Gastrointestinal bleeding is also a factor in the anemia. The bilirubin
and aminotransferases are elevated, the latter usually mildly so. Hypoalbuminemia is marked because of alcohol impairment of albumin synthesis in the
liver. Serum ammonia is often increased because of decreased liver transformation of ammonia to urea. Hypokalemia results from the hyperaldosteronism.

Abstinence from alcohol is the essential component of management for the patient with cirrhosis from alcohol excess and has been demonstrated in most studies to prolong life. However, there are other studies the results of which indicate
that once this stage of alcoholic liver disease has been attained, abstinence from
alcohol has little influence on further progression of the disease or on life expectancy. Differences in outcome between various studies may relate to economic
and social differences in the study populations. Other components of management such as an adequate diet may be helpful, but only provided the patient ab-
stains from alcohol altogether; nothing protects the liver against it and continued
intake renders all other aspects of management futile.

Portal Hypertension

Portal hypertension is defined as a portal venous pressure of greater than 25–30 cmH$_2$O. It is the result of obstruction to the flow of blood between the veins supplying the portal vein, and the inferior vena cava. This obstruction may occur at different levels within the portal circuit, and may develop from a number of causes. However, a block to blood flow within the liver itself, as a result of cirrhosis, is the most common cause in industrialized countries, and most cirrhosis occurs in alcoholics. Probably over half the patients with cirrhosis have portal hypertension.

Figure 12-3 shows the major routes of blood flow into and out of the liver. About ⅓ to ¼ of blood entering the liver does so via the hepatic artery; the major ⅔ to ¾ of liver blood flow is derived from the portal vein; blood leaves the liver through the hepatic vein which enters the inferior vena cava. Normally the inflow and outflow is balanced in such a way that the portal system of vessels maintains a stable quite low-pressure flow. However, destruction of or obstruction to portions of the venous bed within the liver will cause an increasing resistance to flow between portal and hepatic vein, with resulting elevation of pressure throughout vessels of the portal system. The elevated pressure, in turn, leads to the development of venous collateral channels between portal and systemic circuits, sluggish flow throughout the involved vessels, and vascular congestion within the viscera.

In addition to the increased resistance to blood flow out of the portal system because of vascular obstruction in the liver, studies indicate that in many patients with cirrhosis and portal hypertension, there is markedly elevated splanch-

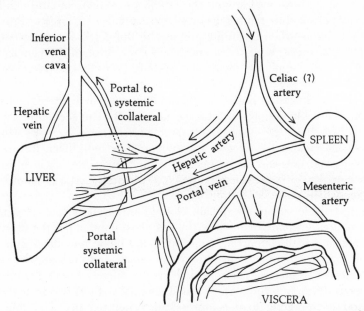

Figure 12-3. The major routes of blood flow into and out of the liver. Blood enters the liver via the hepatic artery and portal vein, flows through the intrahepatic vessels and liver sinusoids, and leaves through the hepatic vein which empties into the inferior vena cava. In portal hypertension from cirrhosis, collateral vessels open between the portal vein and vessels going to the inferior vena cava, because of high pressure in the portal circuit.

nic blood flow. There are probably several reasons for the increased flow of blood through the visceral circulation into the portal vein in cirrhosis, not all of which are known. Two proposed mechanisms are (1) the production of a systemic vasodilator, perhaps by the liver, as a response to progressive obliteration and obstruction of its blood flow; and (2) the development of numerous arteriovenous shunts or small fistulas within the visceral blood circuit, which, since they bypass a considerable amount of capillary resistance, would result in markedly elevated total splanchnic blood flow. It is known, for example, that splenic arteriovenous fistules (from some other cause than cirrhosis) can lead to portal hypertension even in the absence of any evidence of liver disease and intraheptic obstruction to blood flow. It is also known that hypertension and myocardial infarctions have an extremely low incidence in alcoholic cirrhosis, possibly indicating an as yet unidentified systemic vasodilator.

Liver cirrhosis and the resulting portal hypertension cause a number of abnormalities of which the four most characteristic are (1) development of collateral blood flow between vessels of the portal and the systemic venous system; (2) vascular congestion of the spleen with enlargement; (3) the development of ascites; (4) portal–systemic encephalopathy; and (5) systemic edema.

Portal to Systemic Collateral Vessels

As long as there is no obstruction to the flow of blood through the liver from the portal vein to the hepatic vein, the collateral circulation which normally connects the portal and systemic circuits remains nonfunctional. The three sites of such potential connections are at the esophagastric junction, in the lower rectum, and in the abdominal wall around the umbilicus. When flow through the liver sinusoids is blocked by the mechanical obstructions of cirrhosis—fibrosis and nodular regeneration—then mounting pressure in the portal system forces open the collaterals in these three areas, and blood flows through the venous channels from the vessels supplying the portal system, into the systemic veins, therefore bypassing the liver.

The esophagastric region is drained by veins which enter the left gastric vein; from there blood flows into the portal vessels. The section of the lower esophagus just above the esophagastric junction is drained by veins which empty into the vena cava via the azygous and hemiazygous veins. Thus the area between the lower esophagus and the esophagastric junction is one in which the systemic and the portal vein systems come into close proximity. At this point there are small veins which make connection between the two venous systems; in the normal subject these collaterals remain closed. As portal system pressure rises, however, pressure mounts in all of the vessels supplying the portal vasculature; this forces the small connecting veins open and blood now flows in a reverse direction through them, leaving the portal vessels and entering the systemic veins. The lower esophageal veins become greatly dilated, forming varices. Similar collaterals develop in the rectum and abdominal wall. This is in a sense an adaptive response operating to decompress the congested portal system, but it has a number of unfortunate consequences among the most frequent and serious of which is hemorrhage from rupture of the esophageal varices which form as a result of the abnormal blood flow. Most patients survive the first bleed, but rebleeding frequently occurs, and there are few survivors of the second.

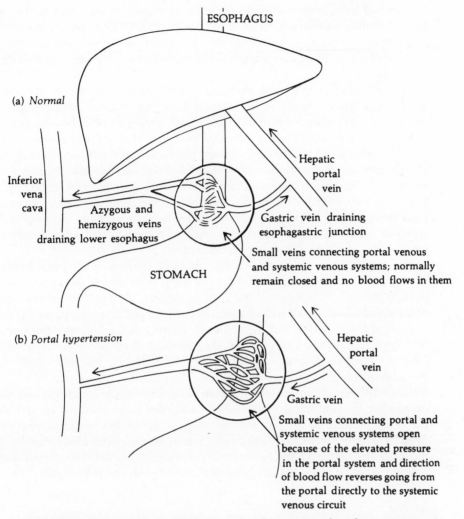

ESOPHAGUS

(a) *Normal*

Inferior
vena
cava

Azygous and
hemizygous veins
draining lower esophagus

STOMACH

Hepatic
portal
vein

Gastric vein draining
esophagastric junction

Small veins connecting portal venous
and systemic venous systems; normally
remain closed and no blood flows in them

(b) *Portal hypertension*

Hepatic
portal
vein

Gastric vein

Small veins connecting portal and
systemic venous systems open
because of the elevated pressure
in the portal system and direction
of blood flow reverses going from
the portal directly to the systemic
venous circuit

Figure 12-4. (a) *Normal.* Lower esophagus venous drainage is to the inferior vena cava via the azygous and hemizygous veins. The esophagastric junction is drained by veins entering the left gastric vein from which blood flows into the hepatic portal vein. Small venous channels, which normally remain closed, connect the portal and systemic circuits in this region. Arrows show direction of normal blood flow. (b) *Portal hypertension.* In portal hypertension, pressure in the portal circuit is greatly elevated, forcing open the venous channels indicated in a. The direction of blood flow now becomes: from the portal vein, through the gastric vein in a reversed direction, through the collaterals, into the veins draining the lower esophagus, and thence via azygous and hemizygous veins into the inferior vena cava. Pressure increases in the connecting venous channels producing esophageal varices.

Upper gastric varices are also frequently present. It should be emphasized that there is evidence that these varices come and go rather than being continuously present, or they may worsen and then ameliorate; their fluctuating nature appears to correlate very considerably with degrees of fluctuation in liver function. There are suggestions that a marked decrease in compensation of the liver disease (caused by intake of alcohol) is the major factor which precipitates hemorrhage from esophageal varices. Mortality rate in patients with esophageal varices that have been confirmed by endoscopy varies widely in reported studies, depending on characteristics of the study populations as concerns associated signs of liver disease (jaundice, ascites, precoma) and other factors; a five-year survival of about 2% has been reported at one extreme, as compared with 22% at the other.

The effects of prophylactic shunting operations such as the portacaval and splenorenal shunts, done in an attempt to forestall initial hemorrhage or to prevent a recurrence, result in a decreased incidence of hemorrhage but an increased incidence of hepatic encephalopathy, so that survival in operated and control patients is not different, though the causes of death are. In fact, some studies indicate that prophylactic portacaval shunt may actually shorten life expectancy rather than increase it. The higher death rate in the operated patients is largely accounted for by the development of hepatic encephalopathy and hepatic coma by about five years after the operation. In addition, the patients who received the shunt surgery have been reported to be hospitalized more often and for longer periods than the unoperated controls.

It is important to emphasize that in alcoholic cirrhosis with portal hypertension, copious bleeding may and often does occur from sites in the upper gastrointestinal tract other than esophageal varices, namely, from gastritis or from gastric or duodenal ulcer. About half of alcoholic cirrhotic patients with portal hypertension bleed from varices, and the others do so from gastric inflammations or peptic ulcers. The source can often be identified by fiberoptic endoscopy. Where bleeding esophageal varices have been demonstrated by this procedure, use of the Blakemore tube, and intravenous and intraarterial (mesentric) pitressin infusions, with blood transfusions, vitamin K, and neomycin by mouth and enema (to combat the additional blood ammonia burden from bacterial breakdown of the blood proteins in the gut; see following) comprise the conservative management. The effectiveness of vasopressin, which lowers portal blood flow by causing vasoconstriction of the splanchnic vasculature, is uncertain. Some authors conclude that its value has not been demonstrated in controlled trials.

Ascites

Ascites is a collection of abnormal quantities of fluid in the peritoneal cavity as a consequence of liver parenchyma destruction and portal hypertension. It often is accompanied by generalized edema from hypoproteinemia and complex disorders of fluid, electrolyte, and protein balance (Chapter 1).

Vascular obstruction in the liver can occur in three areas: presinusoidal, sinusoidal, and postsinusoidal—that is, on the portal side of the liver sinusoids, within the sinusoids themselves, or on the hepatic vein side of the sinusoids. Probably all are involved to some degree in the ascites of alcoholic cirrhosis, but the fact that ascites in this disease is relatively low in protein (around 3.5 g/100 ml) compared with that from certain other causes is taken by some authors to indicate that the major block may be presinusoidal.

A number of factors, both local and systemic, are involved in the development of ascites. The colloidal osmotic pressure of the plasma is a function primarily of the level of serum albumin. Albumin is synthesized by the liver; in chronic destruction of liver parenchyma this function is markedly impaired leading to abnormally low serum albumin. Since it is the colloidal osmotic pressure of the blood that is largely responsible for the return into the capillaries of the venule end, of ECF which filtered out at the arteriole end (Figure 1-7) the return fails to occur in normal amounts, and so interstitial fluid accumulates. In the systemic tissues as a whole this leads to increased interstitial fluid: generalized edema. In the liver, the result is a greatly increased flow of interstitial fluid into the liver lymphatics—more than the lymphatics can drain away—and the excess leaks out of the surface of the liver through the small blebs which cover its surface in this condition. Ascites may markedly increase following a gastrointestinal bleed from varices or an ulcer, because of the further decline in plasma protein caused by the blood loss.

The elevated hydrostatic pressure in the portal circuit and within vessels of portions of the liver itself also induces an excessive filtration of fluid throughout splanchnic, portal, and liver capillaries into the peritoneal cavity, and this high pressure exerts an additive effect with the low plasma colloidal osmotic pressure to increase capillary fluid loss.

When inflammation is present in the cirrhotic liver from acute hepatitis induced by a bout of alcoholism, the inflammation causes a greatly increased flow of high protein lymph, which increases the protein content of the ascites fluid, lowers the protein content of the blood, and may induce exacerbations of ascites.

Patients with low plasma colloid osmotic pressure and ascites have a decreased effective blood perfusion pressure to the kidneys. This low effective perfusion activates the renin–angiotensin–aldosterone system (Chapter 1). The resulting secondary hyperaldosteronism stimulates increased distal renal tubule Na^+ resorption, and as a consequence, water retention. This results in a chronically expanded ECF volume in patients with severe cirrhosis, and to the increased tendency to lose intravascular ECF through the capillaries. Since the liver is the main route of degradation and elimination of circulating aldosterone, hepatocellular destruction contributes to the high plasma aldosterone content.

An additional cause of the expanded ECF volume is the impaired ability of the poorly perfused kidneys to excrete excess free water, so that, although total body Na^+ concentration is increased, water is retained in excess of Na^+, producing dilutional hyponatremia. Abnormally increased ADH secretion may contribute to the water retention, but decreased glomerular filtration rate in cirrhosis and acites is probably a major factor.

Signs and symptoms of ascites usually become apparent when the volume of ascites fluid exceeds 500 ml. As the volume increases it becomes uncomfortable for the patient, compresses abdominal organs and elevates the diaphragm, and impairs respiratory excursions. Bulging flanks, shifting dullness, central tympany, and elevated diaphragms with decreased inspiratory lowering, may all be evident on physical examination.

Management of ascites involves conservative measures. Often a week of bed rest will promote diuresis. Dietary intake of salt is restricted, and fluid intake may be reduced to an amount equal to the previous day's urinary output. The aldosterone antagonist diuretic spironolactone may be used alone or combined with hydrochlorothiazide. The goal of management is to promote return of ascites fluid and interstitial edema fluid into the vascular compartment where it can be eliminated by the kidneys. A daily weight loss of 0.5–1.0 kg indicates that this goal is being met. Attempts to produce a more rapid water loss with strong diuretics may imperil renal perfusion and lead to hepatorenal syndrome and renal failure. Paracentesis is avoided because of the protein loss it incurs, and because of the threat of third-space losses and hypovolemia as fluid from the intravascular ECF rapidly reenters the peritoneal cavity.

Hepatorenal Syndrome

Hepatorenal syndrome is a serious complication of cirrhosis and ascites. It is characterized by acute renal failure in the presence of histologically normal kidneys; and azotemia, oliguria, very low urinary Na^+, marked increase in Na^+ retention, and severe intractable ascites. It may be precipitated by a gastrointestinal bleed, sepsis, paracentesis, and excess diuretics. The mechanisms involved in the cause are not known, but in some patients it may result from a rapid decline in plasma volume and hypotension; in other patients it appears to be associated with peripheral vasodilation (decreased peripheral resistance) and elevated cardiac output. The changes in renal function resemble those of prerenal azotemia (Chapter 10).

Hepatic Encephalopathy

Hepatic encephalopathy is a form of metabolic brain disease—abnormal central nervous system function occurring as a consequence of a systemic metabolic disorder, in this case liver failure. It can occur in either an acute or chronic form, and is characterized by altered mental status, depressed levels of consciousness, and fluctuating neurologic signs. Apparently both extensive destruction of liver parenchyma, resulting in hepatic insufficiency; and extensive shunting of portal blood into the system circulation, bypassing the liver, are essential for its development. This combination of prerequisites for its occurrence indicates that the normal liver and intact liver blood flow function either to remove some substance(s) from the blood which is deleterious to brain function, or to add some substance(s) to the blood which is essential for normal brain function. More likely both are involved.

Although there are probably a number of metabolic abnormalities underlying the two forms of hepatic encephalopathy, much evidence indicates that disordered ammonia metabolism is a significant factor in both the acute and chronic brain derangements.

Normal Ammonia (NH_3) Metabolism

Proteins are made up of amino acids; during digestion in the gastrointestinal tract, dietary proteins (exogenous proteins) are hydrolyzed into their constituent amino acids and absorbed into the blood of the vessels which join to form the hepatic portal system. In addition, the proteins comprising the structures of the body itself (endogenous proteins) are continually in the process of turnover—breakdown and resynthesis—a process which occurs to a large extent in the intestinal mucosa. The amino acids from both sources comprise the body's amino acid pool which supplies the components for protein synthesis and the variety of other metabolic uses of amino acids.

Amino acids undergo a number of metabolic conversions, three of which are transamination, oxidative deamination, and amination. (1) *Transamination* is the conversion of one amino acid to its corresponding keto acid, by removal of an amino group (NH_2) and then transfer of that amino group to a different ketoacid, which converts it to its corresponding amino acid. The enzymes which catalyze the transamination reactions are the serum aminotransferases: aspartate aminotransferase (AST; formerly GOT) and alanine aminotransferase (ALT; formerly GPT). Examples of this type of reaction are:

$$\text{alanine} + \alpha\text{-ketoglutaric acid} \overset{\text{ALT}}{\rightleftharpoons} \text{pyruvic acid} + \text{glutamic acid} \tag{1}$$

and

$$\text{aspartic acid} + \alpha\text{-ketoglutaric acid} \overset{\text{AST}}{\rightleftharpoons} \text{glutamic acid and oxaloacetic acid} \tag{2}$$

(2) *Oxidative deamination* of amino acids is a process occurring in the liver; a hydrogen is removed from an amino acid, converting it to an imino acid. The latter is then combined with water to form its corresponding keto acid, and in the reaction ammonia (NH_3) is formed. An example of this reaction is the removal of hydrogen from alanine, which converts that amino acid to its imino acid; then water combines with the imino acid, forming the corresponding keto acid, pyruvic acid, plus ammonia:

$$\text{alanine} \nearrow \overset{H^+}{} \searrow \text{imino acid} + H_2O \nearrow \text{pyruvic acid} \searrow NH_3$$

In the liver the ammonia (NH_3) formed as a result of the process of deamination of amino acids is converted into urea by combination with CO_2; it enters the blood draining the liver and is carried to the kidneys where it is eliminated in the urine. In the liver $NH_3 + CO_2 \rightarrow$ urea $\rightarrow$ kidney (eliminated in the urine). In severe hepatocellular degeneration this removal of NH_3 from the blood by the liver and its conversion to urea cannot occur at a rate necessary to keep blood NH_3 within normal limits; serum NH_3 levels rise, and if renal function is normal, BUN will decline because of decreased urea production.

(3) *Amination* is the third type of reaction which an amino acid can undergo; in this process an amino acid takes up ammonia, NH_3, and becomes an amine: amino acid + $NH_3 \rightarrow$ amine. One of the most important places in the body where this reaction occurs is in the brain; the amino acid glutamic acid joins with NH_3 and is converted to glutamine: glutamic acid + $NH_3 \rightarrow$ glutamine. The brain takes up large quantities of glutamic acid for binding with NH_3; this uptake is balanced by an about equivalent output of glutamine. It is likely that this is the most important process for binding and eliminating NH_3 from the brain; ammonia has a high toxicity for neurons, and the reaction glutamic acid + $NH_3 \rightarrow$ glutamine is thought to be the most significant mechanism for protecting the brain from NH_3 in the blood, to which it is very susceptible.

Ammonia that is detoxified in this way in the brain, is eliminated at the kidney by the reverse reaction—glutamine is converted back to glutamic acid by the removal of NH_3—glutamine $\rightarrow$ glutamic acid + NH_3. This reaction occurs in the cells of the proximal and distal renal tubules and collecting ducts. The NH_3

diffuses from the tubular cells into the tubular fluid; here it joins with H^+'s, which have been secreted from the tubular cells into tubular fluid, to form ammonium ions: NH^+, which are eliminated in the urine. In the kidney

$$\text{glutamine} \rightarrow NH_3 + H^+ \rightarrow NH^+ \text{ (eliminated in the urine)}$$
$$\searrow \text{glutamic acid}$$

In alkalemia and hypokalemia there is an inadequate H^+ concentration to supply the H^+'s necessary to join with NH_3 to form NH_4^+ for elimination in the urine. Therefore in hypokalemic alkalosis, as from diuretic excess or other cause, the renal mechanism for ridding the body of NH_3 is markedly impaired, which may lead to elevated serum NH_3 levels.

Ammonia (NH_3) is a lipid-soluble substance and all biologic membranes are exceedingly permeable to it, so that it crosses all cell boundaries, including the blood–brain barrier (Chapter 18) and neuron membranes, with the greatest of ease. However, the ammonium ion (NH_4^+) is lipid-insoluble and most cell membranes are highly impermeable to it. Therefore, once the reaction $NH_3 + H^+ \rightarrow NH_{4+}$ has occurred in the kidney tubule, that ammonia has effectively been tied up; i.e., the ion leaves the body instead of diffusing back into the blood. NH_4^+ does not itself, as such, pass the blood–brain barrier. Instead it may dissociate in the blood into H^+ and NH_3, which does enter the brain. This reaction is facilitated in alkalemia, because of the low H^+ content of the ECF available for converting NH_3 to NH_4^+.

Derangements of Ammonia Metabolism in Hepatocellular Destruction and Portal-to-Systemic Shunting

A combination of factors, involving abnormalities in a number of aspects of protein, amino acid, ammonia, ammonium, and urea metabolism, no doubt are involved in the causative processes in hepatic encephalopathy. In addition, it appears certain that other metabolic abnormalities are involved besides excess ammonia in blood perfusing the brain; in the normal subject substances which are toxic to the central nervous system are formed, probably in the gut, and the fact that in cirrhosis and portal hypertension most blood from the gut bypasses the liver means that the liver is unable to remove and detoxify them. The nature and source of these compounds is uncertain at this time, but their importance is attested to by the fact that blood NH_3 levels are often poorly correlated with the presence and degree of severity of hepatic encephalopathy.

However, it is probably the case that it is the *brain* content of NH_3 that is the relevant factor in NH_3 neurotoxicity, rather than the NH_3 content in the *systemic* circulation. The degree to which these two NH_3 pools parallel each other is not clear. Studies have shown that glutamine content of the cerebrospinal fluid appears to be rather well correlated with the presence and severity of hepatic encephalopathy. Therefore, CSF glutamine content, rather than serum NH_3, may be an index of brain NH_3 content, since the reaction glutamic acid + NH_3 $\rightarrow$ glutamine is the brain's main NH_3-detoxifying reaction and would be expected to proceed at an accelerated rate when there are high brain NH_3 levels. Brain glutamic acid content could be a rate-limiting factor in this protective process.

At any rate, as concerns the role of ammonia in hepatic encephalopathy, the major factor in its development appears to be an inadequate removal by the liver of the ammonia which is produced in the gut by the action of intestinal bacteria on amino acids; removal of NH_3 is inadequate because most of this blood fails to pass through the liver. Because of hepatocyte destruction, the ammonia in blood which does pass through the liver is inadequately removed and converted to urea. Therefore, serum NH_3 levels are often elevated. This effect is made more severe by gastrointestinal bleeding, which adds blood proteins to the intestinal lumen; and the breakdown of body proteins (muscle wasting) characteristic of cirrhosis. The excess serum NH_3 overtaxes both the protective brain mechanisms for handling NH_3, and the renal processes for removing it. Hypokalemia, characteristic of the patient with cirrhosis, edema, and ascites (because of the secondary aldosteronism; Chapters 1, 2, and 13) promotes the development of alkalemia, since if there is not enough K^+ to exchange for Na^+ at the distal tubule cation exchange site, then more H^+ will be eliminated. With inadequate plasma H^+ not enough is secreted into the tubule to bind NH_3 into NH_4^+ for excretion, so serum NH_3 increases.

Throughout the body, the equilibrium $NH_3 + H^+ \rightleftharpoons NH_4^+$ is omnipresent. NH_3 is the brain-toxic form; removing H^+ from the equation (alkalemia) shifts it in the direction of increased ammonia production, while adding H^+ (acidemia) to the equation shifts the equilibrium in the direction of the nontoxic ammonium ions, which are unable to penetrate the blood–brain barrier.

Experimental animals (rats) which have had surgical portacaval anastomoses are considered to be laboratory "models" of human chronic liver disease. They may manifest the metabolic abnormalities of hepatic encephalopathy. Recent studies show that the transport of neutral amino acids (such as tryptophan) across the blood–brain barrier and into brain ECF is markedly increased in these animals. This increase may result in the production of abnormal amounts or types of neurotransmitters by neurons. This, in turn, may be responsible for at least some of the central nervous system abnormalities characteristic of hepatic encephalopathy.

Assessment in Hepatic Encephalopathy

This development may be anticipated in a patient with liver disease susceptible to it as a result of a number of precipitating factors: increased protein intake, gastrointestinal bleeding; excess diuretic use; paracentesis; sepsis; the use of sedatives, tranquilizers, and narcotic analgesics; hypoxia; anemia; hypokalemia and alkalemia; and other systemic derangements. Serum NH_3 level may be above the normal 150 mg/100 ml. Early signs are altered mental status: euphoria, depression, restlessness, and agitation; or decreased levels of consciousness: lethargy or obtundation. Higher mental functions such as orientation, recent memory, judgment, and the capacity for abstract thought may show impairment. Behavior may become inappropriate. As encephalopathy progresses mental status may alter further into delerium; or stupor and coma may develop, and neurologic signs appear: muscular rigidity, exaggerated deep tendon reflexes, extensor plantar response, asterixis (a flapping tremor or clonus of the hand at the wrist when the arm is extended), multifocal myoclonus, or seizures. The electroencephalogram shows characteristic changes: bilaterally symmetric bursts of high voltage slow waves at 3–4 cps. Early in hepatic encephalopathy the brain may show few or no histologic changes, but its metabolism is abnormal as shown by decreased oxygen uptake and deranged glucose metabolism. In the chronic hepatic encephalopathy which often develops as a result of a surgical shunt procedure, structural alterations occur in brain tissue which correlate with the progressive mental manifestations.

Management of Hepatic Encephalopathy

This consists of measures to reduce the serum levels of NH_3 and other end-products of protein metabolism. Early recognition of the condition is of first importance, since the prognosis becomes poorer as neurologic deterioration progresses.

In the case of gastrointestinal bleeding, blood is removed by ice-water lavage. Regardless of cause, neomycin is given by mouth and retention enema to eliminate the bacteria which convert amino acids to NH_3. A low protein diet is important to decrease amino acids in the intestine available for this conversion. Potassium supplements may be indicated to combat hypokalemic alkalemia. Lactulose may be given by mouth and enema; its mechanism of action appears to be that of acidification of colon contents so that less NH_3 is formed, and that which is formed is kept in the NH_4^+ form by the acid.

DISORDERS OF THE GALLBLADDER AND BILE DUCTS

Gallstones (Cholelithiasis)

Gallstones are very prevalent, more common in females than males, and the likelihood of their developing increases as one gets older; they may be asymptomatic in perhaps half of all persons who have them. Some studies indicate that persons with gallstones tend to have blood relatives similarly afflicted, thus there is some evidence of a genetic predisposition. They appear to be less common in blacks than whites, and the incidence in American Indians is very high. Certain disorders such as liver cirrhosis, diabetes mellitus, sickle cell disease, and ileitis appear to predispose to gallstones, as do oral contraceptives and cholesterol-lowering diets and medications (clofibrate). Inflammatory injury to the gallbladder, such as from a bacterial infection, appears to promote the formation of gallstones; the inflammatory exudate may act as a nucleus for precipitation of bile salts from their often supersaturated solution in the gallbladder, and bacterial action on bile compounds may alter their chemical composition such that they become less readily held in solution.

In the United States probably three quarters of the gallstones are comprised primarily of cholesterol. Other ingredients of stones are calcium and bile pigments (bilirubin). In oriental cultures stones tend more to be comprised of calcium bilirubinate than cholesterol, perhaps because of the lower cholesterol diet among those populations.

Processes Involved in Gallstone Formation

The basic cause is not known. However, cholesterol stones are reported to form in an orderly sequence of, first, production of bile supersaturated with cholesterol. This occurs during fasting and at night in the normal subject, when the gallbladder stores bile for long periods instead of emptying it into the duodenum, from which it is then resorbed into portal vein blood. It is then returned to the liver, and enters the enterohepatic circulation as described earlier. Second, the precipitation of cholesterol as crystals from the supersaturated solution of bile stored in the gallbladder occurs. Third, those precipitated cholesterol crystals act as nuclei upon which bile constituents of low solubility deposit, so that gradual growth by accretion occurs. The factors initiating the process, as well as perpetuating it once it has begun, may be absence or insufficient amounts of substances in the bile which act as solubilizing agents; or presence within the bile of excess amounts of some substances which reduce the solubility of cholesterol and other compounds of low solubility, such as calcium bilirubinate.

Normally the liver takes cholesterol from the blood and transforms large amounts of it into bile salts and bile acids (the salts and acids are in chemical equilibrium with each other). Then these bile salts, together with untransformed cholesterol, and lecithin (a phospholipid) are secreted into the bile, which itself is largely water. Cholesterol is quite insoluble in water but the bile salts and lecithin, in proper proportions, together form a complicated physicochemical structure which permits large amounts of cholesterol to be held and stored within this structure, and therefore, in a sense, in solution, instead of precipitating out. If the ratio between lecithin and bile salts is abnormal, such that not enough of the complexes are formed; or if the concentration of cholesterol is too high for the complexes to bind it all, then it may precipitate out and initiate gallstone formation.

Another factor which apparently influences these processes by which cholesterol is kept from precipitating out of solution in bile is the process of bile recirculation in the enterohepatic circulation. Bile entering the duodenum via the common duct is to some extent resorbed from the duodenum, enters the portal circuit blood and flows back to the liver. Bile salts in the duodenum are acted upon by intestinal bacteria which modify their composition, thus the chemical composition of bile salts returning to the liver from the duodenum via the portal blood is different from those initially synthesized by the liver. This different composition therefore has an influence upon the nature and solubilizing action of bile released by the liver when there is an active enterohepatic bile recirculation.

There is no doubt but that the activity of the gallbladder itself enters into and probably very importantly influences the relationship between the above processes and the actual formation of gallstones. The two major gallbladder functions are (1) to receive hepatic bile and rapidly resorb from it large amounts of electrolytes and water, thus concentrating it; and (2) to store the resulting concentrated bile until food is ingested, at which time the stimuli from the gastrointestinal tract discussed earlier activate it to contract. In so doing, it delivers the concentrated bile into the duodenum where it promotes fat digestion. The frequency of gallbladder emptying influences the amount of bile entering the enterohepatic circulation and in turn affects the composition of subsequent bile formed by the liver.

The composition of bile from persons with gallstones is sometimes different from that of persons without them; normal bile has a higher cholesterol solubility and fewer precipitated cholesterol crystals. On the other hand there is a very low correlation, if any, between the level of free cholesterol in the blood and the cholesterol content of bile. Thus the processes involved in gallstone formation appear to have to do with the solubilizers bile salts and lecithin. And the three factors involved in this relationship are the nature of the bile secreted by the liver, the concentration and emptying functions of the gallbladder, and the activity of the enterohepatic bile circulation and its total bile salt pool. Persons with gallstones appear to have, in many cases, a diminished total bile salt pool available for solubilizing bile cholesterol. Liver, gallbladder, and enterohepatic circulation are probably all involved in the abnormal relationship between the amounts of cholesterol and the quantity of solubilizing agents which lead to gallstone formation.

Assessment

Subjective

There appears to be a wide spectrum of abdominal discomfort associated with the presence of gallstones, from no symptoms at all through a vague sense of fullness in the upper right quadrant made worse by jolting movements, to severe right upper quadrant pain and tenderness. It is probably the case that gallstones alone do not produce signs or symptoms but do so only when they either cause obstruction of the cystic or common duct, or are associated with inflammatory reactions in the gallbladder. In either of these two cases, inflammation or obstruction, the pain which occurs is often severe, is located usually in the right upper qudrant, and is steady rather than waxing and waning in a "colicky" fashion. The pain is brought on and made worse by food intake, which stimulates gallbladder contractions by processes described earlier. It may last up to four hours, as the gallbladder maintains its contractions in an attempt to empty its contents, often forcing a stone into an occluding position in the cystic duct. When and if the stone enters the common duct, pain becomes more severe, may be accompanied by vomiting, and may radiate to the back.

Symptoms of dyspepsia, pyrosis, water brash, and flatulence, especially associated with ingestion of fatty foods, have traditionally been considered to be symptoms of gallbladder disease. However, well-controlled studies of large numbers of subjects with or without gallstones as confirmed by cholecystogram, demonstrated that dyspeptic symptoms are neither correlated with objectively confirmed gallbladder disease nor are they relieved by cholecystectomy. It has, however, been demonstrated that reflux of bile into the stomach does occur in patients with gallstones, and since bile may have an irritating effect there, does seem to be associated with gastritis. However, it is considered unlikely that this gastritis produces symptoms.

Objective

Right upper quadrant tenderness to palpation, accompanied by inspiratory arrest during deep subhepatic palpation (Murphy's sign) is a sign of gallbladder disease. The gallbladder may be palpable. Jaundice is also a sign, and usually points to obstruction by a stone of the common bile duct or sometimes only edema of the duct. X-ray of the abdomen may reveal stones in a distended gallbladder.

Management of Gallstones

One of the areas of controversy in the management of gallstones revolves around the question of whether it is appropriate to remove the gallbladder of a person who has been discovered incidentally to have gallstones but is devoid of any signs or symptoms from them. There is a dearth of studies concerning the future course of groups of patients with completely asymptomatic gallstones. Conversely, there is general agreement that even a single attack of acute cholecystitis with cholelithiasis is indication for removal of the gallbladder, almost regardless of the age of the patient. The medical management of symptomatic cholelitiasis with a low-fat diet and anticholinergic medication has not proven satisfactory. It does not prevent recurrent attacks of acute cholecystitis nor does it control the complications: chronic cholcystitis, common duct stones (choledocholithiasis), pancreatitis, and biliary colic.

The administration of chenodeoxycholic acid expands the bile salt pool and results in the resorption of cholesterol gallstones, with a reduction in size of some stones and sometimes their eventual disappearance. The compound suppresses cholesterol synthesis and secretion, and it inhibits the synthesis of all bile salts from cholesterol. As a result of its administration there is inhibition of endogenous bile salts, most of the salts consist of the exogenous chenodeoxycholic acid salts, and there is a high concentration of these relative to the concentration of cholesterol. In other words, it increases the ratio of bile salts to cholesterol in the bile. The normal ratio is about 25:1; the ratio in patients with gallstones is about 8:1. When chenodeoxycholic acid is given, the ratio is reported to increase to upward of 12:1. Depending on the size of the stones, one to two years of treatment is generally required for complete resorption. When the drug is stopped, the bile tends to revert to its previous abnormal cholesterol to bile salt–acid ratio and formation of stones resumes. Diarrhea is a side effect, and one of the degradation products of the compound is toxic to the liver, but so far this effect has not been observed in the human, although it ocurs in the other primates. The treatment is not effective in nonfunctioning gallbladders nor in other than cholesterol stones. Even following the dissolution of stones, gallbladder function does not appear to return to normal. Since the bile becomes cholesterol-saturated following stopping the drug, stones may recur. Knowledge of long-term effects of taking this substance await the results of prospective controlled trials.

Acute Cholecystitis

Most often acute inflammation of the gallbladder occurs in association with cholelithiasis; it is a very common disorder with a peak occurrence during middle age.

Cause and Pathologic Changes

When there are stones present in the gallbladder, and that organ contracts to expel its contents into the duodenum, an event activated by food intake, the contraction may force a gallstone against the opening of or even into the cystic duct. The gallbladder contractions continue, and in fact increase in forcefulness; the stone may become impacted in the cystic duct. The gallbladder becomes distended, and the strong contractions compress the arterial supply and the venous and lymphatic drainage.

Bacterial growth probably occurs in the trapped bile, leading to inflammation of the gallbladder lining, infiltration with inflammatory cells, and damge to the submucosal layers. Abnormalities often occur in the lymphatic drainage system of the gallbladder and hepatic ducts, some of which indicate that bile has entered this sytem. As the inflammatory process develops it may include the outer serosa layer and spread to the adjoining peritoneum, causing the more diffuse constant pain of well-established acute cholecystitis. The presence of bile, combined with the impaired circulation in the gallbladder because of elevated pressure and distention, causes a further chemical inflammation of gallbladder tissue. The impairment of circulation may be severe enough to produce pressure necrosis of the wall, and perforation. This may cause peritonitis but more often the leak is contained by surrounding tissue and an abscess develops.

Thus the development of acute cholecystitis appears to develop in two phases: first, the mechanical obstruction, forceful contraction, and distention—the biliary colic phase; and second, the ischemia, inflammation, bacterial proliferation, and chemical irritation phase.

Assessment

Subjective

Pain is the outstanding symptom. It is in the right upper quadrant, of sudden onset, rapidly increases in severity, and is steady rather than colicky. Its duration may be 2 to 4 hours and it may radiate to the back between the level of T6 to T10. As the duration increases it may spread to the midepigastrium.

Objective

Direct tenderness to palpation and to percussion, and muscle spasm and rebound tenderness indicating peritoneal inflammation, may be present. Tenderness becomes more diffuse as the attack progresses. Guarding and rigidity may be marked and the pain may be made worse by coughing or a deep breath. Jaundice which is usually mild may occur in the minority of patients. There may be vomiting. Pain lasting longer than four hours, especially if associated with persistent vomiting, is said to indicate the development of pancreatitis from obstruction of pancreatic outflow caused by a gallstone in the common bile duct. In about half of patients the distended gallbladder may be palpable as a tender mass. There may be fever and an elevated white blood count with a shift to the left. The serum amylase, lipase, and aminotransferase may be elevated. X-ray of the abdomen may reveal a gallstone. Intravenous cholangiogram may reveal nonfilling of the gallbladder; if the gallbladder fills, then an obstructed cystic duct and acute cholecystitis are unlikely and acute pancreatitis more so. Ultrasonography is occasionally ordered. As is often the case in older patients, the signs and symptoms resulting from the obstructive and inflammatory process may be markedly reduced or atypical.

Management

Signs and symptoms subside in most patients in 4 to 5 days with conservative management. Pain control is generally achieved with meperidine and atropine. Nasogastric suction and intravenous fluid and electrolytes may be indicated. Antibiotics may be used. Early surgical consultation is appropriate, especially if the paitent appears to be having a severe attack or one which does not resolve within a short time. A major concern is gangrene of the gallbladder with perforation.

Chronic Cholecystitis

This refers to the condition of repeated attacks of acute cholecystitis. The gallbladder undergoes progressive fibrotic changes with thickening of the layers and chronic infiltration with inflammatory cells. The oral cholecystogram may show a failure to opacify after two doses of contrast medium, and when such a gallbladder is removed it is found to contain stones and to show reduced vascularity. Biliary cirrhosis may be an eventual complication.

DISORDERS OF THE EXOCRINE PANCREAS

Acute Pancreatitis

Acute pancreatitis is defined as an inflammation of the pancreas which, depending on the severity of the attack, is accompanied by varying degrees of pancreatic edema, necrosis, and bleeding, but following which there is a complete return to normal in function of both exocrine and endocrine portions. The two main causes of acute pancreatitis are the chronic pancreatitis of alcoholism and biliary tract disease.

Some authors describe two major forms of acute pancreatitis depending on the cause. Small-duct pancreatitis is said to be the most common form and is associated with obstruction of the small terminal pancreatic ducts that drain the exocrine acini; it is almost always caused by chronic excess alcohol intake. In this form it is usually the case that the acute attack of pancreatitis is superimposed on an already quite well-established chronic pancreatitis. The basic chronic pancreatitis involves irreversible histologic changes in the gland, although pancreatic function, as determined by serum enzyme levels, is still within normal limits between attacks.

Large-duct pancreatitis is said to be brought about by obstruction to the outflow of pancreatic secretions from the major pancreatic ducts usually caused by a gallstone. It is a less common form than the alcohol-caused small-duct disease.

In addition to the two major forms, associated with the two causes alcoholism and biliary tract disease, perhaps in one sixth or more of patients with acute pancreatitis no clear-cut predisposing or causative factor can be demonstrated. In these patients the "idiopathic" pancreatitis has been suggested to be induced by functional (edema, inflammation, or spasm) or structural (stricture or stenosis) narrowing at the sphincter of Oddi. The narrowing may be congenital, or secondary to inflammatory bowel disease, scarring from the passage of gallstones, vascular insufficiency (especially in the elderly), abdominal trauma, or systemic and metabolic disorders such as hyperlipidemia or hyperparathyroidism. Pancreatitis also may be drug-induced (thiazides, oral contraceptive agents).

In addition to the pancreatic damage caused by the mechanical effects of small or large duct obstruction to the outflow of pancreatic enzymes, there appears also to be chemical damage to pancreatic tissue caused by activation of lipolytic and proteolytic enzymes within the gland which results in chemical injury to and autodigestion of acini, ducts, blood vessels, and lymphatics.

Alcohol-Induced Acute Pancreatitis (Small-Duct Pancreatitis)

As is the case with alcohol-induced hepatitis and cirrhosis, there is apparently a strong genetically determined range of individual susceptibility to pancreatic damage from chronic alcohol excess. In certain individuals, alcohol seems to exert a direct toxic effect on pancreatic tissue. This toxic effect is manifested at the cellular level by swelling of mitochondria and degeneration of cytoplasm and cellular organelles resembling the changes induced in hepatocytes exposed to alcohol. Chronic alcohol intake leads to the same abnormal pancreatic changes in laboratory animals as occur in the human alcoholic. The primary factor is suggested by some workers to be precipitation of a protein material in the small pancreatic ducts. The proteinaceous substance may result from self-digestion of pancreas tissue by activation within the pancreas of strong protein and fat hydrolyzing enzymes. Once the material is produced it apparently is too thick to flow through the small ducts to exit from the pancreas, but rather remains within them and causes multiple sites of small duct obstruction. Then when the pancreas is stimulated to secrete by food intake, the acini release more pancreatic enzymes; but these are trapped within the small ducts by the protein material. The enzymes become activated, perhaps by the action of trypsin on the proteolytic zymogens and lipase precursors, because of either a lack of an inhibition substance such as pancreatic trypsin inhibitors, or the presence of a substance which facilitates the conversion of trypsinogen to trypsin. Further chemical autodigestion within the pancreas occurs, and a vicious cycle is established.

In an attack of acute pancreatitis in the alcoholic, the assumption is that the acute manifestations are superimposed on an underlying chronic pancreatitis, which is not yet severe enough to produce signs, symptoms, and laboratory evidence of chronic disease between acute attacks, but is still severe enough to readily result in an acute attack following a bout of increased alcohol intake. Once a baseline of subclinical chronic pancreatitis has developed, then susceptibility of the pancreas to the toxic effects of alcohol becomes markedly increased. In other words, alcohol appears to cause acute attacks of pancreatitis because its long-term use in excess has produced a chronic pancreatitis.

Acute Pancreatitis Resulting from Gallbladder and Biliary Tract Disease (Large-Duct Pancreatitis)

The precise mechanisms by which biliary tract disease precipitates an attack of acute pancreatitis are not understood. Reflux of bile from the common bile duct into the pancreatic duct has been proposed as one explanation. The entrance points of both the common bile duct and the pancreatic duct into the duodenum are close together; in fact, in most persons the two ducts fuse shortly before joining the duodenum and thus enter together, and bile and pancreatic secretions are mixed in this fused segment.

Some evidence indicates that the mixing of these two secretions leads to chemical reactions that produce substances which are destructive to cell membranes. Reflux of such mixtures into the pancreatic duct could cause pancreatitis, and in fact does so in experimental animals, producing a reaction which closely resembles the large-duct (biliary) pancreatitis of the human. When a gallstone is expelled from the gallbladder or common bile duct it could, and probably does, produce obstruction at the sphincter of Oddi. Then, because of continued bile and pancreatic secretion in the presence of large-duct outflow obstruction because of the stone, a head of pressure from secretions builds up behind the obstruction, dilating the large pancreatic ducts and refluxing into pancreatic tissue, causing edema and inflammation. The stone usually passes rapidly, and this is correlated with the fact that biliary-caused pancreatitis almost always resolves quickly and completely. Whether this corresponds with the actual sequence of events in pancreatitis from gallbladder disease is not known.

Changes within the Gland in Acute Pancreatitis

There is a spectrum of severity of pathologic changes in the gland in an acute attack of pancreatitis. The spectrum ranges from edema and inflammation in the milder attack, to necrosis and hemorrhage in the more severe. The former is called interstitial pancreatitis, and the latter is termed hemorrhagic pancreatitis. Interstitial pancreatitis is usually manifested as abdominal pain and an elevated serum amylase (the normal is 40–180 U/100 ml) which returns to normal as the pain subsides within 1 to 3 days. There is edema and an inflammatory infiltrate confined largely to the interstitial tissue of the pancreas in a patchy distribution. Hemorrhagic pancreatitis is characterized by a longer more severe clinical course and more widespread bleeding and cell destruction within the gland. It is likely that the destruction of pancreatic parenchyma in this form is caused by release and activation of strong proteolytic and lipolytic enzymes within the gland itself. The gland becomes greatly swollen and there is bleeding and necrosis of acini, ducts, blood vessels, and interstitium. As healing eventually takes place there is extensive fibrous tissue scar formation with dilation of acini and ducts. It is suggested that the milder interstitial and edematous form is correlated with the large-duct pancreatitis of biliary tract disease, and the more severe hemorrhagic-necrotic form is associated more with the small duct pancreatitis of chronic alcoholism.

In the milder interstitial edema form of acute pancreatitis the attack usually subsides with treatment in under a week. In the more severe hemorrhagic form recovery with treatment may require two weeks or longer. The most common complication is a pancreatic pseudocyst (see following).

In the very severe form which is characterized by extensive destruction of the pancreas and accompanied by shock, the mortality rate is often high. If the patient survives, the convalescence may be long and accompanied by complications such as sepsis. The severe attack may be complicated by the respiratory distress syndrome, acute renal failure, disseminated fat necrosis from the high content of pancreatic lipase in the circulation, prolonged hypotension because of vasodilation, and increased capillary permeability with loss of intravascular ECF into the peritoneum.

These systemic vascular effects probably are caused by the release of kinins from the pancreas into the circulation. Prekallikrein is a substance contained in the pancreas and is also present in the serum; it is activated by a blood clotting factor and transformed into kallikrein. Kallikrein then acts on a plasma globulin to form bradykinin, one of the mediators of the inflammatory reaction. Its actions are strong and widespread vasodilation, stimulation of pain nerve receptors, attraction of leukocyte migration into the area, and increased capillary permeability. Systemic vasodilation and extravasation of intravascular ECF from capillaries leads to hypotension and low-resistance (vasodilated) shock.

Assessment

There is a wide range of severity of signs and symptoms, associated with the equally broad range of pathologic change within the gland.

Subjective

The oustanding symptom is often severe, steady upper abdominal pain, which may be centered in the right upper quadrant, above the umbilicus, or in the left upper quadrant, depending on whether the major site of inflammation is in the head, the body, or the tail of the pancreas. The pain often radiates to the back at the level of the lower thoracic and upper lumbar vertebrae (T10 to L2). Nausea is common.

Objective

Vomiting may be persistent and does not relieve the pain. The patient is restless and in evident distress. The upper abdomen is tender to palpation and there may be muscle guarding. There may be hypoactive bowel sounds, and the paralytic ileus may lead to abdominal distention. If the attack is severe, the release of vasoactive substances from enzymic chemical damage to the pancreas, and even the peritoneum, may cause widespread vasodilation and hypotension (see above). Chemical injury to the pancreas, to surrounding tissues, and to the peritoneum may promote marked extravasation of intravascular ECF into the interstitial spaces and peritoneal cavity (third-spacing). The intravascular fluid loss combined with systemic vasodilation may lead to severe hypotension, shock, prerenal azotemia, and oliguria.

Laboratory. The white blood count may be elevated. Elevation of levels of pancreatic enzymes in the serum provides the definitive assessment in pancreatitis. In the normal individual a small portion of the enzymes from the exocrine pancreas, especially amylase and lipase, continually diffuse out of the duct system of the pancreas, and are also absorbed into the blood from the duodenum. The normal level of amylase produced by this diffusion is about 50 to 175 U/100 ml. When the outflow of enzymes is obstructed because of inflammation, edema or cellular debris, then their entry into the blood is greatly increased and serum levels rise sometimes very high, to over 3000 U/100 ml. Serum amylase rises within a few hours of the onset of symptoms and signs in most patients, often to or above 500 U/100 ml, and usually has subsided to normal after 48 hr. The level of serum lipase rises more slowly and remains elevated longer. The height of the serum amylase level appears not to correlate with the severity of the attack.

In cases where there has been a large release of pancreatic enzymes with dissolution of intraperitoneal fat stores the serum Ca^{2+} levels decline because of the reaction of fatty acids with ionized calcium to form soaps.

Urinary amylase levels also increase in pancreatitis and remain elevated for over a week; 1000 U/hr or more is the usual value in acute pancreatitis, and excretion of more than 300 U/hr is considered abnormally high.

X-ray of the abdomen may reveal calcifications in the pancreas—their presence indicates underlying chronic pancreatitis—and distended loops of intestine evidencing the accompanying paralytic ileus.

Management

Regardless of the cause of the acute pancreatitis, the management of the acute attack tends to be the same. Control of the often severe pain is necessary; meperidine is usually used in preference to morphine because the latter tends to produce more spasm in the smooth muscle of the sphincter of Oddi, and therefore increases obstruction. If there is hypovolemia and hypotension, then fluid and electrolyte replacement is obviously required. Suppression of pancreatic secretion is important to reduce pressure in the acini and ducts behind the obstruction and to minimize the production of the digestive enzymes which destroy pancreatic tissue. This is accomplished by eliminating oral intake and by removing the acid gastric secretions (which stimulate pancreatic secretions) by means of nasogastric suction. The suction also relieves gastrointestinal distention. Some authors suggest that the anticholinergics atropine or propantheline are useful to decrease the gastric acid secretion which promotes pancreatic secretion by stimulating secretin release, and to directly suppress pancreatic secretion via vagal cholinergic inhibition. Others believe that the disadvantage of increased paralytic ileus caused by anticholinergics more than offsets the advantage of decreased secretions. They also cause tachycardia and drying of pulmonary secretions, predisposing to respiratory tree obstruction. Antibiotics are advocated by some workers to prevent infection and abscess formation in the necrotic tissue, but are usually not necessary.

Once the pain, abdominal distention, and tenderness have resolved, the patient may be given oral antacids while the nasogastric tube is closed off at increasing intervals. Later, hourly antacids are continued and a low-fat bland diet begun. The antacids buffer gastric acid, reducing the acid stimulation of the duodenum which activates secretin and pancreatic enzyme release. If the patient is a known alcoholic, abstinence should be urged. Such admonitions are generally to no avail. Where abstinence does occur, it has a good chance of diminishing or eliminating further attacks. However, with each recurrent acute attack destruction of functional pancreatic tissue and fibrosis progress, worsening the underlying chronic disease process. If there is no indication of alcoholism, then gallbladder disease or one of the other less usual causes of pancreatitis will be sought.

Later Complications of Acute Pancreatitis

In a few patients there may be continued fever and abdominal pain which prolongs the course of an attack of acute pancreatitis. This most often occurs in the alcoholic patient and results from an unusually slow resolution of the inflammatory process; or from the development of one of the complications of acute pancreatitis: a pancreatic pseudocyst or a retention cyst. Both contain inflammatory cells, pancreatic secretions, and necrotic products of the acute inflammation. These cysts are said to be quite common and probably occur frequently in the course of development of chronic pancreatitis. They may be large enough to produce a tender palpable abdominal mass and may be accompanied by fever and pain; or at the other extreme the patient may be afebrile and feel quite well. In such patients the serum amylase and lipase may remain elevated for many weeks. It is reported that, given abstinence from alcohol, a continued bland low-fat diet, and hourly antacids, many cysts will eventually resolve without any additional treatment.

Chronic Pancreatitis

Cause

Chronic progressive pancreatitis is most often a disease of persons who have had a high alcohol intake for perhaps five to ten years. During this time, functional and structural damage to the pancreas has occurred, usually without marked appearance of signs or symptoms. In most cases chronic pancreatitis manifests itself insidiously with intermittent relatively mild upper abdominal pain. Then at some point the chronic progressive damage becomes severe enough that, given an episode of increased alcohol intake, an attack of acute pancreatitis occurs. As stated earlier it is probable that in the alcoholic, by the time an episode of acute pancreatitis occurs, the chronic progressive disease is already well established. If the patient continues alcohol intake, the chronic process is often punctuated by acute exacerbations. In chronic pancreatitis, return to normal functional and anatomic status does not occur between acute attacks.

Abnormalities

The processes by which alcohol leads to the development of chronic pancreatitis are probably direct cytotoxic action of alcohol on pancreatic cells, as evidenced by characteristic cytologic changes in pancreas cells exposed to alcohol, in persons susceptible to this cytotoxic effect on the basis of genetic predisposition. In addition, it is suggested that alcohol may stimulate pancreatic secretion at the same time that it obstructs the outflow of the secretions by inducing spasm of smooth muscle within the duct system and sphincter of Oddi. Finally, as discussed previously, evidence indicates that alcohol causes deposition of proteinaceous material, perhaps derived from degenerating pancreatic parenchyma, within the small-duct system of the pancreas, the larger ducts remaining normal and intact until the disease is well advanced. Later the larger ducts and main duct do become fibrotic, cystic, and distorted.

In chronic pancreatitis the whole gland is often diffusely involved in fibrotic changes; acinar cells are atrophic and replaced by fibrous scar tissue; there are areas of focal inflammation, necrosis, hemorrhage and edema; the ducts are filled with a thick protein substance and sometimes calculi, and are fibrotic and distorted. The islets may be preserved.

Assessment in Chronic Pancreatitis

Subjective

A history of prolonged excess intake of alcohol and increasingly frequent and severe episodes of vomiting and acute attacks of pancreatitis with severe abdominal pain can often be elicited. Abdominal pain is the outstanding chief complaint of patients with chronic pancreatitis. Early in the progressive course the pain occurs with the acute attacks and may resolve altogether as they subside. With the passage of time, if the patient continues alcohol intake, the acute attacks become more frequent and more severe and eventually the pain may be continuous. This progression may occur within a few months or over several years. The pain resembles that of the acute attack with respect to locale, severity, and radiation. It is brought on and made worse by food intake, because of the stimulus to exocrine secretion induced by food, which results in the acini releasing digestive enzymes into occluded small ducts, with resulting increased pressure and chemical damage. In the short term the pain is relieved by alcohol because of its anesthetic action; in the longer term, of course, alcohol intake promotes severe exacerbations and progression of the chronic disease.

Diarrhea may be a relatively frequent complaint, and may be caused by the alcohol intake itself, or by the azotorrhea and steatorrhea resulting from the impaired digestion of protein and fat with a consequent malabsorption syndrome induced by the chronic pancreatic exocrine insufficiency. The stools tend to be copious, oily, and foul smelling. Because of the large caloric loss, weight loss is common.

Objective

Abnormalities of blood glucose homeostasis may gradually develop in chronic pancreatitis, because of impairment of the endocrine functions of the pancreas as concerns both insulin and glucagon secretion. Both alpha (glucagon-secreting) and beta (insulin-secreting) islets are progressively destroyed in patients with chronic pancreatitis of long duration, but apparently the beta cell destruction often predominates, since diabetic hyperglycemia is said to be a more frequent development than hypoglycemia.

The patient may have the manifestations of alcoholic liver disease discussed previously: hepatomegaly, cirrhosis with portal hypertension, jaundice, esophageal varices and/or a peptic ulcer, and an enlarged spleen.

Elevated serum amylase and lipase will often be found; however, in far advanced chronic pancreatitis so much functioning tissue may have been destroyed that the serum enzymes may be within normal levels or low. Blood glucose determinations may reveal hypoglycemia with fasting, and postprandial hyperglycemia, and a glucose tolerance test is useful in evaluating the degree of endocrine impairment and islet cell destruction. Stool fat determination is an index of degree of exocrine (digestive enzyme) impairment. X-ray of the abdomen often reveals areas of calcification in the pancreas.

Management of Chronic Pancreatitis

Total abstinence from alcohol is the essential, but infrequently attained, component of management of this disorder. Replacement of the pancreatic enzymes, mainly lipases and proteases, by oral administration of concentrated pancreatic extracts, helps control the impaired digestion and assimilation caused by exocrine insufficiency in some patients. The extracts are usually taken with meals, and with antacids to minimize the inhibition of their action produced by gastric acid. A diet low in fat and high in protein and carbohydrate may be useful, and supplements of medium-chain triglycerides help maintain caloric intake and improve fat absorption.

Management of the often severe pain of chronic pancreatitis comprises a difficult problem, particularly in the patient who continues alcohol intake. Some authors have reported that pancreatic enzyme supplements appear to reduce pain in some patients; even those in whom pancreatic exocrine insufficiency is not yet marked; it is said that the presence of pancreatic enzymes in the duodenum exerts a feedback inhibition of the stimuli for pancreatic secretion, thus blocking the sequence of pain-producing processes. A variety of surgical procedures for the purported function of pain relief in chronic pancreatitis have been recommended, but in the patient who continues alcohol intake, their long-term value seems questionable at best. Attempts at pharmacologic pain control may produce a second addiction.

REFERENCES

Beeson PB and McDermott W, editors: *Textbook of Medicine*. 14th ed. Philadelphia, Pa.: Saunders, 1975.

Bennion, LJ & Grundy, SM: Risk factors for the development of cholelithiasis in man. *N. Engl. J. Med.* 299:1161–1167, 1978.

Chen TS and Chen PS: *Essential Hepatology*. Woburn, Mass.: Butterworth, 1977.

Davenport HW: *Physiology of the Digestive Tract: An Introductory Text*. 4th ed. Chicago, Ill.: Yearbook Medical Publishers, 1977.

Dietschy JM, editor: *Disorders of the Gastrointestinal Tract. Disorders of the Liver. Nutritional Disorders*. New York: Grune and Stratton, 1976.

Fisher MM and Rankin JG: *Alcohol and the Liver. Hepatology*, v. 3. Research and Clinical Issues. New York: Plenum, 1977.

Frolich ED, editor: *Pathophysiology*. Philadelphia, Pa.: Lippincott, 1976.

Ganong WF: *Review of Medical Physiology*. 8th ed. Los Altos, Calif.: Lange Medical Publications, 1977.

Guyton AC: *Textbook of Medical Physiology*. 5th ed. Philadelphia, Pa.: Saunders, 1976.

Hill RB and Kern F: *The Gastrointestinal Tract*. Baltimore, Md.: Williams and Wilkins, 1977.

James JH et al: Blood–brain neutral amino acid transport activity is increased after portacaval anastomosis. *Science* 200:1395–1397, 1978.

Johnson LR, editor: *Gastrointestinal Physiology.* St. Louis, Mo.: Mosby, 1977.

Lindner AE, editor: *Emotional Factors in Gastrointestinal Illness.* New York: Elsevier, 1973. Amsterdam, Excerpta Medica.

Peterson WL, et al.: Healing of duodenal ulcer with an antacid regimen. *N. Engl. J. Med.* 297:341–345, 1977.

Sklar D and Liang MH: Antacids: Cost, taste and buffering. *N. Engl. J. Med.* 296:1007, 1977.

Spiro HM: *Clinical Gastroenterology.* 2nd ed. New York: Macmillan, 1977.

Sabesin SM and Levinson MJ: Acute and chronic hepatitis: multisystemic involvement related to immunologic disease. *Adv. Intern. Med.* 22:424–454, 1977.

Thorn GW, et al, editors: *Harrison's Principles of Internal Medicine.* 8th ed. New York: McGraw-Hill, 1977.

Endocrine Disorders

ANTERIOR PITUITARY

Six hormones are secreted by the anterior pituitary: adrenocorticotropic hormone (ACTH); thyroid stimulating hormone (thyrotropic hormone, TSH); the gonad stimulating hormones: follicle stimulating hormone (FSH) and luteinizing hormone (LH); growth hormone (GH); and prolactin. The function of prolactin is to stimulate breast milk secretion; the other five secretions all stimulate the production and release of hormones from their target organs: the adrenal cortex; thyroid; gonadal tissue; and in the case of growth hormone, somatomedins from the liver, kidneys, and possibly other organs.

Growth hormone itself is an anabolic hormone which produces a positive nitrogen balance and increased protein synthesis. The somatomedins have a number of complex effects on growth, including the production of cartilage at the ends of long bones and growth of soft tissues including viscera and nerves.

ACTH, FSH, LH, and TSH are probably secreted by the pituitary basophils, while the acidophiles secrete prolactin and GH; the chromophobes may be a nonsecretory cell type.

The median eminence of the hypothalamus, which is located at the base of the brain in the area of the 3rd ventricle and optic chiasm, and just above the pituitary, elaborates several distinct hormonal releasing factors which travel to the pituitary in the hypothalamicohypophysial portal veins and influence the production of the pituitary hormones. The releasing factors stimulate TSH, FSH and LH, GH, and possibly ACTH, although this last factor has not yet been isolated. The inhibitory factors are somatostatin, which inhibits the release of GH; and a prolactin-inhibiting factor. It is probable that the rate of secretion of these stimulating and inhibiting hypothalamic hormones is under feedback control from hor-

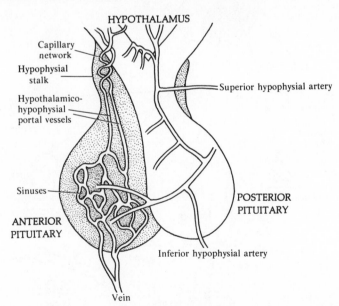

Figure 13-1. Diagram of the relationships between lower hypothalamus and pituitary, indicating the hypothalamicohypophysial portal system. The pituitary lies in the sella turcica of the sphenoid bone. The anterior pituitary is comprised of three cell types: eosinophils, basophils, and chromophobes.

mones of the target endocrine glands rather than from the anterior pituitary tropic hormones. However, recent studies on blood flow to, through, or from the pituitary suggest that pituitary hormones may be transported directly to the brain to influence its function.

Anterior Pituitary Tumors

Approximately 10% of intracranial tumors are derived from the pituitary, and of these the nonsecreting chromophobe adenoma is the most common, accounting for 95% of such tumors. Although chromophobe adenomas produce no secretions, they exert compression on the gland as a whole as they enlarge, and interfere with its blood supply, so that destruction of the secretory tissue may occur resulting in widespread endocrine hypofunction because of inadequate secretion of tropic hormones. In addition they cause neurologic abnormalities as they grow, and may compress the hypothalamus and optic chiasm resulting in impaired vision and disturbances in functions regulated by the hypothalamus: appetite and satiety, body temperature regulation, and other visceral and autonomic activities.

Tumors of the secretory cells of the pituitary generally involve only one secretion. Growth hormone-secreting tumors—eosinophil adenomas—lead to gigan-

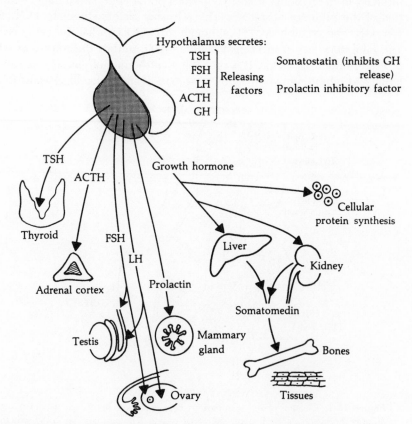

Figure 13-2. Diagram illustrating the relationship of the major hypothalamic releasing and inhibitory factors, the pituitary tropic hormones, and their target organs and tissues.

tism if the tumor develops before the epiphyses of the long bones close, or acromegaly if the age of onset is later. In acromegaly there is overgrowth of bone, soft tissue including viscera, and the connective tissues. In both gigantism and acromegaly, pituitary insufficiency tends to develop later in the course as the tumor destroys the cells that secrete tropic hormones. The result is hypogonadism, hypothyroidism, and adrenal insufficiency.

Pituitary basophilic adenomas which secrete excess ACTH may cause bilateral adrenal hyperplasia and Cushing's disease. Apparently thyrotropin-secreting tumors of the pituitary are rare; patients with thyrotoxicosis seldom have elevated TSH, and in fact more often TSH is low because of feedback suppression of the tropic hormone caused by the excess circulating thyroid hormone.

The treatment of pituitary tumors is by pituitary irradiation or surgical excision. The former is often ineffective and the mortality rate for surgical removal is high.

Panhypopituitarism (Pituitary Insufficiency, Simmonds' Disease)

There are a number of causes of pituitary insufficiency. A chromophobe adenoma which destroys the pituitary by compression is the most frequent; others are craniopharyngioma (Rathke's pouch tumor), eosinophilic adenoma associated with acromegaly, and postpartum pituitary necrosis from intrapartal blood loss and hypotensive shock. This form is called Sheehan's disease. Generally, the first signs of hypopituitarism are failure to lactate and menstruate in females, a decline in libido, and vague symptoms of easy fatigability, lethargy, and lack of energy. Gradually there is loss of axillary and pubic hair, genital and breast atrophy; development of intolerance to cold, bradycardia, and other signs of hypothyroidism; and eventually signs and symptoms of adrenal insufficiency: hypotension, thin atrophic skin, low blood volume, asthenia, and weakness. These changes develop as the gonads, thyroid, and adrenals atrophy and production of their hormones declines.

The onset is insidious, and since the decline in pituitary function is most often gradual over a period of years, the signs and symptoms develop slowly. Laboratory studies show a decrease in both the tropic hormones from the pituitary and hormones from the target glands. Management is the replacement of the target gland hormones starting with cortisol, because of the danger of Addisonian crisis (extreme adrenal insufficiency with circulatory collapse) and then thyroid hormone.

Empty sella syndrome is a special form of pituitary insufficiency seen most often in obese females who have borne many children. Enlargement of the pituitary fossa is seen on skull films and special studies show little or no pituitary tissue. It is thought that there has been ischemic necrosis of an enlarged pituitary. The range of signs and symptoms is wide, depending on the amount of functioning pituitary tissue remaining, from minimal to widespread endocrine deficits.

POSTERIOR PITUITARY (NEUROHYPOPHYSIS)

Vasopressin (ADH), diabetes insipidus (DI), and syndrome of inappropriate secretion of ADH are discussed in Chapter 1.

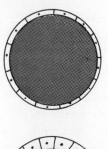

Thyroid follicle from inactive gland showing squamous (flat) epithelium and large storage of colloid

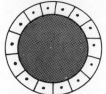

Thyroid follicle from normal gland showing cuboidal epithelium and moderate amount of colloid

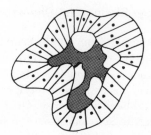

Thyroid follicle from overactive gland showing columnar epithelium, sparse colloid, and vacuoles in colloid from rapid mobilization and secretion of hormone in blood

Figure 13-3. Diagram of a follicle from a thyroid gland under three conditions of activity: hypo-, normal, and hyperactivity. The hypo- and hyperactive states could result from inadequate or excessive stimulation by pituitary TSH, respectively, or from other abnormal states (see text).

THYROID

The thyroid gland is made up of multiple acini or follicles, each bounded by a single layer of cells and containing colloid, the storage form of the hormone. When the gland is actively synthesizing and secreting the hormone the cells are cuboidal or even columnar, and the colloid content of the follicle is decreased because of rapid resorption of the storage form and release into the blood; when the gland is relatively inactive the cells are squamous (flat) and the follicles are filled with colloid. The level of thyroid function is controlled by TSH from the anterior pituitary, which in turn is regulated by TRH from the hypothalamus. Both TSH and TRH are influenced by feedback from the levels of thyroid hormone circulating in the blood; the more hormone, the greater the suppression of the stimulating processes. TSH is essential for maintenance of the structure and function of the thyroid, and the synthesis and secretion of the hormones; TSH acts on thyroid cells by stimulating adenyl cyclase, which causes an increase in intracellular cAMP and consequent increased rate of synthesis and secretion of the two hormones. Correlated with this stimulation is increased vascularity, hypertrophy, and hyperplasia of the gland as a whole.

The two principle hormones from the thyroid are iodine-containing compounds triiodothyronine (T3) and thyroxine (T4), most of which are carried in the blood bound to a plasma globulin. The hormones are stored in the colloid in bound form with thyroglobulin; when secretion of the hormones from colloid occurs the link with thyroglobulin is broken and triiodothyronine and thyroxine are resorbed by thyroid cells and then secreted into the blood. Iodine is required for thyroid hormone synthesis. The actions of the hormones include stimulating the rate of O_2 consumption by cells and regulation of protein synthesis.

Nontoxic Goiter (Simple Goiter)

Simple goiter probably represents a compensatory hypertrophy of the gland resulting originally from a level of hormone synthesis inadequate to meet the needs of the organism. The causes of the original impairment of hormone synthesis are debatable; in some instances the cause is inadequate dietary intake of iodide, but in most cases no cause can be discovered. Initially the low hormone output may lead to a removal of feedback suppression of TSH from the anterior pituitary with resulting increased TSH output. However, in most patients with simple goiter TSH levels are within normal limits. It has been speculated that, in cases where there is not a deficient intake of iodide as the causal process, some poorly understood impairment of iodide trapping by the gland cells has led to defective hormone synthesis, which in turn increases the sensitivity of the thyroid to normal levels of circulating TSH. The increased sensitivity to the stimulating TSH then leads to hypertrophy and hyperplasia of the gland, with increased hormone synthesis, which then becomes adequate to meet metabolic requirements. In some cases, if the compensatory hypertrophy is still inadequate to maintain hormone output at adequate levels, then TSH secretion may increase above normal. If the gland is still unable to produce sufficient hormone under the added stimulation, hypothyroidism may develop.

The gland becomes diffusely enlarged, producing an obvious tumor in the neck which may cause compression of the esophagus and trachea. At late stages the goiter may become nodular. The patient may be euthyroid or hypothyroid. Management is by small iodide supplements where deficiency has been the cause, and regression in size may occur. In the majority of instances where no cause is known, daily administration of thyroid supplements (levothyroxine), especially if begun early in the course, will lead to regression. Results are less satisfactory late in the course.

Hypothyroidism and Myxedema

Inadequate production of thyroid hormone leads to a gradual and progressive slowing of most metabolic functions; myxedema represents the most severe form in which the skin and other tissues become infiltrated with a nonpitting collection of mucopolysaccharides.

One of the most common causes is overtreatment of hyperthroidism, either surgically or with radioactive iodine. If too much functional tissue is removed or destroyed, then the remainder may undergo involution. Another common cause is advanced Hashimoto's thyroiditis (see following). Pituitary insufficiency is a less common cause. Regardless of the cause, the results are the same: depression of most cellular enzyme systems and oxidative metabolism.

The onset is insidious with the gradual development of cold intolerance, dry skin, lethargy, mental slowing, sluggishness, puffiness of face and extremities, sparseness of hair, bradycardia, hypertension, and delayed relaxation time of the deep tendon reflexes ("hung reflexes"). Hoarseness of the voice, cardiac dilation and pericardial effusion, adynamic ileus, and eventually psychoemotional disorders may develop. Myxedema coma is an exaggeration of all abnormalities and is characterized by hypotension, hypoventilation, hypoglycemia, and hypothermia. The mortality rate is high—often 50 to 70% or more.

Management of hypothyroidism consists of returning circulating thyroid hormone level to normal limits with levothyroxine, thyroid extract, or some other replacement medication, such as a synthetic mixture of T3 and T4. Reversal of all of the abnormalities occurs. Elevation of the metabolic rate should be accomplished gradually, especially in the elderly and/or patients with organic heart disease.

Hashimoto's Thyroiditis

This is a chronic immune disorder,·most common in females during middle age, and characterized by changes in the gland involving inflammation, infiltration with lymphocytes, areas of hyperplasia and atrophy, and eventual replacement of increasing amounts of the gland by fibrous scar tissue and the development of hypothyroidism.

The disease probably involves both antibody-mediated and cell-mediated immunity; patients with Hashimoto's have antibodies against thyroid cell cytoplasm, microsomes, and thyroglobulin; and lymphocytes sensitized to a variety of thyroid antigens. There appears to be a strong genetic predisposition.

The gland is enlarged, painful, tender, and often asymmetric. T3–T4 levels may be depressed and TSH elevated, indicating inadequate hormone synthesis with gradually developing hypothyroidism and undersuppression of TSH. Management is replacement with levothyroxine.

Thyrotoxicosis (Graves' Disease, Hyperthyroidism)

Cause

The cause of this increased activity of the thyroid which results in excessive hormone production is not known, although there are several theories. Although hyperthyroidism can be caused by excess hormone production from a single or multiple autonomous adenomas, or excessive TSH production by the pituitary, the usual form is a diffuse hypertrophy, hyperplasia, and generalized hormone oversynthesis and hypersecretion. This is a very common disease and is said to account for more than three quarters of all endocrine abnormalities, excluding only diabetes mellitus. It is more common in females than males, shows a strong familial predisposition and may be associated with Hashimoto's thyroiditis. Graves' disease often has two abnormalities, exophthalmos and dermatologic conditions, associated to varying degrees with the thyrotoxicosis.

Approximately half of patients with diffuse thyrotoxicosis have in their blood a humoral antibody immunoglobulin (IgG), the antigen for which is not known but which is suspected to be one or more components of thyroid cells; the factor is called long-acting thyroid stimulator (LATS). Its action stimulates thyroid adenyl cyclase, increases I_2 uptake by the gland, causes thyroid hyperplasia and increases hormone synthesis and secretion. However, it is not present in all patients with thyrotoxicosis, it is present in some persons without, and its level is poorly correlated with the severity of the thyrotoxicosis.

A still higher percentage of Graves' patients have an additional IgG which also acts as a thyroid stimulator and which is called LATS protector. These substances form part of the basis for a theory of Graves' disease as one of humoral or antibody-mediated immunity.

There is other evidence indicating that cell-mediated immune processes are involved in Graves' (cell-mediated immunity means that there are lymphocytes that are sensitized to a particular tissue, in this case the thyroid, and which attack and destroy the cells by cytotoxic processes; see Chapter 22) in addition to the antibody or humorally mediated immune processes. Some workers hold that Graves' disease and Hashimoto's thyroiditis represent two aspects of a single autoimmune disorder, and that Graves' disease represents a balance between the stimulating and inhibiting effects of antibodies such as LATS and LATS protector; and the destructive effects of cell-mediated cytotoxic processes.

Structural Abnormalities

The gland is soft, enlarged, hypervascular, and histologically shows cellular hypertrophy and hyperplasia. The epithelium is cuboidal or columnar depending on the severity; the extent of the boundary epithelium of each follicle is greatly increased and infolded upon itself; and the colloid is markedly decreased in amount with numerous empty spaces indicating the rapid resorption and secretion of hormone and decreased storage. There is infiltration of lymphycytes, which may be a sign of the degree of cell-mediated cytotoxicity proceeding.

Exophthalmos is often present; in patients who have it there is a factor in the serum which when injected into experimental animals induces exophthalmos. The substance is not LATS. Gamma globulin is bound to antigens of orbital tissue; there are inflammatory cellular infiltrates involving mast cells, lymphocytes, and plasma cells; and the orbital muscles are hypertrophied early, but later may become fibrotic. Some authors believe that these changes are the result of cell-mediated immunity directed against orbital antigens.

Changes in other organs also occur in some patients with Graves', including generalized lymph node hyperplasia and infiltration, enlargement of the thymus and/or spleen, cardiomegaly, striated muscle fiber degeneration, osteoporosis, and structural alterations in the liver. Studies have shown that Graves' disease of long duration gradually progresses to hypothyroidism, probably as a consequence of the inflammatory and immunologic processes described above. The course of the disease in the long term is characterized by remissions and exacerbations. Causes of death in untreated or inadequately treated thyrotoxicosis are congestive heart failure and inanition.

Assessment

Subjective

Complaints of palpitations, nervousness, irritability, and anxiety; shortness of breath on exertion; heat intolerance and sweating; weakness, fatigue, insomnia, and tremulousness; diarrhea and weight loss, are common.

Objective

Common signs of thyrotoxicosis are gland enlargement; a fine tremor of the extended hands and fingers; protruding eyes with inability to converge; there may be lid lag and sclera visible below and above the iris on vertical gaze testing, and a widened palpebral fissure; hyperdynamic circulation and tachycardia; ankle edema; and marked muscle weakness on strength testing. The patient appears nervous and fidgety, and overly compliant. The skin is warm and moist. There may be palpable supraclavicular lymph nodes.

The heart is markedly affected in hyperthyroidism, particularly in the elderly patient or one with ischemic or other organic heart disease. Because of the elevated O_2 consumption in most tissues induced by the excess thyroid hormone, a high cardiac output is required to meet peripheral O_2 needs. In addition the thyroid hormones appear to increase myocardial contractility; there is increased force of contraction, heart rate, and spontaneous impulse formation, leading to arrhythmias. All of these factors, combined with the peripheral vasodilation and decreased peripheral resistance, produce a markedly elevated cardiac output and increased workload on the myocardium which is poorly tolerated in the elderly and in patients with organic heart disease.

In many respects the cardiovascular actions of the catecholamines epinephrine and norepinephrine, and the thyroid hormones T3 and T4, are similar, and they appear to have a synergistic action. Although catecholamine production is normal in most patients with thyrotoxicosis, it may be that high levels of thyroid hormones act to increase the effects of the catecholamines. Note that many of the cardiovascular effects characteristic of the hyperthyroid state are β adrenergic effects; it is reported that sympathectomy or β adrenergic blockade reduce the cardiovascular and some other autonomic effects of excess thyroid hormone, and these effects of excessive T3 and T4 may be mediated via β adrenergic stimulation. For these reasons, cardiovascular assessment is of particular importance in hyperthyroidism. Atrial tachycardia or fibrillation and sinus tachycardia are the common arrhythmias. There may be a systolic murmur, hyperactive PMI, intensified heart sounds, and signs of congestive heart failure such as bibasilar pulmonary rales and pitting ankle edema. The patient's exercise tolerance should be assessed in the interview, as well as incidence of dyspnea on exertion, chest pain, orthopnea, and paroxysmal nocturnal dyspnea.

Thyroid crisis or thyroid storm is a complication of hyperthyroidism which may develop spontaneously; may occur postoperatively, especially in patients who have been inadequately prepared; or may occur in inadequately controlled hyperthyroid patients who are receiving medical management. In the latter case the complication may be precipitated by an accident involving trauma, other surgery, or a systemic illness. Signs of thyroid crisis are delirium, tachycardia, hyperthermia, vomiting and diarrhea, restlessness, dehydration, and hypotension. The mortality rate is high and early recognition is important. Management includes fluid, electrolyte and glucose infusion, cooling blanket, O_2 inhalation, antithyroid medication, and iodides.

Management

Surgery

The aim of treatment is to decrease the synthesis and release of the thyroid hormones. In younger persons up to age 40 subtotal thyroidectomy is often appropriate; as it is also for patients with a markedly enlarged gland, those who do not tolerate antithyroid medication, and for recurrence following a course of antithyroid medication. The operation has a low mortality rate in skilled hands where preparation for surgery has been adequate. Antithyroid medication (propylthiouracil or methimazole) is given until thyroid hormone levels have subsided to normal. This reduces the incidence of intra- and postoperative cardiac arrhythmias, thyrotoxicosis, and thyroid crisis. Iodine in the form of Lugol's solution is then added. The purpose of these measures is to reduce gland vascularity, size, and friability. Complications of surgery, now rare, are injury to the recurrent laryngeal nerve, causing hoarseness; and inadvertent removal of the parathyroids, causing hypocalcemia and tetany. Recurrence of thyrotoxicosis is low, about 5%; development of hypothyroidism is higher (reported to be between 5 and 40%) but lower than in radioactive iodine treatment.

Radioactive Iodine ($^{131}I_2$, RAI)

This is an inexpensive, safe and easy method of reducing the amount of functioning thyroid tissue and hence hormone output. However, incidence of later progression to hypothyroidism is quite high over a period of 5 to 10 years: 40 to 70%. Incidence of cancer is reported not to be increased. Studies indicate that a more prolonged treatment with lower doses reduces the incidence of thyroid failure, but this method results in a delay in lowering hormone production to safer levels.

Antithyroid Agents

Propylthiouracil or methimazole may be employed; they produce a chemical block of the biosynthetic pathways for hormone production. The main side effect is leukopenia; skin rash, pruritis, and epigastric distress are others. In most patients for whom this treatment is selected, satisfactory control is obtained. Higher doses are given until the patient becomes euthyroid, and then the amount of drug is decreased to the dose just sufficient to yield good control. The symptoms of thyrotoxicosis usually abate following three to five weeks of treatment. Hypothyroidism may also develop with this course, in which case the gland will hypertrophy because of increased TSH output resulting from a too great reduction in feedback suppression by T3 and T4. Antithyroid drugs are often given with iodides, which act to suppress T3 and T4 release. Treatment is continued for one to two years and then stopped; about half of patients will then maintain long or indefinite remissions. The remainder may have recurrences within 1 to 12 months; in these another course or a different treatment may be elected.

Exophthalmos usually resolves with treatment of the hyperthyroidism, mode of treatment is said to be unrelated to the course of the exophthalmos.

ADRENAL CORTEX

There are three types of hormones secreted from the adrenal cortex: (1) gluco-corticoids, mainly cortisol but also some corticosterone, which have effects on carbohydrate metabolism and protein synthesis; (2) mineralocorticoids, mainly aldosterone but also some deoxycorticosterone, which regulate Na^+ and K^+ balance via the kidney; and (3) the adrenal androgens, mainly dehydroepiandrosterone.

The secretion of the glucocorticoids is under the control of ACTH from the anterior pituitary and probably an ACTH releasing hormone from the hypothalamus. There is a periodicity in ACTH secretion, and therefore a diurnal variation in cortisol release; it is highest in the early morning prior to awakening in subjects synchronized to a normal day–night schedule. ACTH secretion is also stimulated by physiologic stress; in fact "stress" is defined biologically as any stimulus which increases pituitary release of ACTH and hence increased adrenal glucocorticoid production. This effect is mediated via the effects of stress on the limbic system which may activate increased hypothalamic corticotropin releasing factor. Administration of exogenous glucocorticoids leads to marked suppression of pituitary output of ACTH and adrenocortical function; if steroids are withdrawn suddenly after prolonged administration the patient may experience severe adrenal insufficiency, since during the exogenous steroid treatment the pituitary loses its capacity to synthesize ACTH, and the adrenal cortices become atrophic and hypofunctional.

Mineralocorticoid secretion is controlled to some extent by ACTH but also by the renin–angiotensin system and serum K^+ levels as described in Chapter 1. Other steroidal hormones are secreted by the adrenal cortex, but these are the major ones in the human.

All adrenal steroids are produced from cholesterol along complex interrelated biosynthetic pathways consisting of numerous steps; each conversion is catalyzed by a specific enzyme, and the presence and amount of each enzyme is under the control of a specific gene. For this reason, certain genetic disorders result in inadequate secretion of some normal adrenal hormones, especially cortisol, and excess secretion of some abnormal ones (see following, adrenogenital syndromes).

Glucocorticoids have a number of physiologic actions: they increase the production of glucose from amino acids; stimulate the breakdown of liver glycogen to yield glucose; promote the catabolism of body proteins; are essential for liver synthesis of glycogen; are necessary for the normal responsiveness of blood vessels to circulating catecholamines; maintain normal capillary permeability; stabilize lysozomal membranes; and increase glomerular filtration rate and promote normal renal tubular and collecting duct function. They also exert a feedback suppression on the release of ACTH. The actions of aldosterone have been described in Chapter 1.

Adrenocortical Hypofunction

There are two basic types of adrenocortical hypofunction: that which is caused by an inability of the adrenal cortex itself to produce sufficient cortisol and aldosterone, even under normal stimulation of ACTH (primary); and that which is caused by a failure of anterior pituitary ACTH secretion, with resulting inadequate stimulation to the adrenal cortex (secondary). Primary and secondary forms of adrenocortical insufficiency can be distinguished on the basis of the patient's history as well as by plasma ACTH titer determinations. In the primary form the ACTH levels are high; in the secondary type, plasma ACTH is absent or abnormally low.

Primary Adrenocortical Insufficiency (Addison's Disease)

This is a relatively rare disorder in which there is a deficiency of both glucocorticoid and mineralocorticoid synthesis resulting from atrophy or destruction of the adrenal cortices. Marked deficiency of these hormones is said not to occur until about 80% of both cortices have been eliminated. Formerly tuberculosis was the most common cause but at present the majority of cases appear to result from an immune disorder in which cortical tissue is destroyed by cell-mediated or antibody-mediated autoimmune responses, with activation of the complement system. Fungal infections of the adrenals are a less common cause; and severe injury such as catastrophic burns and extreme systemic illnesses such as septicemia sometimes result in an acute bilateral adrenocortical hemorrhagic necrosis.

The abnormalities which result from deficiency of cortisol are hypoglycemia; inability of the kidneys to eliminate a water load, which may promote dilutional hyponatremia (see Chapter 1); loss of the normal vasoconstrictive response to catecholamines; anorexia, listlessness, fatigability and weakness; and inability to withstand the physiologic stress of injury, surgery, or systemic illness. In addition, the low circulating cortisol removes feedback suppression to ACTH output, so that plasma ACTH increases markedly; the increase of this hormone and an accompanying elevation in melanocyte-stimulating hormone from the intermediate lobe, produces the pigmentation of the skin often seen in patients with Addison's.

The deficiency of aldosterone leads to abnormal function of the distal renal tubule cation exchange site (Chapter 1); there is insufficient resorption of Na^+ from the tubular filtrate, and excess retention of K^+, with resulting hyponatremia and hyperkalemia. The loss of Na^+ leads to a decreased circulating ECF volume, since when Na^+ is lost, H_2O is lost with it. (This is not in conflict with the inability to excrete a free-water load, mentioned above; the loss of Na^+ and H_2O with decline in circulating blood volume is a *gradual chronic* development. When such a patient then drinks, or receives by infusion, large amounts of hypotonic fluids, the chronically depressed GFR reduces the ability of the kidney to eliminate rapidly and effectively the free water—water unaccompanied by Na^+—and acute dilution of ECF Na^+ occurs.) As the ECF volume falls heart size and blood pressure decline, and inadequate vasoconstrictive response to catecholamines promotes a decreased peripheral resistance from vasodilation. Hypovolemia and low peripheral resistance predispose to postural hypotension and syncope; or if severe, to peripheral vascular collapse and hypotensive shock, especially following physiologic stress such as injury, surgery, or systemic illness. Hyperkalemia may promote abnormal cardiac impulse formation leading to EKG changes and arrhythmias.

Other changes are altered mental status because of abnormal brain function caused by steroid deficts (irritability, apathy, restlessness, anxiety, mental confusion) and gastrointestinal complaints: nausea and vomiting, diarrhea, and abdominal distress.

Laboratory values may be within normal limits in mild Addison's, but if severe there is hyponatremia, hyperkalemia, hypochloremia, low bicarbonate, and acidemia. A laboratory test for Addison's is stimulation of the adrenals by intramuscular injection of ACTH; serum cortisol and aldosterone levels are measured prior to and an hour after ACTH administration. If preinjection levels of the adrenal steroids are abnormally low but increase adquately after ACTH injection this indicates a failure of normal adrenal ACTH stimulation. If preinjection levels are low and remain low after injection, then the deficit represents primary adrenal failure.

A test for adequate pituitary ACTH output is the metyrapone suppression test. Metyrapone is a compound which inhibits the enzyme responsibile for the ultimate step in the biosynthesis of cortisol from its precursors; it therefore reduces cortisol production when administered, removing feedback suppression of pituitary ACTH production by cortisol; if pituitary ACTH production is normal, metyrapone injection will therefore result in elevation of pituitary ACTH levels.

Management of Addison's consists of replacement of both cortisol and aldosterone. Cortisol is replaced with cortisone, hydrocortisone or prednisone, and aldosterone with fluorohydrocortisone. Replacement is started with low doses and then gradually built up, with close monitoring of blood pressure, body weight, electrolytes, and cardiac and mental status. Occasionally physiologic stress necessitates an increase in the glucocorticoid dosage. Education of these patients is of major importance. They should be encouraged to wear a Medic Alert bracelet and carry an injectible gluococorticoid in case of emergency. Oral glucocorticoids are irritating to gastric mucosa, predisposing to ulcer formation and gastrointestinal bleeding, and should therefore be taken with an effective liquid antacid such as Mylanta.

Secondary Adrenocortical Insufficiency

This is a slowly developing disorder which is among the abnormalities present in chronic pituitary insufficiency described previously. In secondary adrenocortical insufficiency, aldosterone levels may be within normal limits; this is so because in the case of aldosterone other factors (serum K^+ levels and renin–angiotensin) are responsible for its control in addition to ACTH. Therefore the primarily mineralocorticoid-deficiency effects of adrenal insufficiency (fluid, electrolyte, ECF osmotic and volume abnormalities) occurring in Addison's are less prominent in secondary adrenal hypfunction.

Protracted exogenous adrenal steroids, given, for example, for immunosuppression in transplant patients, or for the control if inflammatory reactions in rheumatoid arthritis; are well known to cause iatrogenic Cushing's (see following). But in addition they chronically suppress pitutitary ACTH and perhaps hypothalamic ACTH releasing factor, and decrease for extended periods the ability of the pituitary to synthesize and release ACTH in response to stress, after the steroids are withdrawn. The prolonged lack of ACTH stimulation to the adrenal cortex leads gradually to an atrophy of the cortisol-producing cells and to a decline in the capacity of these cells to respond to ACTH stimulation once it is resumed, which may persist for months after exogenous steroid withdrawal. Redevelopment of hypothalamic releasing hormone and pituitary ACTH synthesizing capacity, and reinstatement of responsiveness of adrenal cortisol-producing cells to ACTH stimulation, may be very slow to develop, and meanwhile the patinet is chronically and perhaps severely cortisol-deprived. In the interim gradually decreasing amounts of replacement glucocorticoids must be supplied.

Adrenocortical Hyperfunction

Cushing's Syndrome

Causes

Cushing's is a group of physiologic abnormalities caused by an excess of adrenal glucocorticoids, primarily cortisol. Mineralocorticoid hypersecretion is not involved. There are several types, the most common of which is bilateral adrenal gland hyperplasia most often caused by an excess secretion of ACTH from the anterior pituitary. Usually the abnormally high secretion of ACTH comes from a generalized overproduction of the hormone by the whole group of pituitary basophils, but occasionally it is from a basophilic adenoma. A second cause of Cushing's is one or more adenomas of the adrenal cortex which may hypersecrete autonomously or may respond excessively to normal pituitary ACTH output. Some of these adenomas are malignant. A third cause is the production of a compound resembling ACTH in every respect by a nonpituitary neoplasm of nonendocrine tissue; the pancreas, lungs, or thymus may be the source, and the adrenals respond to the substance exactly as though it were pituitary ACTH, by hyperplasia and hypersecretion.

Physiologic Abnormalities

Abnormalities induced by excess cortisol, whether from one of the above causes or from iatrogenic Cushing's (adrenal steroid administration) include catabolism of tissue proteins leading to muscle weakness and muscle wasting; stimulation of deamination of amino acids by the liver, causing a negative nitrogen balance; thinning of the skin; breakdown of the matrix of bone leading to osteoporosis; suppression of all components of physiologic response to injury and infection, including immune system responses; deposition of adipose tissue on the torso, causing striae; stimulation of gluconeogenesis promoting hyperglycemia; and electrolyte abnormalities, caused by excessive Na^+ retention and K^+ elimination, resulting from stimulation of the distal renal tubule cation exchange site. This electrolyte effect is a normal action of aldosterone, but cortisol also produces it when present in excessive amounts. The Na^+ retention causes expansion of the ECF and hypertension and may predispose to strokes, edema, and congestive heart failure.

Assessment

Subjective. There are few or no complaints beyond easy fatigability, except those related to the objective changes, and sometimes to the psychoemotional effects of excess glucocorticoids: emotional instability and irritability, and mood swings between mania and depression. Oligomenorrhea is frequent in females.

Objective. Altered bodily configuration is marked in severe steroid excess: moon face, buffalo hump, truncal obesity with increased abdominal panniculus, and appendicular muscle wasting. The skin is thin, with easy bruising and ecchymoses, lowered resistance to infection, and a ruddy complexion, often with acne, and in females, hirsutism. "Flame" (purplish) striae are present over the lower torso and thighs. The patient is overweight and hypertensive. X-rays may show osteoporosis, and there is decreased glucose tolerance resulting from excess liver gluconeogenesis and insulin resistance, which impairs entry of glucose into cells. Since gluococorticoids suppress eosinophils, there may be eosinopenia. There are increased plasma and urinary steroids; and hypokalemia, hypochloremia, and metabolic alkalemia (see Chapters 1 and 2).

Management

The treatment for Cushing's depends on which of the several causes listed above is responsibile in a given patient. There are a number of special laboratory procedures which aid in differentiating among the possible causes. If an administered dose of dexamethasone suppresses the plasma cortisol levels, this suggests excess pituitary ACTH stimulation as the cause; if cortisol remains unchanged it is assumed that either an ectopic production of ACTH is present or there is autonomous adrenocortical hypersecretion. An ACTH infusion with analysis of subsequent urinary metabolites of cortisol or plasma cortisol levels, as well as other tests, aid in defining the nature of the abnormality.

Cushing's resulting from a bilateral adrenal hyperplasia (where there is no evidence of a basophile adenoma) is usually caused by generalized hypersecretion of anterior pituitary ACTH and may respond to irradiation of the pituitary with proton beam, alpha particles, or implantation of ^{90}Y via a transphenoidal or sterotactic procedure. This treatment has drawbacks in that it is said to be effective in only about one half of patients with Cushing's from pituitary ACTH excess, and there is a quite long delay until decline of adrenal hypersecretion occurs. For this reason in patients who are hypertensive, have steroid diabetes mellitus, severe osteoporosis, or adverse psychoemotional changes, pituitary irradiation may bring too slow an amelioration of abnormalities. Occasionally panhypopituitarism may develop as a longer term consequence of pituitary irradiation.

Bilateral adrenalectomy with lifelong hormonal replacements for cortisol and aldosterone is the recommended treatment at some centers. A compound, mitotane, related to DDT, blocks the secretion of adrenal steroids by causing selective necrosis of cortisol-producing adrenal cells and thus induces a remission. This substance is sometimes used for patients who refuse surgery or who are candidates for total bilateral adrenalectomy but require a period of preoperative reversal of debility prior to and in preparation for surgery. Some patients who have had bilateral adrenalectomy develop pituitary tumors, and in these cases pituitary irradiation may be required subsequently.

It is reported that in some patients the use of the serotonin antagonist cyproheptadine reverses the adrenal hyperplasia; the effect is apparently mediated via suppression of the hypothalamic serotoninergic pathways which stimulate corticotropin releasing factor.

Cushing's from an adrenal adenoma, benign or malignant, requires exploratory surgery and removal of the adrenal having the tumor; most tumors are single and unilateral. Often the gland without the tumor is atrophic and hyposecretory from pituitary ACTH suppression by the hyperactive adenoma, so that cortisol replacement is required when the hyperactive adrenal is removed. If the tumor is malignant, mitotane suppression may be used; although it is primarily effective against cortisol synthesis, aldosterone production is also sometimes suppressed by this compound.

Where a pituitary basophilic adenoma is the cause of the Cushing's then pituitary irradiation or hypophysectomy is necessary. In ectopic ACTH production by a neoplasm, a search for and removal of the tumor is undertaken. Where this is not possible, metyrapone or mitotane suppression of cortisol synthesis may be appropriate.

Aldosterone Hypersecretion (Aldosteronism)

Aldosterone is the main mineralocorticoid, although corticosterone has similar but lesser effects, as does deoxycorticosterone, the latter being secreted in significant amounts only in adrenal disorders. Mineralocorticoids stimulate the distal renal tubule cation exchange site thus promoting the retention of Na^+ and the elimination of K^+ and H^+. As Na^+ is retained, water is retained with it; therefore, there is usually not much increase in Na^+ relative to H_2O (hypernatremia) but there is an expansion of the ECF, which is isosmotic, and total body Na^+ is elevated. Serum K^+ is low and if hypokalemia is marked, then intracellular K^+ is depleted as well. If long continued, hypokalemia leads to abnormal renal function with a loss of renal concentrating ability, polyuria, and azotemia. Once hypokalemic nephropathy has evolved then hypernatremia and hyperosmolarity may supervene because of the inability of the kidneys adequately to resorb water from the tubular filtrate. Muscle weakness and easy fatigability, and EKG abnormalities are also results of hypokalemia. H^+ is eliminated in excess in exchange for Na^+ retention, so that metabolic alkalemia may be present.

There are two forms of aldosteronism: primary, in which the cause of the excess secretion originates in the gland itself, and secondary, in which the stimulus to hypersecretion originates outside the adrenal, usually as a result of increased renin production by the juxtaglomerular apparatus in the kidney (from nephrosis, liver cirrhosis, or congestive heart failure, see Chapter 1; or in conjunction with the increased renin production associated with accelerated or malignant hypertension, see Chapter 3).

Primary Aldosteronism

The usual cause of primary aldosteronism, which is rare, is an aldosterone-secreting adenoma of the adrenal cortex (Conn's syndrome) but occasionally excess aldosterone output occurs from normal-appearing adrenals or in bilateral nodular adrenal hyperplasia. The adenoma of Conn's syndrome is usually small and most often single and unilateral.

The patient is often mildly hypertensive, hypokalemic, alkalemic, and occasionally edema may be present. The reason that edema seldom occurs is that under the continued aldosterone excess of primary aldosteronism an "escape" phenomenon develops once a certain level of Na^+ retention and ECF volume expansion has been reached, so that the Na^+ retention tends to level off. The processes responsbile for this Na^+ escape from aldosterone influence are not known.

Laboratory studies reveal a high plasma aldosterone and low plasma renin because of feedback suppression of renin by the elevated aldosterone levels; plasma renin fails to rise as it normally would in response to Na^+ restriction, dehydration, or diuretics. Normally, serum aldosterone declines when a subject is volume loaded with isotonic saline, but in Conn's syndrome the expected degree of suppression of serum aldosterone does not occur. Urinary K^+ is high because of continued stimulation of the distal renal tubule cation exchange site; and this correlates with the hypokalemia; urinary K^+ loss continues in spite of it and a high Na^+ intake promotes further K^+ loss.

Complications of long-continued aldosterone excess are a worsening hypertension, left ventricular overload with eventual congestive heart failure, chronic renal failure, and strokes. After unilateral adrenalectomy the blood pressure lowers but seldom to the normal range. It has been suggested that the actions of aldosterone excess in causing hypertension include a direct effect on the blood vessels themselves, in addition to the Na^+ retention, and that this alteration of vascular reactivity may be only partially reversible.

Management of Conn's is surgical exploration and removal of the adenomatous adrenal; attempts to locate the tumor preoperatively may be made by catheterization of the adrenal veins via the femorals, with assay of the blood for aldosterone, and adrenal venography. In patients who decline surgery or who are for other reasons not candidates for operative treatment, suppression of the action of aldosterone on the distal renal tubule with the aldosterone antagonist spironolactone will reverse most of the abnormalities and maintain good control for long periods. Side effects of this agent are a decreased libido, impotence, and gynecomastia.

Secondary Aldosteronism

The group of disorders known as secondary aldosteronism develop as a result of activation of the renin–angiotensin system which in turn may be caused by reduced effective perfusion pressure to the kidney characteristic of congestive heart failure, cirrhosis of the liver, and nephrosis; edema is almost invariably present in these disorders. The "escape" of the Na^+ retention processes from excess aldosterone that occurs in primary aldosteronism does not occur in these conditions; the reason is not known. These conditions and their relationship to secondary aldosterone hypersecretion are described in Chapter 1. Secondary hyperaldosteronism also occurs in the accelerated phase of either essential hypertension or hypertension secondary to conditions which cause impaired renal blood flow (see Chapter 3). Aldosterone levels are said to be higher in all forms of secondary than in primary aldosteronism.

The treatment of secondary aldosteronism consists mainly in management of the underlying disorder, whatever it may be.

Adrenogenital Syndrome (Congenital Adrenal Hyperplasia)

There are a number of adrenal syndromes which result in virilization because of excess output of adrenal androgens; some are associated with a deficiency of cor-

(a) Normal

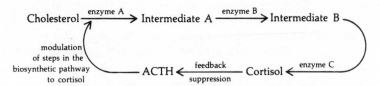

(b) Adrenogenital Syndrome

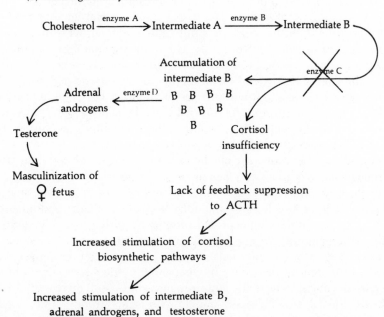

Figure 13-4. Diagram of the sequence of abnormal events in one form of congenital adrenal hyperplasia and adrenogenital syndrome (b). The gene responsible for controlling the enzyme (enzyme C) which catalyzes the transformation of intermediate compound B to cortisol is defective, resulting in inadequate amounts of enzyme C. This deficit has two consequences. 1) Cortisol synthesis is impaired and adrenal glucocorticoid insufficiency develops; there is a lack of feedback suppression to pituitary ACTH secretion, so it increases, further stimulating the biosynthetic steps ahead of the block and leading to increased androgen production. 2) Intermediate compounds accumulate ahead of the blocked step; these are converted along unblocked alternate biosynthetic pathways to adrenal androgens and then to testosterone, leading to masculinization of the female fetus and premature sexual maturation of both male and female child.

tisol and aldosterone. As described earlier, the hormones of the adrenal cortex are synthesized from cholesterol through a series of steps each of which yields a specific intermediate product and is under the control of a specific enzyme, the presence and amount of which, in turn, is regulated by a specific gene (Figure 13-4a). A gene defect may produce an enzyme deficiency that will impair the biosynthetic conversion at that step, resulting both in a deficiency of the end-product hormone (either aldosterone or cortisol) being manufactured by that pathway, and an accumulation of intermediates in the steps ahead of the block.

Intermediates may then be converted along alternate unblocked pathways in some cases to adrenal androgens which may be transformed into testosterone.

Where cortisol synthesis is impaired, the lack of feedback suppression of ACTH will cause an increase in its secretion, excessive stimulation to the adrenals resulting in hyperplasia, a further acceleration of the synthetic steps preceding the block, greater increase of intermediates, and more androgens (Figure 13-4b). In cases where aldosterone synthesis is impaired, removal of feedback suppression to the renin–angiotensin system will cause similar excess stimulation to the gland. In addition, the consequences of cortisol and/or aldosterone deficiency, as described above, will appear to varying degrees depending on the completeness of the blocks and their location along the biosynthetic pathways.

Although this group of disorders is more common in infancy and childhood, it may not appear until later in life; it may affect several family members, and in this event the defective enzyme is the same one in all. Of course the effects are more evident in females than males. The most common form is deficiency of the enzyme 21-hydroxylase. The degree of the block may range from slight to severe; the effects are dependent on the degree of enzyme deficiency. Where the deficiency develops in intrauterine life in a female fetus, the internal sex organs will be normal female, but the external genitalia may be ambiguous, resulting in female pseudohermaphrodism: hypertrophy of the clitoris and fusion of the labioscrotal folds; so that at birth the infant may appear to be a cryptorchid male with hypospadias. The sequence of abnormalities in the biosynthetic pathways in adrenogenital syndrome are diagramed in Figure 13-4.

If the endocrine deficits are mild enough to permit survival then the child, whether male or female, grows rapidly, becomes muscular and hirsute, and has precocious sexual development and progressive virilization. The androgens promote early epiphyseal closure so that such patients have short stature. In case of a lesser degree of enzyme deficiency the changes may not appear until adulthood. In the female there may be deepening of the voice, clitoral hypertrophy, increased clitoral sensitivity and responsiveness and increased sexual libido, growth of facial hair, increased muscle size, acne, atrophy of the female sex accessories and secondary sex characteristics, and amenorrhea.

Note that the status of the clitoris and the sexual libido appear to be "masculine" characteristics in that they, unlike the female reproductive equipment, are responsive to the effects of the male sex hormone testosterone and other androgenic steroids, instead of to estrogen and progestrone. (Incidentally, intrauterine differentiation of the female genital and reproductive apparatus is not under the control of any sex hormones at all. In the total absence of all fetal gonadal hormones—both estrogens and androgens—which is the normal condtion in the female fetus, female internal and external genitalia develop. In the case of a genetically male (XY) embryo, where secretion of fetal testicular androgens fails for some reason, the embryo differentiates as a perfect anatomical female both internally and externally.) Other causes of virilization in the female are an androgen-producing tumor of the ovary (arrhenoblastoma), or a neoplasm of the adrenal. In these cases the onset of virilization may be more abrupt.

Management of congenital adrenal hyperplasia is the maintenance administration of cortisol, and if aldosterone deficiency is present, of fluorohydrocortisone. The cortisol will suppress the excessive secretion of pituitary ACTH, remove excessive stimulation to the adrenal, decrease the synthesis and accumulation of biosynthetic intermediates and reduce the production of adrenal androgens and the abnormalities resulting from it. Of course the congenital structural hermaphroditism of the female remains and is dealt with in other ways, depending on a number of variables, such as the patient's core gender identity, the degree of the anomalies, and the sex of rearing.

ENDOCRINE PANCREAS

The islets of the pancreas are distributed throughout the gland; they are comprised of clusters of three types of cells: the majority are the beta cells that secrete insulin, fewer are the glucagon-synthesizing alpha cells, and the least numerous are cells which contain somatostatin.

Islet Hormones

Insulin

Insulin is a polypeptide hormone which is synthesized in the cytoplasmic reticulum of the beta cells, stored in granules, and, during secretion, is transferred across the beta cell membrane into surrounding capillary blood. Insulin secretion is controlled primarily by the direct effect of blood glucose levels on the beta cells; any increase in blood glucose stimulates increased insulin release, whereas low blood sugar inhibits its release. In addition, the presence of glucose in the gastrointestinal tract stimulates increased beta cell release of insulin by a reaction which is probably mediated by one of the gastrointestinal hormones. Insulin enters the portal vein and therefore flows directly to the liver, producing a considerably higher concentration there than in peripheral tissues; much insulin is bound to liver cells. Excess insulin that is not bound by peripheral cells is degraded rapidly by kidneys and liver, accounting for its relatively short half-life in the blood of about 15 min.

Insulin exerts its effects on peripheral cells by binding to specific glycoprotein insulin receptors on the surface of cell membranes. Several recent studies demonstrate that the insulin which is bound to cell membrane receptors of its target organs then enters the cell interior; there it becomes associated with a number of intracellular organelles, where it exerts its various regulatory functions. A major effect of insulin on cells is facilitation of the transport of primarily glucose, but also amino acids, from the blood into the cell interior. Glucose and amino acid entry into cells is essential to supply metabolic substrate for energy metabolism and protein synthesis. Insulin receptors are particularly numerous in the membranes of liver, kidneys, adipose, muscle (smooth, striated, and cardiac), and white blood cells.

It has been reported that the numbers of insulin receptors are greatly reduced in diabetic and insulin-resistant obese subjects and experimental animals; the result is a marked reduction in the binding of insulin to such cells and therefore an impairment of its metabolic effects. Other studies show that in patients with adult-onset diabetes mellitus, and in obese insulin-resistant individuals, there is an inverse relationship between the titers of circulating insulin and the number of insulin receptors; that is, the higher the concentration of plasma insulin, the fewer the insulin receptors. This relationship does not hold for juvenile-onset diabetics. The significance of these findings is still controversial, but serves to emphasize the apparently different physiologic processes involved in juvenile and adult forms of diabetes.

The basic metabolic actions of insulin on peripheral cells are several: it promotes the entry of glucose into cells, especially those of muscle and adipose tissue; it promotes the storage of glucose as glycogen (glycogenesis) in the liver and inhibits its breakdown to glucose (glycogenolysis); it inhibits the conversion of amino acids to glucose (gluconeogenesis); it facilitates the entry of amino acids into cells, thereby fostering protein synthesis; and it inhibits the breakdown of fat in adipose cells and its release as fatty acids (lipolysis). In the light of these primary metabolic actions of insulin, therefore, it is evident that a deficiency of insulin would result in an impaired entry of glucose into cells and an increased breakdown of liver glycogen with resulting excessive release of glucose into the blood. These two effects, impaired cellular uptake of glucose, and increased liver output of glucose, produce the extracellular hyperglycemia, and the intracellular glucose deficit, which are characteristic of diabetes. In addition there will be decreased protein synthesis and elevated lipolysis. Resulting abnormalities in the patient with diabetes are direct consequences of the above metabolic aberrations.

Glucagon

Just as insulin is an anabolic hormone, serving to promote the buildup of carbohydrates, proteins, and fats, so glucagon is a catabolic one, facilitating their breakdown. Glucagon is synthesized and released not only by the alpha cells of the pancreas but also by the gastrointestinal tract. Many studies indicate that glucagon excess is as intimately involved in the cause and pathologic changes of diabetes as is insulin deficiency. Increased glucagon always accompanies hyperglycemia, and has been shown to be part of the cause of hyperglycemia rather than a consequence. Serum glucagon levels are elevated in diabetes, and unlike the situation in the normal subject, where increasing blood sugar levels suppress glucagon secretion, in diabetic subjects this suppression fails to occur and high output of glucagon continues. Glucagon stimulates the breakdown of glycogen in the liver and its release as glucose. It promotes the conversion of amino acids to glucose (gluconeogenesis) and facilitates the mobilization of free fatty acids from adipose tissue. The enzyme which catalyzes the breakdown of fat and release of free fatty acids into the blood is called hormone-sensitive lipase; it is activated by glucagon and inhibited by insulin. Glucagon activates it by increasing the cAMP content of adipocytes which in turn increases the lipolytic activity of hormone-sensitive lipase and mobilizes the breakdown of fat and release of its breakdown products into the blood.

There is evidence of a dual control for glucagon secretion as there is for insulin. Glucagon secretion is inhibited by increased plasma glucose (in the presence of insulin) and is stimulated by a decline; and the presence of digesting food in the gastrointestinal tract, especially amino acids, appears to stimulate glucagon release, an effect that is probably mediated by a gastrointestinal hormone. There appears to be an equilibrium type of interaction between insulin secretion and glucagon secretion which takes the form of an inverse relationship. High concentrations of insulin suppress glucagon release and low insulin levels promote glucagon release. Hyperglucagonemia is associated with all forms of hypoinsulinism, both that occurring spontaneously in human diabetes, and that produced experimentally in laboratory animals. Thus it appears that glucagon excess contributes to the metabolic abnormalities induced by the insulin deficiency of diabetes, and in fact excess glucagon is probably responsible for much of the hyperglycemia in this disorder.

Moreover, glucagon appears to be closely associated with the development of ketoacidosis, a life-threatening complication in diabetes. Glucagon is involved in the regulation of the oxidation of fatty acids in the liver; the development of ketoacidosis, in which there is increased production of ketone bodies (see following), is correlated with increased concentration of glucagon in the blood. It has been shown that infusion of somatostatin (see below) protects the insulin-deprived diabetic against the development of ketoacidosis. Although the standard treatment for diabetic ketoacidosis is insulin, it appears that much of the effectiveness of insulin in this situation may be to suppress the blood levels of glucagon, thus inhibiting ketogenesis by the liver.

Somatostatin

Somatostatin is present in the third type of cells of the pancreatic islets; it is also called somatotropin inhibiting factor. It is also produced by the hypothalamus and certain cells of the gastrointestinal mucosa; its first described action was the inhibition of the release of somatotropin (growth hormone) from the pituitary gland. Somatostatin acts on the alpha and beta cells to inhibit the release of both glucagon and insulin; somatostatin lowers the plasma glucose to normal levels in an insulin-deprived hyperglycemic subject even when no insulin is given, indicating the significant role played by glucagon excess in the hyperglycemia of human diabetes mellitus.

Diabetes Mellitus

Metabolic Abnormalities

Diabetes is characterized by a number of systemic derangements leading to signs and symptoms among which the most marked are hyperglycemia, glycosuria, polyuria, polydipsia, and hyperphagia.

Glucose Metabolism

Hyperglycemia in diabetes mellitus is the consequence of several abnormalities; two major ones are impaired uptake of glucose from the blood and storage as glycogen, and decreased ability of glucose to enter peripheral cells. In the normal subject a rise in blood glucose prompts a rapid release of insulin from the beta cells; insulin then attaches to insulin receptors on the cell membrane and promotes cell uptake of glucose. Excess blood glucose above that required for immediate metabolic needs is withdrawn from the blood by the cells of several different tissue and converted to compounds representing stored metabolic substrate. Glucose is taken up by muscle cells and stored as glycogen. Glucose is absorbed by adipose tissue, converted to triglyceride, and deposited in the adipocytes as fat droplets. And the liver takes up much excess glucose; part is converted to glycogen and stored, but more is converted to hepatic triglyceride, most of which reenters the blood as lipoproteins and is ultimately deposited in adipose tissue in the form of fat. These routes of blood glucose uptake and conversion are diagramed in Figure 13-5. In diabetics all of these storage processes are impaired. Instead, the metabolic derangements produced by insufficient insulin, combined with the glycogenolytic and lipolytic effects of glucagon, promote hyperglycemia as well as hypertriglyceridemia.

The hyperglycemia then causes an elevation in the osmolarity of the blood; if the blood glucose levels exceed the capacity of the renal tubular transport processes to resorb it from the glomerular filtrate, glucose is retained in the tubular filtrate, elevating the osmotic pressure of this fluid as well, and causing an osmotic diuresis in which large amounts of body water are excreted, leading to dehydration. In osmotic diuresis, a failure of adequate tubular resorption of Na^+ and K^+ occurs; these ions are lost in the urine, and electrolyte deficits develop. A combination of water loss and high osmolarity stimulates the thirst centers, resulting in increased water intake. Since much glucose exits in the urine, this represents a major caloric loss which stimulates the hunger centers in the hypothalamus, resulting in hyperphagia.

The continuous sensations of hunger are also a result of the failure of glucose to enter cells. Subjective appetite is regulated by the interplay between a pair of centers in the hypothalamus. The feeding center in nuclei of the lateral hypothalamus generates eating behavior; the satiety center in the ventromedial nuclei generates sensations of repletion when their glucose content is normal, and suppresses the feeding center. But because of the low intracellular glucose content, suppression of the feeding by the satiety center is impaired and the former becomes tonically active, causing hyperphagia. The overeating increases blood sugar, and a vicious cycle is perpetuated.

In summary: in the normal subject after a meal, simple sugars, amino acids,

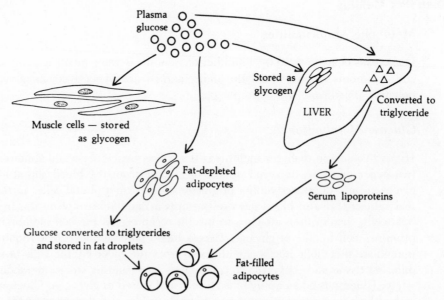

Figure 13-5. Sites of uptake and storage of blood glucose in the presence of normal levels of insulin and glucagon.

fatty acids, and triglycerides are absorbed into the blood from the intestinal mucosa in large amounts. In the case of simple sugars, which are hydrolyzed to glucose, some are promptly taken up by fat and muscle cells, both to meet the metabolic energy requirements of the cells, and for storage as glycogen in muscle and fat in adipocytes. Also, the liver takes up large amounts of glucose, and stores it for future use as glycogen. Adequate quantities of insulin are required for all three of these processes, and in insulin deficit the processes fail. In addition, in the diabetic, oversecretion of glucagon promotes excessive degradation of body stores of glycogen, proteins, and fats, further flooding the circulation with their breakdown products.

The inability of glucose to enter cells deprives them of their major metabolic substrate, and necessitates the intracellular metabolic breakdown of proteins and fats as sources of energy for cellular activities.

Protein Metabolism

As mentioned above, insulin is essential for the transport of amino acids across cell membranes from the blood so that these may be used in protein synthesis. In addition, insulin appears to activate the cells' protein-synthesizing enzyme systems. Both of these processes are impaired by insulin deficit, and glucagon excess promotes still further breakdown of proteins already stored. The amino acids which are able to enter cells from the blood are metabolized to meet the cells' energy requirements as a substitute for the deficient intracellular glucose, and thus are lost to the body's overall protein reserves. Enhanced conversion of amino acids to glucose by the liver, fostered both by insulin deficit and glucagon excess, accentuates protein depletion and negative nitrogen balance, leading to tissue wasting and failure of the several growth and body defense processes, including immunologic ones, all of which are dependent on adequate protein synthesis.

Fat Metabolism

The enzyme hormone-sensitive lipase is inhibited by insulin; in insulin deficit this enzyme is activated leading to fat breakdown and release of fatty acids and triglycerides. Also in combined insulin deficit and glucagon excess there is decreased fat synthesis and further fat hydrolysis.

Fat entering the blood following a meal, and triglycerides synthesized in the liver from glucose and then released into the blood, are normally taken up by the fat cells of adipose tissue with the aid of the enzyme lipoprotein lipase; insulin in adequate amounts is required for the normal action of this enzyme. Therefore, in insulin deficiency the fat products from both dietary sources and liver lipoprotein synthesis fail to be taken up in sufficient quantities by adipocytes and stored as fat droplets. In addition, the intracellular process of fat storage requires the compound glycerol phosphate, which in the normal subject is provided by cellular glucose metabolism; because of intracellular glucose deficits, the amount of this essential compound is inadequate to permit normal fat storage.

A combination of decreased synthesis and especially storage of fats, and increased fat breakdown, both resulting from glucagon hypersecretion and insulin deficit, promotes chronically elevated blood levels of free fatty acids and trigly-cerides; blood levels of these compounds tend to be correlated with the degree of hyperglycemia.

It is of importance to note that hyperinsulinism has been consistently demonstrated to be a correlate of obesity. Obese individuals show elevated plasma insulin levels both in the fasting state and after meals. The elevated insulin levels are the consequence, rather than the cause, of the obesity; positive caloric balance (overeating with weight gain) leads to an increase in plasma insulin. Evidence suggests that chronic overeating (and underexercise) leads to an adaptive hyperplasia and hypersecretion of beta cells so that excess insulin is secreted both during fasting and after food ingestion. Obesity and excess insulin secretion is furthermore correlated with increased peripheral resistance to insulin, and it is suggested that this results from a decrease in the number of insulin receptors in the plasma membranes of peripheral cells. The insulin resistance then increases the requirement for more insulin secretion, with possible overstimulation and eventual exhaustion atrophy of the beta cell insulin-secreting processes. Some authors consider these interrelations to be the underlying sequence of events leading to adult-onset diabetes.

Ketogenesis

Fatty acids are converted in the liver to the compound acetyl coenzyme A (CoA); some of this is metabolized, but because of the elevated blood lipids more is synthesized in the liver than can be utilized by cells, and the excess acetyl CoA is converted (again by the liver) to acetoacetic acid, and then to acetone and β-hydroxybutyric acid. These ketone bodies are also used as energy substrate, but more are produced than can be utilized and the excess accumulates in the blood, causing ketonemia.

These ketone bodies are organic acids, and therefore they also lead to acidemia. The kidneys eliminate large amounts of the organic acids and much Na^+ and K^+ are lost in the urine with them. The renal Na^+ loss takes water with it; the water loss worsens the dehydration already present from the osmotic diuresis caused by hyperglycemia. The patient becomes hypovolemic, hypotensive, and hypokalemic. The acidemia stimulates the respiratory center to produce respiratory compensation for metabolic acidemia and so the patient hyperventilates (Kussmaul's respirations). The inadequate tissue perfusion caused by hypovolemia and hypotension leads to anaerobic cellular metabolism and lactic acidemia. The hyperosmolar acidic body fluids dehydrate brain neurons, impairing their function, and produces altered mental status, decreased levels of consciousness, and impaired regulation of vital functions.

Clinical Characteristics

Diabetes mellitus is a common disorder. There is a strong hereditary predisposition, but life-style factors appear to be closely involved, especially overeating and obesity. It is more common in females than males in cultures in which middle-aged females have a higher incidence of obesity—that is, in western cultures. There are two forms: juvenile onset, which is more severe, is ketosis prone and the pancreas contains and secretes little or no insulin; and adult onset, which is milder, ketosis resistant, and the pancreas contains about half of the normal amount of insulin but secretes it more slowly and in insufficient amounts. Juvenile onset comprises about 10% of diabetes and always requires insulin. Adult onset is most common after age 45; often can be controlled by weight loss, dietary management, and a regular exercise program; and may remain almost completely asymptomatic for many years. It may be revealed only by the discovery of glycosuria or hyperglycemia on routine laboratory tests or not until the vascular complications characteristic of diabetes have manifested themselves in, for example, ischemic heart disease or peripheral vascular insufficiency.

Adult-onset diabetes exists in a spectrum of degrees of severity which correlates with the number of beta cells in the pancreas, their insulin content, and their capacity to release insulin in response to a glucose challenge. Latent diabetes refers to the condition in which the patient has had hyperglycemia and glycosuria under previous circumstances: while obese or pregnant, or during an infection or some other illness or injury. Asymptomatic diabetes is the term applied to patients who have no symptoms but show an abnormal glucose tolerance test, who develop an elevated postprandial blood sugar, but whose fasting blood sugar may be within normal limits. Although patients of this category are asymptomatic, appropriate studies reveal the development and progression of blood vessel abnormalities characteristic of diabetes. Overt diabetes is the classification for patients who manifest glycosuria and hyperglycemia, have signs and symptoms resulting from these, and who have elevated random and fasting blood glucose values.

Chronic Pathologic Changes

The question of the cause of cellular abnormalities which develop as a correlate of diabetes mellitus has long been controversial. Recent studies indicate that glucose in the blood of these patients becomes bound to various protein constituents of cells, alters the molecular characteristics of these proteins, and therefore leads to structural and physiological alterations in the cells. In the presence of elevated serum glucose, glucose enters the cells of blood vessel endothelium and nerve tissue, may bind irreversibly to cellular proteins, and may lead to abnormalities of cell metabolism and production of damaging intermediates such as sorbitol. Whether better control of blood sugar levels in diabetics reduces cellular abnormalities, however, remains unknown.

Large Blood Vessels

Atherosclerosis is accelerated in all diabetics; the basic processes involved appear to be the same as or similar to atherosclerotic changes occurring in nondiabetics (see Chapter 4) but develop more rapidly, are more severe, and occur equally in diabetic males and females. Premature ischemic heart disease and atherosclerotic cerebrovascular disease commonly develop and are frequent causes of death. Peripheral vascular occlusion is also common and may cause intermittent claudication and gangrene of the feet.

Small Blood Vessels (Microangiopathy)

Abnormalities of the small blood vessels characteristic of diabetes are thickened basement membranes resulting from deposition of glycoproteins, and other abnormalities characteristic for specific organs involved. There is some evidence that rigorous control of blood glucose levels through more frequent insulin injections and rigid dietary restriction may retard, though it does not prevent, the small blood vessel abnormalities and their consequences in diabetes.

Eye.   Probably more than 15% of blindness is caused by diabetic retinopathy; microaneurysms, narrowed arterioles, dilated veins, small hemorrhages, and capillary degeneration leading to edema formation and exudation of blood components ("waxy" and "cotton" exudates) are characteristic funduscopic findings in patients who have been symptomatic diabetics for 10 to 20 years. Hypertension, atherosclerosis, and chronic diabetic renal insufficiency accelerate and worsen the eye changes. Other visual disturbances characteristic of diabetes are palsies of the oculomotor nerve (CN III·) leading to strabismus with diplopia; visual blurring; impaired accommodation; and a high incidence of cataracts. Retinal and preretinal hemorrhages and proliferative retinopathy and neovascularization occur leading to fibrosis and retinal detachment in some patients. Whether rigid control of blood sugar levels with appropriate insulin, diet, and exercise results in a better visual prognosis remains unsettled.

Kidney.   The kidneys appear to be markedly susceptible to diabetes-induced abnormalities. Diabetic kidneys show a number of lesions including thickening of the capillary basement membrane of the glomeruli; and glomerulosclerosis in which there are exudates and deposition of abnormal glycoproteins and other material in nodules and fibrils in the capillaries. Proteinuria appears in most patients who have had overt diabetes for 15 or 20 years; this sign of abnormal glomerular membrane permeability then often evolves into progressive renal insufficiency with azotemia and uremia over the next few years. It is said that 40% of juvenile-onset diabetics die of chronic renal failure. Pyelonephritis is a frequent occurrence in many diabetics.

Nervous System.   The early and severe atherosclerosis predisposes the diabetic patient to infarction or hemorrhage, most commonly cerebral but also in the brainstem and spinal cord. Autonomic neuropathy also occurs and may involve both the sympathetic and parasympathetic divisions; consequences are impotence and other sexual malfunction; orthostatic hypotension; abnormal gastrointestinal motility with constipation, noctural diarrhea, or delayed gastric emptying; abnormal neural control of peripheral blood vessel reactivity; difficulty emptying the bladder; and abnormal pupillary reflexes.

Peripheral neuropathy is the most common form of neural abnormality in the diabetic, and involves both sensory and motor nerves resulting in loss of deep tendon reflexes and motor weakness; loss of pain, temperature, and pressure sense; impaired proprioception with resulting ataxia and disequilibrium; hypoesthesia and anesthesia for skin, muscle and joint sensation (which may lead to the Charcot joint) and foot injuries which go unattended; paresthesias; and spontaneous pain and hyperesthesias, usually of the extremities. Recent studies indicate that some neural impairment in diabetics results from slowed nerve conduction caused by impairment of the myelin sheath by high serum glucose levels.

Skin. Disorders of the skin characteristic of the symptomatic diabetic are the result of a number of underlying abnormalities: the large and small blood vessel disease, described above, which markedly affects blood supply to and blood flow in the skin; the predisposition to infection caused by impaired immune responses and glucose and lipid-rich body fluids (a good culture medium); and the peripheral neuropathy which predisposes to injury and then lack of awareness of and attention to it. Skin and mucous membrane infections are common, often staphylococcal or streptococcal, and occur most often at sites of chronic irritation or in ischemic areas. Vulvovaginitis is common in diabetic females. Atrophic skin areas are found most often in the lower legs; the skin is thin, hairless, pigmented, and bordered by telangiectases; it is usually devoid of sensation.

Acute Complications

Aside from acute manifestations of the chronic cardiovascular abnormalities in diabetes, such as myocardial infarction and stroke, the two acute complications are ketoacidemic coma and hyperosmolar coma.

Ketoacidosis and Coma

The sequence of physiologic changes leading to ketoacidemia have been described above. Occasionally the event occurs in a previously undiagnosed, and therefore untreated, diabetic; but more often it is the result of omitting insulin or not taking enough at times of increased requirements such as during a respiratory or other infection, injury, or a related illness such as myocardial infarction.

Gastrointestinal symptoms and signs are common in diabetic ketoacidemia, especially nausea, vomiting, and abdominal pain. Laboratory tests will show an elevated blood glucose and ketones and low HCO_3^-; K^+ may be low; total body Na^+ will be low but because of the dehydration, the Na^+ to H_2O ratio may be normal; BUN and serum lipids are often elevated. Urinalysis reveals ketones, glucose, and often protein. Hyperglycemia has caused osmotic diuresis and dehydration; and the accumulation of keto acids and lactic acid has produced acidemia with electrolyte loss: Na^+, K^+, Cl^-, and HCO_3^-. Therefore reversal of the hyperglycemia, acidemia, and hypovolemia are the major concerns. Assessment of these conditions is described in Chapters 1 and 2. Management consists of fluid and electrolyte replacement—often large amounts are required; insulin and K^+, and HCO_3^-. Other supportive and assessment measures may be indicated: attention to a clear airway, O_2 supplements and monitoring of the EKG and central venous pressure.

Hyperosmolar Coma

Serum hyperosmolarity is discussed in Chapter 1. In the specific case of the diabetic, the patient is often elderly, frequently with impaired renal function, severely hyperglycemic (blood glucose of perhaps 500 to 1000 mg/100 ml), not severely ketotic, but dehydrated, and with a high serum osmolarity (normal is around 300 mosm/L). The BUN is usually somewhat elevated but the creatinine normal (prerenal azotemia, see Chapter 10). The patient may be hyperventilating and serum pH and HCO_3^- may be low, not from ketosis but from the lactic acidemia of poor tissue perfusion resulting from dehydration and hypovolemia.

Often there is a prior history, from the patient or relatives, of a period of increasing glycosuria, polyuria, and polydipsia prior to the acute onset of the illness. Ketosis usually does not develop in this situation because the patient is an adult-onset type of diabetic with reduced but not absent insulin and excessive (but not severely so) output of glucagon; the balance between the insulin deficiency and the hyperglucagonemia has been such that the greatly exaggerated lipolysis necessary to generate the ketoacidotic state has not developed.

Assessment in hyperosmolar states has been described in Chapter 1. Management consists of insulin administration and careful gradual rehydration with precautions described in Chapter 1 to avoid ECF overload, which is a likely development in view of the hyperosmolarity of both the ECF and ICF. Occasionally during rehydration and after insulin administration the patient may rouse from coma and appear improved, only to deteriorate rapidly and lapse back into coma. In this case the cause has probably been the following sequence: (1) insulin causes rapid movement of glucose into cells; (2) the intracellular environment is already hyperosmolar; (3) as fluid and electrolyte are infused which are markedly lower in osmolarity than the patient's ECF and ICF, osmotic concentration of the ECF declines; (4) but glucose does not diffuse readily out of cells along the now-reversed osmotic gradient; (5) water, on the other hand, moves very rapidly along osmotic gradients into the hypertonic intracellular space, causing the cells to take up water and swell; the result is swelling of the neurons of the brainstem regulating consciousness and vital functions.

Assessment and Management of the Ambulatory Diabetic

Signs and symptoms of adult onset diabetes are polydipsia, polyuria, polyphagia, and either weight loss or weight gain. A family history of diabetes is often present. Other indicative factors are onset of nocturia, impotence in males, vulvar pruritis in females, urinary tract infections, complaint of blurred vision or decreased visual acuity, fatigue, or other complaints relating to the pathologic changes in diabetes discussed previously. Periodic regular evaluation of the major areas of complications as described above are necessary for monitoring progression of the disease and the results of the management regimen. There is no disorder in which patient education is as crucial, and in which patients must learn so thoroughly to be their own health care agents, as diabetes.

Weight loss, dietary control, and a regular exercise program are the central components of management in adult-onset diabetes. The value of most oral hypogycemic agents remains controversial. Insulin may be required where conservative measures fail to bring adequate control. Prevention of infection is important in maintaining regulation. Periodic monitoring of laboratory values—blood and urine glucose, cholesterol and triglycerides, electrolytes, BUN and creatinine; and body weight and blood pressure—should be performed at regular intervals.

PARATHYROIDS, CALCIUM, AND 1,25-DIHYDROXYCHOLECALCIFEROL

Only about 2% of Ca^{2+} in the body is in the body fluids; its concentration is 10 mg/100 ml (5 meq/L); 98% of Ca^{2+} is in the skeleton, primarily as a complex salt called hydroxyapatite, comprised of Ca^{2+}, PO_4^{3-}, and OH^-. Of the Ca^{2+} in the ECF, about half is bound to plasma proteins and the other half is ionized; it is the latter portion that meets physiologic requirements for Ca^{2+} in blood coagulation; neural excitation, conduction, and synaptic transmission; muscle excitation and contraction; and other essential functions.

Ca^{2+} in the ECF is in dynamic equilibrium with Ca^{2+} in the skeleton. Cells in the skeleton which are concerned with bone formation and resorption exist in three forms: osteocytes are bone cells enclosed by calcified collagen; osteoblasts are the bone-forming cells which secrete the collagen and calcify it; and osteoclasts break down bone and release its Ca^{2+}. Osteocytes are also capable of breaking down bone.

A low serum Ca^{2+} causes increased neuromuscular excitability, tetany, carpal and pedal spasm, laryngospasm, bronchospasm, anxiety, circumoral and acral paresthesias, EKG changes, and seizures. Carpopedal spasm, acral paresthesias, anxiety, altered mental status, and even seizures are not infrequent events in patients with severe anxiety hyperventilation. The processes underlying these developments are the result of respiratory alkalemia produced by the hyperventilation. As the $Paco_2$ falls, the pH rises and the alkalemia promotes increased ionization of the Ca^{2+}-binding plasma proteins. The protein anions then rapidly bind more Ca^{2+}, and ionized Ca^{2+} levels fall, causing neuromuscular hyperexcitability. (The effect of hypocapnia on the cerebral vasculature, which accounts for the mental status and level of consciousness alterations in hyperventilation, is discussed in Chapter 2.)

Hypercalcemia may cause anorexia, nausea and vomiting, weakness and lethargy, muscle hypotonia and hyporeflexia, and constipation. A high serum Ca^{2+}, if chronic, leads to polyuria and polydipsia from lesions in the nephron, and causes deposits of Ca^{2+} and PO_4^{3-} in blood vessels, joints, cornea, kidney, and gastric mucosa.

Blood levels of Ca^{2+} are maintained within a normal range by Ca^{2+} absorption and excretion via the intestine, urinary retention or excretions by the kidney, and deposition in or release from bone. These equilibria are under the control of three hormones: parathyroid hormone, calcitonin, and 1,25-dihydroxycholecalciferol which is synthesized in the kidney.

Phosphorus, mainly as inorganic phosphate, is among the most abundant elements in the body, is concerned with essentially all metabolic functions, and is present in the ECF at around 3.5 mg of P/100 ml. Most of it is unbound to plasma proteins. Hyper- or hypophosphatemia seldom occur and when they do are rarely symptomatic. Phosphate is readily absorbed from the intestine and its balance in the ECF is regulated primarily at the kidney, in part by parathyroid hormone. There is usually an inverse relationship between Ca^+ and PO_4^{3-} in the ECF; as PO_4^{3-} concentration increases above a certain level in body fluids, Ca^{2+} concentration declines, and vice versa.

Regulation of Serum Calcium and Phosphorus Levels

Parathyroid Hormone (PTH)

This hormone secreted by the four parathyroid glands embedded in the thyroid increases serum Ca^{2+} and decreases serum PO_4^{3-}. PTH acts on the kidney tubules to decrease tubular resorption (and therefore increase renal elimination) of PO_4^{3-} and increase renal tubular resorption of Ca^{2+}; it acts on bone to mobilize Ca^{2+} and PO_4^{3-} from it thereby elevating serum levels of these ions; and it increases the formation of 1,25-dihydroxycholecalciferol. Secretion of PTH is regulated by a direct effect of serum Ca^{2+} levels on the parathyroid glands; as ionized Ca^{2+} concentration declines in the blood the synthesis and release of the hormone is stimulated; as ionized Ca^{2+} rises above certain levels, PTH secretion is suppressed and its actions which serve to elevate serum Ca^{2+} are thereby inhibited. Elevation of serum PO_4^{3-} stimulates PTH release indirectly via its direct effect of lowering serum Ca^{2+}.

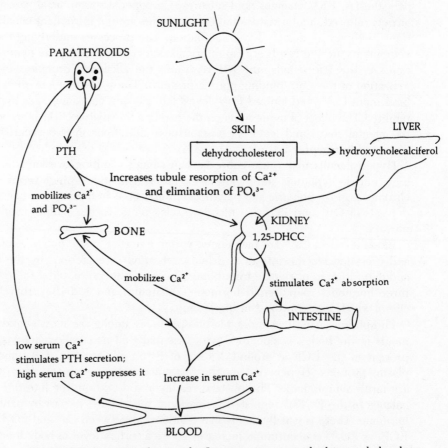

Figure 13-6. Factors regulating and influencing serum ionized calcium and phosphate.

Calcitonin

The hormone calcitonin, secreted by special cells of the thyroid, exerts a Ca^{2+} lowering influence by means of effects on bone and kidney that are the reverse of those produced by PTH. Like PTH its secretion is regulated by Ca^{2+} concentration of the ECF, being inhibited by a decline, and stimulated by an increase in serum Ca^{2+}. It also lowers serum PO_4^{3-} by its action in inhibiting bone resorption. The physiologic function, if any, in adults is not known, and neither increases of the hormone, as occurs in thyroid medullary carcinoma, nor decreases as a result of thyroidectomy, produce any known physiologic alterations. It is said to be of some therapeutic value in reducing bone turnover in Paget's disease, and is being evaluated in the management of osteoporosis.

1,25-dehydroxycholecalciferol (1,25-DHCC)

The precursor of vitamin D_3, cholecalciferol, is a substance (7-dehydrocholesterol) produced and stored in large amounts in the skin; it is transformed into vitamin D_3 by the action of ultraviolet light. Vitamin D_2 is present in the diet in foods enriched with irradiated ergosterol, and D_3 is present in rradiated yeast and cod and other fish liver oils. Vitamin D itself is not biologically active; it is transformed by enzymes in the liver to 25-hydroxycholecalciferol, and then by enzymes in the kidney to the active form 1,25-DHCC. All of the precursors of 1,25-DHCC, and the end product itself, have special transport systems in the blood comprised of specific carrier proteins which combine with each intermediate and transport it to the site of the next conversion and ultimately to the target organs. 1-25-DHCC has two known sites of action. It stimulates the active absorption of Ca^{2+} by the mucosa of the small intestine and it mobilizes Ca^{2+} from bone.

Disorders of the Parathyroids

Hyperparathyroidism

Primary Hyperparathyroidism

Reports indicate that this disorder is more common than formerly thought; symptoms are minimal in most cases, and it may be present, unsuspected for long periods. It is primarily a disorder of adults with highest incidence in the years from 30 to 50. In most patients the excessive secretion of PTH is from an adenoma of one gland, but less frequently there is hyperplasia of all, and malignancy occurs rarely. Parathyroid adenomas sometimes occur in unusual sites: the thymus or the mediastinum. The hyperplasia may be a portion of the multiple endocrine adenomatosis syndromes. These are genetic disorders which may take several forms, in one of which there is hyperparathyroidism and pancreatic islet and pituitary tumors that may be associated with gastric hypersecretion and peptic ulcer. Adenomas when present can seldom be palpated, and there are no specific physical signs aside from the effects of hypercalcemia.

Kidney involvement includes stone formation, which predisposes to urinary tract obstruction and/or infection, and calcium deposits in renal parenchyma that may lead to renal insufficiency and failure. X-ray evidences of bone involvement include a finding of irregularities in the bone outline in the phalanges called subperiosteal resorption, bone cysts, and small punched-out lesions in the skull. In the extreme form of skeletal involvement, osteitis fibrosa cystica, there are multiple areas of resorption with cyst formation. Symptoms of hypercalcemia include anorexia, nausea, and vomiting; polyuria and polydipsia; mental changes; muscle weakness and atrophy. Pancreatitis is reported to occur in greater frequency in hyperparathyroidism. Serum Ca^{2+} determinations and assay of parathyroid hormone levels by radioimmunoassay are used in diagnosis.

Secondary Hyperparathyroidism

Secondary hyperparathyroidism is a form of metabolic bone disease in which there is excessive production of PTH secondary to some systemic disorder which results in a chronically depressed serum Ca^{2+} level. The low ionized Ca^{2+} stimulates parathyroid hyperplasia and high PTH output with resulting demineralization of the skeleton. In chronic renal failure, Ca^{2+} is low primarily because the diseased kidneys are unable to synthesize 1,25-DHCC, but also because the high serum PO_4^{3-} depresses the ionization of Ca^{2+}. (Management of chronic renal failure is discussed in Chapter 10.) Specifically, for secondary hyperparathyroidism, treatment with vitamin D, reducing serum PO_4^{3-} with dietary restriction and the use of antacids, improved dialysis, and a successful transplant, are methods of control. Occasionally the parathyroids appear to become autonomously hypersecreting, and subtotal parathyroidectomy may be required. Some authors suggest that a resistance to the action of PTH on the part of the target organs is responsible for the continued hypocalcemia, in spite of hypersecretion of PTH, which is seen in various types of metabolic bone diseases.

Hypoparathyroidism

Hypoparathyroidism results from a deficiency of PTH with resulting hypocalcemia and the signs and symptoms of neuromuscular hyperexcitability. The most common cause is inadvertent removal of or damage to the vascular supply to the parathyroids during subtotal thyroidectomy, radical neck dissection for malignancy, or surgery for hyperparathyroidism. Signs and symptoms may develop within a few hours after thyroidectomy, or not until days or weeks, or even longer. Idiopathic hypothyroidism also sometimes occurs in conjunction with other endocrine deficiencies, in which case antiendocrine gland antibodies may be present, indicating an autoimmune basis. Pseudohypoparathyroidism is a rare hereditary disorder in which there is insensitivity of the target organs to the actions of PTH.

Signs of hypoparathyroidism include muscle cramps, tetany, and hypocalcemic seizures. Tests for latent tetany include Chvostek's sign, in which a tap on the face in the area of the facial nerve produces a facial muscle twitch; and Trousseau's sign, in which a blood pressure cuff is inflated on the arm and a carpal spasm develops; carpal spasm typically involves tonic contraction of the thumb and wrist flexors and the finger extensors.

In chronic hypoparathyroidism there may be calcium deposits in soft tissues. Complaints of malaise, easy fatigability and acral paresthesias are typical. Treatment includes dietary Ca^{2+} and vitamin D supplements, but regulation of serum Ca^{2+} may entail difficulties because of continued excessive urinary Ca^{2+} output resulting from the lack of PTH stimulation to renal Ca^{2+} resorption. Nephrolithiasis, vitamin D toxicity, and hypercalcemia may develop. Also, without PTH, sensitivity to vitamin D is markedly reduced. Management requires frequent monitoring of serum and urinary Ca^{2+} levels. Mg^{2+} is sometimes added to the regimen and is said to improve maintenance in some patients who were not doing well, apparently by improving responsiveness to the vitamin D, but the underlying process involved is not known.

REFERENCES

Beach FA, editor: *Human Sexuality in Four Perspectives*. Baltimore, Md.: Johns Hopkins University Press, 1977.

Beeson PB and McDermott W, editors: *Textbook of Medicine*. 14th ed. Philadelphia, Pa.: Saunders, 1975.

Bergland RM, and Page RB: Pituitary–brain vascular relations: A new paradigm. *Science* 204:18–24, 1979.

Ezrin C, et al, editors: *Clinical Endocrinology: A Survey of Current Practice*. New York: Appleton-Century-Crofts, 1977.

Frohlich ED, editor: *Pathophysiology*. Philadelphia, Pa.: Lippincott, 1976.

Ganong WF: *Review of Medical Physiology*. 8th ed. Los Altos, Calif.: Lange Medical Publications, 1977.

Goldfine ID, et al: Entry of insulin into human cultured lymphocytes: Electron microscope autoradiographic analysis. *Science* 202:760–763, 1978.

Guyton AC: *Textbook of Medical Physiology*. 5th ed. Philadelphia, Pa.: Saunders, 1976.

Kolata GB: Controversy over Study of Diabetes drugs continues for nearly a decade. *Science* 203:986–990, 1979.

Kolata GB: Blood sugar and the complications of diabetes. *Science* 203:1098–1099, 1979.

Solomon DH and Kleeman KE: Concepts of pathogenesis of Graves' disease. *Adv. Int. Med.* 22:273–299, 1977.

Thorn GW, et al, editors: *Harrison's Principles of Internal Medicine*. 8th ed. New York: McGraw-Hill, 1977.

CHAPTER FOURTEEN

Disorders of Consciousness and Mental Status

NORMAL CONSCIOUSNESS AND MENTAL STATUS

Basic Scheme of Brain Structure and Function

The primary structural divisions of the brain are: (1) the forebrain, which includes the cerebral hemispheres and the diencephalon (the diencephalon, in turn, is made up of the thalamus and the hypothalamus); (2) the midbrain, comprised of the corpora quadrigemina and cerebral peduncles; and (3) the hindbrain, the parts of which are the pons, medulla, and cerebellum.

The Cerebral Cortex

The outer layer of the cerebral hemispheres is the cortex, approximately 5 mm in depth and composed of six sublayers, each of which has a slightly different appearance microscopically, correlated with the different types of cells and portions of cells in each sublayer. The cerebral cortex is considered to be the site for the higher mental functions of the central nervous system: language, capacity for abstract thought, judgment, learning and memory, and intelligence and creativity, however these may be defined. These are the qualities of human mental function which together form the basis for the collection of attributes known as the mental status.

Certain higher mental functions may be localized to different areas of the cerebral cortex, and there are cortical areas having specific motor and sensory functions. For example, the sensory receiving areas for vision are localized to the occipital lobes; a strip in front of the central fissure comprises centers for voluntary motor activity; and a comparable area behind the central fissure is the receiving area for sensations from the body surface. Other areas of the cortex are considered to serve as "intrinsic" areas with more general integrative functions. Presently, however, the classical view of brain localization is undergoing marked revision.

The two cerebral hemispheres are lateralized; that is they are specialized for different functions. They are connected at the base in the midline by the corpus callosum and anterior commissures, which contain fiber tracts that mediate interaction and communication between them. For the most part the right side of the body is controlled by and gives input into the left cerebral hemisphere. Likewise the left body half is controlled by and sends input into the right cerebral hemisphere. In normal intact individuals both cerebral hemispheres interact

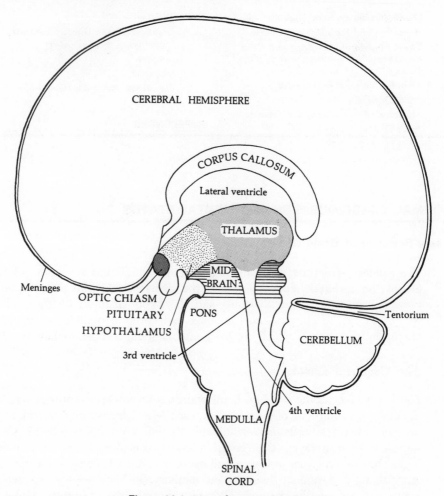

Figure 14-1. Major divisions of the brain.

via these connections and participate together in the integration and control of most aspects of cognition, sensation, and behavior. Although some similar functions motor activity are represented in both hemispheres, nevertheless in the normal processes of development of the human the two cerebral hemispheres tend to differentiate their respective activities along different lines and with different capacities and emphases. That is, they specialize for different and to some extent mutually contradictory and sometimes inhibitory mechanisms. In most persons the right cerebral hemisphere, connected most strongly to the left body half, is specialized for visual–spatial–tactile perception, integration, and response; mental imagery; musical skill and appreciation; artistic production; analogical thinking and a gestalt (holistic) mode of thought. It is the intuitive, subjective brain half. Conversely in most individuals the left cerebral hemisphere, related more to the right body half, is specialized for verbal, logical, sequential thinking, involving analysis, mathematical calculation, and temporal organization. It is the "rational" objective brain half. Research on hemisphere interaction indicates that in fact ongoing verbal–analytic activity in the left cerebral hemisphere tends to inhibit, across the corpus callosum, the holistic, intui-

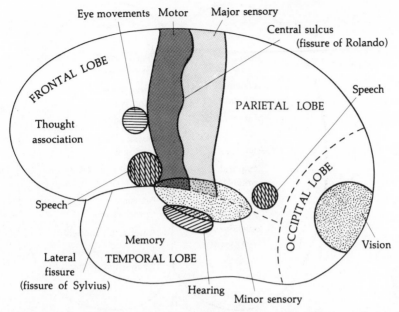

Figure 14-2. Lateral view of a cerebral hemisphere indicating lobes, fissures, and areas for special functions. (Localization theory is now undergoing major modifications.)

tive, emotional functions of the right cerebral hemisphere. Some evidence indicates that the right hemisphere may have functionally closer ties to the deeper-lying brain structures of the limbic system, which are responsible for emotional responses and instinctual behavior, than does the left.

The Basal Ganglia and Thalamus

Beneath the cerebral cortex and about at the level of the lateral and third ventricles of the brain, and surrounding them, are the thalamus and basal ganglia. The thalamus is composed of groups of nuclei (collections of nerve cell bodies) through which motor and sensory nerve impulses are conveyed between the cerebral cortex and lower brain centers; and via which flow impulses concerned with more complex integration and association between cortex and other centers. All areas of the cerebral cortex have direct connections, both afferent and efferent, with the thalamus, and in many respects the thalamus and its specific projection areas in the cortex function together as a unit. The basal ganglia (Figure 20-1) appear to be concerned with the basic control systems for bodily movements.

The Hypothalamus and Limbic System

The hypothalamus is located below and to the front of the thalamus and in the approximate center of a group of related structures toward the base of the brain: a small rim of the lowermost section of the cerebral hemispheres, the amygdala, hippocampus, and septum. Together, the hypothalamus and these structures comprise the limbic system; they are the neural basis of the emotional and instinctual functions. They regulate such behavior as feeding, fighting, running

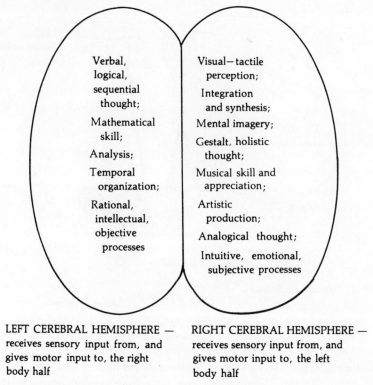

LEFT CEREBRAL HEMISPHERE —
receives sensory input from, and
gives motor input to, the right
body half

RIGHT CEREBRAL HEMISPHERE —
receives sensory input from, and
gives motor input to, the left
body half

Figure 14-3. Diagram of the left and right cerebral hemispheres showing lateralization of specialization for higher mental function as it occurs in most persons.

away; emotions related to sexual activity and erotic sensations; genital functions such as penile erection; feelings of intense pleasure; and terror and dread. They are concerned with the primitive interplay of oral, aggressive, and sexual motivation; emotional responses; feelings of pleasure and aversion; and conflict generated by competing neural activity in various lower and higher brain centers.

Other functions of the hypothalamus include regulation of body temperature, control of secretions of the endocrine glands, regulation of water balance, influences on the sleep cycle and other physiologic periodicities; it also contains centers which influence the activity of the autonomic nervous system.

The Brainstem

Brainstem is the term applied to the structures of the central portion of the lower brain, extending from the thalamus to the beginning of the spinal cord; it includes the thalamus and hypothalamus, the midbrain, the pons, and the medulla. The midbrain is comprised of the corpora quadrigemina and the cerebral peduncles; these structures contain the nuclei of the 3rd and 4th cranial nerves, visual and auditory pathways between the sense organs and the cerebral cortex, and large bundles of neural connections running between the cerebral hemispheres and lower structures, i.e., pons, medulla, and spinal cord. The pons contains neural centers which influence respiration; pathways between the cerebellum and other parts of the brain; and nuclei for the 5th, 6th, and 7th, and

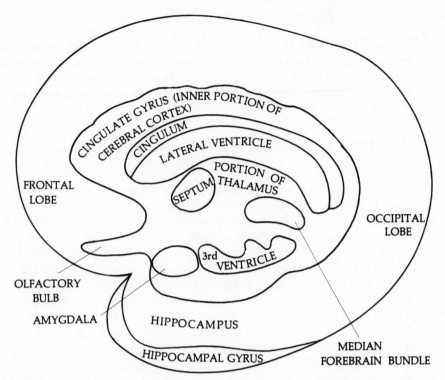

Figure 14-4. Diagram of the limbic system, including the median forebrain bundle, a pathway involved in sensations of pleasure.

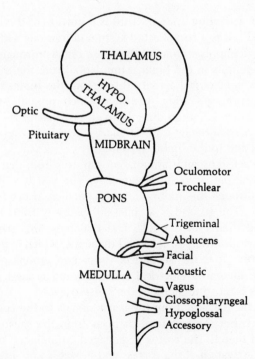

Figure 14-5. Diagram of the brainstem (some authors do not include the thalamus as a portion of the brainstem) showing approximate sites of origin of the cranial nerves. The basal ganglia (nuclei) are located around and close to portions of the thalamus.

the cochlear division of the 8th cranial nerves. The medulla contains the vital centers which are concerned with reflex autonomic regulation of vasomotor tone, respiration, and heart rate; centers for swallow, gag, cough, vomit, and sneeze reflexes; and nuclei for the auditory division of the 8th cranial nerves as well as for cranial nerves 9 through 12.

The Brainstem Reticular Formation

The reticular formation is a collection of extensively branching neurons having numerous synaptic interconnections within itself and with adjacent brain structures. It lies within the brainstem, forming its core, and continues throughout the inner portions of the hypothalamus, midbrain, pons, and medulla. It has a number of functions, but those relevant to this discussion relate to its role in regulating the level of electrical activity in the cerebral cortex and hence the level of conscious arousal of the brain. Since it is also the location of the vital centers which regulate blood pressure, influence heart rate, rhythm, and force of contraction, control respiration, and affect other vegetative functions, it is evident that many of the abnormalities of the central nervous system that cause altered levels of consciousness will also produce changes in the vital signs and other visceral activities.

Brain Function Basic to Level of Consciousness and Mental Status

The Reticular Activating System

The reticular activating system (RAS) is a portion of the brainstem reticular formation (BSRF); it is a complicated system of neurons with many synapses which receives nerve impulses from all the sense organs throughout the body as well as from higher centers in the brain. Stimulation from these sources produces a diffuse increase in electrical activity throughout the brainstem reticular formation. There are neural activating pathways which project from the RAS to other areas of the brain; some go directly to all portions of the cerebral cortex, while others go to several nuclei in the thalamus and from there on up to both the cerebral cortex and to the limbic system.

When any sense organ is stimulated impulses from that sense organ travel two different neural pathways simultaneously. The first is a direct pathway from the sense organ through the midbrain, to its specific sensory receiving area in the cerebral cortex. The second is a collateral pathway from the sense organ to the midbrain and then into the RAS and thalamus; this stimulation increases the level of electrical activity in RAS and thalamus, which is then projected up to the cerebral cortex. It is the second of these two groups of neural impulses that produces the increased electrical activation and arousal of the cerebral cortex, which results from stimulation of the sense organs.

If the specific pathway from the sense organs to the cortical sensory receiving areas is intact, but the collateral pathway from the sense organ to the thalamus and RAS and then to the cortex is damaged, stimulation of the sense organs will not produce activation of the cortex, and in fact is not "perceived" by the cortex. Thus the collateral RAS–thalamic pathways are essential for cortical perception of, activation by, and reaction to, all sensory stimuli, whether the stimuli origi-

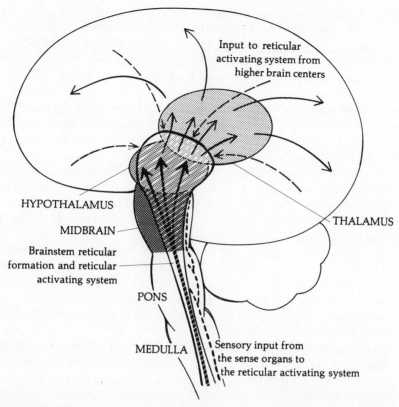

Figure 14-6. Diagram of the brainstem reticular formation and reticular activating system indicating afferent input to it from the organs of special sense and higher brain centers, and its action in arousal of the whole brain.

nate from within the body (pain, hunger, thirst, muscle activity) or from outside (sound, smell, sight, touch).

In addition to stimulation of RAS–thalamic pathways from the sense organs there are also systems of nerve fibers from the cerebral cortex itself to the RAS and thalamus which increase electrical activity in the RAS. This then feeds back to further increase cortical activation and arousal. This is the process responsible for the familiar fact that internal brain states such as intellectual activity, emotional arousal, worry and anxiety, and other mental and emotional states produce increased cortical activation and increased level of consciousness.

The Electrical Activity of the Cortex: EEG

The EEG is discussed more fully in Chapter 15, Disorders of Sleep, but for the present discussion it is necessary to describe briefly the neural basis for the electrical activity of the brain as measured from the scalp surface by the EEG, and to point out the correlation between the electrical activity of the brain and the level of consciousness.

In the mentally and physically quiescent person the electrical activity of the brain is of a type called synchronized: quite slow brain waves of moderate amplitude, indicating that very large numbers of neural structures toward the surface of the brain are undergoing a similar type of rhythmic electrical activity in harmony. The individual feels relaxed and possibly drowsy. If the subject is then stimulated by a noise, visual input, pain, or disturbing mental content, the electrical activity of the brain changes to a lower amplitude faster waveform; this is called a desynchronized EEG, and it correlates with increased level of mental activity, increased arousal and awareness, and an increased level of consciousness. Desynchronization is the replacement of a relatively high amplitude, slow wave, synchronized electrical activity in the brain; with a lower amplitude, faster wave, irregular electrical activity; electrical desynchronization accompanies increased cerebral activation and alertness.

In experimental animals a lesion in the RAS will result in a coma of long duration and unresponsiveness to sensory stimuli of any sort; the animal is unarousable. Conversely, stimulation of the RAS of an intact sleeping animal, by means of implanted electrodes, results in rapid desynchronization of the EEG and prompt awakening and behavioral alertness.

Anesthetics and hypnotic and tranquilizing drugs probably produce decreased levels of consciousness and/or unconsciousness by blocking neural transmission in the multisynaptic pathways of the reticular activating system. Patients with lesions in the upper portions of the reticular core of the brainstem, or with diffuse metabolic depression of these areas because of systemic disorders, are stuporous or comatose (see following).

There is some evidence that there is a degree of differentiation in function of various parts of the RAS relative to level of consciousness. It appears that the upper portions of the reticular formation in the region of the diencephalon (thalamus and hypothalamus) may be concerned with more rapidly shifting levels of conscious arousal, having to do with selective attention to specific components of experience and mental activity; while the more caudal portions of the reticular formation in the pons and medulla may be involved with more basic sleep–wakefulness cycles.

As mentioned above the source of the electrical activity measured and recorded in the EEG is the most superficial layers of the gray matter of the cortex. These first few layers are made up primarily of masses of dendrites, the cell bodies of which are located in the deeper layers of the cortex beneath the dendrites. Unlike the cell body and axon of a neuron, the dendrites seldom show the propagated waves of excitation (action potentials) which comprise the nerve impulse occurring in the cell body and axon as it transmits a stimulus (Chapter 17). Rather, the dendrites, which are covered with many synaptic knobs of terminals from axons of other neurons, undergo phasic changes in transmembrane potential above and below the resting about -80 mV, in response to excitatory and inhibitory influences from the axon terminals of these other neurons. When the transmembrane potential increases, the outside of the dendrites becomes more positive with respect to the inside. This is called hyperpolarization. When the potential difference across the membrane decreases (but still remains above threshold) this is called hypopolarization.

As masses of dendrites hyper- and hypopolarize together in synchronous and rhythmic fashion they become positive or negative, respectively, with respect to their cell bodies deeper in the cortex and with respect to other nearby masses of dendrites with similar phasic changes having a slightly different timing. The differences in electrical potential between dendrites and cell bodies and between one mass of dendrites and another can be recorded from the scalp electrodes of the EEG. The greater the degree of activation of the cortex by the RAS arousal system, the more desynchronized are the waveforms of the EEG, and the more alert the individual. The less the stimulation from the RAS, the more synchronized are the waves of the EEG, and the less alert the subject.

The Motivational Systems of the Brain

Certain neural structures in the region of the hypothalamus and limbic system concerned with pleasure and aversion appear to bear close functional relationships to the RAS arousal system and cortical activation. In persons with normal levels of conscious awareness, within this state of normal consciousness there can be a very wide range of variation in the degree of mental activation under a

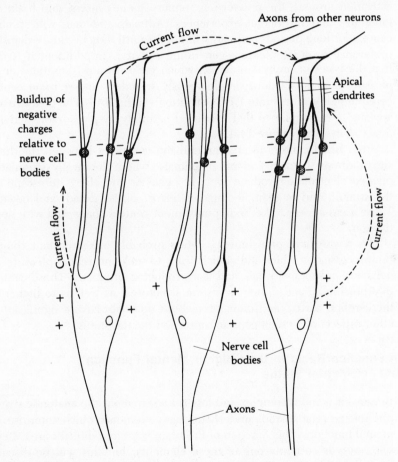

Figure 14-7. Neurons in superficial layers of cerebral cortex. The upper layer of apical dendrites receives many axon terminals from neurons elsewhere in the brain. Impulses from these axons cause hyper- and hypopolarizing changes in the transmembrane potentials of the apical dendrites. These influences cause apical dendrites to become electronegative, for example relative to their nerve cell bodies, or relative to other masses of apical dendrites in another area of the cerebral cortex. These differences in electrical charge cause current to flow in the ECF around the neurons; the variations in current flow are recorded from the scalp surface as the EEG.

variety of circumstances. Part of this range includes selective attention to a single aspect of inner mental activity or to an element of the environment; overall vigilance; intense concentration; the extreme arousal accompanying strong emotional states; or the very low levels of arousal characteristic of apathy, boredom, and depression.

The motivational systems appearing to be related to cortical arousal are brain centers concerned with reward and punishment or pleasure and displeasure, respectively. In animals and humans in which electrodes have been implanted in certain brain structures, electrical stimulation of regions in the area of the septum and median forebrain bundle in the limbic–hypothalamic region is pleasurable or rewarding. The median forebrain bundle is a major pathway for impulses traveling both ways between the limbic system and the brainstem reticular formation and thus constitutes a central component in the linkage between cortical activation–arousal, the pleasure or reinforcement centers, and brain centers for emotional and instinctual experiences. Animals and man will stimulate these centers for long periods (animals will persist until they become exhausted, and in preference to other pleasure-generating activity). In addition, it is now known that the types of brain stimulation which yield reward (sensations or feelings of pleasure and satisfaction) simultaneously stimulate higher brain centers in the cerebral hemispheres into EEG activation via the RAS. The pleasure and arousal appears to be similar to that produced naturally by pleasurable activities in the intact individual (Figure 14-4).

Other brain centers located around the ventricles between the diencephalon and midbrain in man and other animals, when electrically stimulated by implanted electrodes, produce aversive behavior and efforts to escape or shut off the stimuli; and in man, feelings of terror, panic, dread, and negative affect. These areas appear to be brain punishment centers concerned with negative motivation.

The reward and punishment centers probably are important components of the processes by which individuals learn to seek and repeat pleasure-generating behavior and to avoid pain and fear-producing situations. These centers project to other limbic and upper brainstem structures, as well as to higher centers in the cerebral cortex, and their interactions no doubt have a significant impact on other aspects of level of consciousness and mental status.

Brain Function Basic to the "Higher Mental Function" Aspects of Mental Status

Because it is more complex and less is known about the anatomic structures and physiologic relationships underlying many elements which comprise the higher mental functions, this function of the brain is a more difficult area. Level of consciousness is certainly one of these elements, but this will be discussed separately because of its central importance in numerous disorders of the brain, and because clinically it is sometimes assessed as a component independent of the other aspects of mental status.

Mental status has been referred to as the sum total of the contents of consciousness. It includes a number of components: (1) perception, defined as the act of acquiring sensory information originating both from the environment and from one's own self; (2) the intellectual processes: memory, judgment, abstract reasoning, logic, the store of information, symbolization, and association; (3) mood, affect, and temperament; (4) motivation to thought and action; and (5) insight into one's self, the behavior of others, and the meaning of external objects and events. Observable behavior is the outward manifestation of the mental status. Neural substrates underlying the various aspects of mental status, however, are multiple, complex, and in most cases incompletely understood.

DECREASED LEVEL OF CONSCIOUSNESS

A decreased level of consciousness is always the consequence of some type of impairment of brain function. The outer manifestations of the depressed brain function may range in degree from mere inattentiveness or mild and unobvious mental confusion, through drowsiness, lethargy, and stupor, to light or deep coma. It may be brief or prolonged.

The causes of decreased alertness or lack of arousal fall into two major categories: (1) those resulting from an abnormality within the brain itself, such as head trauma, seizures, elevated intracranial pressure, or specific brain lesions such as a tumor, cerebral infarction, or hemorrhage; and (2) those resulting from the adverse effects on the brain of general systemic disorders outside the brain, including fluid, electrolyte, and acid–base disturbances; hypoglycemia; hypoxemia or hypercapnia; toxic products resulting from liver or kidney failure; toxic drugs such as alcohol; or inadequate brain perfusion from hypotension or a cardiac arrhythmia. It is evident that the two categories of abnormality producing decreased consciousness, therefore, are (1) structural lesions originating within the brain; and (2) metabolic disorders originating elsewhere in the body. A third category of disorder, neuron metabolic or microstructural abnormalities originating within the brain, tends to produce dementia long before the level of consciousness is affected, and will be discussed in the following section on altered mental status.

The brain is an exceedingly fragile organ. It tends rapidly to undergo irreversible damage under adverse circumstances, particularly if they are prolonged. Brain tissue does not regenerate. Since life loses its meaning in direct proportion as brain function is impaired, and since all of the conditions which produce decreased levels of consciousness are capable of resulting in permanent brain damage, then obviously early recognition and prompt intervention to arrest or, if possible, reverse the causative disorder is essential.

Normal consciousness may be defined as a state of being behaviorally awake, with awareness of the self and the environment, and with the ability to respond to external stimuli (although the response may be inappropriate). Although I have drawn an apparently rigid line of distinction between level of consciousness and mental status, it needs to be emphasized that the portions of the brain underlying the higher mental functions related to mental status, and the brain structures subserving cortical activation and therefore level of consciousness, function together as a unit. Therefore when a patient is inattentive or lethargic it is difficult to conceive that his thought processes, and the verbal and other behavioral manifestations of them, could be unaltered. In fact varying degrees of mental confusion are characteristic accompaniments of decreased levels of consciousness, so much so that inattention, mental confusion, and stupor are regarded by some authors as being closely related points on a continuum, since patients lapsing into and arousing from comatose states often pass through these stages in sequence. However, the nature of the *mental confusion* accompanying decreased levels of consciousness appears different in most cases from the *delirium* of certain metabolic brain disorders on the one hand, and the *dementia* of degenerative brain disease on the other (see following).

So it appears that normal consciousness depends on a close interaction between *arousal*—that is, wakefulness—which is the product of a normally functioning brainstem reticular activating system; and the *contents of consciousness* contributed by intact cerebral hemispheres.

Levels of Consciousness

Confusional State

At the confusional level of reduced consciousness patients manifest an incapacity to follow simple commands, are unable to form short-term memories, and are disoriented as to person, place, and time. They misinterpret stimuli from the environment and have a short attention span.

Lethargy or Obtundation

Lethargy is a more advanced state of behavioral apathy, inattention, and blunted alertness in which patients appear unaware of what is going on around them and are unable to think and speak coherently when aroused. Their responsiveness is reduced, they appear drowsy, and sleep most of the time.

Stupor

Stupor is defined as minimal mental and physical activity; patients open their eyes in response to verbal or physical stimulation, although they may fail to react further. When the stimulus is withdrawn they lapse back into torpor.

Coma

Coma is a state in which patients appear to be asleep and are unable to respond either to normal external stimuli or their own internal needs. In light coma they may make semiappropriate movements such as partial withdrawal or a grimace in response to a vigorous painful stimulus. Deep tendon and plantar, as well as brainstem reflexes: corneal, pupillary, ocular, and pharyngeal are generally preserved. In deep coma, vigorous painful stimuli may elicit either no response, or a primitive level of inappropriate response such as decerebrate or decorticate posturing (see following). Reflexes may be absent.

Causes and Processes Involved in Stupor and Coma

Disorders which result in a marked decrease in level of consciousness form three categories: (1) visible structural lesions of, in, or closely adjacent to those portions of the brainstem regulating consciousness (diencephalon, midbrain, and upper pons) which compress or directly disrupt the brainstem reticular system; (2) visible structural lesions of the cerebral hemispheres which cause elevated intracranial pressure of a degree sufficient to compress and distort the brainstem reticular system; and (3) systemic disorders which cause diffuse metabolic depression affecting both the cerebral hemispheres and the brainstem reticular system.

Lesions in the Region of the Reticular Activating System

Bilateral lesions of the diencephalon (thalamus and hypothalamus), midbrain, and pons, impair conscious arousal by directly destroying the activating mechanisms of the brain. Lesions confined to these areas are rare but may include brain tumor, brain abscess, hemorrhage, or ischemic infarction.

Lesions of the Cerebral Hemispheres

Damage to the cerebral hemispheres, either acutely from head injury, cerebral hemorrhage, or infarction, or less acutely from a brain tumor or abscess, must be very extensive to produce stupor and coma. Lesions confined to the cerebral hemispheres, unless they are very extensive and destroy large masses of cerebral tissue, instead of causing stupor or coma, lead to focal neurologic deficits which are to some degree related to the region of the hemispheres affected: motor weakness or paralysis; sensory disturbances such as paresthesia or anesthesia; defects of speech, hearing, and vision; or alteration in the higher mental functions of memory, reason, and language.

Therefore, rather than causing stupor and coma directly, cerebral hemisphere destructive lesions may produce them indirectly via changes that lead to expansion of the intracranial contents by blood, edema fluid, a tumor mass or other abnormality, with resulting distortion of the upper brainstem and compression of its reticular formation and reticular activating system. The processes involved in these conditions are mechanical and circulatory ones which may produce the process known as transtentorial herniation.

The posterior portion of the brain, in the region of the occipital lobes, and at the level of the margin between the midbrain and pons, is separated from the cerebellum by double infolding of the meninges called the tentorium (Figure 14-1). All the structures of the brain above this fold of tissue are called supratentorial; they include the cerebral hemispheres, diencephalon, and midbrain. All the structures below the fold—cerebellum, pons, and medulla—are termed infratentorial.

Structures of the supratentorial compartment lie within the confines of a nonexpansible container, the cranium. Therefore, when a rapidly growing brain tumor, an accumulation of blood from a brain hemorrhage, or cerebral edema increases the volume of, and therefore the pressure within, the supratentorial region, the resulting expansion exerts pressure through the only opening available, namely, downward through the space frontal or ventral to the tentorial fold. This space is called the tentorial notch, and displacement of supratentorial brain structures toward and through the notch is transtentorial herniation. The compression of the upper brainstem resulting from this shift of intracranial contents impairs the function of the brainstem reticular formation, resulting in ob-

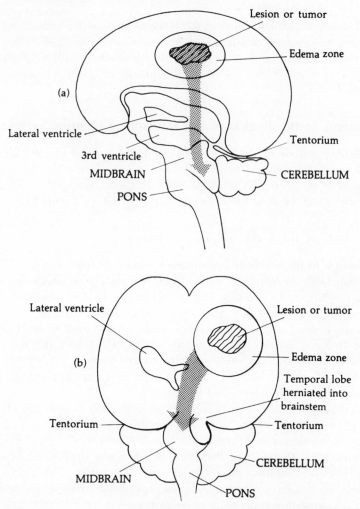

Figure 14-8. (a) Diagram of cross section of brain having an expanding mass lesion and a surrounding zone of edema. Pressure is exerted downward, compressing and distorting ventricles and brainstem structures. (b) Coronal section of (a).

tundation and stupor. The increased pressure and distortion of the structures in this area of the brain then compress the blood supply to it, and ischemia and hypoxia from impaired circulation further depress its functions. If the process continues, infarction of these structures results in irreversible coma and death.

In addition to decreasing levels of consciousness, brainstem compression and distortion are very frequently accompanied by alterations in respiratory and heart rate and rhythm, fluctuations in blood pressure, skeletal muscle activity, and neurologic signs relating to cranial nerve function (see following).

Diffuse Metabolic Depression of Cerebrum and Brainstem

Stupor and coma resulting from systemic disorders that diffusely impair the metabolism of cerebral and brainstem neurons is sometimes called metabolic encephalopathy. The range of systemic disorders which lead to depressed levels of consciousness is very broad and little is known of the precise mechanisms involved at the cellular level in the production of stupor and coma in each case. Decreased cerebral oxygen consumption is a correlate of such encephalopathies.

Basically, normal neuron function is dependent on processes at the cell membrane level that maintain a differential distribution of ions, and therefore of electrical charges, on the two sides of the neuron cell membrane. The inside of the cell is electronegative with respect to the outside by about -80 mV; this difference is called the transmembrane potential, and its basis is primarily active transport mechanisms within the cell membrane itself which maintain a high internal concentration of K^+ relative to Na^+, and a high external concentration of Na^+ relative to K^+. The active transport processes require an energy substrate, primarily glucose; an adequate supply of O_2; a normal range of temperature and pH, ionic composition, and osmotic concentration; and the absence of toxic substances, in order to function adequately. When the neuron is stimulated to transmit an impulse, membrane permeability rapidly alters, movement of ions across the membrane occurs, and a propagated wave of electrical charge which is self-sustaining, sweeps along the neuron. Immediately behind it, recovery occurs and the resting condition is restored, again through energy- and O_2-consuming active transport processes. The wave of excitation and the recovery are together termed the action potential (Chapter 17).

Therefore, in order for normal neuron function to occur, the prerequisites for neural activity listed above—glucose, O_2, acid-base, ionic and osmotic balance, and an absence of toxic materials—must be met. Metabolic brain depression represents the consequences of an imbalance in one or more of these requirements.

Systemic metabolic disorders such as uremic renal failure, hepatic insufficiency, diabetic ketoacidosis, and severe infections, probably interfere with normal levels of consciousness primarily by producing metabolic intermediates and end products such as organic acids, ammonia, and toxins which adversely affect neurons and suppress the metabolic processes necessary to normal membrane excitation and recovery.

Hypoxemia, hypoglycemia, acid- or alkalemia; and hyper- or hypoosmolar states and electrolyte abnormalities result either in inadequate metabolic substrate (glucose) and O_2 necessary for neuron metabolism; or else physical and chemical alterations in pH, osmotic pressure, temperature, and ionic balance, outside the range within which the enzyme systems responsible for neuron metabolism can operate. These enzymes also require coenzymes in order to function, which explains why deficiencies in such substances as thiamine and other cofactors may produce coma.

Correlates of Stupor and Coma

Cerebral oxygen consumption and cerebral metabolic rate are reported to be reduced in conditions producing stupor and coma. In some of these states cerebral blood flow is also below normal. Most conditions which produce unconsciousness also alter the EEG. In the case of a large lesion of a cerebral hemisphere, focal or unilateral slowing occurs; as compression of the upper midbrain develops and level of consciousness decreases, the amplitude increases and the slowing becomes bilateral and generalized. Lesions within the reticular formation itself also cause generalized high amplitude slow activity. Metabolic brain depression is reported to produce a symmetrical and diffuse slowing of the EEG, with a quite direct correlation between the degree of lethargy, stupor or coma; and the degree of slowing. In moderate to deep coma, a high voltage slow activity of 1–4 cps predominates and the EEG may resemble that of stage 4 slow wave sleep (see Chapter 15, Disorders of Sleep).

Central Nervous System Assessment

A general guideline in assessment of the central nervous system is that the presence of stupor or coma without focal neurologic abnormalities indicates a metabolic disorder.

Responses to Stimulation

Level of consciousness may be assessed by the degree of stimulation necessary to elicit a response. In decreasing consciousness, a vocal response is said to be the first to be lost. Calling patients by name, requesting them to execute a simple command such as opening their eyes or squeezing the examiner's hand, or producing stimuli which cause pain, such as pinching the neck or applying supraorbital or suprasternal pressure, in a gradually increasing fashion, gives an estimate of the patient's degree of depressed consciousness. Appropriate reactions such as a response to the command; or in the case of pain stimuli, semiappropriate responses such as a moan, grimace, or partial withdrawal; or inappropriate ones such as decerebrate posturing; indicate progressively depressed levels of consciousness.

Respiratory Rate and Rhythm

Lesions of various portions of the brain have different effects on respiration, since breathing is under the control of structures at several levels. This relationship may give an indication of the location of the disorder in focal lesions producing stupor and coma.

Posthyperventilation Apnea

In a normal subject, hyperventilating for several breaths will seldom lead to a period of apnea but merely to a reduced tidal volume for a few breaths until the $PaCO_2$ returns to normal. In patients with metabolic depression or focal lesions of the cerebrum or diencephalon, taking several deep breaths (if they are awake enough to cooperate) culminates in a brief respiratory arrest until the $PaCO_2$ returns to normal.

Cheyne-Stokes Respirations

Alternating hyperpnea and apnea with a gradual buildup and then decline in respiratory depth before and after the apnea, may occur in metabolic depression or bilateral lesions in the deep areas of the hemispheres and basal ganglia. The mechanisms producing this pattern have been discussed in Chapter 7, Heart Failure.

Central Neurogenic Hyperventilation

This pattern is said to occur in lesions which have destroyed the reticular formation in the area of the 4th ventricle in the lower midbrain and upper pons; it is produced by hemorrhage or infarction of that area, by transtentorial herniation from cerebral edema, or in hypoxemic or hypoglycemic coma. Respirations are regular, deep and rapid, with rates of 60/min or more. Such patients develop marked respiratory alkalemia. It appears to result from a hypersensitivity of the brainstem to normal CO_2 levels.

Apneustic Breathing

Prolonged deep inspirations with a pause at the end of each may result from removal of inhibition from the brainstem apneustic center. It is seen in structural or metabolic impairment at the level of the pons. The lesions may be in the upper medulla or low pons.

Biot's Respirations (Cluster Breathing)

This pattern resembles Cheyne-Stokes, with intermittent periods of apnea, but the clusters of breaths in between apneic periods fluctuate randomly in depth.

Nonpatterned Respirations

This is sometimes referred to as ataxic breathing, and there are random alterations in rate and depth. This form may occur in metabolic or structural impairment of the medulla. Both of the latter patterns often presage respiratory arrest.

Pupillary Reactions

Hutchinson's Pupil

This is unilateral dilation of a pupil which is unreactive to light. It occurs during transtentorial herniation when a portion of the temporal lobe is pushed against the edge of the tentorium and compresses CN III (oculomotor). The parasympathetic fibers of that nerve are more susceptible to pressure block than the sympathetic; therefore, the latter operate unopposed and the pupil becomes widely dilated and fixed to light.

Horner's Syndrome

Unilateral lesions of the brainstem at either the level of the hypothalamus or the medulla may interfere with sympathetic pathways and result in the triad of eyelid ptosis and enophthalmos, miosis, and anhidrosis, on the same side. It may be an early sign of impending transtentorial herniation.

Midposition (5 mm) Pupils Unreactive to Light

This type may indicate damage to the midbrain which is the center for pupillary dilating and constricting reflexes. If the midbrain undergoes ischemic necrosis, however, then both pupils dilate widely and are unresponsive, but may be slightly unequal (aniscoria) and irregular rather than smoothly round. In this case, both sympathetic and parasympathetic innervation to the pupils have been destroyed.

Bilateral Constricted Pupils Slightly Reactive to Strong Light

Lesions of the pons usually interrupt the sympathetic pathways and therefore miosis occurs, but slight reactiveness to light is still visible with a strong stimulus.

Bilateral Pupillary Size and Responsiveness

PERRLA stands for pupils equal, round, regular, and reactive to light and accommodation. Normal pupil responsiveness in the presence of stupor or coma almost always rules out structural brainstem lesions and indicates metabolic brainstem depression, except terminally. The exceptions are atropine overdose, which produces fixed dilated pupils (mydriasis), glutethimide which causes medium and unreactive pupils, and the opiate alkaloids which produce miosis.

Ocular Movements

Action of the extraocular muscles (EOMs) which control eye movements are integrated in brainstem nuclei and neural pathways lying in the midbrain and pons near the brainstem reticular activating system; for this reason lesions which impair consciousness also often produce abnormalities of eye movements.

In the conscious cooperative patient the integrity of the EOMs is tested by asking the patient to follow with his eyes the examiner's finger move through the cardinal positions of gaze, the traditional wide "H": ├────┤ . However, the obtunded, stuporous, or comatose patient is incapable of this; therefore, the EOMs are tested via the oculocephalic and oculovestibular reflexes.

Unilateral abnormalities in eye position or eye movement indicate a structural lesion rather than metabolic depression as the cause of the reduced level of consciousness. Moreover, most structural lesions which produce stupor or coma, including brain herniation, impair conjugate eye movements, while most metabolic brain depression does not.

Oculocephalic Reflex (Doll's Eyes)

The comatose patient's head is grasped between the examiner's hands in such a way that the little fingers hold the lids open so that the response of the eyes can be observed. The head is turned briskly to the right and to the left alternately. (The examiner first makes certain that there is no cervical injury or possible dislocation.) A positive response is a horizontal deviation of the eyes rapidly and conjugately in the opposite direction to the head movement, with a prompt return to the resting midline position. The integrity of vertical eye movements is tested by moving the head up and down; again, the response is the same as the above, except it is in the vertical plane. Positive doll's eyes indicate intact EOM brainstem neural pathways. When the eyes remain in the resting position throughout the movements, it is a negative response indicating that the brainstem centers that integrate eye movement with head movements are destroyed. The afferents for this reflex involve both receptors in the vestibular system and proprioreceptors in the neck. The response is negative in the intact awake normal person because of inhibition by higher centers in the cerebral cortex.

Oculovestibular Reflexes (Calorics, Chapter 16)

Each ear is irrigated with cold water. In the normal subject the result is horizontal nystagmus with the slow component toward the irrigated ear and the fast (corrective) component away from it.

In the comatose patient with intact brainstem function, there is no nystagmus but a tonic deviation of the eyes toward the ear irrigated with cold water (or away from an ear irrigated with warm water). The explanation for the difference in response between the normal and comatose patient is that the fast corrective eye movement in nystagmus depends on intact functioning cerebral hemispheres. In stupor or coma the fast component is eliminated, so that the slow component is the only response, and this results in a tonic deviation toward the ear irrigated with cold water. Before testing the other ear, 5 min should elapse.

Irrigation of both ears simultaneously with cold water tests downward eye movement; in the comatose patient with intact brainstem function, the eyes deviate downward. Similarly, irrigating both ears simultaneously with warm water produces upward deviation if the patient is comatose and the brainstem intact.

In light coma, oculocephalic and oculovestibular responses are intact provided there is no structural lesion in the brainstem. In deeper coma the response becomes even more marked and readily elicited. When the brainstem becomes very severely depressed from a metabolic cause, eventually both of these reflex responses become sluggish and more difficult to elicit. They are absent in destructive brainstem lesions. If one eye adducts and the other fails to adduct, this deficit is called internuclear ophthalmoplegia and it indicates a lesion which occurs commonly in brainstem damage: interruption of a special pathway concerned with extraocular muscle control, the medial longitudinal fasciculus. This tract is one of the main connections of the vestibular nuclei with other nuclei in the brainstem; if it is damaged at the level of the pons the lesion results in dissociation of conjugate eye movements and the resulting dissociation is called internuclear ophthalmoplegia.

Conjugate Tonic Deviation of the Eyes

In hemiplegia caused by a large lesion of the cerebral hemispheres, the eyes deviate conjugately toward the side of the lesion, and therefore away from the paralyzed side; in other words, they turn toward the side in which the innervation is still intact. However, if the hemiplegia is caused by a lesion in the pons, then it affects the neural pathways controlling eye movements below the point where they have crossed over (i.e., below the decussation), and in this case the eyes deviate away from the side of the lesion and therefore toward the paralyzed side.

Corneal Reflex

Stimulation of the cornea causes reflex bilateral eyelid closure and upward deviation of the eyes. This reflex response, if intact, indicates intact brainstem pathways from the midbrain to the lower pons, since it involves the brainstem nuclei of both CN VII (facial) in the pons and CN III (oculomotor) in the midbrain.

Lower Brainstem Reflexes: Cough, Gag, Swallow, Spontaneous Respirations

Lower brainstem reflexes are lost only in profound near-terminal metabolic coma and in destructive brainstem lesions so severe as to have resulted in an isoelectric EEG, that is, in brain death.

Skeletal Muscle Activity

Decorticate and Decerebrate Responses

These responses and/or positions are the consequences of lesions that disrupt the neural pathways between higher and lower brain centers that regulate tonic activity in the antigravity muscles.

Decorticate Rigidity. In decorticate rigidity (or decorticate posturing, if the position changes spontaneously or as a result of noxious stimulation) the arm, wrist, and fingers are flexed and adducted, the leg is extended, rotated inward, and the foot is in extension.

Decorticate rigidity may be seen on the affected side in lesions that have damaged brain structures above the level of the thalamus, often hemorrhage or infarction in the area of the internal capsule (a portion of the corticospinal tract in the region between the thalamus and the basal ganglia). It may occur acutely (spontaneously in spasms or in response to noxious stimulation) in severe head injuries and acute cerebral hemorrhage. The tonic neck reflex, normal in infants, may also appear as a portion of decorticate posturing; if the head is turned to one side the arm on that side extends and the opposite one flexes.

Decerebrate Rigidity. The full pattern of decerebrate rigidity includes clenched teeth; opisthotonos; arms extended, adducted, and hyperpronated; and the legs extended with feet extended, as in decorticate rigidity. Where this motor pattern occurs, there is a functional separation between the cerebral hemispheres, basal ganglia, and thalamus above and the midbrain and pons below. It results from a diffuse facilitation of the muscle stretch reflexes resulting from removal of the normal inhibition exerted by higher brain centers. It occurs

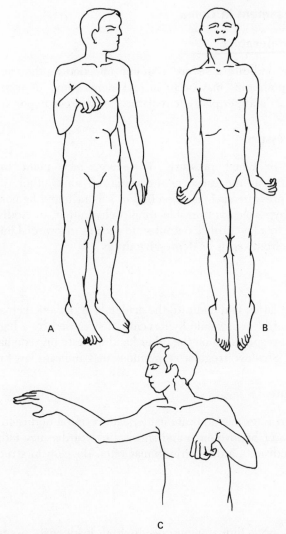

Figure 14-9. (A) Decorticate posture on right side, normal on left. (B) Decerebrate rigidity bilaterally. (C) Tonic neck reflex.

in massive head injury, large intracerebral hemorrhages and infarctions, and brain herniation with edema and hypoxia. In less severe lesions fragments of the response may occur either spontaneously or more often in response to a painful stimulus. Also a patient may show decerebrate responses on one side and decorticate on the other, or a shift between decorticate and decerebrate responses. These shifting motor reactions appear to correlate with fluctuations in blood flow to various portions of the brain.

Lack of Response to Painful Stimulation

This indicates severe metabolic depression of, or a destructive lesion in, the brainstem reticular activating system, or a bilateral interruption of the corticospinal tracts at the level of the brainstem.

General Assessment in Coma

Body Temperature

Fever may indicate a severe systemic infection as the cause of the stupor or coma. Hypothermia may occur in myxedema coma, depressive drug poisoning, hypovolemia and peripheral circulatory collapse, or hypoglycemia.

Blood Pressure

Elevation of blood pressure, if severe, may point to hypertensive encephalopathy as the cause of the coma, or some other cause of elevated intracranial pressure such as a cerebral or subarachnoid hemorrhage. Hypotension indicates hypovolemia from bleeding, dehydration, or Addisonian crisis. It also may point to a low cardiac output state such as myocardial infarction, or a vasodilated state from sepsis or depressive drugs.

Respiration

Hyperventilation may indicate the acidemia of diabetic ketoacidosis or renal failure; or central neurogenic hyperventilation caused by a high brainstem lesion. Depressed respirations on the other hand indicate myxedema or depressive drug poisoning. Shallow irregular respirations may indicate low brainstem lesion.

Heart Rate

Rapid heart rates may indicate inadequate cerebral perfusion caused by a cardiac arrhythmia or hypovolemia and shock; bradycardia may indicate heart block or hypothyroidism. Cardiac arrhythmias often develop in structural lesions of the brainstem.

Skin

Central cyanosis (lips, tongue) results from inadequate oxygenation of hemoglobin from respiratory failure or heart failure. Spiders and palmar erythema suggest alcoholism. Pink color may indicate carbon monoxide poisoning. Pallor is associated with blood loss and compensatory vasoconstriction. Sweating occurs in hypoglycemia and hemorrhagic shock, while in uremia and diabetic ketoacidosis the skin is dry.

Optic Fundi

Hypertensive or diabetic retinopathy may indicate the cause of the coma. Papilledema and decreased venous pulsations point to elevated intracranial pressure.

Management

The usual supportive measures of a clear airway, adequate ventilation, heart action, and blood pressure, and administration of oxygen and fluids take precedence over diagnostic procedures. Since hypoxemia and hypoglycemia are the two metabolic causes of coma most likely to result in permanent brain damage, O_2 is given immediately and glucose is administered after blood chemistries have been drawn.

Altered Mental Status

There are four major categories of disorders of the central nervous system which may produce altered mental status, with or without accompanying changes in the level of consciousness. These categories include (1) acute or chronic visible structural lesions of the brain: cerebral infarction, intracerebral or subdural hemorrhage or hematoma, a brain tumor or a brain abscess, or traumatic destruction of specific motor, sensory, or association areas of the cerebral cortex; (2) so-called functional brain disease: the psychoneuroses and psychoses; (3) metabolic or exogenous brain syndromes resulting from systemic disorders which produce mental confusion and/or delirium; and (4) degenerative or endogenous brain diseases which lead to progressive dementia.

Assessment may pose a difficult problem in patients with altered mental status, because these four categories of cause very frequently produce similar signs and symptoms during various stages in their development and evolution. Management and future course in each category may be quite different; therefore, determination of the underlying cause in a given instance becomes a matter of great practical importance. Especially in the cases of altered mental status caused by metabolic (exogenous) brain disease, or by a rapidly evolving brain lesion, accurate assessment and appropriate management can mean the difference between reversal or arrest of the process on the one hand, or permanent mental and physical disability, or death, on the other.

Confusion is a term often employed for the altered mental status accompanying disorders of the brain. The meanings of the word confusion used in this sense include perplexity, bewilderment, befuddlement, and mental jumbling; in addition, there is the connotation of a disorderly mixing of mental contents, a mistaking of one idea or object for another, misinterpretation of external events, and easy distractibility. In a broader sense, confusion refers to a lack of normal speed and clarity of thought, with accompanying inappropriateness of behavior.

Careful assessment of the quality of thought and accompanying behavior of patients manifesting altered mental status may reveal that the term mental confusion may be divided into three categories which, although they often blend or overlap, nevertheless have certain distinguishing characteristics. The first category is sometimes referred to as *mental clouding*, in which conscious awareness or alertness, perception, psychomotor activity, and responsiveness, appears to be depressed; this category is the quiet confusion associated with descent into and recovery from stupor and coma. This form of mental confusion has been discussed in the preceding section.

The second category of confusion is *delirium*, sometimes called toxic psychosis, which is of acute onset and relatively brief duration; is accompanied by agitation, tremulousness, and hyperarousal; and is characterized by illusions and hallucinations, complete disorientation, psychomotor overactivity, and autonomic activation. The third category of confusion is *dementia* in which the major deficits appear to be in intellectual function, with impairment of psychomotor activity, the ability to calculate, reason abstractly, form new memory traces, and apply appropriate judgment. In general, although there are major exceptions, delirium is caused by systemic metabolic disorders originating outside the brain and is readily reversible when the underlying abnormality is corrected; dementia is often progressive and irreversible and results from degenerative processes within the cells of the brain. For these reasons delirium and the associated metabolic brain disease is called exogenous, while dementia and the associated degenerative brain disease is termed endogenous. However, classifications shift as new knowledge accumulates, and one form of degenerative brain disease leading to irreversible dementia, Creutzfeldt-Jakob disease, long classified as an endogenous disorder, is now known to be caused by a transmissible agent and is therefore now classed as an infectious slow virus disease.

Metabolic (Exogenous) Brain Disease and Delirium

As discussed above, systemic metabolic disorders often lead to quiet mental confusion, physical hypoactivity, and decreased levels of consciousness. However, some patients with brain function impairment from systemic abnormalities manifest mental changes characterized by auditory, tactile, and visual hallucinations, illusions and persistent delusions, alertness and vigilance coupled with incoherent thinking and speech, inaccessibility to normal environmental interactions, and inability to sleep.

The most common causes of a vivid and dramatic delirium are said to be the withdrawal of alcohol, barbiturates, or other depressive drugs following a period of severe intoxication. Other causes may be an overdose of a drug with psychoactive properties, acute liver failure, bacterial toxins in severe infections, a high fever, or thyrotoxicosis.

In some patients a more quiet type of delirium may resemble, or alternate with, metabolic mental confusion and stupor. A common form of altered mental status that may incorporate various aspects of delirium, simple mental confusion, and dementia is seen in elderly patients with cerebral atherosclerosis or senile dementia, who develop, or have an exacerbation of, an underlying systemic disorder. Although the patient's pre–illness mental status may have been only minimally and unevidently impaired, the imposition of one or more metabolic derangements may serve to amplify the impairment and lead to marked mental, emotional, and behavioral aberrations. Anemia, hypoxemia from congestive heart failure or lung disease, hypovolemia from dehydration, a systemic infection, or any one or a combination of other disorders, may dramatically illustrate the marginal nature of a person's cerebral function. This condition has been termed beclouded dementia; the mental status returns to baseline values when the metabolic abnormality is reversed unless permanent brain damage occurred during the episode.

Degenerative (Endogenous) Brain Disease and Dementia

Dementia is defined as a usually irreversible deterioration of intellectual functioning from an organic brain disorder and is often accompanied by emotional disturbances. Unlike the altered mental status resulting from systemic metabolic abnormalities, the onset tends to be gradual and insidious and may resemble depression, boredom or fatigue. As it evolves it comes to impair every component of behavior: use of language, judgment, reason, and problem-solving ability. Impairment of recent memory is often the earliest sign. Apathy, indifference to the environment, and lack of self-care, together with irritability and depression, develop later.

Loss of specific mental faculties, as occurs in the various forms of aphasias, or other isolated neurologic deficits resulting from focal damage to the cerebral hemispheres, are not considered to be forms of dementia. Also the intellectual deficits occurring in severe hypothyroidism and other endocrine disorders are often excluded because of their ready reversibility with appropriate treatment, and because the decline in mental status is secondary to an abnormal process originating outside the brain. So the former group of disorders would be considered focal neurologic deficits from localized lesions, and the latter would be classed as metabolic (exogenous) brain disease.

Reversible or Arrestible Disorders Producing the Signs and Symptoms of Dementia

Hypothyroidism

This disorder, characterized by generalized mental and physical slowing from lack of thyroid hormone, is discussed in Chapter 13.

General Paresis (Neurosyphilis)

There is a long latent period, more than 20 years, from the time of infection to the appearance of signs and symptoms. There is diffuse brain degeneration accompanied by intellectual deficits involving memory, orientation, insight, and judgment; emotional disturbances accompanied by delusions, hallucinations and illusions; and neurologic signs including hyperactive reflexes and Argyll-Robertson pupils (small, irregular, and reactive to accommodation but not to light). Penicillin is the management and leads to arrest of progression but not reversal.

Occult (Normal Pressure) Hydrocephalus

This disorder may be the consequence of an old head injury which produced subarachnoid bleeding, inflammation of the subarachnoid space with scar formation, and eventual partial obstruction to the flow of cerebrospinal fluid from the ventricles through the subarachnoid space to the area where it is reasorbed in the arachnoid villi.

An individual with this disorder manifests progressive intellectual deterioration, motor slowing, ataxia, and other deficits. The CSF pressure is normal or near normal and the patients do not complain of headaches or show signs of elevated intracranial pressure. However, the ventricles are enlarged and special studies show impaired flow of CSF out of the ventricles into the subarachnoid space, and a thinning of the cerebral hemispheres. This is a potentially arrestable dementing syndrome; the management is surgical placement of a shunt to convey CSF from the ventricles to the atrium or peritoneum.

Wernicke's and Korsakoff's Syndromes

These disorders are the consequence of thiamine deficiency and are most often seen in chronic alcoholics. The dementia is accompanied by disturbances of function of the extraocular muscles and severe ataxia; and is characterized by disorientation, apathy, lack of insight, irrationality, and incoherence. In Korsakoff's, defective memory for both recent and past events is the outstanding characteristic of the intellectual deficits. Cerebellar, thalamic, and upper brainstem lesions are found at autopsy. When the ocular and gait abnormalities appear before the memory and other intellectual deficits, prompt treatment with thiamine may prevent the appearance of the latter. While the neurologic abnormalities clear with thiamine administration, the memory deficits, once developed, resolve slowly, partially, or more often not at all. Institutional care is usually necessary.

Chronic Subdural Hematoma and Other Focal Neurologic Lesions, Such as Brain Tumors

These are, at least in some cases, potentially correctable causes of mental and neurologic impairment.

Progressive Irreversible Dementia

Senile Dementia

This is a common disorder of aging consisting of diffuse cerebral atrophy correlated with variable degrees of dementia. It may be associated with diffuse cerebrovascular disease, but the cause is not known beyond the fact that some degree of declining brain mass and weight appears inevitably to occur with advancing age. In many individuals there are few associated signs or symptoms.

Alzheimer's Disease (Presenile Dementia)

The onset is in middle or late life and manifests as progressive intellectual deterioration. Earliest signs are impairment of recent memory and slight disorientation, often accompanied by depression or anxiety. The progression is slow over many years. Later, lack of self-care, mutism, aimless hyperactivity, and delusions may develop. In advanced stages there may be ataxia and other neurologic deficits.

At autopsy the brain shows atrophy of the cortex, shrunken convolutions, and enlargement of the ventricles. Microscopically there is a marked loss of neurons with proliferation of glia cells and structural abnormalities of the neuron cytoplasm.

There is no treatment beyond supportive care and the prevention or correction of metabolic systemic disorders, which make the mental status much worse.

Pick's Disease

This disorder is much less common than the above. There is severe atrophy of the frontal and temporal lobes as well as the thalamus and basal ganglia, with a decrease in white matter (tracts) being more marked than that of gray (nerve cell bodies). Characteristics of the patient and course are similar to that of Alzheimer's.

Huntington's Chorea

This is an hereditary disorder occurring mainly in middle life, which is slowly progressive and long in duration before resulting in death, sometimes from infection but often by suicide. There are characteristic uncontrollable movements affecting the trunk, shoulder girdle, and lower extremities which result in a bizarre dancelike gait, as well as grimacing, irregular respirations, and dysarthria. Emotional changes are marked, and often there is a manic-depressive type of mood change pattern, alternating with profound apathy. The dementia is progressive and severe, and in most cases the intellectual deterioration develops in parallel with the motor disorders.

The brain shows atrophy most marked in the frontal lobes and basal ganglia, with loss of nerve cells and deficiencies in the synthesis of neurotransmitter substances.

Creutzfeldt-Jakob Disease (Subacute Spongiform Encephalopathy)

This disorder appears to be caused by a transmissible agent of the slow virus variety, and runs a shorter course of a few months to two years. The dementia is rapidly progressive and is accompanied by emotional manifestations and neurologic symptoms and signs: ataxia, aphasia, seizures, and paralysis. There is severe neuron destruction of the cortex, basal ganglia, and cerebellum. Inoculation of brain and other tissues from affected patients produces the disease in other primates after a long latent period. There is no treatment.

Assessment

Diagnosis

The search for a treatable cause in dementia is crucial, since similar signs and symptoms can result from correctable, or at least arrestable, disorders as from the incurable and inexorably progressive ones. The search will therefore include a general as well as a neurologic examination, laboratory tests to rule out systemic metabolic disorders, and special neurologic diagnostic procedures: skull films, EEG, brain scan, computerized tomography (CT) scan, and possibly others.

The Mental Status Examination for Dementia

The most useful elements of assessment include (1) orientation to person, place and time; (2) language use: naming of objects and understanding of verbal commands; (3) the fund of knowledge: capital cities, presidents, rivers; (4) recent memory: giving the patient three objects to be remembered immediately, at 30 minutes, and at 1 hour; (5) the attention span and calculation; serial 7's or 3's subtracted from 100; (6) drawing: a man, house, clock face; and (7) abstract thought: interpretation of proverbs or asking for characteristics that two objects have in common, for example, a car and a bicycle, an apple and an orange, a table and a chair.

A good bit of tact is often required in administering these tests; even quite evidently impaired individuals may be angry or insulted and accuse the examiner of thinking they are "crazy" or "dumb" unless an explanation is given, or the questions are subtly phrased. One valuable opening statement is: "I just arrived and don't yet know the circumstances of your illness and how you came to be in the clinic (or in the hospital) today. Could you tell me what has happened, why you are here, and how you got here?" The nature of the response provides important information concerning the patient's mental status.

In patient assessment there is no aid so valuable as that which can be obtained from an intelligent, reliable friend or relative who has had close association with the patient for a considerable time as well as the recent past, and who is able to give an orderly sequential account of the nature, degree, and timing of the observed changes. Obtaining information as to the ability of the patient to find his way around town, make change during a purchase, balance a checkbook, dress and behave appropriately, yield valuable information about the patient's mental status and the course of the disorder.

REFERENCES

Beeson PB and McDermott W, editors: *Textbook of Medicine.* 14th ed. Philadelphia, Pa.: Saunders, 1975.

DeMeyer WE: The clinical interview and the screening neurological examination. In: Toole JF, editor: *Clinical Concepts of Neurological Disorders.* Baltimore, Md.: Williams and Wilkins, 1977.

Dimond SF and Beaumont JG, editors: *Hemisphere Function in the Human Brain.* New York: Halstead Press, Wiley, 1974.

Eccles JC: *The Understanding of the Brain.* New York: McGraw-Hill, 1973.

Frohlich ED, editor: *Pathophysiology.* Philadelphia, Pa.: Lippincott, 1976.

Galin D and Ornstein RE: Hemispheric specialization and the duality of consciousness. In: Widroe HM, editor: *Human Behavior and Brain Function.* Springfield, Ohio: Charles C Thomas, 1975.

Ganong WF: *Review of Medical Physiology,* 8th ed. Los Altos, Calif.: Lang Medical Publications, 1977.

Gazzaniga MS and LeDoux JE: The integrated mind. New York: Plenum, 1978.

Goldensohn ES and Appel SH, editors: *Scientific Approaches to Clinical Neurology,* 2 vols. Philadelphia, Pa.: Lea & Febiger, 1977.

Guyton AC: *Textbook of Medical Physiology.* 5th ed. Philadelphia, Pa.: Saunders, 1976.

Heath R: Pleasure and brain activity in man. *J. Nerv. and Ment. Dis.* 154:3–18, 1972.

Maclean PD: Edited by Boag TJ and Campbell D: *A Triune Concept of the Brain and Behaviour.* Toronto: University of Toronto Press, 1973.

Matthews WB: *Practical Neurology,* 3rd ed. London: Blackwell Scientific Publications, 1975.

Merritt HH: *A Textbook of Neurology.* 5th ed. Philadelphia, Pa.: Lea & Febiger, 1973.

Olds J: Drives and reinforcements. Behavioral studies of hypothalamic functions. New York: Raven, 1977.

Penfield, Wilder: *The Mystery of the Mind. A Critical Study of Consciousness and the Human Brain.* Princeton, N.J.: Princeton University Press, 1975.

Plum F and Posner JB: *The Diagnosis of Stupor and Coma.* 2nd ed. Philadelphia, Pa., F.A. Davis Co., 1972.

Popper KR and Eccles JC: *The Self and Its Brain.* New York Springer Int. 1977.

Rolls ET: The neural basis of brain-stimulation reward. *Progr. Neurobiol.* 3:73–160, 1974.

Schwartz GE, et al: Right hemisphere lateralization for emotion in the human brain: interaction with cognition. *Science* 190:286–288, 1975.

ter Meulen V and Katz M, editors: *Slow Virus Infections of the Central Nervous System.* New York: Springer-Verlag, 1977.

Thorn GW, et al, editors: *Harrison's Principles of Internal Medicine,* 8th ed. New York: McGraw-Hill, 1977.

Toole JF, editor: *Clinical Concepts of Neurological Disorders.* Baltimore, Md.: Williams & Wilkins, 1977.

Uttal, WR. *The psychobiology of mind.* Hillsdale, N.J.: Lawrence Erlbaum Associates, 1978.

Sleep Disorders

NORMAL SLEEP

Knowledge concerning human sleep has been obtained primarily from research on normal subjects who spend two or more nights in sleep laboratories where they are monitored continuously throughout the night. In a number of centers there are laboratories for the study of sleep disorders where monitoring and trials of treatment are undertaken with individuals presenting a variety of disturbances of sleep. Several variables are recorded with the multichannel polygraph: the scalp electroencephalogram (EEG), which records the electrical activity occurring in superficial portions of the brain; the electromyogram (EMG) of the chin muscles, which measures the degree of muscle tone; and the electrooculogram (EOG), which records the direction, frequency, and magnitude of eye movements. Other parameters such as the EKG, respiratory rate and depth, O_2 saturation (with the ear oximeter), and additional ones may also be monitored and recorded for correlation with the standard sleep research variables.

EEG Waveforms; Correlates in Consciousness and Behavior

Wakefulness

In general in the normal EEG there tends to be an inverse relationship between amplitude of a waveform (measured in microvolts, μV) and its frequency (measured in cycles per second, cps). The greater the amplitude, the lower the frequency; high-amplitude low-frequency waves in the EEG are called high voltage slow (HVS). Waves of low amplitude with high frequencies are termed low voltage fast (LVF). Most EEG recordings show mixed frequencies and are therefore evaluated on the basis of the percentages of the dominant waveforms at successive time intervals. Probable neural processes underlying the electrical activity recorded from the scalp are discussed in Chapters 14 and 17 and diagramed in Figure 14-7.

The alpha rhythm has an amplitude of approximately 50 μV, a frequency of 8–14 cps, and is the predominant waveform recorded from individuals who are in a quiet environment and a state of relaxed wakefulness with the eyes closed. The alpha rhythm is most marked over the parietooccipital area and first becomes established during adolescence. Muscle tone is usually rather high unless the subject is practiced in progressive relaxation, yoga, or meditation, and eye movements usually occur in random fashion.

Beta waves are of lower amplitude (voltage) and a higher frequency of about 18–30 cps; they are most prominent over the frontal region. This is the typical waveform recorded from mentally alert individuals with the eyes open and is called desynchronization. When a quiescent person showing predominant alpha rhythm opens his eyes, hears a sudden loud noise or, with eyes closed, performs a mental task involving concentration or visualization, the EEG waves shift suddenly from alpha to beta; this shift is called alpha blocking or the alerting or orienting response.

Theta waves, or a theta rhythm, are of a higher amplitude and slower frequency than the alpha—about 4–7 cps. As a person resting quietly with the eyes closed and in alpha rhythm becomes drowsy, the alpha waves become increasingly interspersed with these slower waves.

Delta waves are the waveform recorded during deep sleep, barbiturate and other anesthesia, and coma. They are of high amplitude (over 75 μV) and slow frequency—0.5 to about 3 cps. Although the EEG waveforms of natural deep sleep and coma may resemble each other, nevertheless it should be emphasized that the two conditions are quite distinct metabolically. During sleep the O_2 consumption of brain tissue remains at or above that of waking levels, while in coma and anesthesia it is always reduced.

Sleep States and Sleep Stages

Sleep States: REM and N-REM

The sleep states, rapid eye movement (REM) and nonrapid eye movement (N-REM), and the sleep stages (N-REM stages 1–4) are differentiated on the basis of the data obtained from the three parameters monitored during studies of sleep: the EEG, the EMG, and the EOG. The two sleep states, REM and N-REM, are completely different, physiologically distinct conditions which differ from each other in a number of basic ways including the neural processes underlying them.

In N-REM sleep the EEG shows high voltage slow waves (theta and delta) sometimes with sleep spindles and K complexes (see following); the EMG of the chin muscles records tone decreasing as a person falls asleep, but it never declines to very low levels. The EOG indicates few eye movements except slow brief ones as the subject falls asleep, at which time the eyes deviate conjugately upward. There are occasional changes of body position; the respirations are regular and deep; blood pressure is stable at below waking levels, and the heart rate is regular and slow. Subjects wakened from N-REM sleep report mental activity which tends to be verbal, repetitive, and resembles thoughts rather than images.

Studies of sleeping subjects with all-night automated time lapse photography, correlated with EEG recordings, show that postural immobility begins in descending stage 2 and lasts through stage 3 or 4, just before the sleep begins to "lighten" back up to stage 2. At that time major whole body movements occur. These studies show that persons who rate themselves as "good" sleepers have fewer of these postural shifts during the night than do subjects who rate themselves as "poor" sleepers.

REM sleep is characterized by an EEG showing predominantly low amplitude and mixed frequency waveforms; the alpha rhythm comprises less than 50% of the record, which is mainly beta with some theta (in other words, mainly LVF) resembling the state of alert wakefulness. The EOG reveals frequent rapid conjugate eye movements in all directions, and the chin muscle EMG indicates very low muscle tone, sometimes approaching zero—that is, deep relaxation. Generalized profound relaxation of the skeletal musculature is a prominent feature of the REM state in both humans and other animals. Apparently the single muscle group excepted is the muscles of mastication; bruxism (teeth grinding) occurs during REM sleep. There are occasional minor muscle twitches, the respirations are shallow and of a variable rate; the heart rate is rapid and fluctuates markedly; the blood pressure is likewise variable and on occasion rises to very high levels. In the male there are frequent penile erections—nocturnal penile tumescence (NPT). Subjects awakened from REM sleep describe vivid pictorial visual images, often with a storylike dramatic content.

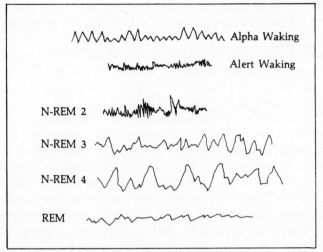

Figure 15-1. Waveforms of the EEG in alert and restful (eyes closed) waking (alpha); stages 2, 3, and 4 N-REM sleep; and in REM sleep.

N-REM Sleep Stages

Stage 1 N-REM is characterized by less than 50% alpha rhythm; the waveform is primarily beta (LVF) with some theta. There are occasional slow roving eye movements. Stage 2 N-REM is defined as mainly beta and theta waves, with less than 20% delta, and with sleep spindles (brief bursts of synchronous 12–15 cps waves lasting less than a half second) and K complexes (a high amplitude nega-tive wave followed by a positive one). K complexes sometimes follow sensory stimulation such as a noise from the environment, or an internal sensation such as a smooth muscle bladder, stomach, or intestinal contraction. There are no eye movements, and the eyes are turned upward. Stage 3 and 4 are sometimes called slow wave sleep (SWS) because they are characterized by the appearance of the high voltage (75 μV or above) slow (0.5–3) delta waves; when the recording is comprised of 20–50% delta it is stage 3, and stage 4 is comprised of more than half delta. There may be sleep spindles in both 3 and 4 but there are no eye movements.

Unlike the states of REM and N-REM, which are two physiologically distinct conditions, the stages of N-REM are somewhat arbitrarily defined subdivisions of a single physiologic condition.

N-REM and REM Sequence

During a typical night's sleep there is an orderly and quite stable (from night to night) sequence of alternating N-REM and REM states. As the subject rests quietly in bed and then starts to become drowsy the predominant alpha pattern gives way to increasing amounts of theta and LVF, muscle activity declines, there are slow roving eye movements, and the subject enters N-REM stage 1, with the characteristics described above. This first period of N-REM lasts about an hour and a half and during this time the sleeper passes through stages 2 and 3 to the deep stage 4; then the stages reverse to progressive lighter levels until, after 90 min or so, there is often a burst of theta waves. The sleeper then enters a REM period with its characteristic EEG change to the lower voltage faster mixed frequencies described above, the profound skeletal muscle relaxation, and the marked autonomic activation; within about 60 sec the rapid conjugate eye movements in all directions appear. The REM state lasts about 15 min, and at its conclusion the subject returns to N-REM stage 2, and then on to 3 and sometimes 4.

Following the initial REM period of the night, REM and N-REM episodes then alternate throughout the remainder of the night, with the REMs recurring approximately every 90 min. The first REM period tends to be the shortest and has fewest eye movements; both REM duration and number of eye movements increase as the night progresses. Conversely, most of the SWS occurs in the initial periods and decreases toward morning; stage 2 increases proportionately as SWS declines. About one fourth of total sleep time per night is spent in REM; stage 2 comprises about 50%, with stages 3 and 4 accounting for 10% each, and stage 1, 5%. With aging, overall sleep time declines, stage 4 decreases markedly, and REM decreases somewhat. Correspondingly, there are more periods of wakefulness and more lighter stages 1 and 2. At all ages, females sleep more than do males.

REM sleep has often been called paradoxical sleep; there are two reasons for this. The sleeper is profoundly unconscious and may be more difficult to awaken than in the deep sleep of stages 3 and 4, yet the brain shows electrical activity of an awake alert individual. And the skeletal musculature is profoundly relaxed, yet there is fluctuating and increased activation of the autonomic nervous system; in the awake subject, autonomic activation usually is accomplished by high levels of skeletal muscle tension.

Mental Activity During Sleep

Knowledge about the types of mental activity characteristic of the two sleep states, REM and N-REM, and the stages of N-REM sleep, is obtained by an investigator in a sleep laboratory observing the sleep state and stage being recorded on the polygraph and then awakening subjects from the specific condition being studied and asking them what was going through their mind just before the awakening. If the subject is awakened from N-REM stages 2, 3, and 4 the reports usually describe specific verbal thoughtlike, usually nonemotional, mental activity largely devoid of visual images or storylike content. Awakenings from stage 2 sleep yield more reports of mental activity than from stage 3, and stage 3 in turn yields more than from stage 4. Awakenings from REM episodes elicit the vivid visual-pictorial active "playlets", often bizarre and emotionally tinged, with which we are all familiar as dreams. Mental activity from the stage 1 of sleep onset is reported to resemble one or the other type. When it is of the pictorial experience variety it is called hypnogogic imagery. During REM periods intensity of the eye movements is correlated positively with the amount of behavioral activity of the dream content and the vividness of the visual imagery.

It has been speculated that the mental activity characteristic of N-REM represents processes primarily occuring in the left hemisphere, since that, in most persons, is the so-called dominant hemisphere primarily concerned with verbal ideational activity; while the sleep mentation (dreams) characteristic of the REM state may be primarily the product of the nondominant right (in most persons) hemisphere, which is concerned mainly with visual-spatial imagery, and which apparently has closer ties to the limbic system of the brain—the structures concerned with emotional and instinctual phenomena (Chapter 14).

Sleep Deprivation, Total or Selective

The subjective responses to relatively minor sleep loss are the feelings of irritability, fatigue, inability to concentrate, thought disturbance, and poor performance, with which all are familiar. More prolonged total sleep deprivation (60 hr or more) is reported to lead to increased oral behavior including smoking, drinking, and eating; motor incoordination; dysarthria; hand tremor; short attention span; nystagmus, ptosis, and weakened neck flexion. Some subjects also report visual illusions or hallucinations, paranoid ideation, and increased feelings of hostility and aggression. In patients who are seizure prone, EEGs following protracted wakefulness may show increased spike discharges. During total sleep deprivation the quiescent EEG shows a decline in the amount of alpha, and closing the eyes is reported to bring about less alpha than in the nonsleep-deprived subject. Laboratory studies show increased plasma cortisol and blood glucose levels. In recovery from sleep deprivation there is increased total sleep time, increased percentage of time spent in stages 3 and 4 on the first recovery night, and increased REM percentage following the first night. This indicates that making up lost SWS is the first, and repairing REM deficit is the second, priority. Overall increased sleep times does not ever equal the total amount lost.

Selective sleep state or sleep stage deprivation is accomplished by monitoring the subject's polygraph parameters and arousing him at the onset of the state or stage under investigation. Deprivation of either SWS or REM over several successive nights results in an increased frequency of onset of that stage, so that the sleeper must be roused more and more often. During subsequent recovery nights the percentage of the deprived state is greatly increased. Selective SWS deprivation may cause a state of hyporesponsiveness and apathy during wakefulness.

Early reports indicated that selective REM deprivation resulted in severe psychoemotional abnormalities, but later reports showed that there were few consistent changes which could be uncovered by standard cognitive-type psychologic tests. However, some studies suggest that projective tests better measure the effects and that there may be increased introversion and withdrawal, impaired reality testing, altered levels of aggression, increased hypochondriasis, and, in males, increased homosexual fantasies and drive. REM-deprived subjects also have been reported to show hyperactivity. Probably the nature of the subjects' predeprivation personality is an important determinant of the alterations, or lack thereof, produced by selective REM deprivation. Some more recent work indicates that REM suppression may be of value in the treatment of depressed patients.

Brainstem Regulation of Sleep States

The probable neural processes involved in maintaining consciousness and in generating the electrical activity recorded from the scalp in the EEG, together with their correlation with levels of consciousness, were discussed in the preceding chapter. Because of the close involvement of these processes with wakefulness, sleep states, and sleep stages, it is appropriate to consider them again here in somewhat greater detail, together with a mention of some relevant neurotransmitter pathways. The relationships are extremely complicated and as yet incompletely known. Most of the information presently available is the result of studies with experimental animals and the degree of applicability to the human is still conjectural.

There are two general categories of waveforms generated by the brain and recorded in the EEG: (1) desynchronized activity, which is called beta, is a low amplitude and high frequency or low voltage fast (LVF) rhythm and is usually characterized by alert wakefulness accompanied by mental activity, but is also seen in REM sleep and N-REM stage 1 sleep; and (2) synchronized activity seen in a spectrum of three waveforms of increasing amplitude and decreasing frequency: alpha, theta, and delta, the latter of which is called high voltage slow (HVS), and is correlated with decreasing mental activity and levels of consciousness.

The alpha, theta, and delta forms of synchronized electrical activity result from the simultaneous rhythmic electrical changes occurring synchronously in increasingly larger populations of neural elements in the cerebral cortex. The beta or desynchronized type of rhythm indicates a breakup of simultaneity with different neural populations engaged in disparate electrical changes.

One important process responsible for the synchronized type of higher amplitude lower frequency waveforms is the slow rhythmic discharge of neural impulses projecting upward to the cerebral cortex from the thalamus. The thalamus can therefore be considered as a kind of neural pacemaker for the synchronous cortical electrical activity characteristic of relaxed, quiet, eyes-closed wakefulness; drowsiness; and N-REM sleep. Studies indicate that a unilateral lesion in a certain area of the thalamus results in desynchronization of the cortical EEG on the same side.

However, this slow rhythmic pacemaker function of the thalamus in generating electrical synchrony in neural elements of the cerebral cortex is importantly influenced, in turn, by neural impulses ascending to the thalamus from lower areas of the brainstem in the pons and medulla. Low-frequency electrical stimulation of core structures in this portion of the brainstem produces both a markedly synchronous HVS EEG and N-REM sleep. If the synchronizing influences of these lower brainstem areas on the thalamus are blocked by transection of the brainstem at mid-pons level, the result is constant electrical desynchronization of the cortical EEG. Lesions in this area of the mid-pons cause cessation of all sleep; and disruption of the ascending serotoninergic pathways from the mid-pons leads to insomnia (see following).

Neural Regulation of Conscious Wakefulness

The state of awakeness, in contrast with the sleep states of REM and N-REM, appears to depend on at least three different neural systems in the brainstem and cerebrum which have as their neurotransmitters acetylcholine, norepinephrine, and dopamine, respectively.

Electrical stimulation of the brainstem reticular formation activating system (RAS) produces desynchronization (LVF, activation) in the EEG, behavioral arousal, and the release of increased amounts of acetylcholine (ACh) in the cerebral cortex of experimental animals. Injection of ACh (but not saline) into sleeping animals leads to EEG desynchronization and behavioral wakefulness; and chemicals which cause increased levels of ACh in the cerebral cortex, by blocking the enzyme (cholinesterase) that degrades it, decrease sleeping time in animals. These pathways having ACh as the neurotransmitter are called cholinergic tracts; there are reported to be two major ones: one centered in the dorsal midbrain and pons which projects to the thalamus, and the other centered in the ventral midbrain with radiations to the hypothalamus and portions of the limbic system. Both cholinergic tracts have projections to higher areas in the cerebral hemispheres.

Another neural pathway subserving cortical electrical activation and therefore EEG desynchronization and arousal has as its neurotransmitter norepinephrine, and is referred to as a noradrenergic tract. This pathway is a portion of the reticular formation in the central core of the midbrain and pons.

The possible third neuron system is suggested to be one subserving behavioral wakefulness and conscious mental arousal; it appears to be centered in the ventral layers of the midbrain, has as its neurotransmitter dopamine, and is therefore a dopaminergic tract. It is reported that lesions in this fiber system lead to an activated or desynchronized EEG, but a lack of behavioral wakefulness or mental arousal, so that in this situation there would be a discongruity between cortical electrical activity and behavioral alertness.

Neural Regulation of N-REM Sleep: The Serotonin System

The onset of N-REM sleep appears to be partially the result of a decrease in neural desynchronizing influences transmitted upward to the cerebral hemispheres along the activating system. This decrease in desynchronization stimuli is at least in part the consequence of active inhibition of the RAS by another neural system, which has serotonin (5-hydroxytryptamine, 5-HT) as its neurotransmitter, and is therefore a serotoninergic system.

Neurons which contain, and secrete at their terminals, serotonin are reported to be localized in the inner (medial) portion of an area in the lower midbrain and upper pons called the raphe nuclei. Fibers from the nerve cell bodies of this system travel anteriorly to the hypothalamus and thalamus (which together make up the diencephalon, the uppermost portion of the brainstem), to portions of the frontal cortex and to the limbic system. Electrical stimulation of this serotonin tract in experimental animals produces markedly increased sleep of both the N-REM and REM states. It also inhibits the electrical activity in the activating system which, as described above, mediate mental alertness, behavioral arousal, and EEG desynchronization. Conversely, destruction of this area by a large lesion results in a total lack of sleep. If the lesion is smaller, so that a portion of the raphe nuclei remains, then there will be some N-REM and occasional REM. These destructive lesions cause decreased content of serotonin in the cerebral hemispheres. Similarly, suppression of neurosecretion by these nerve cells by serotonin antagonists, or administration of pharmacologic agents which deplete brain serotonin, produces insomnia with a decline in both N-REM and REM states. Giving chemicals which causes serotonin content to return to normal permits the return of sleep.

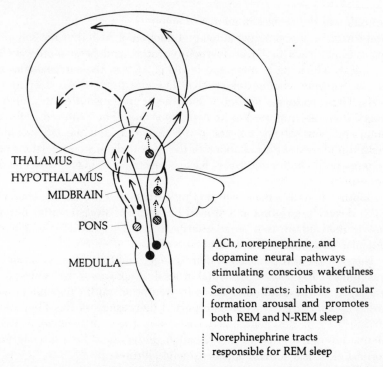

THALAMUS
HYPOTHALAMUS
MIDBRAIN

PONS

MEDULLA

ACh, norepinephrine, and
dopamine neural pathways
stimulating conscious wakefulness

Serotonin tracts; inhibits reticular
formation arousal and promotes
both REM and N-REM sleep

Norephinephrine tracts
responsible for REM sleep

Figure 15-2. Proposed neural pathways underlying the sleep-wakefulness and N-REM-REM cycles. 1) Mediates conscious wakefulness; neurotransmitters are acetylcholine, norepinephrine and dopamine; 2) inhibits the reticular activating-wakefulness systems and promotes both REM and N-REM sleep, the neurotransmitter is serotonin; and 3) responsible for periodically generating REM sleep, the neurotransmitter is norepinephrine.

Some workers believe there is a localization of function concerning sleep control in the raphe nuclei. The anterior portions of this structure may be more concerned with the regulation of both the EEG and other physiologic characteristics of N-REM sleep described earlier. The posterior portion of the raphe nuclei may be more involved in influencing the area in the dorsal pons which appears to be the center of control for the REM state: the locus ceruleus. Neurons from the posterior portion of the raphe nuclei pass to the locus ceruleus and these fibers therefore form a connection between the N-REM sleep system of the posterior raphe nuclei and the REM sleep system of the locus ceruleus; they may in some way prepare for the onset of initiation of the REM periods which follow a phase of N-REM. In this way, in the normal subject, REM sleep is always preceded by a period of N-REM sleep.

It must be emphasized that the neural structures and processes proposed as the substrates of the sleep states and stages are as yet not well worked out. Therefore this discussion is is but a portion of several theories accounting for sleep mechanisms, and the diagram at Figure 15-2 is very hypothetical.

Whatever physiologic processes underlying the two sleep states may be, they seem to interact closely under normal circumstances. But as stated, the neural processes responsible for the origin of, and orderly interaction between, N-REM and REM sleep are not known. In the disorder of sleep called narcolepsy (see following) the normal relation between N-REM and REM is disrupted so that not only do frequent REM periods develop spontaneously during times of usual wakefulness without the normal prior N-REM phase, but various of the components of REM sleep: profound muscle relaxation, rapid eye movements, vivid visual imagery, loss of consciousness, and EEG desynchronization; may become dissociated from each other and occur separately.

The proposed serotoninergic neural system that controls the several aspects of N-REM sleep, that prepares for and initiates REM sleep, and that inhibits the RAS (thus suppressing cortical arousal, EEG desynchronization and behavioral wakefulness) is postulated by some investigators to, in turn, be activated by the presence of some compound—a neurohumor—which acts as a sleep-promoting substance. This factor may be some product of fatigue which is formed during a long period of wakefulness. Conversely the serotoninergic N-REM system may be activated by the depletion of some factor which is used up during wakefulness and replenished during sleep and which once it attains a certain concentration, leads to feelings of fatigue and the initiation of sleep. There are reports that some substances extracted from the blood and cerebrospinal fluid of sleep-deprived or somnolent animals will, when injected into awake animals, induce N-REM sleep.

The pacemaker function of the thalamus in generating the spectrum of synchronized EEG rhythms of increasing amplitude and decreasing frequency in the order: alpha, theta, delta, has been described above. In the genesis of N-REM sleep the pacemaker role of the thalamus appears to come under the influence of ascending neural impulses coming to it from this serotoninergic N-REM system centered in the raphe nuclei of the central region of the pons.

Neural Regulation of REM Sleep: The Noradrenergic System

The various physiologic, behavioral, and EEG components of REM sleep may be regulated by systems of brainstem neurons having norepinephrine, and others possibly dopamine, as their neurotransmitters; therefore these would be noradrenergic and dopaminergic tracts. Such systems of neurons are widely distributed through the reticular formation of the brainstem (BSRF) but have major concentrations in the locus ceruleus, an area in the dorsolateral aspect of the pons near the 4th ventricle; in the substantia nigra of the dorsolateral areas of the midbrain; and in the hypothalamus. Some evidence indicates that this noradrenergic, and possibly also a dopaminergic, system is necessary for the REM state. Onset of a REM period is preceded by a marked electrical activation in the nuclei of the pons which are the centers for this noradrenergic system. Electrical stimulation of these areas increases REM sleep; lesions in these structures, or pharmacologic inhibition by norepinephrine antagonists, decreases or eliminates REM. The REM suppression is correlated with a decline in norepinephrine content in regions of the brain anterior to the lesion or pharmacologic blockade. (An apparent paradox is the fact that, in the intact human or other animal, monoamine oxidase inhibitors such as phenelzine, which increase brain norepinephrine content by interfering with its enzymic degradation by monoamine oxidase, decrease REM or eliminate it altogether, depending on the dosage.)

Some authors suggest that the various components of REM sleep may be controlled by different areas of the locus ceruleus. Medial portions of the noradrenergic REM system may regulate the rapid eye movements and the desynchronized (LVF) EEG, while more posterior sites may control the marked decrease in skeletal muscle tone characteristic of the REM state. This structural localization of control of the different aspects of REM may explain how it can be that in narcolepsy there occurs a dissociation or fragmentation of the physiologic components of REM: loss of consciousness, eye movements, activated EEG, vivid dream imagery (hypnogogic hallucinations), and absence of muscle tone (cataplexy and sleep paralysis).

Pharmacologic Agents and Sleep

Alcohol

Alcohol is the most widely used of all psychoactive agents, and probably more persons are dependent on or addicted to it than to all other sedatives, hypnotics, tranquilizers, and mood modifiers combined. The effects of short-term alcohol intake upon sleep in normal subjects are to decrease the latency to sleep onset, to slightly increase or produce no change in the overall sleep time, and to cause a marked and consistent suppression of the REM state. The decreased percentage of REM sleep following alcohol intake seems to result from a decrease in the duration of each individual REM episode, rather than to a depression in the number of such episodes, although some studies where alcohol was administered for a longer study period also indicate fewer as well as shorter REM periods.

When alcohol is taken for a longer period by normal subjects, the percentage of REM gradually returns to the normal baseline prealcohol level. Then when alcohol is acutely withdrawn there is a marked REM rebound characterized by increased number, duration, and vividness of imagery of REM periods. This REM rebound effect is found with many other drugs (see following), but it is greater in the case of alcohol than with any other. After alcohol withdrawal in these normal subjects who have taken it regularly for several days, there is also a strong suppression of SWS stage 4.

Chronic long-term use of alcohol leads to chronic suppression of REM and stage 4 SWS. The decreases in REM and stage 4 are made up by an increase in stages 1 and 2 (that is, there is "lighter" sleep); and in chronic alcoholics there appears to develop a sustained abnormal pattern of sleep control, called fractured sleep, with suppressed SWS, suppressed REM, increased stages 1 and 2, and increased shifting among stages. Acute withdrawal following long-term chronic excess in alcoholics results in a further fragmentation of the sleep pattern with large REM rebound, vivid imagery, further decreases in SWS, and more frequent shifting between states and stages. In alcoholics who develop delirium tremens and other psychotic manifestations during withdrawal, REM frequency and length increase greatly, and it has been suggested that there is a correlation between degree of REM rebound in acute withdrawal and the hallucinations and delirium that develop in some alcoholic patients.

Chronic alcoholics who have been "dry" for at least three weeks have been reported to show more REM and stages 1 and 2 and less SWS than nonalcoholic control subjects; the increased REM percentage resulted from more, rather than increased length of, REM periods. There are also multiple awakenings. Alcoholics who have been abstinent for as long as one or two years continue to show decreased stages 3 and 4, increased REM and the lighter stages 1 and 2, and an increased number of stage changes and many awakenings, indicating markedly abnormal sleep patterns. There are reports that as long as four years of abstinence may be required to restore SWS to the normal about 20% in such subjects.

Barbiturates

Commonly used and abused, barbiturates are among the most frequently prescribed drugs, and are the most common pharmacologic agents used for suicide. The effects of barbiturates on normal subjects have been studied extensively in many sleep laboratories and all have been found to have the same characteristic effects on sleep patterns. In the first few to about 14 days of nightly barbiturate administration, they decrease sleep latency (the time to sleep onset after retiring), decrease the number of awakenings and body movements during the night, increase the amount of N-REM sleep (distributing it among the 4 N-REM stages), and markedly and consistently decrease the amount of time spent in REM sleep. With continued nightly use at the same dosage (for beyond about 2 weeks), the percentage of REM time returns to close to the normal baseline levels (as is the case with continued alcohol administration in normal nonalcoholic subjects); and the drug's effect of decreasing sleep latency, body movements and number of awakenings, is reported to return to predrug baseline levels. Then if the dosage is increased, once again REM suppression occurs and once again, if the drug is continued, REM and other parameters tend to return to baseline level. When the barbiturate is ultimately withdrawn, marked REM overshoot or rebound to greatly increased levels occurs and is maintained for extended periods. The incidence of nightmares seems to be high in REM overshoot. After slightly over two weeks of nightly barbiturate intake in moderate doses, followed by abrupt withdrawal, REM percentage remains markedly increased for over five weeks.

Patients who have been using barbiturates and other sleep medications such as glutethimide, methaqualone, chloral hydrate, and others, have been studied in sleep laboratories while they continue their drugs and it has been found that they have difficulty falling asleep, have many awakenings, and little SWS. Chronic use of multiple doses of these medications over long periods results in ultimately greatly reduced percentage of both REM and N-REM stages 3 and 4; in some cases there is no SWS at all. When the drugs are gradually withdrawn there is a large increase in frequency, vividness, and frightening content of dreaming sleep. Stages 3 and 4 return gradually to normal baseline levels without overshoot. Once patients are weaned from the drug the quality of their sleep is not poorer than, and is often improved over, that of their drug-taking periods.

In spite of this demonstrated lack of prolonged effectiveness in promoting sleep (ineffective after about 14 days) their adverse effects upon the normal sleep cycle, and their known dangers, studies report that 27 million prescriptions per year are written for hypnotics, many of these for barbiturates, and many for large numbers (between 30 and 60).

Morphine, Heroin, and Other Opiate Alkaloids

Opiate alkaloids are reported to produce effects on sleep similar to those of alcohol and barbiturates, prompting the speculation that all drugs which produce physiologic tolerance and addiction have similar effects upon the brain processes which regulate sleep states and stages.

Benzodiazepine Tranquilizers

Nitrazepam, flunitrazepam, and triazolam, short-acting benzodiazepine tranquilizers, have been shown to result in markedly worsened sleep (rebound insomnia), on withdrawal following nightly administration of a single dose for 14 nights. Increased anxiety may also accompany the insomnia.

Amphetamines

Amphetamines decrease total sleep time as well as decreasing REM percentage; withdrawal then results in marked REM rebound.

Phenelzine

Phenelzine is a monoamine oxidase inhibitor and so-called antidepressant; it has the unique effect of completely abolishing the REM state during the whole time it is administered. No tolerance develops, that is, with continued administration its complete REM suppressing effects continue; however, strong REM rebound does occur upon withdrawal.

Lysergic Acid Diethylamide (LSD).

Unlike the above agents, LSD is reported to facilitate the REM state by shortening the time to the first REM period, lengthening the first few REM periods, and overall increasing REM percentage.

Diazepam, Thorazine, Diphenylhydantoin, and Phenobarbital

Diazepam (tranquilizer), thorazine (antipsychotic), diphenylhydantoin (phenytoin—anticonvulsant) and phenobarbital have in common the effect of consistently decreasing the amount of Stage 4 delta sleep.

Flurazepam

Flurazepam is a hypnotic agent that shortens the latency to sleep onset, decreases the number of awakenings during the night, and increases total sleep duration. However, it is reported to decrease the percentage of SWS stages 3 and 4 and correspondingly increase stage 2. The decrease in stage 4 SWS is profound and is accompanied by a decline in number and amplitude of delta waves. At dosages of 15 or 30 mg, studies indicate that it does not cause suppression of REM percentage, or REM rebound when it is withdrawn, but it does decrease the number of rapid eye movements during REM periods. A dose of 60 mg does appear to result in REM suppression. Unlike the barbiturates and other hypnotics discussed above, flurazepam appears to maintain its sleep-facilitating effects when continued for periods beyond two weeks; the upper limits of the duration of effectiveness for this drug are apparently not yet known. A recent report indicates that a remarkably large percentage of all prescriptions written are for flurazepam, and that as its use increases the prescribing of barbiturates is declining. A serious side effect of flurazepam is the accumulation of long–acting metabolites in the blood.

SLEEP AND DISEASE STATES

Cardiovascular Disease

As mentioned earlier, REM state sleep is associated with a high level of autonomic activation. Rapid fluctuations in such autonomically influenced parameters as heart rate, blood pressure, respiratory rate and depth, and an elevation of adrenocorticosteroid hormones in the blood and urine, are characteristic of REM sleep. Myocardial infarctions more commonly occur during sleep at night, than during daytime active wakefulness. Some all-night sleep laboratory monitoring studies have shown that nocturnal angina and significant S-T segment depression often occur during a REM period. In addition, other research indicates that cardiac arrhythmias may develop more frequently during REM than N-REM sleep. So in some studies acute cardiac events appear to correlate with the marked autonomic activation of the REM state. In these abnormalities REM onset begins before the various changes.

Patients with ischemic heart disease have markedly increased latency to sleep onset and diminished amounts of stages 3 and 4 SWS—less than half of normal— as compared with that of age-matched controls. Also their sleep tends to be fragmented, in the sense that they have frequent nocturnal awakenings and then tend to take longer to return to sleep than comparable subjects without coronary artery atherosclerosis. Whether these sleep abnormalities revealed by some (but not all) research studies in patients with ischemic heart disease are a portion of the physiologic conditions that predispose to heart disease, or are a consequence of the abnormalities resulting from it, is not known.

Some studies show that in patients with essential hypertension the total peripheral resistance increases during REM periods.

Seizure Disorders

Sleep-laboratory studies of patients with epilepsy reveal that most of these patients have reduced percentage of stage 4 sleep. It is well-known that seizure discharges (grand mal, focal epilepsy and temporal lobe seizures) are markedly increased during N-REM sleep, especially the lighter stages 1 and 2, during morning drowsiness and dozing prior to sleep onset at night or in an afternoon nap. Such epileptic discharges decrease or disappear altogether during REM periods. A period of sleep deprivation increases the frequency and severity of seizures in epileptic patients.

Peptic Ulcer Disease

In control subjects gastric acid secretion does not increase during REM episodes, but in patients with peptic ulcer disease REM episodes are correlated with a large increase (up to 20-fold) in acid production as compared with matched normal controls. The increase is not as great during N-REM sleep. Gastrin secretion is reported to occur in periodic bursts during the night in some patients with PUD.

Hypo- and Hyperthyroidism

Hypothyroidism is a well known cause of hypersomnia; conversely, hyperthyroidism is often associated with insomnia. In addition, hypothyroidism is associated with decreased levels of SWS stages 3 and 4; this situation is reversed following thyroid supplements once the subject becomes euthyroid. On the other hand, patients with thyrotoxicosis have amounts of SWS above that of controls, and following treatment with an antithyroid drug such as propylthiouracil, stage 3 and 4 percentages return to normal gradually over several months.

Adult Asthma

Asthma in adults is largely of the intrinsic type. In one study patients were shown to have reduced stage 4 sleep percentage, increased number of awakenings during the night, but no observable correlation between onset of asthmatic attacks and sleep stage or state. In another study asthmatic attacks appeared to correlate strongly with REM periods; to a lesser extent they occured in N-REM stages 1 and 2, and not at all in N-REM 3 and 4.

Others

Both the cluster and the migraine types of vascular headaches are said to have their onset during REM periods. Atherosclerotic cerebrovascular disease with accompanying dementia is said to be associated with greatly reduced REM, stage 4, and overall sleep time, as compared with normal age-matched controls.

ABNORMALITIES OF SLEEP

Insomnia in Otherwise Normal Subjects ("Idiopathic" insomnia)

Types of insomnia

Some surveys of outpatients of private physicians have indicated that between one third and one half are taking prescribed hypnotic drugs. Insomnia may take one or a combination of three forms: increased latency to sleep onset at night, frequent awakenings or protracted wakeful periods during the night, or early morning awakenings with inability to go back to sleep. It is the most common of all disorders of sleep and a frequent chief complaint in the adult ambulatory clinical setting.

It is important to emphasize that insomnia is a patient complaint of inability to sleep, or an unsatisfying quality or quantity of sleep, and is therefore a subjective experience. It cannot be called an objective disorder until one or more of the various forms of insomnia has been demonstrated objectively with appropriate monitoring in a sleep research laboratory. Some authors differentiate primary from secondary insomnia. The latter is associated with other medical or psychiatric conditions such as the pain of arthritis or peptic ulcer disease; the respiratory distress of COPD or chronic congestive heart failure; or such psychoemotional states as worry, anxiety, or general "nervousness"; and depression resulting from adverse life circumstances. Primary or idiopathic insomnia, on the other hand, is that occurring in otherwise healthy subjects where the disorder has tended to be of long standing and unassociated with other physical or psychoemotional abnormalities.

In the United States various surveys of the general population report complaints of chronic sleep difficulty in from 15 to 20% of persons responding; more females than males report long-standing inability to obtain sleep of satisfying quality or quantity. Several all-night monitoring studies have been done with such subjects and in some of these the results show that, in comparison with age-matched controls who describe themselves as good sleepers, self-described poor sleepers have decreased amounts of REM sleep, more stage 2 and less SWS stages 3 and 4, more awakenings and body movements, more switching between stages, faster heart rate, higher rectal temperature, and more peripheral vasoconstriction, both before and during sleep. Other studies have demonstrated entirely normal sleep in "poor sleepers." Increasing age is correlated with decreased sleep depth and duration in all individuals.

Insomnia and Psychologic Characteristics

Some studies indicate that most patients with insomnia have psychoemotional disturbances as indicated by scores in the pathologic range on MMPI testing. The implication in such conclusions is that the insomnia is secondary to psychopathology; however, it seems equally logical to conjecture that where such a correlation exists, both the insomnia and abnormal test results could occur on the basis of subtle poorly understood abnormalities of brain function involving the upper brainstem, limbic system, and their cortical projections. Most abnormal scores were found on the scales for schizophrenic tendencies, sociopathic features, obsessive-compulsive qualities, and depression. Interviews with patients revealed that, while younger subjects readily admit that subjective psychoemotional problems seem to be related to their insomnia, older ones appear to be unwilling or unable to make such a connection (if, indeed, it exists at all).

Some investigators prominent in sleep research contend that by far the most frequent cause of insomnia in otherwise healthy subjects is psychoemotional disorders—that is, insomnia is considered to be secondary to psychiatric disturbances of various types. Other researchers, equally prominent in the field of sleep studies, are convinced that most instances of persistent insomnia result from abnormalities of the physiologic processes underlying the two sleep states—such disorders as sleep apnea, nocturnal myoclonus and many still-unknown dysfunctions (see following). This group of workers state that their investigations have failed to reveal a significant correlation between insomnia and psychopathology. A review of the literature relating a number of personality variables to quality of sleep (subjective and objective) suggests that psychologic characteristics do not appear to bear any clear cut relationship to subjective complaints of poor sleep, or to objective sleep characteristics as measured in the laboratory.

Insomnia and Hypnotic Agents

All sleep researchers seem to be in agreement that hypnotics are greatly over-prescribed and probably do more harm than good. The frequently prescribed sedatives and hypnotics: barbiturates, meprobamate, glutethimide, methaqualone, and others (with the exception of flurazepam in small doses), produce REM suppression and tolerance (more has to be taken to achieve the same soporific effect), the sleep-promoting effects wear off within 10 to 14 days, and quality and quantity of sleep often becomes poorer than it was prior to starting the drugs, with marked decrease in both REM and deep sleep stages 3 and 4. Then withdrawal of the drug leads to longer latency to sleep onset, marked REM rebound (with the content being increasingly vivid and nightmarish) and increased awakenings. The patient experiences worse insomnia and obtains a prescription refill. One might conclude that hypnotic drugs are a major *cause* of sleep disturbances, their use constitutes iatrogenic addiction, and the resulting worsening of sleep is iatrogenic insomnia. The suggestion has been made that barbiturates should be banned altogether. In response to controversy arising from this proposal, the National Institute of Drug Abuse contracted with the Institute of Medicine for a study of the medical use of barbiturates and other hypnotics. Recommendations from the committee conducting this study include the following points: (1) that increased recognition be given to the adverse effects of accumulation of long-acting metabolites of the benzodiazepines, especially flurazepam and nitrazepam; (2) that there be improved education of health practitioners concerning sleep disorders and the adverse effects of medications for their management; and (3) that there be increased research on sleep complaints and alternatives to pharmacologic treatment of them including life style changes.

Insomnia and Life Style

It is remarkable that there are few (if any) studies exploring the relationship of elements of the patient's life style to complaints of insomnia, and to the objective quality of sleep as evaluated by sleep laboratory monitoring. A single study has reported increase of deep SWS stage 4 sleep to result from a regimen of regular exercise in conditioned subjects. It would seem that in a complaint of insomnia it is logical first to inquire what if anything the patients does during the day to become physically tired. For most patients it is almost certainly more appropriate first to investigate the events of the day before complicating the difficulties of the night with hypnotic medication. The management of insomnia in reasonably healthy subjects should be directed at changes in the life style based on discussions with patients of their dissatisfactions; development of new interests and hobbies to make the day more satisfying; guiding the development of a daily program of exercise training, and noting its consequences for the sleep pattern once the program is well established; and providing training in progressive relaxation by the Jacobson or similar method.

Of course it is easier and less time consuming to write a prescription than it is to deliver effective patient education, and unfortunately it is the prescription which many patients seem to want, in spite of the fact that in so doing they are turning over the control of a significant aspect of their lives to an agency outside themselves.

Insomnia and Biofeedback Training

For patients with chronic "idiopathic" insomnia for whom these alterations of life style appear to be of insufficient benefit, or are rejected, more formal programs of training with biofeedback techniques may be considered. Such training may be effective in decreasing the chronic levels of hyperarousal and increased muscle tension which have been reported for many subjects with chronic insomnia. Three types of biofeedback relaxation training have been studied in some detail in patients with insomnia but without physical or psychiatric disorders. The first method attempts to help the subject reduce his generalized muscle tension by teaching relaxation of the frontalis muscle (forehead) electromyogram (EMG). This approach resulted in subjective reports from patients, who kept daily sleep logs, of improved sleep at home; however, objective sleep-testing did not show marked change in monitored sleep characteristics in the laboratory setting.

The second category of biofeedback training was that directed at teaching patients to reduce the frontalis EMG and simultaneously to increase the amount of theta waves (3–7 cps—the "drowsiness" rhythm) in the EEG. Learning to increase theta is apparently quite difficult. Results of this combined frontalis EMG and EEG theta training yielded no changes in subjective or objective sleep quality aside from an increase in REM.

The third type of biofeedback training tested for effectiveness in this study concerns training patients to augment the EEG sensorimotor rhythm (SMR). This is a 12–14 cps sleep spindle rhythm from the sensory and motor areas of the cortex which is of low amplitude during waking. Training of this rhythm appears to reduce seizure frequency in some epileptics; therefore it is suggested to be related to some process in the brain which inhibits phasic motor activity. The training improved various measures of sleep quality in the laboratory, and the degree to which patients were able to increase their SMR correlated positively with this improvement. (Training this rhythm is also said to be quite difficult.)

On the basis of their sleep-laboratory evaluations of the well patients with complaints of insomnia, these investigatory distinguished three major classes of insomniacs: (1) patients with excessive psychologic and/or neuromuscular tension and long latencies to sleep onset; (2) those judged to have a "poor sleep system" on the basis of low degree of arousal, excessive nocturnal awakenings, and poor sleep spindling during stage 2; and (3) those subjects who do not clearly belong in either category. It is suggested that a different type of biofeedback training may be appropriate for each group.

Insomnia and Aging

Research reports from a number of sleep laboratories confirm the impression of elderly subjects and their health care providers that advancing age is correlated with a decrease in amount and soundness of nocturnal sleep. In the EEG characteristic alterations with increasing age are a decline in the alpha rhythm; depressed amplitude, frequency and altered form of the stage 2 sleep spindles; and a decrease in amount and amplitude of the delta waves of stages 3 and 4 (slow wave sleep). The overall amount of nocturnal wakefulness and the lighter stages 1 and 2 increase, and REM and stage 4 undergo marked diminution as senescence progresses. Otherwise healthy elderly subjects subjectively experience these objectively demonstrated changes as poor, unsatisfying sleep as concerns both quality and quantity. It is of interest to note that scores on tests of higher mental function are reported to be correlated with monitored sleep variables in the elderly; REM quantity and intelligence scores vary in parallel.

A physiologic correlate of the above alterations has been shown to be a decrease in cerebral blood flow and brain oxygen consumption. In elderly subjects in whom the alpha rhythm, the REM state, and stage 4 N-REM are well preserved, cerebral blood flow tends to be maintained at levels approaching the normal for younger individuals. Some studies suggest that structural alterations in the brainstem of senescent individuals may be correlated with the subjective and objective changes, specifically, degeneration and loss of neurons in brainstem structives underlying the normal sleep-wakefulness cycle.

Management of the normal decline in quantity and quality of sleep with advancing age in the well elderly ideally includes the modifications of life style suggested above, namely, measures to increase the sources of satisfaction and self-fulfillment during the day such as work they enjoy, pursuit of hobbies, and involvement with social activities such as a retired senior volunteer program; a regular program of age-and-health appropriate physical exercise such as daily long walks, swimming, bowling, and similar sports; the health practitioner's teaching of patients concerning the normal alteration in sleep quality and quantity accompanying aging, and techniques of progressive relaxation such as the Jacobson method; and reassurance that well individuals will naturally get the amount of sleep they require provided they avoid chronic use of hypnotic medication and provided the elements of their life style are suitable (including regular adequate meals, increased daytime activity levels, and control of daytime boredom, sedentariness, and the habit of napping or dozing).

Narcolepsy

Narcolepsy, or Gelineau's syndrome, is a disorder comprised of four components which are called the narcoleptic tetrad: brief irresistible attacks of sleep of about 10–15 minutes' duration at intervals throughout the 24 hours; cataplexy; hypnagogic hallucinations; and sleep paralysis. When the sleep attacks occur alone, as they do in some patients, the sleep is thought by some workers to be N-REM; when the sleep attacks occur in conjunction with one or more of the other manifestations (cataplexy, hypnogogic hallucinations and sleep paralysis) it is thought to be REM sleep. The four manifestations are dissociated components of the REM state. Nocturnal sleep is said to be abnormal in some patients because it begins with a REM period instead of the usual 90 to 120 minutes of N-REM. Nighttime sleep is reported to show increased body movements and decreased stages 3 and 4.

Cataplexy is a sudden muscular weakness—an actual loss of postural tonus in the skeletal muscles throughout the body—which may last for a few seconds to several minutes. The loss of tone may be so complete that the patient falls to the ground paralyzed, or only partial in that his head sags or knees buckle so that he must seek support to keep from falling. These cataplectic episodes are usually induced by an emotional response such as sudden anger, laughter, excitement, or a conflict situation. Cataplexy as the sole manifestation of narcolepsy is exceedingly rare.

Hypnagogic hallucinations are extremely vivid REM imagery at sleep onset, usually only at night, which may have a remarkable air of reality and which may be frightening. Some patients also have these experiences on awakening in the morning, when they are called hypnopompic imagery.

Sleep paralysis is a loss of tonus in the skeletal muscles which may occur either at sleep onset, on awakening from sleep, or both. The patient is mentally alert and often finds the paralysis, which may last only a few seconds or many minutes, anxiety-inducing or actually terrifying. Sleep paralysis and hypnogogic or hypnopompic hallucinations sometimes occur together. Sleep paralysis occurs as the sole manifestation of narcolepsy in the minority of narcoleptic patients—less than 6%.

The sleep attacks sometimes occur without warning while others describe a premonitory overwhelming sleepiness or sense of fatigue. Some patients are able to prevent or delay the sleep by various strategies such as mental concentration or physical activity, while others seem to be simply stopped in their tracks no matter what they are doing. They increase in frequency as the day progresses and tend to occur most often after meals and in boring circumstances. Approximately a quarter of patients with narcolepsy manifest only the sleep attacks without the other three components. In these patients the sleep is said to be N-REM, although this may be controversial.

Most patients with narcolepsy manifest two or more of these four elements of the narcoleptic tetrad. The association of the sleep attacks and cataplexy is the most common form. Sleep paralysis and hypnogogic hallucinations are reported to occur only in approximately one-fourth of narcoleptic patients, and about 10% of patients have all four components.

Narcolepsy is relatively rare—perhaps 100,000 persons in the United States are afflicted, and as stated, not all those have all four components of the tetrad. There appears to be a familial tendency. Age at onset is reported to be usually between 10–20 years and both sexes are affected; the disorder tends to be lifelong. The cause is not known, although it is suspected to involve derangements in the REM-regulating neural structures in the brainstem which results in fragmentation or dissociation of the components of the REM state: visual imagery with rapid eye movement, profound muscle relaxation, and "activated"—that is, low voltage fast—EEG, and unconsciousness, with intrusion of those dissociated components into wakefulness.

Management of narcolepsy should include arrangement of patients' life circumstances so that they are able to take brief naps during the day when they feel the need. Methylphenidate and phenmetrazine are effective in suppressing REM attacks but apparently do not control the other components of the tetrad. Imipramine and amitryptiline are reported to reduce the incidence of these other abnormalities but to have no influence on the sleep attacks. Some workers use both types of drugs in the management of narcolepsy for control of the various components. Phenelzine, a monoamine oxidase inhibitor, is reported to to reduce REM attacks and cataplexy, but the safety of such MAO-suppressing agents is not established and their use is reserved for severely symptomatic patients.

N-REM Hypersomnias

Pickwickian Syndrome

Pickwickian syndrome refers to an associated group of abnormalities: obesity, excessive appetite, daytime somnolence, and alveolar hypoventilation; the latter may lead to erythrocytosis, and the signs and symptoms of cor pulmonale because of the chronic arterial hypoxemia and hypercapnia (Chapter 9). The lungs are normal, but intraabdominal pressure is increased because of the obesity; the increased pressure elevates the diaphragm into the chest and decreases pulmonary excursions during breathing; this is markedly worsened at night when the patient reclines. The work of breathing is additionally increased by the energy required to move the heavy chest wall. These patients have an abnormal tolerance to the deranged blood gases; their hypoxemic and hypercapneic ventilatory drives appear to be greatly reduced. Some of these patients also have sleep apnea (see following). Although some workers have postulated a hypothalamic disorder which would produce all three manifestations: depressed ventilatory drive, hyperphagia, and somnolence, it is reported that weight loss leads to marked improvement in ventilatory status and a decreased somnolence in some patients.

Sleep Apnea Syndromes

Apnea is cessation of respirations. In normal subjects there is marked variability in rate and depth of respirations during REM periods. In REM phases where the eye movements and dreaming are especially intense, breathing amplitude and rate decline to low levels and periods of apnea lasting 15 sec or more may occur. In general, these are not associated with sleep disturbance. However, in adults with daytime somnolence (excessive daytime sleepiness; EDS) and nocturnal sleep apnea, the apneic episodes are more frequent, and longer, and seem to occur in both of the sleep states REM and N-REM and all N-REM sleep stages. They may be associated with nocturnal insomnia in some patients, and with daytime hypersomnia in many. The patients are sluggish and mentally confused on morning awakening. The periods of apnea lead to multiple brief awakenings—as many as 400–500—of which the subject may have no recollection the following day, but which often leave him in a state of chronic sleep deficit. Sleep apnea frequently appears to be present in association with the Pickwickian syndrome, has been reported to occur in a few patients with narcolepsy, and is seen in some patients with chronic insomnia. EDS and sleep apnea affect primarily males. It is a surprisingly common cause of sleep disorders, and may have a genetic basis.

Three categories of sleep apnea have been described: a central, a peripheral, and a mixed type. In the central form, defined as cessation of air flow and respirating movements lasting >10 sec, spontaneous periods of respiratory arrest of variable duration appear to occur as a result of some failure of the ventilatory control processes in the brainstem associated with the sleep state; rhythmic breathing movements of the diaphragm and intercostal muscles cease for perids of up to, or even longer than, one minute. The apnea causes arterial O_2 desaturation and marked elevation of $Paco_2$ which results in powerful stimulation to the respiratory control centers and sudden respiratory effort with arousal from sleep. The patient startles into wakefulness and breathing resumes with a gasp for air. This sequence may be repeated several hundred times each night with the result that nocturnal sleep is markedly deficient in both quantity and quality, producing daytime lethargy and hypersomnia.

The peripheral (obstructive) form of sleep apnea appears to occur in association with, or secondary to, upper airway obstruction in which the muscles of the oropharynx and the tongue become profoundly relaxed during sleep, occluding the airway. During the airway obstruction alveolar ventilation becomes depressed with resulting arterial hypoxemia and hypercapnia. Sinus bradycardia and systemic arterial and pulmonary artery hypertension often develop during the apneic episodes. The blood gas alterations stimulate vigorous rhythmic movements of the muscles of breathing, but air exchange does not occur until the patient suddenly startles briefly into wakefulness, oropharyngeal muscle tonus increases relieving the airway obstruction, normal breathing resumes and the patient goes back to sleep, only to have the whole sequence repeated again in a short time. Mixed sleep apnea is described as arrest of airflow and respiratory excursions in the first part of each episode, with breathing movements unaccompanied by airflow occurring toward its conclusion. Often patients manifest the three types during a night's sleep in the laboratory with one form predominating.

Patients usually have no recollection or conscious awareness of these conditions and so regard the daytime somnolence as a mystery, often seeking medical consultation for several years before a proper assessment is made. As stated, central and peripheral types of sleep apnea may occur together, and there is speculation that the underlying etiologies of the two may be related. However, it has been reported that the central form of sleep apnea tends more often to produce insomnia, with fewer complaints of daytime somnolence; while the obstructive upper airway type of sleep apnea is more often associated with lack of awareness of the disturbed nature of nocturnal sleep and greater difficulties with diurnal hypersomnia. Accompanying symptoms may be chronically depressed intellectual function, frequent severe headaches, psychiatric syndromes, loud snoring and bizarre nocturnal motor activity.

Treatments used for sleep apnea included dietary weight loss where indicated, doxapram or medroxyprogesterone (respiratory stimulants), clomipramine, surgical removal of adenoids and partial soft palate resection, and tracheostomy with a permanent tracheal valve placement. The treatments selected depend upon careful assessment in the sleep laboratory of the type of apnea present.

Hypersomnias Secondary to Neurologic and Systemic Disorders

Chronic hypersomnia may be the consequence of a number of neurologic abnormalities. It is said to be one of the forms of migraine; it occurs in brain tumors; after head trauma; in atherosclerotic cerebrovascular disease; and in metabolic encephalopathies associated with uremia, hypoglycemia, hypothyroidism, severe anemia, congestive heart failure, chronic obstructive pulmonary disease, and drug abuse, including alcohol. Hypersomnia is a frequent correlate of psychiatric depression (as is also insomnia).

Other Disorders of N-REM Sleep

Somnambulism (Sleep walking)

Sleepwalking usually begins in childhood, is more common in males than females, and appears to be familial in incidence. The subject or his relatives
awaken in the morning and see evidences of nocturnal activity, such as clothing
strewn about or items in the room rearranged, for which the sleeper has no recollection. On occasion the sleeper is seen sleepwalking by family members. The
episodes are said to go on for several minutes.

Sleepwalking is confined exclusively to the N-REM state, particularly stages 3
and 4. EEG monitoring shows that each episode begins with a sudden onset of
high amplitude and slow frequency (HVS) waves. The actual motor activity may
be accompanied by a higher frequency lower amplitude waveform. During the
actual sleepwalking the subjects are remarkably unaware of stimuli from the environment, such as being spoken to, and are confused and disoriented if aroused.
Some reports have suggested that sleepwalking patients are able to carry out
complex motor skills such as unlocking a door, while others indicate that motor
performance is markedly reduced. There is always complete amnesia for the episode. An interesting reported fact is that sleepwalking can be initiated in a subject known to have the disorder by standing him on his feet during sleep; this is
not the case for a nonsomnambulist. Most sleepwalkers have a decreased incidence of these occurrences as they grow older and it usually disappears eventually. Sleepwalking has been less well characterized in adults than in children;
some studies report that adult somnambulists appear on testing to have associated psychiatric abnormalities, while in children this seems not to be the
case.

Nocturnal Enuresis

Although considerably less common in adults than in children, young adults may
have a prevalence of occasional or even frequent enuresis of 2–3%. As in sleepwalking, there is a familial incidence. Organic disorders such as benign prostatic
hypertrophy, urethral diverticulum, epispadias, urinary tract infections, the polyuria of diabetes mellitus or insipidus, and metabolic or degenerative neurologic
abnormalities, may be the cause and should be sought for in an adult with
frequent or even occasional enuresis. Most enuresis occurs in stage 4 sleep and
more often early in the night than later. The actual micturition follows a burst of
HVS, associated with changes of body position, and is accompanied by an EEG
characteristic of stage 1 or 2 with a good bit of alpha. In children the management should be directed at counseling the parents to patience and forbearance of
overreaction rather than directed at interventions with the child. There is some
indication that psychoemotional abnormalities may be associated with enuresis in
adults, but this is not the case with children.

Night Terrors

Night terrors should be distinguished from nightmares, which are frightening or
unpleasant dream contents associated with a REM period. A night terror occurs

during stage 4 SWS, often during the first stage 4 episode of the night. They are more common in children than adults. Autonomic activation is marked: tachycardia, hyperpnea, and elevation of blood pressure. Emotional accompaniments are often intense, as the name implies: feeling of suffocation, anxiety and apprehension, and profound fright. The subject usually can describe no dream content beyond sometimes a single terrifying image; in one case the subject described a sheet wadded up on the ceiling which was about to fall on her face and suffocate her.

The whole episode is not longer than a couple of minutes and is heralded by a sudden onset of a predominantly waking alpha-type EEG, and accompanied by motor activity, vocalizations—often a scream—and not infrequently, sleepwalking. Psychoemotional disturbances are not characteristic of children with night terrors unless the episodes are frequent and persist; more often they tend to be simply outgrown. In adults, however, daytime anxiety and other manifestations of psychiatric disorders are more frequent. In the adult who describes "bad dreams" the first thought should be of unpleasant REM mentation accompanying the REM rebound of alcohol or other drug withdrawal states, as described in previous sections.

Nocturnal Myoclonus

Nocturnal myoclonus phenomenon appears to be the underlying disorder in some complaints of insomnia. These subjects are reported to have a stereotyped form of abnormal leg movements involving the quadriceps femoris and anterior tibialis muscles which occur during N-REM sleep. These movements occur throughout the night at about half-minute intervals and last up to 4 sec each. Each of the frequent muscular contractions rouses the patient, as shown by the appearance of a more desynchronized EEG waveform during and immediately following them; he is not aware of them but reports nights of poor quality sleep from which he arises still fatigued. This is not the same as the restless legs syndrome, which is a phenomenon associated with delayed sleep onset, and in which the subject feels a vague nagging discomfort in his legs that causes him to shift them about frequently.

REFERENCES

Beeson PB and McDermott W, editors: *Textbook of Medicine*. 14th ed. Philadelphia, Pa.: Saunders, 1975.

Benson H: *The Relaxation Response*. New York: Avon Books, and Morrow, 1975.

Feinberg I, et al: Flurazepam effects on slow-wave sleep: Stage 4 suppressed but number of delta waves constant. *Science* 198:847–848, 1977.

Freemon FR: *Sleep Research. A Critical Review*. Springfield, Ill.: C C Thomas, 1972.

Frohlich ED, editor: *Pathophysiology*. Philadelphia, Pa.: Lippincott, 1976.

Ganong WF: *Review of Medical Physiology*. 8th ed. Los Altos, Calif.: Lange Medical Publications, 1977.

Guilleminault C and Dement WC: *Sleep Apnea Syndromes*. Kroc Foundation Series, v. 11. New York: Alan R. Liss, Inc., 1978.

Guilleminault C, Dement WC, and Passouant P: Narcolepsy. *Advances in Sleep Research*, v. 3. New York: Spectrum, 1976.

Guyton AC: *Textbook of Medical Physiology*. 5th ed. Philadelphia, Pa.: Saunders, 1976.

Hobson JA, et al: Ethology of sleep studied with time-lapse photography: Postural immobility and sleep-cycle phases in humans. *Science* 201:1251–1253, 1978.

Holman RB, Dement WC, and Guilleminault C: Sleep disorders and neurotransmitters. In: Usdin E, et al, editors: *Neuroregulators and Psychiatric Disorders*. New York: Oxford University Press, 1977.

Jacobson E: *Anxiety and Tension Control: A Physiologic Approach*. Philadelphia, Pa.: Lippincott, 1964.

Kales A, editor: Sleep. *Physiology and Pathology*. Philadelphia, Pa.: Lippincott, 1969.

Kales A, et al: Rebound insomnia: a new clinical syndrome. *Science* 201:1039–1041, 1978.

Kales A and Kales JD: Recent findings in the diagnosis and treatment of disturbed sleep. *N. Engl. J. Med.* 290:487–499, 1974.

Mendelson WB, et al: *Human Sleep and Its Disorders*. New York: Plenum, 1977.

Solomon F, et al: Special report. Sleeping pills, insomnia, and medical practice. *N. Engl. J. Med.* 300:803–808, 1979.

Thorn GW, et al, editors: *Harrison's Principles of Internal Medicine*. 8th ed. New York: McGraw-Hill, 1977.

Williams, RL and Karacan, I, editors: *Sleep Disorders, Diagnosis and Treatment*. New York: Wiley, 1978.

CHAPTER SIXTEEN

Vertigo, Dizziness, and Syncope

ASSESSMENT IN COMPLAINTS OF VERTIGO, DIZZINESS, AND SYNCOPE

The Chief Complaint

A common group of patient complaints in the ambulatory setting relates to disturbing experiences which patients describe with such terms as dizzy spells, lightheadedness, blackouts, wooziness, weakness, and the like. Often the terms are used interchangeably, with dizziness being the most frequent. The word, as patients use it, includes the full range of subjective sensations from vertigo, through loss of balance or loss of consciousness, to ill-defined lightheadedness.

The first and perhaps most important aspect of assessment in such complaints is to determine the actual nature of the subjective experience, and whether it is characterized by a sense of spinning or rotation: either the environment (room) spinning around the patient in one direction, or the patient feeling that he is whirling in the opposite direction. This would seem to be a straightforward kind of distinction to make: between rotational sensations and nonrotatory ones such as swaying, faintness, loss of balance, dimming of vision, and so on. But apparently it is not, because patients often have great difficulty in describing the exact quality of the sensation. One of the reasons this is so is the fact that studies have shown that after an attack of true vertigo the patient may have continuing sensations of disturbed spatial relations to the environment, some unsteadiness or wavering of gait on walking, a vague sense of swaying or movement of the surroundings, feelings of precarious balance, and instability of head movement and position, which may last several hours. Therefore all these sensations are closely related to actual vertigo and may constitute minor forms of vertigo attacks in many patients. And all these sensations also may occur to varying degrees in conditions which lead to an impending syncope, a loss of balance, or the disorders associated with lightheadedness.

The History of Present Illness

Of all the aspects of assessment, a careful and inclusive history is the most important. Letting the patient talk freely, and encouraging him fully to describe in detail a recent typical episode, together with premonitory and accompanying sensations such as nausea, loss of balance, palpitations, shortness of breath, impending faint, and dimming of vision, is the second step in assessment. Obtaining an eyewitness account of an episode from a friend or relative, if possible, with statements of accompanying events such as pallor, motor activity, unsteadiness of gait, slurring of speech, possible loss of consciousness and its duration, and circumstances under which the attacks occur, is most helpful.

The descriptions by the patient, supplemented by information from a companion, may help to place the occurrences into one of several categories: (1) true vertigo; (2) impending or actual syncope; (3) loss of balance with impending or actual fall; (4) vague lightheadedness, often resulting from an anxiety attack with hyperventilation; or (5) a seizure. A study of the etiology in a large group of patients presenting with a chief complaint of dizziness at an adult walk-in clinic revealed that vestibular disorders were the cause in 38%; hyperventilation syndrome in 23%; multiple sensory deficits in 13%; brainstem ischemia in 5%; cardiovascular disorders in 4%; psychoemotional disorders in 9%; and assorted neurologic abnormalities such as multiple sclerosis, brain tumor, and autonomic neuropathy, in the remainder, with a few remaining of uncertain etiology.

If the patient's spontaneous account has failed to clarify the nature of the subjective experience, it may be helpful to ask a number of key questions appropriate to such complaints: (1) Do you feel that you or the room are whirling around?; (2) Do you feel as though you might pass out?; (3) Does it seem as if you are about to lose your balance, and do you have to take hold of some object to steady yourself?; (4) Do you feel that you're not getting enough air?; (5) Do things seem to be getting far away, dim, or dark?; (6) Do you feel panicky, nervous, or frightened?; (7) When was your last meal prior to the attack?; What did you eat?; (8) Had you been standing up prior to the attack, or was it brought on by a change of position?

Other descriptors or qualifiers of the experiences which aid in placing the complaint into one of the five categories listed above include: (1) what the patient is doing when the attack begins; (2) what is the first thing he notices as it starts; (3) how often the attacks come and how long they last (if they are discrete episodes) or whether the feelings are more or less continuous but vary in degree; (4) suddenness vs. gradualness of onset; (5) accompanying symptoms and signs (nausea, palpitations, numbness and tingling, tinnitus, visual disturbances, etc.); and (6) relation to physical exertion, change of whole body position or head position, walking, stooping over, long standing, and food intake.

In addition, the patient's age, sex, presence of other health disorders (psychoemotional as well as physiologic), e.g., hypertension, atherosclerosis, diabetes mellitus, organic heart disease, a seizure disorder, or osteoarthritis, or a recent illness causing anorexia, vomiting, diarrhea, or blood loss are of value in helping to place the episode into one of the five etiologic categories. Inquiry as to the use of alcohol and other drugs, and complete information concerning medications, is crucial.

The Physical Examination

A screening physical examination with emphasis on the neurologic, cardiovascular, and respiratory systems is essential, with the addition of active range of motion of the cervical spine for evidence of degenerative joint disease. Blood pressure and pulse should be taken in both arms. In addition, there are a number of special tests that can be rapidly and easily performed which help to assess the probable cause of the attacks. After each of these maneuvers the patient should be questioned closely as to whether the test has produced symptoms resembling the experiences of which he complains. One instance of successfully reproducing the sensations by a controlled test is worth a hundred words.

These tests are presented without reference to whether the chief complaint was resolved into the category of a rotational sensation (true vertigo) or a nonrotational one (pseudovertigo; "dizziness," loss of balance, syncope, seizure, etc.), since it most often occurs that, at the beginning of the physical examination, the examiner is still uncertain in which category the complaint belongs.

Hyperventilation

The patient is asked to breathe deeply and rapidly through the mouth while the examiner times 3 min and to signal the onset of any of the symptoms of which he complains. This test, which induces hypocapnia, respiratory alkalemia, and cerebrovascular constriction, is described more fully in Chapter 2. If the patient is a younger person, especially female, without accompanying or recent systemic illness, and appears nervous or anxious, this is an appropriate first test to try.

Descriptors of the episode which tend to point to hyperventilation as the etiology of the complaint include the feeling that he is unable to get enough air, headache, numbness and tingling about the mouth and in the hands, weakness of the hands and arms, and feeling that things are getting far away.

Postural Blood Pressure Measurements

For a patient of any age who is having or has recently had a systemic illness which caused anorexia, nausea, vomiting, diarrhea, or sweating, or for an older person receiving diuretics, vasodilators, or antihypertensive agents, this is an appropriate first test.

Descriptors pointing to postural hypotension as the cause of the complaint include onset of the symptoms occurring immediately upon rising from a sitting to standing position, palpitations or tachycardia, dimming of vision, or roaring in the ears, feeling that he is about to faint, and associated weakness.

The blood pressure and heart rate are taken reclining, sitting up, immediately after standing up, and after standing 3 min. The postural change on assuming the upright position causes a gravitational shift of blood from the head. In a normal subject the decline in perfusion pressure to the head, neck, and upper thorax is sensed by the baroreceptors of the aortic arch and carotid sinus. Afferent nerve impulses from these pressure sensors to the vasomotor and cardioregulatory centers in the brainstem elicit reflex vasoconstriction and tachycardia, mediated by the sympathetic adrenergic division of the autonomic nervous system, which promptly restores cerebral perfusion pressure to normal. In most subjects with normal ECF volume these compensatory responses are rapid and effective, so that there is little difference between reclining and standing values.

An immediate decline in blood pressure from recumbency to standing of 20/10 mmHg, with an over 15 bpm elevation in heart rate, may indicate hypovolemia, and an inability of the reflex responses rapidly and fully to compensate for gravitational shifts and a reduced blood volume. When the pressure and heart rate are measured again after a minute or two in the standing position (or sitting, if the patient is unable to stand) and are found to have returned to closer to the recumbent values, this indicates that, given a bit of time, the adrenergic reflexes have been able to compensate for the blood shifts induced by the gravitational effects of postural change, and therefore that the hypovolemia is not severe. If the blood pressure remains low and the heart rate rapid after one to two minutes in the upright position, this indicates a more severe degree of hypovolemia for which the reflex adrenergic responses are unable to compensate.

A fall in blood pressure from reclining to sitting or standing which is unaccompanied by an increase in heart rate indicates a failure of the baroreceptor–brainstem–adrenergic reflex compensation for reduced cerebral perfusion. In this case there may or may not also be hypovolemia, but the failure of the heart rate to rise immediately, and the blood pressure to increase within a minute or two, indicates postural hypotension. This may be on the basis of inadequate responsiveness of the baroreceptors, the brainstem nuclei, or the peripheral adrenergic effectors, to a decreased perfusion pressure. Possible causes include vasodilator agents, tranquilizers, adrenergic blocking agents, antihypertensive drugs, or the adrenergic autonomic disorder idiopathic postural hypotension.

Occasionally the immediate compensatory response to standing (elevated heart rate and vasoconstriction) is normal, but if the patient is asked to stand quietly for 3 min, the blood pressure may gradually decline enough to lower cerebral perfusion, and "dizziness" in the sense of faintness or impending loss of consciousness, may occur. In this case a decline in venous return to the right heart because of lack of pumping action from skeletal muscle contraction, combined with the effects of gravity on blood distribution, and an apparent sluggishness or "fatigue" of the compensatory circulatory reflexes, lowers cerebral perfusion pressure to inadequate levels and faintness or syncope may occur.

Other causes of postural hypotension, in addition to hypovolemia, vasodilation from pharmacologic agents, and sympathetic autonomic insufficiency, are alcoholic or diabetic autonomic neuropathy, and physical deconditioning in the elderly, in patients who have been at bed rest, and in flabby sedentary individuals.

Carotid Sinus Stimulation

Gentle unilateral, alternating, and nonocclusive massage of the region of the carotid sinus below the angle of the jaw may reveal a hypersensitivity of the carotid sinus circulatory reflexes referred to above. The test should not be performed on a patient with organic heart disease or one with known atherosclerotic cerebral vascular disease. The danger in such patients is that of inducing a bradycardia or complete heart block; or of displacing or dislodging an atheromatous plaque in the carotid system which could embolize to the cerebrum, or produce occlusion at the level of the internal carotid with a resulting infarction. The test should be performed with EKG monitoring; the patient reclines, alternating unilateral pressure is applied, and the monitor watched for bradycardia or brief sinus arrest.

In patients with hyperresponsiveness of the carotid sinuses, the pressure may induce exaggerated responses of bradycardia, asystole, or marked peripheral vasodilation, all of which may cause hypotension. Some patients with carotid sinus syndrome have the profound bradycardia response, which can be blocked by the anticholinergic, antivagal drug atropine. Other patients manifest the strong vasodepressor–hypotensive response without bradycardia, which can be blocked by vasopressor agents but not atropine. In either case perfusion pressure to the brain declines and faintness or syncope may occur especially when the patient is upright. Tight collars, turning the head, or other events which apply pressure to the carotid sinus area may bring on the syncope.

Valsalva Maneuver

When a subject coughs, strains to lift a heavy object, or attempts to defecate or empty the bladder, he closes the glottis and compresses the abdomen by muscle contraction; this elevates intrathoracic pressure. The result is a marked fall in venous return to the right heart and an abrupt decline in cardiac output. If there is borderline adequacy of cerebral circulation because of atherosclerosis, the further drop in blood flow to the brain may result in a feeling of lightheadedness or actual syncope. The test for this type of "dizziness" is to ask the patient to blow into the tube of a blood pressure manometer and try to elevate the mercury to 30 mm or so for several seconds.

Cardiac Rate and Rhythm

The patient may have periodic cardiac arrhythmias such as sudden bradycardia, a run of supraventricular tachycardia, or brief heart block, yet be completely unaware of any palpitations, sense of heart irregularity, or shortness of breath. However, the marked reduction in cardiac output caused by these arrhythmias may produce what is called cardiac dizziness: faintness or a brief loss of consciousness. The effect of arrhythmias on the brain is made worse by cerebral atherosclerosis, anemia, or organic heart disease. If auscultation or a rhythm strip indicate frequent irregularities, or even if they do not, depending on the patient's age and physical condition, 24-hr Holter monitoring may be appropriate.

Head Turning

The patient is seated in a chair, asked to tilt the head back and turn (rotate) the head first to one side for a few seconds and then to the other. If the patient has degenerative disease of the cervical spine, then osteophytes on the cervical vertebrae or narrowing of the foramina may compress the vertebral artery and produce sensations of dizziness, faintness, or vertigo on the basis of decreased blood flow to the brainstem, especially in the presence of vertebral–basilar atherosclerosis (Chapter 18).

In addition to reduced brain blood flow, cervical spondylosis may lead to vertigo during this maneuver because of abnormal sensory input to the brainstem vestibular system from the diseased joints and the frequently associated muscle spasm. Proprioceptors in the neck provide significant afferent impulses to the brainstem pathways which integrate eye movements (oculocephalic reflexes) and maintain equilibrium, so that abnormalities in the cervical receptors for this system can lead to the condition called cervicogenic dizziness, with vertigo, nausea, vomiting, loss of balance, and unsteadiness of gait.

Postural Test for Benign Positional Vertigo

The patient is asked to lie down on a bed or examining table and then, keeping his eyes open, to turn his body so that he lies first on one side for a few moments, and then on the other. In one or two seconds after lying down, or turning over, as the case may be, he may experience and complain of vertigo, and one should watch carefully for the accompanying nystagmus; vertigo and nystagmus, if induced by this maneuver, last about 30 sec and then fade. When the patient turns over again it may recur for a shorter duration but then ceases; in other words, the reaction fatigues after several trials. After a period of rest it may be inducible again. The condition is postural vertigo.

Walk and Turn Quickly

The patient is requested to walk away a few paces, stop abruptly, turn rapidly 180° and face the examiner. Unsteadiness or loss of balance and complaint of dizziness may be elicited in this way in patients with multisensory deficits from degenerative or atherosclerotic brain disease; diabetic or alcoholic neuropathy;

cataract removal, who are having difficulty adjusting to their corrective lenses; cervical spine degenerative joint disease; and impaired proprioceptive, vestibular, or cerebellar function.

TRUE VERTIGO

Accurate awareness of the orientation of the head and body in space, and the rate and direction of head and body movements, including rotation, depends on three closely integrated systems of position and motion receptors, their afferent neural pathways to the brainstem, and their nuclei and interconnecting tracts within the brain. These are (1) the vestibular organs of the inner ear; (2) the visual system from the retina of the eye; and (3) the system of proprioceptors in the joints, muscles, tendons, and skin. Of the musculoskeletal proprioceptor system, the most important for spatial orientation are afferent impulses from the extraocular muscles of the eye, the muscles and joints of the neck, and kinesthetic sensors of the upper torso and legs.

The maintenance of equilibrium results from the integration within the brain of sensory input from these sources. From the brainstem nuclei receiving sensory information from the vestibular organs, secondary tracts are given off to the brainstem nuclei which control eye movements; to the thalamus, the cerebellum, and the cerebral cortex; and to the spinal cord. The labyrinths supply the most significant afferent input concerned with equilibrium of the three sensory systems, and disturbances in the vestibular system are the cause of the most severe and most definitive vertigo.

The Vestibular Apparatus

The Semicircular Canals and the Vestibule

There are three semicircular canals in each inner ear, oriented in the three mutually perpendicular planes of space. They are comprised of membranes filled with endolymph; the membranous canals lie in similarly shaped canals within the petrous portions of the temporal bones. A fluid layer of perilymph, which is continuous with the subarachnoid space, and therefore with the cerebrospinal fluid, lies between the bony chambers and the membranous canals. The perilymph and endolymph do not communicate, since there is no opening between the semicircular canals and the bony labyrinths in which they are contained. Each semicircular canal has an enlargement at one end called the ampulla, within each of which is a mechanoreceptor organ which senses motion of the endolymph. Each of these three mechanoreceptors is made up of two parts, a basal crista made up of hair cells and an apical cupula. When the head rotates in the plane of one of the semicircular canals, the endolymph of the canal moves in the opposite direction, bulging the cupula in that direction, which stimulates the hair cells of the crista and, thereby, some of the afferent nerve fibers of the vestibular division of CN VIII (acoustic). When rotation stops, the endolymph decelerates and the cupula bulges in the other direction.

The vestibule is located near, and is indirectly continuous with the ampullas of, the semicircular canals. The vestibule is comprised of two parts, the saccule

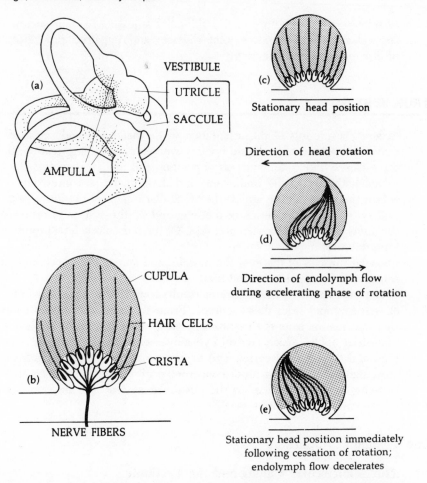

Figure 16-1. Diagram of the (a) semicircular canals, ampullae, saccule and utricle; (b) enlarged diagram of the crista and cupula of the ampulla of one semicircular canal; (c) position of the cupula during stationary head position; (d) position of cupula during accelerating head rotation; (e) position of cupula immediately after head rotation ceases.

and the utricle, which are two membranous sacs also filled with endolymph; each also contains a mechanoreceptor, in this case called the macula, comprised of hair cells, above which is located crystals of calcium carbonate—the otoliths—in a gelatinous matrix. Movement of the endolymph of the saccule and utricle causes the otoliths to be displaced in the opposite direction, which stimulates the hair cells of the maculas. These hair cells are also supplied with fibers from the vestibular division of CN VIII.

Caloric stimulation of the endolymph produced by irrigation of the auditory canals with water above or below body temperature produces convection currents in it and leads thereby to stimulation of the mechanoreceptors of the ampullas and the saccule and utricle similar to the currents in the endolymph produced by head movement. The result is the sensation of rotation (vertigo) accompanied by nystagmus, disturbance of equilibrium, and nausea (for caloric testing see following).

The mechanoreceptors of the ampullae of the semicircular canals signal the

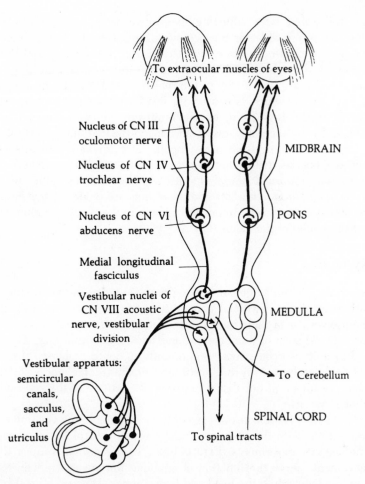

Nucleus of CN III
oculomotor nerve

Nucleus of CN IV
trochlear nerve

Nucleus of CN VI
abducens nerve

Medial longitudinal
fasciculus

Vestibular nuclei of
CN VIII acoustic
nerve, vestibular
division

Vestibular apparatus:
semicircular
canals,
sacculus,
and
utriculus

To extraocular muscles of eyes

MIDBRAIN

PONS

MEDULLA

To Cerebellum

SPINAL CORD

To spinal tracts

Figure 16-2. Diagram of the anatomic relationships among: the vestibular apparatus, the vestibular nuclei in the brainstem, and the brainstem nuclei of the cranial nerves controlling the extraocular muscles. The vestibular nuclei also send connections to nerve centers in the spinal cord controlling postural muscles, and to the cerebellum. Neural connections in the brainstem are shown for one side only, although of course the entire system is bilaterally symmetrical, and has many decussations.

rate of change (acceleration or deceleration) of motions of the head, while the mechanoreceptors of the saccule and utricle relay information concerning the position of the head relative to the force of gravity.

The dendrites supplying these mechanoreceptors have their cell bodies in a vestibular ganglion on each side, from which axons continue to a complex set of vestibular nuclei in the medulla. (Neurons also go from the receptors to portions of the cerebellum.) Then from the vestibular nuclei, second-order neurons travel in two directions. Some neurons travel down the spinal cord in the vestibulospinal tracts and are concerned with postural adjustments. Some neurons pass upward through the medial longitudinal fasciculus to the higher portion of the brainstem: midbrain and pons, in which lie the nuclei of the cranial nerves (CNS III, IV, VI) innervating the extraocular muscles and controlling eye movements. It is these pathways connecting the vestibular and oculomotor nuclei that are concerned with adjusting eye movements as the head is moved, and they are responsible for the oculovestibular reflexes; it is a brainstem lesion in the medial longitudinal fasciculus that causes internuclear opthalmoplegia. These topics are discussed in Chapter 14. Still other neural pathways extend from the brainstem vestibular nuclei to the thalamus and then to the cerebral cortex.

The vertigo which is caused by lesions involving the labyrinth, its afferent nerves to the brainstem, or the brainstem vestibular nuclei, is often accompanied by nystagmus, ataxia, and incoordinated motor activity, and visceral symptoms resulting from parasympathetic autonomic activation: nausea, vomiting, diaphoresis, pallor and sometimes diarrhea. The muscle incoordination results from abnormal neural impulses to the muscles along the vestibulospinal tracts. The autonomic signs and symptoms are evidence that impulses from the vestibular nuclei in the brainstem radiate to the parasympathetic centers including the nuclei of the vagus (CN X).

Nystagmus

Nystagmus is the conjugate jerking movements of the eyes which occurs in disturbances of the vestibular apparatus in the inner ear, of the vestibular nerves themselves, or of their nuclei in the brainstem; it is often accompanied by vertigo, disturbance of equilibrium, and nausea and vomiting. This group of signs and symptoms occurs most prominently in acute unilateral disorders which do not completely destroy the vestibular apparatus, the nerve, or the nuclei, and which result in an imbalance between the activity of the right and the left vestibular systems.

Nystagmus is the consequence of the activation of the vestibular system and its connections with the brainstem nuclei which control the extraocular muscles to produce eye movements (Figure 16-2). In the normal subject these reflex eye movements serve the function of enabling the eyes to remain fixated on a stationary object while the head and body rotates. When the head begins to rotate, as for example when a ballet dancer begins a whirl, the eyes move slowly in the direction opposite the rotation, as though fixated on some object. (The endolymph of the semicircular canal in the plane of rotation also moves in the direction opposite to the rotation.) When the eyes have moved as far as possible in that direction, they make a rapid and brief compensatory swing back to the midline, then again remain fixated on the new point, and so on. The direction of a nystagmus is named on the basis of the fast (compensatory, recovery, or correctional) component. Therefore, during bodily rotation to the right, the slow component of nystagmus is to the left, the fast recovery component is to the right, and it is a right nystagmus. Most nystagmus is horizontal, but there can also be vertical and rotatory nystagmus. Abnormal conditions producing stimulation of the vestibular system, neural pathways, or central connections in the brainstem, lead to spontaneous activation of the nystagmus and vertigo elicited in the normal subject by physical rotation.

Caloric testing, with or without electronystagmography, is sometimes used for the purpose of identifying the side having the hypoactive labyrinth in suspected Ménière's disease or a possible acoustic neurinoma (see following). Both warm and cool water are used alternately to irrigate the external ear canals for 1–2 min, with at least 5 min between each irrigation. The procedure induces a flow

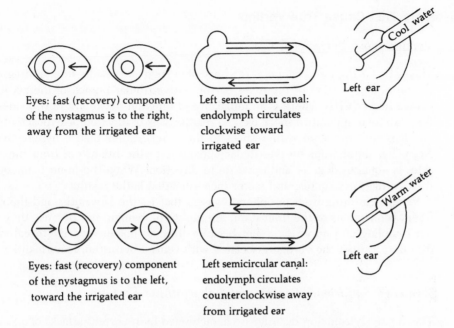

Eyes: fast (recovery) component of the nystagmus is to the right, away from the irrigated ear

Left semicircular canal: endolymph circulates clockwise toward irrigated ear

Left ear

Eyes: fast (recovery) component of the nystagmus is to the left, toward the irrigated ear

Left semicircular canal: endolymph circulates counterclockwise away from irrigated ear

Left ear

With cool and warm water, respectively, to the right ear, the directions of movement of endolymph and eyes are the reverse.

Figure 16-3. Diagram showing the direction of the fast component of nystagmus, and the direction of flow of endolymph in the horizontal semicircular canal, in response to irrigation of the left external ear canal with warm or cool water.

of endolymph in the semicircular canals, and vertigo and nystagmus; when warm water is used the fast component is toward the ear being irrigated; in the case of cool water the fast component is away from the irrigated ear (Figure 16-3). Duration of the nystagmus during each irrigation is timed with a stopwatch.

Paresis (hypoactivity) of the canal on one side (or dominance—that is, relative hyperactivity—of the other) is said to be present when the duration of nystagmus induced by both warm and cool water in one ear is less than that resulting from irrigation of the opposite ear. Directional preponderance is the term applied to a longer nystagmus in one direction than in the other in response to irrigation of either ear with warm and cold water. When the responses are equal in duration in both eyes to all irrigations, then it is concluded that the test is within normal limits even though the overall duration of nystagmus may be unusually long or short. In electronystagmography, the speed of the slow component, the amplitude of the eye deviations, and the precise number of beats in response to each irrigation, is recorded; this permits quantification of the responses and aids in interpretation of the results. Dominance on one side is said to indicate a peripheral vestibular lesion on the opposite side, while a central brainstem lesion may be indicated by a spontaneous nystagmus, without paresis (or dominance) but with directional preponderance, more often toward the side of the lesion.

Disorders That Cause True Vertigo

Vertigo from Peripheral Causes

This is by far the more common category of vertigo and results from a disease of the vestibular portion of the inner ear or the vestibular branch of the auditory cranial nerve (VIII). There is an imbalance of function between the two sides of the vestibular apparatus, more likely a relative lack of function or hypoactivity of one labyrinth or nerve with respect to the other, rather than a hyperactivity. Normally, input from the vestibular apparatus to the brainstem from the two sides is equal in degree, and opposite in direction. When the input is unequal, then vertigo, nystagmus, and motor incoordination is the result.

Vertigo resulting from peripheral causes, that is, the labyrinths and their afferent connections to the brainstem, are said to be benign, not because they are not disabling and unpleasant, but because they do not involve life-threatening disorders as does the vertigo associated with central brainstem abnormalities.

Ménière's Syndrome (Paroxysmal Labyrinthine Vertigo)

This relatively common disorder is characterized by recurrent attacks of a symptom complex comprised of severe vertigo, often nystagmus, progressive loss of hearing, and tinnitus. The symptoms of vertigo and nystagmus are intermittent rather than continuous, but the tinnitus and hearing deficits, although more marked during attacks of vertigo, may be present to a lesser degree between attacks. The cause is not known, although on occasion it is reported to follow head trauma or a middle ear infection. The attacks of vertigo are violent, of a sudden onset, and often are recurrent at quite regular intervals; they may last 15 minutes to 2 hours or more and are often accompanied by diaphoresis, nausea, and vomiting. There may be remissions of weeks or months between periods of several attacks per day. The onset is most often in middle age. Progressive deafness is more often unilateral than bilateral, and deficient response (paresis) of the involved labyrinth to caloric testing is present in about half of affected patients. Attempts to discern characteristic pathologic changes in the vestibular apparatus or nerve have been largely unsuccessful and there is no effective treatment, although antivertigo and antiemetic agents are helpful in controlling the acute attacks.

Postural Vertigo (Benign Positional Vertigo)

This is said to be the most common cause of vertigo. The patient complains of discrete, brief attacks of vertigo when he lies down, turns over in bed, stoops, or gets up in the morning. The attacks are accompanied by nausea and nystagmus and last but seconds or at most a few minutes; the patient is free of symptoms between the brief episodes, and there are no neurologic or other signs aside from nystagmus. The caloric responses are said to be normal. Attacks may persist intermittently for several weeks and then resolve spontaneously. The cause is not known, although on occasion it is reported to follow head injury and be a portion of the postconcussion syndrome (irritability, headache, inability to concentrate, loss of balance on postural change, and "dizzy spells"). It is common in elderly individuals, reportedly more so in females than males. Meclizine may decrease the frequency and severity of the attacks.

Acute Labyrinthitis (Vestibular Neuronitis, Viral Labyrinthitis)

The signs and symptoms are continuous severe vertigo, nystagmus, nausea and vomiting, and disturbances of equilibrium. The vertigo and accompanying signs and symptoms are continuous for days rather than episodic, and the patient appears prostrated, pale, diaphoretic, and concentrates on holding his head very still. The duration is several days to two weeks of marked prostration and disability; balance difficulties and brief vertigo on head movement may persist for weeks or months following subsidence of the acute attack. This disorder is considered by some to be a viral infection of the vestibular branch of CN VIII and there may be a history of a head cold, sore throat, or "flu" in the days or weeks preceding the onset. There is usually no impairment of hearing, but headache and photophobia may be present. Perphenazine or the medications mentioned below may be useful in controlling the vertigo.

Toxic Labyrinthitis

Damage to CN VIII (or the labyrinths) may be caused by a number of pharmacologic agents, including aspirin, quinine, and streptomycin. Accompanying symptoms may be hearing loss, tinnitus, and the other accompaniments to vertigo, which may continue for days or weeks. There may also be blurring of vision on motion because of impairment of the oculovestibular reflexes which adjust eye movement to body and therefore head motion.

Management of Peripheral Vertigo

Although there is no effective treatment for these vertiginous disorders, which though disabling are not life threatening, a number of medications are useful in controlling the symptoms, signs, and subjective responses to vertigo.

Labyrinthine suppressants are basically types of antihistamine drugs that also have anticholinergic and sedative actions. The action appears to be both peripheral, in suppressing vestibular and organ receptors; and central, in inhibiting the activation of parasympathetic cholinergic centers in the brainstem. Pharmacologic agents in this category include cyclizine, meclizine, dimenhydrinate, promethazine, and scopolamine.

Antiemetic agents of the phenothiazine class act to suppress central vestibular pathways. They include prochlorperazine, trimethobenzamide, chlorpromazine, and benzquinamide.

Pure anticholinergic drugs which inhibit the activation of cholinergic centers in the brainstem are atropine and hyoscine.

Some patients react to vertigo with anxiety or depression; in the former case chlordiazepoxide, diazepam, or phenobarbital may be useful; in the latter case amitriptyline is sometimes indicated. Although these agents do not affect the severity or frequency of vertigo, they modify the response to it.

Vertigo from Central (Brainstem) Causes

Acoustic Neurinoma

This tumor of the sheath of the vestibular division of the acoustic nerve (CN VIII) arises in the internal auditory meatus but as it grows it extends intracranially in the posterior fossa to occupy an area between the pons and cerebellum (the cerebellopontine angle). It comprises about 8% of brain tumors, occurs slightly more often in females than males, and the onset of symptoms is usually between ages 30 and 60. The tumors are nonmalignant and slow-growing, but as they enlarge they compress the cerebellum and brainstem, stretch and distort CN V and VI, and envelop CN VII and VIII. Progressive unilateral hearing loss and tinnitus are the chief complaints in about three fourths of the patients and often occur prior to other symptoms by several years. Ataxia of gait, or veering in one direction with walking, vertigo, horizontal nystagmus, facial paresthesias, hypoesthesia, and paresis, incoordination in use of one or both hands, are other symptoms; and signs are diminished corneal reflexes and loss of the vestibular response to caloric testing on the affected side. Diagnosis is made by computed tomography (CT scan), audiometry, CSF analysis (there is protein elevation), and other procedures. Surgical removal of the tumor is necessary as acoustic neurinomas are not radiosensitive.

Brainstem Transient Ischemic Attacks

Vertigo may be a symptom of vertebral–basilar insufficiency and may occur in brief episodes alone or in conjunction with other neurologic signs and symptoms, e.g., dysarthria, ataxia, blurred vision or diplopia, paresis, or paresthesias. Diminution of blood flow to the brainstem vestibular nuclei, or to the vestibular apparatus itself, which may be caused by fluctuations in blood pressure, postural changes, or head and neck movements, result in periods of transient central vertigo. The vertebral arteries ascend through the foramina of the transverse processes of C6 through C1 vertebrae; they may be narrowed by atherosclerosis and/or pressure from the vertebral osteophytes of degenerative joint disease. Turing the head to one side causes mechanical twisting and compression of the vertebral artery on the opposite side. A combination of atherosclerotic vessels and cervical spondylosis may add to this mechanical distortion and result in brainstem ischemia which is associated with vertigo, nystagmus, and sometimes other neurologic signs and symptoms.

Occlusion of the proximal portion of the subclavian arteries, from which the vertebrals arise, may lead to subclavian steal syndrome in which reversal of flow in the vertebral artery occurs, causing blood to be siphoned away from the brain and into the arm. Use of the arms or head movements may accentuate the resulting cerebral ischemia. Blood pressure in the affected arm is reduced and there may be a supraclavicular bruit caused by turbulent flow in the partially occluded subclavian (Figure 16-4).

Brain ischemia is discussed in more detail in Chapter 18.

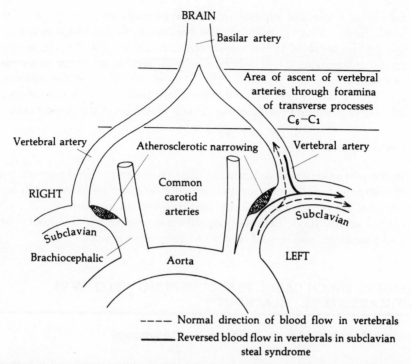

BRAIN

Basilar artery

Area of ascent of vertebral
arteries through foramina
of transverse processes
C_6-C_1

Vertebral artery

Atherosclerotic narrowing

Vertebral artery

RIGHT

Common
carotid
arteries

Subclavian

Subclavian

Brachiocephalic

Aorta

LEFT

- - - - Normal direction of blood flow in vertebrals

———— Reversed blood flow in vertebrals in subclavian
steal syndrome

Figure 16-4. Diagram of the origin of the vertebral arteries from the subclavian arteries, common sites of atherosclerotic narrowing of the subclavians just proximal to origin of the vertebrals; transit of vertebrals through the foramina of the transverse processes of vertebra C6 through C1; and their fusion to form the basilar artery which supplies the brainstem and posterior portion of the cerebral hemispheres. Foraminal narrowing, producing partial occlusion of the vertebrals, made more severe by head turning; and atherosclerotic narrowing of the subclavians, producing partial reversal of blood flow in the vertebrals and causing subclavian steal syndrome, are two processes responsible for brainstem transient ischemic attacks.

Multiple Sclerosis

Attacks of vertigo may be a symptom of multiple sclerosis in some patients. This may result from degeneration and plaque formation in the brainstem, especially the inner reticular core of the pons. It is more often found in early stages of the disease but may be associated with exacerbations. Although it is reported to be brief in most cases, on occasion it may be severe and protracted.

Convulsive Disorders and Migraine

In seizure disorders, the aura may sometimes take the form of an attack of vertigo; this is most likely to occur in the case of epileptic attacks originating in the temporal and parietal lobes. Electrical stimulation of these areas of the brain during surgery in the conscious patient has been reported to induce severe vertigo. In some patients, especially children, the attack of vertigo may itself be the only seizure manifestation. It is probable that these areas of the cortex are the ones receiving the projections from the vestibular nuclei in the brainstem.

Vertigo may also occur in association with migraine headaches, either as an aura or as a migraine equivalent, and occasionally may occur during the actual headache on change of position. The implication in this situation is that some of the arteries involved in the vasoconstriction and vasodilation phases of migraine are those supplying the peripheral vestibular mechanism of the inner ear or their central nuclei in the brainstem (these vessels would be of the vertebral–basilar system); or the vessels supplying the projections in the temporal and parietal lobes of the cerebral cortex (these vessels would be of the carotid system).

Posttraumatic Vertigo

In the postconcussion syndrome, or after more serious head injuries, complaints of vertigo and/or dizziness are the second most common (headache is first). Analysis of these complaints indicates that true vertigo is relatively rare, while feelings of unsteadiness, disturbed equilibrium, impending "blackout," bizarre visual sensations, and mental confusion are more common.

DISORDERS WHICH CAUSE PSEUDOVERTIGO ("DIZZINESS," LIGHTHEADEDNESS, "BLACKOUT")

Disorders Associated with Syncope or Presyncope

Syncope is defined as sudden transient loss of consciousness; it is caused by impaired cerebral metabolism usually resulting from a deficiency of oxygen or glucose. The deficiency may be the consequence of decreased cerebral perfusion because of hypovolemia, hypotension, reduced cardiac output, or intrinsic cerebrovascular alterations; or it may be caused by hypoglycemia.

Vasovagal Syncope

Vasovagal syncope is the common faint that occurs in conjunction with strong emotional reactions which are usually unpleasant or frightening, or with injury, pain, or unpleasant sights. It appears to be a response mediated by parasympathetic centers in the brainstem and the vagus nerves and consists of widespread peripheral vasodilation and sometimes marked bradycardia. As a result of these responses cardiac output and therefore cerebral perfusion drops to a level inadequate to sustain consciousness. The patient falls, which on the basis of gravity induced blood shifts restores adequate blood flow to the brain, and consciousness returns promptly.

Premonitory signs of an impending syncope from any one of the above causes are often dimming or darkening of vision, a sensation of muscle weakness, a feeling that everything is receding far away, seeing spots before the eyes, and ringing or roaring in the ears, nausea or cold sweat, all apparently induced by autonomic discharge and a decline in cerebral blood flow.

Transient Ischemic Attacks

Either carotid or vertebral–basilar artery insufficiency may cause impending or actual loss of consciousness. These disorders are discussed in Chapter 18. Often

the acute attack occurs as a consequence of hypovolemia or hypotension superimposed upon a cerebral vasculature having diffuse atherosclerotic narrowing.
Subclavian steal syndrome and vertebral–basilar syndrome resulting from cervical spondylosis (see above) are other causes of TIA syncope, especially in the
elderly.

Cardiac Arrhythmias

Bradycardia, paroxysmal supraventricular tachycardia, transient complete heart
block producing Adams-Stokes syndrome, Wolff-Parkinson-White syndrome,
and other cardiac arrhythmias that may result in markedly reduced cerebral perfusion, with impending or actual syncope, are discussed in Chapter 6.

Carotid Sinus Hypersensitivity

The processes involved in the group of disorders that comprise carotid sinus
hypersensitivity have been covered in earlier sections of this chapter.

Postural Hypotension

Elderly patients receiving diuretics, antihypertensive agents, and on sodium-re-
stricted diets are particularly prone to develop hypovolemia and postural hypotension. The decreased circulating blood volume decreases venous return to the
right heart, lowers myocardial contractile force, and reduces cardiac output and
cerebral perfusion. Reduced peripheral vascular resistance from systemic vasodilation may be caused by vasodilator medication (nitroglycerine, isosorbide dinitrate, some tranquilizers, such as chlorpromazine) and antihypertensive agents
which reduce the reflex sympathetic adrenergic responses to postural change;
these topics are discussed earlier in the chapter. Dehydration from inadequate
fluid intake or excess fluid loss may themselves, or in combination with the
above factors, produce postural dizziness and syncope. Other causes are autonomic neuropathy of the diabetic or alcoholic. All of these effects are additive
with atherosclerotic cerebrovascular disease in producing syncope or presyn-
cope.

Reactive or Fasting Hypoglycemia

Reactive or fasting hypoglycemia is a rare cause of syncope, although patients
often believe that they have it and that it is responsible for their lightheadedness, giddiness, or feelings of faintness or weakness. A blood sugar determination obtained during a symptomatic period will resolve this question. These patients are often found to have anxiety hyperventilation.

Tussive, Micturition, Defecation Syncope

The mechanism of tussive, micturition, or defecation syncope may be the Valsalva maneuver, described earlier, which causes a drop in cardiac output and
therefore in cerebral perfusion because of elevated intrathoracic pressure. Some
authors have suggested that the elevated intrathoracic pressure produced by

these acts causes a brief elevation in pressure of the cerebrospinal fluid which then briefly exceeds brain perfusion pressure, resulting in a temporary reduction in arterial blood flow sufficient to lead to syncope. Some workers believe that micturition syncope represents a combination of postural hypotension from inadequate compensatory circulatory reflexes and vagally mediated cardioinhibition and vasodilation.

Disorders Associated with Loss of Balance

Multiple Sensory Impairment

Multiple sensory impairment is a very common cause of dizziness, in the sense of a sensation of imbalance, unsteadiness or swaying, in the elderly. Usually a combination of two or more of the following causes are present in such patients: (1) visual difficulties, such as inability to adjust to bifocal or trifocal refraction, or postcataract refractions; (2) diabetic or alcoholic neuropathy; (3) degenerative disease of the cerebral hemispheres, basal ganglia, or vestibular apparatus; (4) orthopedic or arthritic abnormalities; (5) cervical spondylosis; (6) impaired hearing; and (7) degenerative disease of the muscle, joint, and tendon proprioceptors. In cervical spine degenerative joint disease (cervical spondylosis) there is often associated spastic contraction of the muscles of the neck and scalp, abnormal proprioceptive impulses from the neck to the vestibular and ocular nuclei in the brainstem, and impaired blood flow through the vertebral arteries. All of these combine to produce a syndrome of cervicogenic dizziness, cerebrovascular insufficiency, instability of head position, and blurred visual images. A cervical collar, walking cane, and program of balancing exercises may be very helpful. The contribution of overmedication to the multisensory dizziness of the elderly can hardly be overemphasized.

Postconcussion Syndrome

Multiple sensory deficits are probably involved in the post-head trauma symptom complex as described above.

Psychoemotional Disorders

Attacks of anxiety hyperventilation, transient bizarre gait alterations occurring in psychiatric illness, and vague sensations of panic, mental confusion, and inability to concentrate, may all be called dizziness, blackout, or lightheadedness by patients with psychiatric conditions.

Seizures

Absence attacks, vertigo, or feelings of remoteness or unreality, auras of various types, and a sudden fall with loss of consciousness, all may accompany, or themselves be, various types of seizures. Two types of information help separate out the dizziness and blackout associated with seizure disorders from those of other cause. The first is the account of witnesses as to whether there was convulsive motor activity and/or incontinence accompanying the attack; the second is with respect to the patient's feelings and behavior upon regaining consciousness. Most seizures are associated with a postictal state: headache, drowsiness, and mental confusion, which lasts for minutes or an hour or more. Most syncopal episodes are succeeded by a brief feeling of weakness but the mental status is clear and alert. Seizures are discussed in detail in Chapter 17.

REFERENCES

Beeson PB and McDermott W, editors: *Textbook of Medicine.* 14th ed. Philadelphia, Pa.: Saunders, 1975.

Branch WT and Funkenstein H: Clinical evaluation of vertigo. *Primary Care* 4:267–282, 1977.

Clairmont AA et al.: Dizziness. A logical approach to diagnosis and treatment. *Postgrad. Med.* 56:139–144, 1974.

Dix MR: The physiological basis and practical value of head exercises in the treatment of vertigo. *Practitioner* 217:919–924, 1976.

Drachman DA and Hart CW: An approach to the dizzy patient. *Neurology* 22:323–334, 1972.

Facer GW and Baragos NE. The dizzy patient. *Postgrad. Med.* 57:73–77, 1975.

Ganong WF: *Review of Medical Physiology*, 8th ed. Los Altos, Calif.: Lange Medical Publications, 1977.

Guyton AC: *Textbook of Medical Physiology*, 5th ed. Philadelphia, Pa.: Saunders, 1976.

Matthews WB: *Practical Neurology*, 3rd ed. London: Blackwell Scientific Publications, 1975.

Merritt HH: *A Textbook of Neurology*, 5th ed. Philadelphia, Pa.: Lea & Febiger, 1973.

Noble RJ: The patient with syncope. *JAMA* 237:1372–1376, 1977.

Thorn GW et al., editors: *Harrison's Principles of Internal Medicine*, 8th ed. New York: McGraw-Hill, 1977.

Turner JS, Jr: The dizzy patient: diagnosis and treatment. *Drugs* 13:382–387, 1977.

CHAPTER SEVENTEEN

Seizure Disorders

EXCITATION AND CONDUCTION IN NEURAL TISSUE

Neurons

There are many different types of specialized neurons comprising the central, peripheral, and autonomic nervous systems. In general, the major functions of neurons are to receive stimuli; to conduct impulses; to transmit impulses to other neurons and to effector structures such as muscle and gland tissue; and to synthesize and secrete such chemical messengers as neurotransmitters and neuroendocrine substances. A typical motor neuron is composed of: (1) a mass of processes, the dendrites, which are extensions of the cell body or soma and which are specialized for receiving input from the axon terminals of other neurons; (2) the cell body or soma itself, which contains the cell nucleus and other organelles and which is the center of neural functions, including synthesis of proteins for maintenance of the neuron, and the manufacture of neurotransmitters and other chemical effectors; and (3) the axon, with its terminal arborizations, which is an extension of the cell body and which transmits neural impulses away from the receptive dendrites and cell body.

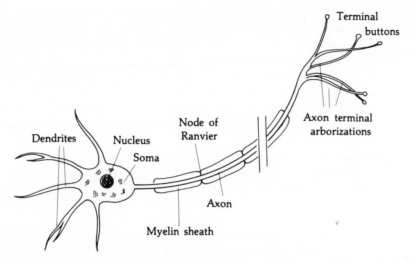

Figure 17-1. Diagram of a typical myelinated motor neuron·showing dendrites, cell body, axon with myelin sheath, axon arborizations, and terminal buttons.

Resting Potential

The reception and conduction of nerve impulses is a metabolically active self-sustaining and self-propagating process within the neuron cell membrane requiring the consumption of O_2 and energy substrate, mainly glucose. In the normal nonactive (resting) neuron there is a difference in electrical potential across the cell membrane of about 70 to 80 mV; the inside of the cell is electronegative with respect to the outside. The resting membrane potential is expressed as -80 mV.

This potential difference between the inside and outside of the cell is correlated with a differential distribution of ions on the two sides of the cell membrane. The concentration of Na^+ is much larger in the ECF outside the cell than within it; the cell membrane is slightly permeable to Na^+ so that the ion tends to diffuse across the membrane along both the chemical concentration gradient (there is more Na^+ outside than inside) and along the electrical gradient (the cell interior is negative relative to the outside). The inside of the cell is maintained low in Na^+ (in spite of these two forces affecting diffusion which would act to permit Na^+ to enter), by virtue of a metabolic pump in the cell membrane which actively transports out of the cell those Na^+ which diffuse in along the gradients. The energy for this pump is supplied by ATP.

Unlike the Na^+ distribution, the concentration of K^+ is much larger inside the cell than outside. The tendency here is for K^+ to diffuse out of the cell into the ECF along its chemical concentration gradient. In this case the electrical gradient is opposite the chemical one: the electrical drive is toward keeping the positive K^+ inside the cell, therefore the tendency for K^+ to leak out is not as great as the tendency for Na^+ to diffuse in. Nevertheless some does, and so the active transport mechanism for extruding Na^+ from the cell is also involved, though to a lesser degree, in pumping some K^+ back into the cell. In fact the two active transport mechanisms are linked and the pump is called the sodium–potassium pump since the transport of Na^+ is coupled to that of K^+, although much more Na^+ is pumped out than K^+ is transported in.

The net result of the differential distribution of the diffusible positively charged ions, and the concentration of intracellular nondiffusible negatively charged ions (which I have not discussed) is the resting transmembrane electrical potential. If cells are deprived of O_2 or metabolic substrate for generating ATP, or if the enzyme systems involved in the active transport process are inactivated by some toxic substance, then Na^+ diffuses into the cell, K^+ diffuses out of it, and the resting potential difference across the membrane declines. When the cell ceases to metabolize altogether (cell death) the potential difference between inside and outside is abolished.

The third major ion involved in the transmembrane potential is Cl^-; the concentration of Cl^- is greater outside the cell in the ECF than it is intracellularly, and therefore its tendency is to diffuse from the ECF across the cell membrane into the cell. However, since Cl^- is a negative ion, and the inside of the cell is

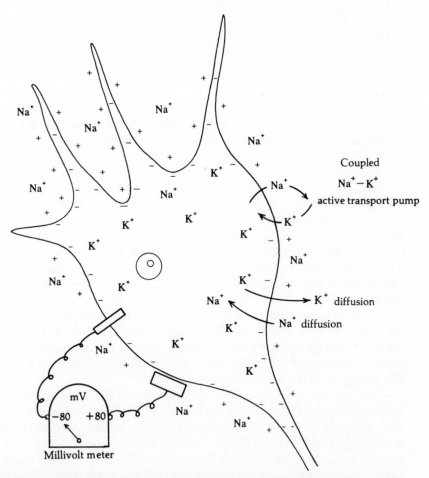

Figure 17-2. Diagram of a portion of a neuron showing a millivoltmeter attached to recording electrodes inside and at the surface of the cell membrane, recording a transmembrane potential of −80 mv. Also indicated is relative distribution of Na^+ and K^+ on the two sides of the membrane, direction of diffusion gradients, and the membrane Na^+−K^+ active transport exchange pump for maintaining differential distribution of ions on the two sides of the cell membrane.

negative relative to the outside, the tendency of Cl⁻ to diffuse in along its chemical concentration gradient is opposed by the tendency for it to diffuse out along the electrical gradient. In the case of Cl⁻ these two opposite gradients are about equal and therefore balance out, so that Cl⁻ efflux and influx remain stable without the necessity for an active transport process in the membrane to be involved in the equilibrium.

Although I have described these processes with special reference to the neuron resting potential, the situation is similar for almost all cells. The difference is that in most other cells, with the exception of muscle, there is no excitability, receptivity, or conductivity.

Action Potential

When a subthreshold excitatory (negative) stimulus is applied to the resting neuron, the about −75 mV transmembrane resting potential is reduced slightly by approximately 6–9 mV. In experimental conditions such a partial depolarization may be produced by application of a stimulus using electrodes; in normal intact neural tissue it may be the result of excitatory stimuli arriving at the dendrites or soma from presynaptic neurons (see following). In either case the subthreshold stimulus, although too weak to produce an impulse, does cause a transient alteration in the cell membrane which is restricted to the localized area in the region of the stimulus. This transient alteration takes two related forms: (1) the magnitude of the transmembrane resting potential is reduced by an amount related to the strength of the excitatory stimulus; and (2) the permeability to Na⁺ of the portion of the neuron membrane in the immediate vicinity of the stimulus increases, so that Na⁺ from the ECF diffuses into the neuron through ionic channels in the membrane opened by the excitatory stimulus. In the case of weak and brief subthreshold stimuli these changes in the membrane are equally transitory and active processes in the membrane promptly restore the resting condition to normal once the stimulus is withdrawn.

However, if the excitatory stimulus impinging on the neuron cell membrane is longer and stronger, enough to reduce the transmembrane resting potential by about 15 mV, then it may be adequate to reach the threshold stimulus value for that neuron. Threshold value for most neurons is a reduction in the transmembrane potential by about 15 mV to approximately −60 mV. A stimulus of threshold magnitude produces a degree of membrane depolarization and an increase in permeability to Na⁺ extensive enough to generate a neuron impulse. The response of a membrane to subthreshold stimuli is largely passive, but threshold stimulation induces an active process in the membrane, whereby the depolarization and permeability changes become self-sustaining and self-propagating. A wave of depolarization sweeps along the neuron in both directions from the point of application of the threshold stimulus; this propagated wave of excitation is called the spike potential.

The entire neuron participates in this active process in an orderly and sequential fashion, which results not only in depolarization of the neuron but in an actual reversal of polarity, so that very briefly, as the wave passes along, the inside of the cell becomes electrically positive by about +30 mV with respect to the outside. The reversal of polarity is the result principally of the large influx of Na⁺ into the cell from the ECF. The wave of excitation is propagated from the point

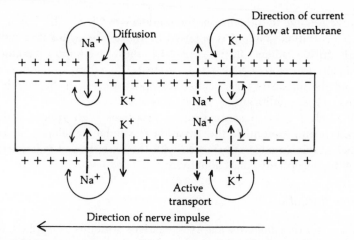

Figure 17-3. Diagram of the events of an action potential in a segment of nerve axon, showing direction of passage of impulse, movement of ions in both excitation (diffusion) and recovery (active transport) phases, and current flow through membrane as the nerve impulse is propagated along.

of stimulus application along the whole length of the neuron; although neurons can conduct an impulse in either direction, synaptic transmission is always unidirectional: from the axon terminals of the presynaptic neuron to the dendrites and soma of the postsynaptic one.

Immediately following the propagated wave of excitation, there is a recovery wave which restores the membrane potential to resting levels. The wave of depolarization and subsequent repolarization are together termed the action potential.

Just as the differential distribution of ions on the two sides of the cell membrane are correlated with the resting membrane potential, so are differential movements of ions across the cell membrane into and out of the cell correlated with the various phases of the action potential. A small decline in resting potential of around 6–9 mV is correlated with altered membrane permeability permitting influx of Na^+ and Cl^- and efflux of K^+. The greater the drop in membrane potential toward the firing level (threshold) caused by the stimulus, the greater the permeability increase to Na^+ with a corresponding increase in Na^+ diffusion from the ECF into the cell. Once threshold level depolarization is attained, the increase in Na^+ permeability is very large and at that point a spike potential is initiated as described above. The reversal in membrane potential (overshoot) is correlated with the large influx of Na^+. During the recovery process (repolarization) the permeability of the membrane returns toward normal, further ion diffusion ceases, and the Na^+–K^+ pump returns the transmembrane ionic concentrations and potential difference to the resting level. Figure 17-3 indicates the main phases of the action potential: depolarization, reversal of polarity, and recovery, in a nonmyelinated nerve.

Electrotonus

As mentioned above, a stimulus which is too weak to reach the threshold or firing level, and thus initiate an action potential, nevertheless does produce an alteration in transmembrane potential and ion permeability. Such stimulation is called subthreshold. If the stimulus is a negatively charged one, as from the negative pole of a stimulating electrode, it decreases the potential difference across the membrane by decreasing the number of positive charges at the surface of the neuron membrane, lowers the transmembrane potential toward the threshold or firing level, and thus increases the excitability and responsiveness of the neuron in the region of the applied stimulus. This effect is termed *catelectrotonus* because the stimulis is negative or cathodal.

If the stimulus is a positively charged one, as from the positive pole of a stimulating electrode, it increases the potential difference across the neuron membrane by causing an accumulation of positive charges at the outside surface and decreases the excitability and responsiveness of the neuron in the region of the applied stimulus. This effect is termed anelectrotonus because the stimulus is positive (anodal). Cathodal (negative) stimuli are termed depolarizing; anodal (positive) stimuli are called hyperpolarizing.

These two types of electrical influence on neurons correspond with the two types of synapses in the central nervous sytem: excitatory and inhibitory, the balance between which determines the level of excitability and responsiveness of parts of the brain, and of the brain as a whole, to a wide range of stimuli, both normal and abnormal. The balance between excitation and inhibition in neural systems of the brain is intimately related to the processes underlying all of the seizure disorders. Figure 17-4a,b shows a diagramatic representation of catelec-

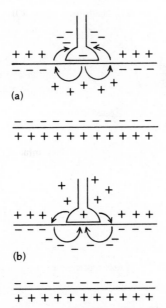

Figure 17-4. (a) Portion of a neuron showing the effect of a negatively charged stimulus applied either by the negative pole of an electrode (cathode) or in an excitatory synaptic button. Negative charges accumulate at the membrane surface, the transmembrane potential is decreased, the membrane is partially depolarized, and the effect of the stimulus is excitatory. (b) Portion of a neuron showing the effect of a positively charged stimulus applied either by the positive pole of an electrode (anode) or an inhibitory synaptic button. Positive charges accumulate at the membrane surface, the transmembrane potential is increased, the membrane is partially hyperpolarized, and the effect of the stimulus is inhibitory.

trotonus, excitation, and partial depolarization; and anelectrotonus, inhibition, and hyperpolarization.

Synapses

A synapse is the area at which the synaptic knobs on the terminal axon arborizations of a presynaptic neuron come into close apposition with the dendrites or soma, or both, of a postsynaptic neuron (Figure 17-5). The number of synaptic knobs of presynaptic axons on each postsynaptic neuron is said to average a few thousand. A nerve cell body with inhibitory terminal buttons from a presynaptic neuron is shown in Figure 17-5a. Figure 17-5b shows an enlarged view of an excitatory snaptic knob and its relation to the membrane of a dendrite of the postsynaptic neuron.

These knobs represent the axon terminals of about a hundred presynaptic neurons; that is, only a portion of the many knobs are contributed by a given neuron, thus many presynaptic neurons give input to each postsynaptic neuron. This is called the principle of *convergence* in the nervous system: many presynaptic neurons converge on each postsynaptic neuron. In turn, the axons of each neuron arborize or divide into many terminals, so that each neuron makes contact with about a hundred other neurons; this is termed the principle of *divergence*. These principles are illustrated in Figure 17-6.

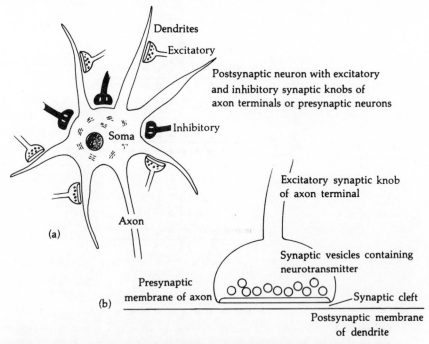

Figure 17-5. (a) Diagram of a nerve cell body with inhibitory and excitatory terminal buttons from a presynaptic neuron. (b) Enlarged view of an excitatory synaptic knob, its relation to the synaptic cleft and the membrane of a dendrite of the post synaptic neuron.

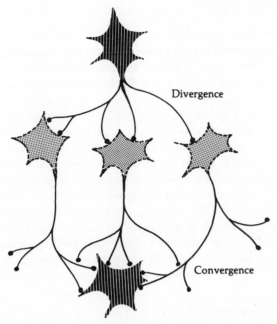

Divergence

Convergence

Figure 17-6. Diagram illustrating divergence and convergence in neurons of the central nervous system. The terminal arborizations of a presynaptic neuron diverge to influence many postsynaptic neurons. Conversely, the axons from many presynaptic neurons converge on one postsynaptic neuron.

Synaptic Transmission

Synapses may be either chemical or electrical or a combination of the two (compound synapses); the great majority are chemical. The propagated wave of excitation (nerve impulse) arrives at the terminal arborizations of the axon and spreads to the synaptic knobs; inside each of the latter, next to the synaptic membrane, are vesicles which contain the neurotransmitter characteristic of each neuron. Each neuron contains only one type of neurotransmitter. The nerve impulse arrives at the synaptic membrane, depolarizes it, and increases the permeability of the membrane to Ca^{2+}. Ca^{2+} enters the synaptic knobs causing the vesicles containing neurotransmitter to fuse to the membrane; the latter then develops channels through which the transmitter diffuses into the synaptic cleft, across it, and into contact with the postsynaptic membrane. The action of the presynaptic neuron on the postsynaptic one depends on whether the synapse is an excitatory or an inhibitory one. In any event the stimulus from a single presynaptic neuron very seldom leads to the initiation of a spike potential in a postsynaptic neuron. Rather it produces a transient alteration in membrane permeability and transmembrane electrical potential which may either increase or decrease the excitability of an area on the postsynaptic neuron, depending upon whether the activated synapse was an excitatory or an inhibitory one. In general, excitatory synapses are more often out on the dendrites of postsynaptic neurons, while inhibitory synapses occur more often on the cell body (soma) of the neuron (Figure 17-5a,b).

Excitatory Synapses

If the synapse is an excitatory one, the neurotransmitter released by the presynaptic knobs acts on the postsynaptic membrane and induces a depolarizing current which flows inward at the synaptic cleft, inducing a decline in transmembrane potential. Correlated with this electrical change is an ionic one. The excitatory neurotransmitter released by the presynaptic knob induces an increase in permeability to Na^+ in the postsynaptic membrane—essentially it opens channels through which Na^+ flows from the ECF into the postsynaptic neuron along the electrical and chemical gradient, and the potential difference across the membrane declines. If this occurs at only a few areas under synaptic knobs the effect is transient and the result is a transient catelectrotonus, which in the case of normal neural transmission at a synaptic junction is called an excitatory postsynaptic potential (EPSP). However, if there is simultaneous activation of many excitatory synaptic knobs then the EPSPs summate and the degree of depolarization of the cell may be sufficient to reach threshold and initiate an impulse in the postsynaptic fiber. The excitatory neurotransmitter at many synapses is acetylcholine; others are serotonin, dopamine, and norepinephrine.

Inhibitory Synapses

If the synapse is an inhibitory one, the result of its activation is a decrease in excitability of the postsynaptic membrane. The decreased excitability is produced by means of one of two types of inhibitory processes: presynaptic inhibition or postsynaptic inhibition. Both presynaptic and postsynaptic inhibition, especially the latter, are crucial for normal function of the central nervous system. When the normal inhibitory processes are disturbed from whatever cause, then abnormal hyperexcitability and seizure discharge may result. Substances such as strychnine and picrotoxin which interfere with the action of inhibitory neurotransmitters produce convulsions.

Presynaptic Inhibition.   The amount of neurotransmitter released by a synapse is correlated with the magnitude of the spike potential arriving at an axon terminal; the larger the impulse in millivolts, the more transmitter is released at the terminal. In presynaptic inhibition, an inhibitory terminal produces partial depolarization of an excitatory terminal, thus reducing the amount of excitatory transmitter released, and therefore the strength of the stimulus received by the postsynaptic neuron. The effect is to reduce the mangitude of the EPSP produced at the excitatory synapse. This form of presynaptic inhibition is illustrated in Figure 17-7a. The neurotransmitter at the inhibitory synapse is probably γ-aminobutyric acid (GABA). This type of synaptic inhibition is more prominent in lower portions of the brain, such as the thalamus and brainstem, than in the cerebral cortex.

Postsynaptic Inhibition.   This is the more important form of inhibition in the cerebral cortex and brain centers above the thalamus. There are several types of postsynaptic inhibition, but in general inhibitory synapses of the postsynaptic variety exert their inhibition of postsynaptic cells by producing an increased charge on the membrane—a hyperpolarization Such hyperpolarizations of neuron mem-

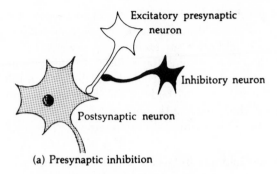

Excitatory presynaptic
neuron

Inhibitory neuron

Postsynaptic neuron

(a) Presynaptic inhibition

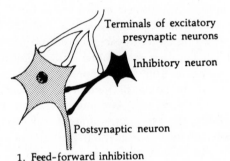

Terminals of excitatory
presynaptic neurons

Inhibitory neuron

Postsynaptic neuron

1. Feed-forward inhibition

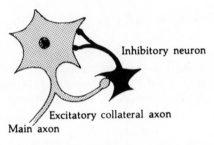

Inhibitory neuron

Excitatory collateral axon

Main axon

2. Feedback inhibition

(b) Postsynaptic inhibition

Figure 17-7. (a) Diagram of presynaptic inhibition. (b) Diagram of postsynaptic inhibition, feedforward and feedback types.

branes reduce their excitability and responsiveness and are called inhibitory postsynaptic potentials (IPSPs); they increase the magnitude of the transmembrane potential. The net inhibitory effect on the postsynaptic neuron depends on the number of such impulses arriving at the various synapses on it, but the overall result tends to be to strongly reduce the responsiveness of the postsynaptic neuron to stimulating impulses coming to it from excitatory synapses. In an IPSP, current flows outward at the synaptic cleft; the ionic correlate of this current flow and altered potential difference across the membrane is the fact that the inhibitory neurotransmitter, GABA, causes channels to open in the postsynaptic membrane which are permeable to K^+ and Cl^- but not to Na^+. Therefore K^+ and Cl^- diffuse out of the cell, increasing the magnitude of the transmembrane potential. Figure 17-7b shows two types of postsynaptic inhibition.

Inhibitory neural pathways may be of either a feedforward or a feedback type. In feedforward inhibition an excitatory presynaptic axon gives off a collateral branch which goes to an inhibitory neuron. In feedback inhibition the postsynaptic neuron itself gives off an excitatory collateral to an inhibitory neuron; this in turn synapses with the cell body of the same postsynaptic neuron. In this case stimulation of the postsynaptic neuron by an excitatory stimulus will then activate inhibition of the same cell; the neuron suppresses its own activity.

Electrotonic Balance Between EPSPs and IPSPs

Whether or not a postsynaptic neuron will reach threshold and initiate a spike potential (nerve impulse) in response to influences from axon terminals impinging on it, depends on the balance between the strengths of the stimulating and the inhibiting forces acting on it. In each neuron in the brain there is a constant fluctuating interaction between stimulating and inhibiting influences from the multitude of axon terminals from other neurons making connections with it; the result is a continuous fluctation in membrane resting potential around the average -75 mV, and therefore a continuous waxing and waning of responsiveness and excitability. As the balance of input shifts in the depolarizing direction, becoming more intensely stimulating, then the neuron initiates repetitive spike potentials; as the balance shifts toward inhibition and hyperpolarization then impulse generation declines and the neuron becomes more quiescent.

Both pre- and postsynaptic inhibition act to modulate the level of excitation and degree of neural firing by influencing the catelectrotonus produced at excitatory synapses. Minor discharges are damped out altogether, and excessively rapid or prolonged neural firing is moderated by inhibitory systems, which serve to shape and direct neural function by appropriate inhibitory anelectrotonus. In many inhibitory neurons, especially in the cerebral cortex, inhibitory transmitter is released at neuron axon terminals by catelectrotonus; that is, depolarization and impulse generation are not essential for many inhibitory neurons to exert their hyperpolarizing, and therefore damping and moderating, effects. It is sufficient if they are partially depolarized by subthreshold stimuli from excitatory neurons; the partial depolarization causes inhibitory transmitter release and a suppression of excessive neural excitability and discharge.

Such tonic inhibitory influences produce enhanced stability of neuron membranes, and promote coherent function of neural systems in the brain and spinal cord. Metabolic and structural abnormalities which interfere with the function of inhibitory neural pathways in the brain predispose to excessive neural excitability and result in the various types of seizure discharges.

The Cerebral Cortex

The cerebral cortex is the outermost layer of the cerebral hemispheres; it is approximately 3–5 mm thick, comprised of gray matter, and contains several billion neurons. There are two main types of neurons in the cortex: (1) the large pyramidal cells whose dendrites form a dense layer of processes at the outermost portion of the cortex (apical dendrites) and whose nerve cell bodies are placed somewhat more deeply in the cortex; and (2) the smaller stellate cells which are of two types, excitatory and inhibitory, and which exert excitatory and inhibitory influences on the dendrites and nerve cell bodies of the pyramidal cells. In addition, axons of nerve cells from deeper structures in the cerebrum, especially the thalamus, enter and leave the cortical layer and make extensive synaptic interconnections with both pyramidal and the two types of stellate cells (Figure 17-8).

Inhibitory synapses on pyramidal cells from the axon terminals of inhibitory stellate cells appear to be located mainly on the somas of the pyramidal cells, and therefore are placed more deeply in the cerebral cortex. Excitatory synapses from the excitatory stellate cells occur primarily on the apical dendrites of the pyramidal cells, and therefore are found at more superficial layers of the cerebral cortex. For this reason, excitatory stimulation of the pyramidal cells of the cerebral cortex occurs mainly in the more superficial areas where the dense masses of apical dendrites are located; in other words, most of the slow electrotonic potentials in the surface layers are EPSPs and therefore electronegative. Conversely, inhibition of neural activity in the pyramidal cells takes place principally in the deeper layers of the cortex where the pyramidal cell bodies are located; i.e., most of the slow electrotonic potentials in the deeper layers are ISPSs and therefore electropositive (Chapter 14, Figure 14-7).

Figure 17-8 is a greatly simplified diagram of (1) a pyramidal cell, with its apical dendrites and more deeply oriented cell body and axon; (2) an afferent axon from the thalamus; (3) inhibitory and excitatory stellate cells; and (4) the interconnections of these various neural elements. The depicted unit is but one of similar millions in the cortex; the units are arranged not only in repeating horizontal arrays but also in repeateing vertical columns. Thus neural activity in the cortex occurs not only in series within each unit, but in parallel, involving huge populations of similar units.

As described earlier, neurons manifest two types of electrical activity: (1) rapid and brief propagated action potentials, which are the conducted nerve impulses; and (2) slow, longer-maintained fluctuations in excitability resulting from the balance between excitatory (EPSPs) and inhibitory (IPSPs) synaptic influences. Normal electrical activity recorded from the surface of the scalp by the EEG (electroenceophalogram) or the pial surface of the cortex by the ECoG (electrocorticogram) is not produced by action potentials (conducted nerve impulses) of individual neurons in the cortex, but rather by the waxing and waning of relative negativity and positivity resulting from postsynaptic potentials (EPSPs and IPSPs) in large masses of dendrites and cell bodies. External electric current flow which can be measured by an EEG can be set up only when electrical potential differences occur between two different regions of entire populations of neurons (for example, between groups of superficial dendrites and groups of deeper cell bodies); or between masses of two different groups of cells (for example, the apical dendrites of a parietal area and the apical dendrites of a frontal site). Therefore, the majority of electrical potentials recorded by the EEG are generated in the most superficial portion of the cerebral hemispheres and are the summations of synchronous and rhythmic multiple partial depolarizations (EPSPs) and hyperpolarizations (IPSPs) in large populations of dendrites and cell bodies.

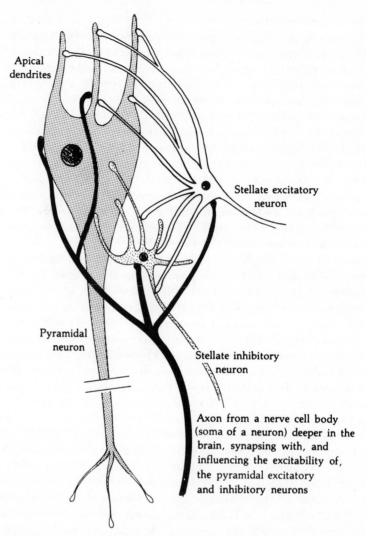

Apical
dendrites

Stellate excitatory
neuron

Pyramidal
neuron

Stellate inhibitory
neuron

Axon from a nerve cell body
(soma of a neuron) deeper in the
brain, synapsing with, and
influencing the excitability of,
the pyramidal excitatory
and inhibitory neurons

Figure 17-8. Diagram of a pyramidal neuron in the cerebral cortex, showing its apical dendrites and deeper cell body and axon; stellate excitatory and inhibitory cells; and the axon from a neuron in lower brain centers projecting to the cerebral cortex. The latter axon synapses with the pyramidal neuron and with both inhibitory and excitatory stellate neurons. The activity in the pyramidal neuron is determined by excitatory and inhibitory influences from the various presynaptic neurons that make contact with it.

SEIZURES, CONVULSIONS, AND EPILEPSY

A seizure may be defined as a sudden transient alteration in mental status, often accompanied by a reduced level of consciousness and convulsive skeletal muscle contractions, resulting from abnormal electrical activity in populations of brain cells. The manifestations of seizure activity in the brain may take the form of paroxysmal loss of consciousness (partial or complete); tonic and/or clonic muscle contraction which is either generalized or occurs in localized areas; periods of behavioral change often associated with diminished awareness of the environment, and amnesia; illusory or hallucinatory sensory manifestations; or alterations in mood and affect.

Seizures of various types may occur occasionally in the course of many general systemic abnormalities such as hypoglycemia, hypoxemia, febrile disorders, endocrine imbalances, drug withdrawal, and other metabolic derangements. They also often are correlated with structural alterations in the brain such as trauma, brain tumor, infarction, and hemorrhage. When a seizure is accompanied by tonic and/or clonic motor activity, either localized or generalized, it is called a convulsion.

The term epilepsy, however, is reserved for a condition in which there are chronically recurring seizures of a similar type over a long period of time; and which appear to be caused by a primary alteration in the excitability of neurons in the brain, rather than occurring secondary to a metabolic or structural abnormality. In true epilepsy it appears that the external manifestations are the consequence of excessive and synchronous discharge of large groups of neurons in the brain. These discharges can usually be recorded in the EEG and many manifest as abnormal patterns in frequency and amplitude of the electrical activity of the cerebral cortex. Each of the various types of epilepsy is correlated with characteristic abnormalities in the EEG. EEG aberrations may appear only during seizures; between-seizure EEGs may or may not be normal. In most cases the causes of these paroxysmal discharges is not known.

Neural Bases of Epilepsy

As has been described previously, in the normal brain a stable balance exists between excitatory and inhibitory synaptic influences on post-synaptic neurons so that areas of excessive depolarization do not develop. However in a portion of the brain which appears to generate abnormal paroxysmal electrical discharge, called an epileptogenic focus, the nerve cells seem to be subjected to an abnormal or imbalanced interplay between excitatory (EPSPs) and inhibitory (IPSPs) synaptic influences. When an epileptogenic focus is produced experimentally in the brain of a laboratory animal, which then goes on to develop recurring seizures of a typical form, measurement of electrical activity in the neurons of that focus show not only characteristic discharges during the seizures, but what are called interictal (between-seizure) spike discharges.

Such interictal spike discharges occur and can be measured and recorded also in patients with epileptogenic foci. The neurons of an epileptogenic focus display an abnormal pattern of electrical activity which is the neural basis for the spike discharge; this electrical change is called a parosysmal depolarization shift (PDS). It appears to be generated by excessive synaptic EPSPs (or inadequate IPSPs) but it is of greater amplitude (about -30 mV) and longer duration than an EPSP. As the PDS develops, the transmembrane electrical potential declines toward threshold and as it does so numerous action potentials are generated in the neurons of the spike focus. But the depolarization increases and persists and as threshold is passed there are no further action potentials but only extreme and prolonged electronegativity which is recorded in the EEG as the epileptogenic spike focus. Electrodes inserted into the cortex of experimental animals with such foci indicate that the negativity is greatest at more superficial levels of the cortex which correspond to the masses of apical dendrites of pyramidal cells described above.

During actual seizure discharge (rather than the interseizure spike discharges) high-amplitude slow waveforms called spike and waves are generated from the cortex. In this case, the spike portion of the spike and wave complex appears to be generated as described above (PDS), but the slow wave portions (which are also negative waves, but slower) between spikes is reported to be the result of IPSPs generated in deeper layers of the cortex occupied by the pyramidal cell bodies. In either case, whether the superficial dendrite portions become strongly electronegative to the deeper cell bodies because of dendritic EPSP's; or whether the deeper soma portions become strongly electropositive with respect to the superficial dendrites because of IPSPs; the electrical current flow measured at the surface by the EEG will still be negative because in both cases the dendrites are negative to the cell bodies, although as a result of two different processes. The spike of the spike and wave complex seen in many seizure EEGs is therefore suggested to result from excessive EPSPs in the apical dendrites while the wave is proposed to develop from excessive IPSPs in the deeper cell bodies.

Deeper structures in the brain, particularly the thalamus and the midbrain, appear also to be involved in not only the initiation of seizure discharges but also in their spread from the site of origin to involve adjacent or even distant brain areas. And some forms of seizures appear to originate and remain localized altogether within brainstem structures, and involve the cortex either not at all or only indirectly or secondarily.

Types of Epilepsy

There is a variety of classification schemes for types of recurring seizure disorders; perhaps the most familiar is that based on the nature of the manifestations occurring during an attack. This is probably a useful scheme because in a seizure the external objective manifestations and the subjective experiences which the patient describes are often characteristic of the areas of the brain involved in the abnormal discharge. In any case, the abnormal discharge may remain localized to the point of origin, it may simultaneously involve the entire brain from the onset, or it may originate in a given area and then generalize to involve a more extensive area or even the whole brain.

Probably a million persons in the United States have recurrent seizures of characteristic form which therefore merit the designation of true epilepsy; incidence rate is highest in early childhood, relatively low between 20 and 70 years, and then rises again in old age. Recurrent seizures are more common in males than females. In most patients no structural leision in the brain can be demonstrated with presently available methods and the cause is usually not known. The role of genetic factors in predisposition to epilepsy remains controversial although most studies indicate that the disorder is familial. Genetic factors appear to be stronger in females and in patients whose epilepsy began in early childhood.

Grand Mal (Generalized Tonic–Clonic Convulsions)

Grand mal is the most familiar and typical form of seizure and occurs at all ages; approximately 90% of patients with epilepsy have attacks of this type. Regardless of the area of the brain in which the discharge originates, it generalizes to involve the entire brain and produces unconsciousness and violent contractions of all the skeletal musculature. The attack usually begins with some type of aura lasting a couple of seconds and often taking the form of weakness, lightheadedness, epigastric sensations or fear; then a vocalization; an abrupt loss of consciousness; and a fall to the ground. The tonic phase is characterized by strong contraction of all musculature; since the extensors are stronger they prevail and so there is rigid extension accompanied by respiratory arrest. Urinary and fecal incontinence may occur. This is followed by the clonic phase in which there is alternating contraction of flexors and extensors producing jerking movements. Respirations resume and are stertorous and irregular. The jerking subsides and consciousness gradually returns. The postictal state is characteristically one of depression, mental confusion, lethargy, headache, weakness and nausea; at times accompanied by neurologic signs of dysphasia, paresis, and paresthesias which may correlate with the brain site of origin of the seizure.

The EEG at onset shows a marked negative deviation followed by a rapid series of high-voltage spikes during the tonic phase. In the clonic phase there are alternating slow waves and spikes, the latter occurring during the clonic jerks. At the end of the clonic phase slow low amplitude activity develops which may persist for long periods. Three quarters of patients with generalized convulsions have abnormal between-seizure EEGs.

It is interesting to note that grand mal seizures may occur at night during sleep and in this case the EEG activity is the same but there is no motor component unless the patient awakens during the seizure whereupon the typical motor convulsions develops.

Most generalized seizures may be reasonably well controlled with diphenylhydantoin and phenobarbital. Occasionally primidone as a substitute for phenobarbital produces better control. Multiple seizures (status epilepticus) are controlled with the benzodiazepine agent diazepam.

Recently, specific receptors (binding sites) for benzodiazepines have been demonstrated in the central nervous system. The number of these receptors in the cerebral cortex increases following experimentally induced seizures in laboratory animals. It is suggested that these membrane binding sites, which appears to mediate the anticonvulsant action of diazepam, may normally be concerned with regulation of nervous excitability and seizure threshold.

Petit Mal

Petit mal is an epilepsy of childhood, more common in females, but since it sometimes persists into adolescence or young adulthood it is mentioned here. On occasion it persists through adult life. Some authors consider that the site of origin of these seizures is in the upper brainstem. The attacks are characterized by transient absences of brief (5–30 sec) duration where loss of contact with the environment occurs. The patient stops what he is doing, stares into space, and may also show eye blinking, facial twitches, arm jerking, or head nodding. The attacks vary from 5 to more than 100 per day. The disorder tends to clear after adolescence. Attention and concentration tend to prevent the attacks and relaxed drowsiness enhances them; they are more frequent on awakening in the morning. They may also be brought on by flickering lights and hyperventilation.

Petit mal seizures are associated with a characteristic EEG pattern of 3 cps high-voltage spike and wave complexes; the interictal EEG is usually normal. Patients with petit mal are of normal or high intelligence and without psychologic disturbances; there is almost never a history of any sort of brain trauma or infection. Control is usually achieved with ethosuximide or trimethadione.

Focal (Partial) Epilepsy

The seizure disorder known as focal epilepsy is most commonly seen in patients with a structural lesion of the cerebral cortex caused by a head injury, brain infection, brain tumor, vascular lesion, birth trauma, or perinatal hypoxia. The lesion may be in any of the lobes of the cortex and may be macroscopic or microscopic.

This disorder often begins with a subclinical epileptogenic spike focus, that is, an EEG abnormality which takes the form of single or multiple spike discharges sometimes followed by a slow wave. Later it may evolve into a focal motor or sensory seizure disorder with overt manifestations. The classical jacksonian seizure is characteristic of focal or partial epilepsy. Where the lesion is in a motor area of the cortex the seizure may begin with a convulsive twitching of fingers of one arm and then spread proximately to the hand, wrist, arm, face, and then the leg on the same side. This progression is called the jacksonian march. If the lesion is in a cortical sensory area then there may be a similar march of sensations such as numbness or tingling of a hand which then spreads in like fashion. In either case the focal seizure may generalize; that is, it spreads to the remainder of the brain on the same side and then across the subcortical structures to the opposite side, at which time the patient loses consciousness and the seizures resembles a grand mal attack.

The EEG during the actual seizure, if it remains focal, shows a series of spike discharges which increase in amplitude; if the seizure generalizes, then the EEG shows the sequence described above for a generalized convulsion. After the clinical seizure subsides there is EEG slowing and flattening which may be correlated with a localized muscle paralysis (Todd's paralysis) indicating the site of origin of the seizure discharge.

Management of focal epilepsy involves suppression of seizure discharge with diphenylhydantoin (now called phenytoin) or mesantoin and phenobarbital.

Psychomotor Epilepsy (Anterior Temporal Lobe Seizure, Limbic Epilepsy)

Psychomotor epilepsy is one special type of focal seizure or partial epilepsy which involves the temporal lobe and the portions of the limbic system (Chapter 14) which underlie it: the hippocampus and amygdala. The disorder occurs most commonly in adults, but is associated in almost two thirds of patients with a structural lesion of the anterior temporal lobe and deeper limbic structures, and a history of head trauma or a brain infection such as encephalitis. The seizures themselves most commonly take the form of alterations of mental function, mood, and affect, and abnormal behavior and motor activity rather than convulsions. In most of these patients there is an interictal EEG abnormality consisting of a negatieve spike focus, often alternating with slow waves, in the anterior temporal lobe; it is most active during sleep. These anterior temporal lobe spikes are persistent, tend not to clear up with advancing age as other focal seizure activity often does, and in fact may become bilateral owing to the development of a "mirror focus" on the contralateral side.

The actual psychomotor seizure often begins with an aura involving visceral sensations such as epigastric distress which ascends into the throat, feelings of dread or anxiety, or hallucinations and illusions. This is succeeded by altered levels of consciousness but not actual unconsciousness, and a change in mental status and emotions: feelings of depersonalization, compulsive thoughts, rage attacks, or déjà vu. Automatic bizarre motor behavior may accompany or follow and take the form of oral activity (lipsmacking, chewing); walking, running, or dancing; fighting; shouting or singing; and other stereotyped activity for which there is usually amnesia following the attack. In many patients the seizure generalizes into a grand mal convulsion. The focal attacks may last seconds to hours.

Many patients with psychomotor epilepsy have psychiatric disorders of various types, and it is said to be not uncommon that when the actual seizures are controlled by anticonvulsant medication the psychoemotional difficulties become more pronounced. It has also been reported by many workers that patients with psychomotor epilepsy are markedly hyposexual or even asexual as far as drive and activity are concerned and that when it is possible for the focal lesion in the brain to be removed surgically, postoperative hypersexuality and compulsive sexual activity may develop and persist. Temporal lobe epilepsy may prove difficult to control; diphenylhydantoin and primidone are the customary drugs.

Diencephalic Seizures

Diencephalic seizures are a sensory experience considered by some authors to be a very common form of epilepsy, while other workers do not categorize it as a class of epilepsy at all, perhaps because the EEG typically remains normal (beta, LVF) during the episodes. Persons with these experiences typically show a characteristic form of EEG sleep pattern called 14 and 6 cps positive spikes (in contrast with other EEG seizure abnormalities in which the spike discharges are negative).

Diencephalic seizures are said to originate in the thalamus and hypothalamus, which are the two brain areas making up the diencephalon (at the uppermost portion of the brainstem). This area encircles the central or periventricular gray matter and surrounds the third ventricle deep in the center of the brain. These areas are intimately concerned, along with the limbic system, with the regulation of mood and affect, visceral and vegetative functions, and sensations.

Diencephalic epilepsy is not a convulsive disorder but rather one involving (1) visceral symptoms and signs: headache, vertigo, nausea and vomiting, diaphoresis, altered rate and rhythm of respirations, and increased rate and force of heart beat; and (2) emotional and instinctual experiences: fear, rage, laughing, crying, and profound negative affect or dread.

Although reported to be very common in children and adolescents, especially those with allergies and duodenal ulcer, it also may occur in adults. It is said often to affect several family members.

REFERENCES

Beeson PB and McDermott W, editors; *Textbook of Medicine*. 14th ed. Philadelphia, Pa.: Saunders, 1975.

Ganong WF: *Review of Medical Physiology*, 8th ed. Los Altos, Calif.: Lange Medical Publications, 1977.

Goldensohn ES and Appel SH, editors: *Scientific Approaches to Clinical Neurology*, 2 vols. Philadelphia, Pa.: Lea & Febiger, 1977.

Guyton AC: *Textbook of Medical Physiology*. 5th ed. Philadelphia, Pa.: Saunders, 1976.

Laidlaw JP: *A Textbook of Epilepsy*. New York: Churchill Livingstone, 1976.

Matthews WB: *Practical Neurology*, 3rd ed. London: Blackwell Scientific Publications, 1975.

Merritt HH: *A Textbook of Neurology*, 5th ed. Philadelphia, Pa.: Lea and Febiger, 1973.

Möhler, H and Okada T: Benzodiazepine receptor: Demonstration in the central nervous system. *Science* 198:849–851, 1977.

Paul SM and Skolnick P: Rapid changes in brain benzodiaepine receptor after experimental seizures. *Science* 202:892–894, 1978.

Sands H: *The Epilepsy Fact Book*. Philadelphia, Pa.: Davis, 1977.

Solomon GE and Plum F: *Clinical Management of Seizures*. Philadelphia, Pa.: Saunders, 1976.

Thorn GW, et al., editors: *Harrison's Principles of Internal Medicine*, 8th ed. New York: McGraw-Hill, 1977.

CHAPTER EIGHTEEN

Cerebrovascular Disease

BLOOD SUPPLY TO THE BRAIN

Arteries and Veins

The brain receives its arterial supply from two sources: the two internal carotid arteries, and the two vertebral arteries; the latter join to form the basilar artery. The circle of Willis, at the base of the brain, is derived from the internal carotids and the basilar, and in turn gives off the six major arteries which supply the brain: the two anterior, two middle, and two posterior, cerebral arteries. These vessels and their relationships are diagramed in Figures 18-1, 18-2, and 18-3.

Blood flow through the brain is about 800 ml/min; of the approximately 75 ml ejected from the left ventricle at each contraction, 15 ml goes to the brain; two thirds of the cardiac output destined to supply the brain enters it through the internal carotid system and one third via the vertebral–basilar system.

At the angle of the jaw the common carotids divide into the internal and external carotids; the latter then ascend in the neck behind the pharynx and pass through the cavernous sinuses in the region of the pituitary gland and sella tur-

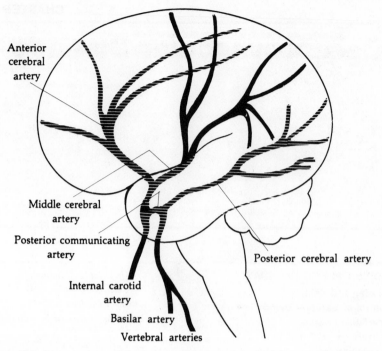

Figure 18-1. Major arteries of the brain. Diagram is of the lateral aspect of a hemisphere. The vessels shown in solid lines lie on the lateral surface of the hemisphere; the vessels shown in broken lines lie along the medial surface.

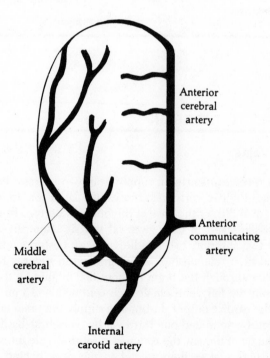

Figure 18-2. Frontal aspect of a cerebral hemisphere showing the major branches of the carotid system.

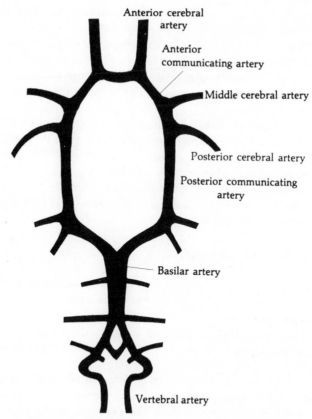

Figure 18-3. The circle of Willis and its major branches.

cica. Then, after giving off the ophthalmic arteries, the external carotids divide into the anterior and middle cerebral arteries. This internal carotid system supplies the eyes and the frontal, parietal, and portions of the temporal lobes.

The two vertebrals, after branching from the two subclavians, ascend toward the head in bony canals (foramina) through the transverse processes on each side of the cervical vertebrae (C6 through C1); they enter the cranial cavity through the foramen magnum, give off branches to the cerebellum, and at the area between the medulla and pons, fuse to form the basilar artery. After giving off a number of branches the basilar artery divides into the two posterior cerebral arteries at the midbrain. The posterior cerebral arteries supply a portion of the thalamus, the brainstem, the acoustic and vestibular structures, the cerebellum, and the upper area of the spinal cord.

There are a number of anastomoses between the carotid and the vertebral–basilar systems which serve to some extent to protect the brain from ischemia in the event of damage to, or gradual obstruction within, one of the major arteries. These interconnections are (1) partially extracranial (between the external carotids and the vertebrals); (2) partly intracranial (within the circle of Willis which connects carotid and vertebral–basilar systems and the right and left carotid supply); and (3) external-to-internal ramifications occurring mainly in the area of the eye and orbit. The anastomoses provide for alternate routes and collateral pathways of bloodflow should flow in a major pathway be compromised. Nevertheless in the normal intact subject these anastomotic channels do not provide for a very large flow, and there is usually little crossing over of blood between right and left internal carotid systems. When, for example, in studies attempting to explore the lateralization of various brain functions between right and left cerebral hemispheres, sodium amytal is injected into the right carotid, it is right cerebral function which becomes briefly impaired; function in the left hemisphere remains intact.

Venous drainage of blood from the brain is accomplished mainly by two large groups of venous channels which lie between layers of the dura: (1) the superior–posterior group of five dural sinuses, which include the superior and inferior sagittal sinuses; and (2) the anterior–inferior group of four paired sinuses, including the cavernous sinuses. Most of the blood from the major sinuses enters the internal jugular veins which descend in the neck together with the internal carotid arteries and the vagus nerves.

Control of Cerebral Blood Flow

The three major factors determining total cerebral blood flow are (1) the perfusion pressure to the brain; (2) the resistance in the cerebral blood vessels; and (3) intracranial pressure.

Perfusion Pressure

The perfusion pressure to an organ is determined by the pressure drop across the vessels of that organ; that is, perfusion pressure is the blood pressure in the arteries entering the organ, minus the pressure in the veins draining it. The greater the arterial pressure, and the lower the venous pressure, the higher the perfusion pressure and the greater the blood flow in the structure. As pressure in the arteries entering the organ declines, or pressure in the veins draining it rises, then perfusion pressure and hence blood flow to the organ will fall, other factors equal. In other words, the greater the pressure drop across the vasculature of the brain, the greater the blood flow to and through it.

The most important factor determining cerebral perfusion pressure is the pressure in the major arteries, especially the carotid arteries, supplying the brain. The pressure in the veins draining the brain approximates central venous pressure; in the normal subject this value is around 5 mmHg and tends to remain stable. It becomes elevated under conditions which increase intrathoracic pressure, such as the expiratory phase of respirations in severe emphysema or an asthmatic attack; and in circumstances where ventricular end-diastolic volume and pressure is increased, such as congestive heart failure. Therefore in normal subjects cerebral arterial pressure is the principal factor in determining perfusion pressure of the brain. Cerebral arterial pressure, in turn, is determined by circulating blood volume, systemic arterial blood pressure, and total peripheral resistance (systemic vasodilation or vasoconstriction). The pressure receptors at the bifurcation of the common carotids and in the aortic arch serve an important function in regulating the blood pressure of the systemic circulation as well as that of the arteries supplying the head (Chapters 3 and 13).

In spite of the known significant function of perfusion pressure in the regulation of total blood flow through most organs, in the case of the brain, studies of the cerebral blood flow indicate that there is a remarkably constant blood flow over a very wide range of perfusion pressures. Some reports indicate constant levels of cerebral blood flow with systemic arterial pressures from a low of around 70 or 80 mmHg to as high as 160 mmHg or more. This indicates that in the case of the brain there are processes in addition to perfusion pressure, or blood pressure in the arteries supplying it, which play an even more critical role in determining cerebral blood flow. That factor appears to be cerebral vascular resistance—the relative degree of vasoconstriction or vasodilation of the vessels within the brain itself.

Cerebrovascular Resistance

The regulation of cerebrovascular resistance in the brain occurs mainly at the level of the smaller arteries and arterioles which arise from the larger more superficial arteries and actually penetrate the brain substance itself. These small vessels are innervated both by parasympathetic cholinergic vasodilator and by sympathetic adrenergic vasoconstrictor fibers. But unlike the important function of vasodilator and vasoconstrictor fibers in regulating both systemic arterial pressure and blood flow through most organs and tissues, there is little evidence that neural vasomotor reflex regulation is a significant factor in controlling cerebrovascular resistance. Rather, the major factors influencing the diameter and tone of small arteries and arterioles in the brain are myogenic (autoregulation) and chemical (CO_2, pH, O_2) influences. These two factors may be closely related.

Autoregulation

Autoregulation is the process whereby blood flow through an organ is maintained within a given normal range by changes in vascular tone (degree of constriction or dilation) in response to variations in perfusion pressure. The blood vessels in the brain appear to respond to an increased intravascular pressure (which would elevate cerebral blood flow above optimum levels) by direct active vasoconstriction, which promptly reduces cerebral blood flow. Conversely, a reduction in perfusion pressure (which would reduce cerebral blood flow to below optimum levels) seems directly to induce a decrease in vessel smooth muscle tone, and results in vasodilation which compensatorily improves cerebral blood flow. Therefore increased pressure induces vasoconstriction, and decreased pressure induces vasodilation. This is considered to be a direct myogenic response, that is, an inherent quality of smooth muscle by which adaptive changes in muscle tone are induced by altered intravascular pressures.

Chemical Influences

CO_2 has a strong direct effect on cerebral arteries and arterioles: increased CO_2 causes cerebral vasodilation, a decline in cerebral vascular resistance, and increased cerebral blood flow. A decreased pH has a similar effect, and it is possible that the effect of CO_2 on cerebral blood flow is mediated indirectly via the lowered pH resulting from elevated CO_2. Conversely, decreased CO_2 or increased pH leads to vasoconstriction and decreased cerebral blood flow. In spite of the decreased cerebral blood flow resulting from the hypocapnia and respiratory alkalemia of hyperventilation (produced by mechanical ventilation, for example, in the treatment of cerebral edema from head trauma; see Chapter 2) still there is little reduction in cerebral oxygen consumption even at a $Paco_2$ of about 20 mmHg, which is reported to reduce cerebral blood flow to half of normal. O_2 levels have a reversed and milder effect on brain blood vessels, low O_2 causing vasodilation and increased cerebral blood flow, and high O_2 a slight vasoconstriction. These influences of CO_2, O_2, and pH on cerebral vasomotor tone are adaptive in that they tend to adjust cerebral blood flow to meet metabolic requirements of the brain.

Intracranial Pressure

Since changes in intracranial pressure occur within a nonexpansible structure, the skull, conditions which produce elevated intracranial pressure, such as cerebral edema, hydrocephalus, or brain tumor, tend to compress the cerebral vessels and cause obstruction within, first, the low pressure veins and sinuses which drain blood from the brain, and later, at increased pressures, the arterial inflow. Therefore as intracranial pressure rises, the consequence is a reduction in perfusion pressure and cerebral blood flow via two changes: elevated outflow pressure and decreased inflow pressure. Elevated intracranial pressure and cerebral edema are discussed in Chapter 14.

Brain Oxygen Requirements

Adequate O_2 supply to the brain is crucial for its normal function. O_2 consumption of brain tissue accounts for about 20% of basal whole-body O_2 consumption, and averages approximately 45 ml/min. Occlusion of the blood supply to the brain as a whole results in EEG abnormalities within a second or two, and unconsciousness within just a few more. Unlike skeletal muscle and some other tissues, O_2 is not stored by neurons and in cardiac arrest, for example, cerebral O_2 supply consists only of that bound to Hb within the capillaries of the brain. Total brain blood volume is reported to be about 75 ml with an oxygen content of only slightly over 10 ml (20 ml O_2 /100 ml fully oxygenated blood); this O_2 would be depleted within slightly over 10 sec after failure of blood flow to brain tissue. Therefore unconsciousness results promptly following arrest of the circulation.

Since the higher brain centers in the cerebral cortex, basal ganglia, and thalamus are less resistant to O_2 deprivation than the brainstem, which controls visceral function, a period of hypoxemia may result in an abolition of all higher mental functions, and severe motor and sensory abnormalities, while the vegetative functions may continue to maintain "life" indefinitely.

Brain ischemia (and therefore hypoxia) localized to specific areas results in focal necrosis (infarction) of brain tissue, and neurological deficits corresponding to the functions served by the destroyed area are the consequence. In addition, both localized and generalized brain hypoxia cause abnormalities in the ability of the brain capillaries and neurons to regulate the passage of ions and water across their membranes, so that focal or generalized cerebral edema is the inevitable result of severe ischemia and hypoxia.

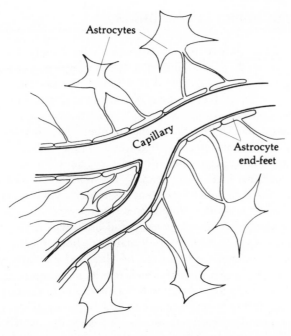

Figure 18-4. Diagram of a longitudinal section of a brain capillary showing the capillary membrane invested with the end feet of astrocytes, which form a protective layer around the capillary, and also wrap around neuron cell bodies (not shown).

Brain Capillaries: The Blood–Brain Barrier

Water, O_2 and CO_2 are the only substances which cross the membranes of brain capillaries with facility in the adult; essentially all other ions and molecules including glucose and Na^+, K^+, and HCO_3^- traverse these membranes much more slowly than those of capillaries elsewhere in the body, and large numbers of substances gain only minimal access to brain tissue. The blood–brain barrier, therefore, is not a special series of structures; the term merely refers to the restrictive permeability characteristics of brain capillaries. They permit ready permeation into the brain of a very limited number of substances; and only slow and limited penetration to a large number of other substances, which are able to cross the capillary membranes of most organs with ease. One of the reasons for this is that the individual cells that make up the capillary membranes of the brain are bound tightly together.

Brain capillaries have another histologic uniqueness which correlates with their special physiologic qualities. Capillaries lie in close proximity to neuron cell bodies; astrocytes join the capillaries to the neurons by means of cell extensions which are wrapped around both capillaries and neurons. These so-called astrocyte end-feet are so numerous that they form a continuous membrane which invests all brain capillaries; it is thought that these structures regulate the flow of substances both ways across the capillary membranes.

VASCULAR DISORDERS OF THE BRAIN

Cerebrovascular disease is common—the most frequent of all neurologic disorders of adults. It is predominantly the consequence of atherosclerosis and/or hypertension. The culmination of cerebrovascular disease is the stroke, which is defined as the rapid development of focal neurologic abnormalities that persist for variable periods of time, as a result of cerebrovascular disease. Evidence indicates that in the United States the number of strokes has markedly declined over the past 25 years, perhaps because of dietary changes, early detection and better control of hypertension, decreased cigaret smoking among the middle-aged, and perhaps increased exercise. The range of severity of strokes is wide, from a minor and relatively transient neurologic symptom or sign (such as darkening of vision; numbness, tingling or weakness of an extremity or one side of the face; or staggering gait) to widespread brain damage leading to coma, loss of motor and sensory function, and ultimately to brain death.

Vascular diseases of the brain can be classified into two main categories. The first category is vascular disease which results in ischemia and infarction of brain tissue; the two principal causes of this type are atherosclerotic thrombus formation in brain arteries, and emboli to the brain usually originating in the left heart. The second category of vascular disease is that which leads to intracranial hemorrhage; in this type there are three main causes: hypertensive vascular disease, in which bleeding is more often into the brain parenchyma itself, that is, it is most often intracerebral; rupture of a saccular aneurysm, which tends to cause subarachnoid bleeding; and rupture of an arteriovenous malformation, which may cause bleeding into either brain parenchyma or the subarachnoid space or both.

About three fourths of strokes are of the ischemia and infarction type, from thrombi or emboli; while approximately a quarter result from intracranial hemorrhage. Of infarction strokes, about 90% are caused by atherothrombosus and 10% by emboli. Of hemorrhagic strokes, over half result from hypertensive vascular disease, about a quarter are caused by rupture of a saccular aneurysm, and perhaps 8% from arteriovenous malformations; the remainder result from neoplasms and other disorders. In some cases no cause for the bleeding can be discerned. If strokes from all causes are combined, the types break down into the following approximate percentages: atherothrombosus 65%; embolism 10%; intracerebral hemorrhage 15%; and subarachnoid hemorrhage 10%.

Ischemia and Infarction

Most instances of ischemia and infarction of the brain result from cerebral atherosclerosis and thrombus formation; the minority are caused by emboli. Interruption of the blood supply to an area of the brain (ischemia) that lasts for 30 sec or more produces a marked alteration in neuron metabolism because of O_2 deprivation. If the blood flow resumes promptly at this ischemic stage, neuron metabolism is restored, CO_2 and lactic acid (from anaerobic metabolism) that accumulated during the decreased blood flow is removed by reperfusion, O_2 supply resumes, and neuron function returns to normal after a variable period, depending on the duration and degree of ischemic hypoxia. If blood flow is not restored within 60 sec, however, neuron metabolism and function may cease;

and after a very few minutes irreversible hypoxic neuron damage occurs (infarction).

Atherosclerotic Thrombosus

Underlying Abnormalities

The process of cerebrovascular atherosclerosis probably begins at an early age with the development of the fatty streak, which consists of deposits of lipid material below the endothelium of cerebral vessels. It is observed at autopsy in infants and children dying of other causes, and is thought by many workers to represent the early stages of atherosclerotic cardiovascular and cerebrovascular disease. With the passage of time, the fatty material increases, the inner intimal layer thickens, and the vessel lumen narrows. Eventually fibrous tissue develops in the area of the lesion, causing irregularities in the intima which may become disrupted leading to bleeding and an ulcerated defect in the vessel lining. The structural and biochemical abnormalities of the vessel lining predispose to the development of mural thrombi; with deposition of fibrin, cholesterol, clumps of platelets, and ultimately calcium. These abnormal collections of material cause progressive narrowing of the lumen via thrombosis and portions may become unstable and break off to form emboli. Therefore actual vascular occlusion sufficient to cause neurologic signs and symptoms may occur either because of clot formation at the site of an ulcerated atherosclerotic lesion in the inner vessel wall, or the shedding of emboli from such a clot which promote platelet aggregation and occlude arteries distal to the lesion. The prevalence of the lesions increases with age and is similar in males and females, although the ulcerations and calcifications are more prominent in men. The atheromatous process appears to be greatly accelerated in patients with hypertension and/or diabetes mellitus: it begins earlier and progresses more rapidly.

These atheromatous plaques occur most commonly at vessel bifurcations and where vessels curve sharply. They occur in the carotid system more than the vertebral–basilar system; in the extracranial arteries much more than the intracranial; and among the intracranial ones, they affect the larger superficial vessels of the brain more than the smaller ones which penetrate into brain parenchyma. In the carotid system the most frequent site is in the internal carotid at the bifurcation near the carotid sinus; in the vertebral–basilar system a prominent location is the point at which the vertebrals join to become the basilar. The anterior, middle and to a lesser extent posterior cerebral arteries are also commonly affected at their branchings and curves.

There appears to be a strong relationship between both organic heart disease and hypertension, and cerebrovascular disease and infarction. Hypertension is known to accelerate atherosclerosis, but in addition it may play the role of precipitating factor in some strokes. A period of rapid elevation of blood pressure, such as occurs during REM (dreaming) periods when the patient is asleep (many strokes occur during sleep); or such as occur during sudden exertion or straining; is suggested by some workers to induce a sudden autoregulative vasoconstriction of brain vessels. If the constriction occurs in a vascular tree which has multifocal organic narrowing, then the resulting pressure drop could be enough to cause ischemia and infarction.

In the case of heart disease, impaired myocardial performance from organic heart disease is known to be present in perhaps half of the patients who sustain a brain infarction. Moreover, following an infarction, reports indicate that in as many as half of such patients heart disease will be the actual cause of death. The way in which heart disease contributes to the brain ischemia and infarction is proposed by some authors to be: episodes of lowered cardiac output, which result in periodic marked hypotension and greatly decreased cerebral perfusion, culminating in ischemia and infarction. The reduced output may result from a run of arrhythmias, congestive heart failure, or a myocardial infarction. As is the case with hypertension, it is suggested that the combination of a hypotensive episode and a focally organically narrowed vasculature together lower perfusion pressure to the brain; the decline may be so large that autoregulative compensation is unable to maintain a cerebral blood flow adequate to prevent ischemia and infarction.

Increasing evidence indicates that a major proportion of brain ischemic events and infarctions result from emboli originating in atheromatous lesions in the large arteries supplying the brain. Such emboli may be comprised of debris which has broken off of an atheroma, or a platelet–fibrin complex formed there; these may travel in the bloodstream to lodge in a smaller more distal artery; there it may stimulate platelet aggregation and thrombus formation. In addition, when platelets aggregate they release vasoactive chemicals; these may cause spasm of arterioles sufficient to produce a critical drop in perfusion pressure across the affected vessels with resulting infarction.

Clinical Manifestations

Studies show that individuals with certain characteristics are more predisposed to strokes than others; among the conditions demonstrated to be associated with clinically evident strokes are a history of transient ischemic attacks; hypertension; organic heart disease; other evidences of atherosclerosis such as claudication, angina, and arterial bruits; impaired glucose tolerance or overt diabetes mellitus; elevated blood lipids (although the relationship of hyperlipidemia to strokes is less marked than it is to myocardial infarction); and cigaret smoking.

Transient Ischemic Attacks (TIAs). *Types.* This term is applied to neurologic signs and symptoms resulting from cerebrovascular insufficiency which resolve completely within 12 hr or less without residual effects; most last from a few seconds to 5 or 10 min. They are much more common in males than females, and in hypertensive persons. The symptoms during a TIA depend upon what portion of the brain is ischemic, but there are two main types, those involving the cerebral hemispheres (cartoid TIAs) and those involving the brainstem (vertebrobasilar TIAs). Carotid TIAs are often characterized by impairment of vision, temporary or monocular blindness on the side of the affected artery, or by paresis or paresthesias of the face or one or both extremities of the opposite side. Vertebral–basilar TIAs often manifest as dysarthria, dysphasia, ataxia, dizziness or vertigo, blurred vision, visual field defects, or diplopia, paresis and paresthesias, or brief loss of consciousness—in various combinations. Commonly patients may have manifestations typical of both types.

Causes. The changes in the brain circulation responsible for producing TIAs is still the subject of speculation. There are three theories; the processes described by each may interact to produce the attacks, so that each may play a part in the cause, or the processes may be different in carotid and vertebral TIAs, or different from patient to patient. (1) The oldest theory suggests that some factor, such as momentarily elevated blood pressure, produces an autoregulative vasospasm which in a normal vasculature would be without effect, but in vessels organically narrowed by atherosclerosis results in localized perfusion defects to specific areas of the brain. (2) A second theory suggests that a periodic focal reduction in perfusion pressure to a portion of the brain, perhaps resulting from a momentary decline in cardiac output or elevated central venous pressure, could combine with the organic vessel narrowing and an inadequate collateral blood flow to produce temporary neurologic signs and symptoms. (3) A newer theory suggests that formation and dissemination of microemboli, comprised of platelets, fibrin, or plaque fragments released from areas of atherosclerotic lesions, produce a temporary reduction of blood flow; microemboli may promote platelet aggregation in a given vascular territory sufficient to cause reversible deficits. In support of this theory is the observation that in patients with TIAs, emboli can sometimes be seen in retinal vessels on funduscopic examination. In addition to the mechanical obstruction produced by platelet aggregates, vascular spasm occurs in response to the release of vasoactive chemicals such as serotonin and prostaglandins from activated platelets.

A recent study of the effects of two antiplatelet agents, aspirin and sulfinpyrazone, alone or in combination, on TIAs, stroke, and death, reports that aspirin but not sulfinpyrazone significantly reduces risk of all three events. These data support platelet microembolic phenomena as a significant causative process in TIAs and strokes.

Other causes of TIAs are two conditions which are known to produce decreased cerebral perfusion in the vertebral–basilar system and to be associated with brief loss of consciousness and other symptoms and signs of brainstem ischemia. These two conditions are subclavian steal syndrome and the vertebral–basilar insufficiency associated with cervical spondylosis. In the most frequently occurring form of the subclavian steal syndrome there is an atherosclerotic narrowing of the left subclavian artery between its takeoff from the aorta and the origin of the left vertebral artery. This partial subclavian stenosis produces a marked pressure drop in the portion of the subclavian distal to the lesion and at the point where the vertebral artery arises. The lowered pressure produces an intermittent reversal of flow in the vertebral artery; instead of blood flowing from vertebral to basilar to brainstem, flow reverses along the pressure gradient: blood is drawn from the brain down the basilar and vertebral arteries into the subclavian artery and then to the left arm. The stenosis of the subclavian is partial, so the symptoms may appear only with muscular exercise in the arms. A delay and decreased amplitude in the left radial artery compared to the right with exertion or a change in arm position in a patient with symptoms of brainstem ischemia point to subclavian steal syndrome as a possible cause (Chapter 16, Figure 16-2).

Cervical spondylosis (degenerative joint disease or osteoarthritis of the cervical spine) may produce narrowing of, and encroachment of osteophytes (bony spurs) into the foramina in the cervical vertebrae through which the vertebral arteries ascend to the head. The result is impeded blood flow to the brainstem, especially with turning of the head, which may be sufficient to produce loss of consciousness or other symptoms and signs of ischemia in the vertebral–basilar circuit. It is a form of vertebral–basilar syndrome, and its effects would be expected to be more severe in a situation where there is widespread atherosclerotic cerebrovascular disease. TIAs caused by cervical spondylosis can sometimes be induced by tilting the head back and then turning the head from side to side (Chapter 16).

Assessment. Patient assessment in complaints which could be interpreted as those of TIAs has two components. The first involves initial steps to distinguish TIAs from conditions which may mimic them and to assess the contribution of systemic abnormalities to their occurrence: cardiac arrhythmias, carotid sinus hypersensitivity, seizures, hypoglycemia, vasovagal syncope, vestibular disorders causing vertigo, Valsalva effects, and so on (Chapter 16).

The second component of assessment in suspected TIAs is other signs and symptoms which may indicate systemic atherosclerotic disease: diminished arterial pulses, the presence of arterial bruits, funduscopic abnormalities, and signs and symptoms or a history of hypertension, organic heart disease, and diabetes mellitus. Cerebral angiography constitutes the definitive evaluation for cerebrovascular disease; it should not be undertaken unless there are strong indications since there is significant morbidity and mortality.

Management. The important aspect of management in TIAs is the attempt to prevent a stroke: control of hypertension, congestive heart failure and/or diabetes mellitus, if present; weight loss and a low fat and cholesterol diet; cessation of smoking; and a graded exercise program after careful diagnostic workup. Vascular surgery is appropriate for some patients.

Studies have indicated that about 5% of persons per year with TIAs will go on to have strokes. The prospective randomized, double-blind trial of aspirin and sulfinpyrazone in patients with threatened stroke conducted by the Canadian Cooperative Study Group revealed that in 585 men and women patients with a history of TIAs, aspirin (but not sulfinpyrazone) 350 mg four times per day reduced the risk of continued TIAs, strokes, and death by 19% and lowered the risk of stroke and death by 31% in an over two-year study period. In males the reduction in stroke or death was 48%, while in females there was no significant effect. Other studies have shown that vasodilators have no, and anticoagulants have questionable, preventive effect in such stroke-prone persons.

Progressing Stroke. This is the term applied to the gradually developing motor, sensory, and other neurologic deficits during a period of several hours from the first onset of symptoms to the point where neurologic deterioration ceases and the patient stabilizes. In the great majority of patients the development of major deficits is preceded for hours, days, or even weeks, by a series of TIAs or by other manifestations: mental confusion, headache, dizziness, or drowsiness. In most patients the onset of the actual thrombotic occlusion is abrupt and the neurologic changes reach their maximum within a few minutes or hours; they may involve several body parts simultaneously, and include paralysis, sen-

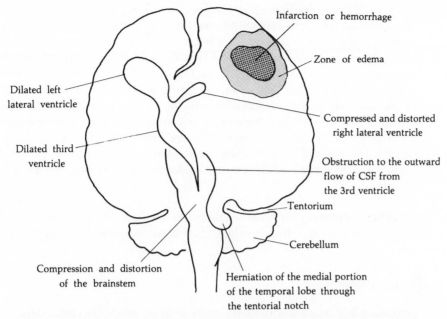

Figure 18-5. Coronal section of brain with right hemisphere cerebral infarction and large surrounding zone of edema producing displacement of brain structures, compression and distortion of brain stem, and obstruction of drainage of cerebrospinal fluid from the lateral and third ventricles. Obstruction to the ventricular system causes CSF to accumulate in them (hydrocephalus), further elevating intracranial pressure.

sory loss, and speech defects. Conversely, they may begin with just one area such as a hand, leg, or side of the face and then evolve, progressively involving more body parts and functions. The kind and severity of neurologic deficits which develop depend on the vascular territory involved and the functions subserved by it.

In addition to the focal neurologic deficits resulting from the ischemic destruction of brain tissue, widespread brain abnormalities result from the cerebral edema which is the inevitable accompaniment to ischemic brain damage. Capillaries lose their selective permeability, and ECF enters the brain interstitial spaces in large quantities. The result is swelling of the affected hemisphere and resulting distortion of intracranial structures. Intracranial pressure becomes elevated and this has two effects: it impairs blood supply to the brain and venous drainage from it, resulting in vascular congestion and further ischemia; and it impedes the normal circulation and resorption of cerebrospinal fluid, so that acute hydrocephalus may develop. This is a vicious cycle because it leads to further vascular congestion, cerebral edema and elevated intracranial pressure (Chapter 14). Eventually the increased pressure compresses the brainstem vital and consciousness centers producing alterations of heart rate, blood pressure, and respiration, and deepening coma.

A stepwise intermittent stroke progression may sometimes go on for several days or even weeks. Generalized signs and symptoms accompanying a progressing stroke may include seizures, headache, vomiting, and coma. Serious complications often occurring during this active evolution of the stroke are severe cerebral edema, elevated intracranial pressure, and brain herniation; management of this stage importantly includes measures to control these often fatal complications. Heparin appears to slow the neurologic deterioration in some instances, but is reported not to influence mortality; adrenal glucocorticoids and oral glycerol, mannitol, or urea; and hypothermia and hyperventilation; may be used to control cerebral edema though their effectiveness has been questioned.

The area of infarction first softens (encephalomalacia). If blood flow is restored to the infarcted area as a result of breakdown or migration of the thrombus then bleeding into the softened tissue may occur. Liquefaction of the infarcted area eventually develops and phagocytes remove most of the debris, leaving a cavity which contains fluid, proliferating blood vessels, glia, and fibrous scar tissue. Such scars may occasionally become epileptogenic foci and initiate a seizure disorder.

Completed Stroke. Optimal rehabilitation and prevention of new strokes (as discussed above) are the important considerations once the patient's condition has stabilized.

Brain Embolism

Embolism is a much less frequent cause of brain infarction than is atherothrombosus. Embolic occlusion of an artery can of course occur in the presence of a normal cerebral vasculature, but if atherosclerotic cerebrovascular disease is present it is likely that an embolus might have more widespread consequences because of already-present areas of marginal perfusion. Most brain emboli develop in the heart; but fat from long bone fracture or lipid tissue trauma, air from lung injury, septic masses from a focus of infection, or fragments of atherosclerotic lesions may embolize to the brain. These emboli then travel until they become lodged at an arterial bifurcation or a site of luminal narrowing and cause focal ischemia and infarction within the tissue supplied by the occluded vessel. The damage will be larger and more complete if the area has poor collateral circulation from adjoining vessels.

Most brain emboli have their origin in the heart. The nonpropulsive turbulence set up by atrial fibrillation promotes clot formation in the left atrium with eventual flow to the left ventricle and brain. Myocardial infarction predisposes to the development of mural thrombi which then embolize, and bacterial endocarditis leads to the formation of multiple septic emboli.

Embolic occlusion of a vessel leads to signs, symptoms, and changes in the brain which are similar to those caused by atherothrombosus, but of all strokes the neurologic deficits of embolic ones are said to evolve most rapidly into the definitive stage at which the patient will stabilize. Therefore the time course of the progressing embolic stroke is more likely to be seconds to minutes rather than hours to days, and there are likely to be few or no premonitory symptoms. Recurrence is likely unless the underlying condition leading to embolus formation is controlled. In most cases the management includes immediate heparin and long-term warfarin. If there is bleeding into the infarct anticoagulation may pose a risk which is said to be less than that from additional newly formed emboli.

Syndromes Caused by Atherothrombotic or Embolic Infarction

Carotid System

In individuals with normal circulation to and through the brain, *unilateral occlusion of either the common or the internal carotid* is said to result in no measurable deficit. The reason for this is the large number of anastamoses between the right and left carotid system and between the carotid and the vertebral–basilar systems. Although these interconnecting channels often do not carry much cross-flow in the normal intact subject, when occlusion occurs gradually, flow in them may develop sufficiently to maintain close to normal perfusion. However, in patients with atherosclerotic cerebrovascular disease, because of the widespread nature of the lesions, the auxiliary flow is usually inadequate to sustain cerebral perfusion. In this situation, then, internal carotid occlusion from an atherothrombus or an embolus often results in an infarction; this may develop in stages and culminate in contralateral hemiparesis or hemiplegia (most marked in the face and upper extremity), hemisensory deficit or loss, and aphasia (if the infarction is in the dominant hemisphere). Occasionally visual field defects may occur. In the extremities which are paretic, deep tendon reflexes are hyperactive, the plantar reflex may be extensor (upgoing toes), and muscle tone is increased producing spasticity and contractures. Sensory impairment includes position sense, two-point discrimination, tactile shape perception, and vibration. The size of the infarct, and therefore the magnitude of the deficits, depend largely on the degree of collateral circulation.

Occlusion of the anterior cerebral artery or one of its major branchings may cause paralysis and loss of sensation mainly of the lower extremity of the opposite side. Additionally aphasia and mental confusion develops if the dominant hemisphere is the one affected.

The middle cerebral artery is very frequently involved in thrombotic or embolic occlusion; and since it supplies the large lateral portion of the cerebral hemisphere the consequence is contralateral hemiplegia and hemianesthesia if the main vessel is occluded. The defects are greatest in the face and upper extremity. In addition it causes the form of bilaterial visual defect called homonymous hemianopia, in which the half of the visual field of both eyes, contralateral to the side of the lesion in the brain, is blind; in other words in a left hemisphere lesion, there are visual field defects in the right half of both eyes because the right visual field in both eyes is supplied by the left hemisphere, and the left half by the right hemisphere. If the infarction is in the dominant hemisphere, again aphasia will result. Obstruction to one branch of the middle cerebral is more common than main trunk blockage, and in this case various subtypes of aphasia alone or in combinations with hemiplegia may result.

Posterior cerebral artery occlusion results in posterior cerebral hemisphere infarctions, as well as variable damage to the thalamus and upper brainstem if the obstruction is near the origin of the vessel. Thalamic syndrome may develop, which produces a chronic burning pain; and there may be transient flaccid hemiparesis or paralysis, marked permanent sensory loss, and disturbances of voluntary movement; all are contralateral.

Vertebral–Basilar System

Infarction in this system is much less common. Basilar artery occlusion, if it develops acutely, causes widespread neurologic deficits and coma. That which develops more gradually may give rise to visual and ocular abnormalities and variable motor and sensory disorders which are more localized because the gradual development of obstruction permits time for some collateral blood flow to develop. The cerebellum and various portions of the brainstem: diencephalon, midbrain, pons and medulla; may be affected depending upon what vessels or branches are occluded. The resulting abnormalities will depend upon what functions were subserved by the affected area. The possible combinations of neurologic abnormalities become extremely complicated and diverse.

Intracranial Hemorrhage

There are three main causes of spontaneous intracranial hemorrhage: (1) intracerebral bleeding from hypertensive cerebrovascular disease; (2) rupture of a saccular aneurysm; or (3) rupture of an arteriovenous malformation. The intracerebral hypertensive hemorrhage probably accounts for more than half of all intracranial hemorrhages.

Hypertensive Intracerebral Hemorrhage

Most authors believe that chronic hypertension causes progressive structural abnormalities in blood vessels: thickening, fibrinoid degeneration, and necrosis of areas of the vessel wall, and the development of microaneurysms along the length of vessels. These changes weaken the vessel wall and permit perforation to occur. Unlike atherosclerosis, which occurs more in the larger vessels outside brain tissue, the structural changes caused by sustained hypertension occur in the smaller arteries and arterioles within brain parenchyma. Cerebral vessels have thinner walls than vessels in other parts of the body and this may enhance their susceptibility to hypertensive degenerative changes. The aneurysms are small, around a millimeter or so, and are frequently found in the area of the basal ganglia and thalamus, central white matter just beneath the gray matter of the cerebral cortex, and in the pons, midbrain, and cerebellum.

In addition to the aneurysms, it is well known that hypertension greatly promotes the development of atherosclerosis, and although this process occurs more in vessels outside brain tissue, it also occurs in parenchymal vessels and may predispose them to hypertensive angiopathy. Similarly, atherosclerosis makes more severe the changes caused by hypertension; the vessels are already thickened by the hypertension and thus more readily narrowed by plaques which may also erode and further weaken the vessel wall.

Hemorrhages into the basal ganglia and internal capsule comprise the great majority of hypertensive intracerebral bleeding. Hemorrhage into this area creates a hematoma which disrupts the main motor and sensory pathways between the cerebral cortex and the deeper motor and sensory control structures in the basal ganglia, thalamus, and upper brainstem. The onset is usually sudden, without premonitory signs or symptoms, and the neurologic deficits are reported to evolve over 1–24 hr. Blood entering brain tissue under pressure

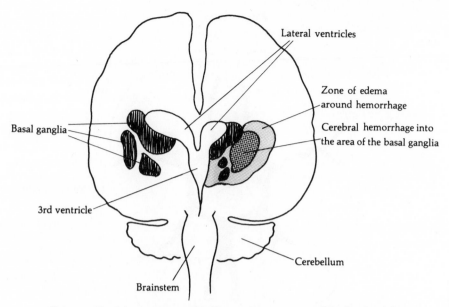

Figure 18-6. Hypertensive cerebral hemorrhage into area of the basal ganglia.

compresses and destroys it, and if the hemorrhage is large the blood may act like a rapidly developing tumor, compressing and distorting adjacent areas of the brain and interfering with their blood supply. Neurologic deficits produced by intracerebral hemorrhage are slow to resolve because it requires a long time for the blood to be resorbed. If the hemorrhage is large, loss of consciousness occurs, with hemiplegia and hemisensory loss. Upper brainstem compression may develop with its accompanying signs: deepening coma; marked abnormalities of vital signs because of compression of the vital centers for respiratory, heart rate and vasomotor control; dilated pupils which are fixed to light; and plantar extensor reflexes. Decerebrate rigidity may occur. In a smaller, slower hemorrhage the sequence may be slowed with mental confusion, dysarthria, hemiparesis, and other changes developing more gradually and less severely (Chapter 14).

Saccular Aneurysm Rupture

Bleeding from the rupture of a saccular aneurym accounts for the majority of subarachnoid hemorrhages. Most aneurysms are the result of a congenital defect in the middle layers of the arteries, the tunica media and elastica, which causes a local weakness so that the intima bulges out through the defect and is covered only by the outer layer, the adventitia. Such defects occur most often at a point of artery bifurcation, and frequently occur on the internal carotid and anterior and middle cerebral arteries in the circle of Willis which lies in the subarachnoid space near the base of the brain. The incidence of these defects is reported to increase with age, so that acquired factors may be implicated in addition to the congenital defects. The subarachnoid space lies between the innermost covering of the brain, the pia mater, and the fine middle meningeal layer, the arachnoid. The space is filled with cerebrospinal fluid, and the pia and arachnoid are loosely connected by a meshwork of delicate fibers. With the passage of time and under

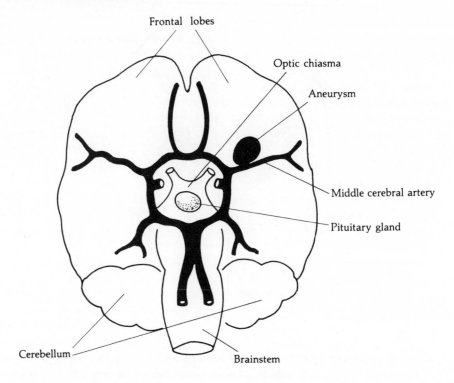

Ventral surface of brain, temporal lobes removed to expose the
middle cerebral artery on both sides

Figure 18-7. Ventral view of the brain and circle of Willis, showing an aneurysm of the middle cerebral artery.

the influence of blood pressure in the vessel, progressive thinning and enlargement of the aneurysm occurs. Aneurysm size may range from a few millimeters to larger than an egg, but the average is about 15 mm; and there may be atheromatous lesions and clots within it. The great majority cause no symptoms or signs prior to rupture; but sometimes if they are large and compress cranial nerves or brain parenchyma, then focal neurologic deficits (most often visual or eye movement abnormalities or occasionally seizures or headaches) may develop.

Rupture of the aneurysm, which usually occurs while the subject is engaged in his usual activities, results in the ejection of blood under high pressure into the subarachnoid space. The manifestations of the rupture depend on its size and the amount and rate of entry of blood into the surrounding area. There may be a complaint of severe headache or localized pain in the head, with maintenance of normal mental status and level of consciousness; there may be extreme head pain followed by prompt loss of consciousness; or coma may develop rapidly with no previous symptoms. This last type of onset is considered to indicate a poor prognosis. Sometimes a generalized seizure is the first sign. If consciousness is not lost the headache becomes generalized, and mental confusion, obtundation, or delirium may develop.

If bleeding is copious the blood itself causes elevated intracranial pressure, distortion of brain structures, and eventually compression of vital centers and of the reticular mechanisms responsible for maintaining consciousness. Also the presence of blood in the subarachnoid space causes meningeal irritation so that within a few hours there may be nuchal rigidity—the patient is unable to flex the head so that the chin touches the chest, and attempts at passive neck flexion elicit reflex muscle spasms. Kernig's and Brudzinski's signs are two indications of meningeal irritation. In Kernig's sign the patient lies on his back with one hip and knee each flexed at 90°; extension of the lower leg by straightening the leg joint causes pain at the back of the upper leg and resistance to the extension. In Brudzinski's sign, passive flexing of the neck elicits involuntary flexing at the hips.

Free blood in the arachnoid space and around brain blood vessels has two other adverse effects. It causes irritation of vital centers in the brainstem, leading to abnormal activity in the autonomic nervous system centers, with elevation of blood pressure and cardiac arrhythmias. And it stimulates smooth muscle in the walls of brain arteries, causing vascular spasm and edema; the spasm and swelling of the vessel walls may be sufficient to cause ischemia and infarction in brain parenchyma itself, especially when there is already atherosclerotic narrowing of the vessels.

The sterile hemogenic meningitis caused by hemolysis and breakdown of blood in the subarachnoid space may have a longer-term consequence; the meningeal inflammation may take the form of an adhesive arachnoiditis and fibrosis of the pia in which there is a thickening and production of exudates by the meninges in the large cerebrospinal fluid channels at the base of the brain, with permanent scarring and formation of adhesions. The adhesions may impede the flow of cerebrospinal fluid from the ventricles to the sites where it is resorbed by the arachnoid villi, causing hydrocephalus and elevated intracranial pressure (Figure 18-8).

Early management consists of absolute bed rest, with the head of the bed somewhat elevated, administration of aminocaproic acid to inhibit clot lysis, low

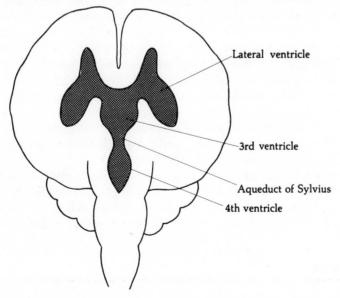

Figure 18-8. Dilation of ventricular system with cerebrospinal fluid caused by an obstruction to the flow of CSF from the ventricular system to the subarachnoid space where it is resorbed.

fluid intake and hyperosmotic agents to minimize brain edema, control of hypertension, and prevention of cerebral infarction from vasospasm. Reserpine and kanamycin have been reported to reduce the incidence of this last complication, but the mechanism of action is unclear.

In patients who survive the acute phase of aneurysm rupture the subsequent course is difficult to predict; the likelihood of a recurrent hemorrhage from the same site is said to be great. The mortality rate in ruptured saccular aneurysms increases with increasing age of the patient and is well correlated with severity of the signs and symptoms during the acute phase; of deaths occurring early, but after the acute phase, most are reported to be due to rebleeding. Because of the high incidence of repeated hemorrhage, surgery is usually performed in a week or so after the patient is well stabilized. Angiographic studies are used in an attempt to determine the site of bleeding, and to identify the configuration of vessels in the circle of Willis. A number of procedures may be appropriate including ligation of the supplying vessel, isolating the aneurysm by placing clips on either side of it, investment or wrapping, or plugging it with some material.

Arteriovenous Malformation Rupture

There are a number of different types of vascular anomalies of the brain, of which the arteriovenous malformation is one. They may occur at any site in the central nervous system but frequently are found in the region of the middle cerebral artery. They are composed of a mass of arterial and venous channels having many dilated areas. They are congenital developmental defects in which capillaries failed to develop between arterial and venous supply to an area; instead, the arterial and venous channels are connected by abnormally thin vessels. They are often wedge-shaped, with the base at the cerebral cortex and the apex deep in cerebral tissue or connecting with the lateral ventricle; but may be small, a few millimeters in diameter, confined to the cortex or underlying white matter. There appears to be a familial tendency and males are affected twice as often as females.

The onset of symptoms may occur in childhood or early adult life and most commonly takes the form of frequent severe headaches or seizures. Most vascular malformations eventually bleed, usually by young adulthood, and intracranial hemorrhage may be the first sign; the bleeding may be intracerebral or subarachnoid or both. It is often accompanied by focal neurologic signs: hemiplegia, hemianesthesia, and hemianopia; if bleeding is severe there may be marked elevation of intracranial pressure with brainstem compression and coma. However, most patients survive the hemorrhage.

Management appears to be controversial. Some workers suggest that prognosis is better with conservative management; while others advocate attempts to locate and ligate the supplying vessels, to obstruct the vessels with some form of artificial embolization, or to reduce the structure with radiation.

REFERENCES

Barnett HJM et al.: The Canadian Cooperative Study Group. A randomized trial of aspirin and sulfinpyrazone in threatened stroke. *N. Engl. J. Med.* 299:53–59, 1978.

Beeson PB and McDermott W, editors: *Textbook of Medicine,* 14th ed. Philadelphia, Pa. Saunders, 1975.

Ganong WF: *Review of Medical Physiology,* 8th ed. Palo Altos, Calif.: Lange Medical Publishers, 1977.

Goldensohn ES and Appel SH, editors: *Scientific Approaches to Clinical Neurology,* 2 vols. Philadelphia, Pa.: Lea & Febiger, 1977.

Guyton AC: *Textbook of Medical Physiology,* 5th ed. Philadelphia, Pa.: Saunders, 1976.

Matthews WB: *Practical Neurology,* 3rd ed. London: Blackwell Scientific Publications, 1975.

Merritt HH: *A Textbook of Neurology,* 5th ed. Philadelphia, Pa.: Lea and Febiger, 1973.

Thorn GW, et al., editors: *Harrison's Principles of Internal Medicine,* 8th ed. New York: McGraw-Hill, 1977.

Weiss HJ: Antiplatelet therapy. *N. Engl. J. Med.,* Part 1, 298:1344–1347, 1978; Part 2, 298:1403–1406, 1978.

Pain

PAIN PATHWAYS

There are gaps in the knowledge of anatomic structures subserving the sensory modality of pain, controversy over the functions of and connections between known structures, and disagreement about nomenclature. Still there are certain areas of general consensus, and the present account is an attempted synthesis of several views of an extremely complicated situation.

Divisions

Peripheral Pain Pathways

Receptors

A sensory unit is a single afferent neuron with its peripheral branches and receptors, its cell body in the dorsal root ganglion, and its central connections in the spinal cord. The receptor for the sensation of pain, both in the skin and in deeper structures such as muscles, bones, joints, and visceral organs, is a fine nonencapsulated, unmyelinated free nerve ending with terminal aborizations which subdivide to supply several square millimeters of tissue. These pain receptors cannot be distinguished on the basis of histologic appearance from receptors for many other senses: pressure and touch, cold and warmth. However, the pain receptors probably have *functional* specificity in that no matter in what way they are stimulated, provided the stimulus is strong enough to reach threshhold and initiate an impulse in the neuron, pain receptors and fibers convey only pain sensations. In addition it appears that no matter at what portion of a pain pathway a stimulus is applied, the perceived sensation is that of a stimulus applied to the part innervated by that particular pathway. This phenomenon is known as *projection*.

In the skin there are large numbers of pain receptors; each area receives the branches of several pain neurons and these branches overlap extensively; therefore a single stimulus affects the receptors of several sensory units. The most sensitive areas are those supplied with large numbers of sensory units, while structures which are relatively insensitive to pain are those having a sparse distribution of sensory units and their peripheral arborizations.

The number of sensory units and their associated pain receptors in a peripheral structure is correlated with the degree of representation of that structure in the central pain pathways of the spinal cord, brainstem, and brain; the greater the number of sensory units supplying a given area, the larger will be the mass of nerve cells in the central nervous system devoted to receiving and integrating that sensory input. In general, the number of pain endings in the visceral and deep somatic structures are fewer than at the body surface.

However, there are other factors influencing the sensitivity of a given structure to pain, some of which are not well understood. A given area of skin, for example, mapped for pain receptors, will show different patterns of sensitivity and responsiveness at different times and under various circumstances, so that the patterns of receptor distribution appear to shift. It is thought that this variability depends not only on changing focal factors in the area being mapped (perhaps blood flow, skin temperature, and the state of receptors for other sensory modalities in the area), but perhaps even more upon central factors within the spinal cord, brainstem, and brain, some of which will be discussed subsequently.

The strength of the applied stimulus is also a significant factor in determining the extent of the response of sensory units; as stimulus strength increases there is activation of the receptors of sensory units adjacent to the area being stimulated so that the effects of stimulation spread out. As more sensory units respond the responding areas of the central pain pathways also increase, so that a strong stimulus results in more extensive activation of the central nervous system than a weak one.

It is proposed that the kinds of pain which result from all forms of tissue injury, including trauma and inflammation, are mediated by the release of certain biochemical substances from injured cells which then either directly stimulate the pain receptors, or lower their thresholds so that they fire spontaneously or with only slight stimulation. The most prominent candidate for this role of neurohumoral mediator of pain is the vasodilator polypeptide bradykinin. The kinins are formed from certain globulins in the blood called kininogens by the action of proteolytic enzymes, the kallikreins. Bradykinin causes pain when injected into tissue, and also promotes vasodilation and increased capillary permeability. Other substances which have been implicated as mediators of pain are histamine and serotonin.

Afferent Fibers and Dorsal Roots

Most peripheral nerves, both somatic and visceral, are mixed nerves; that is they contain both sensory (afferent) fibers, which conduct sensory impulses into the spinal cord through the dorsal roots and dorsal root ganglia; and motor (efferent) fibers, which conduct motor impulses out of the spinal cord along the ventral roots. A short distance from the spinal cord, or brainstem, in the case of the cranial nerves, the ventral and dorsal roots join to form the mixed nerve. These mixed peripheral nerves contain large numbers of fibers of various sizes ranging from about 0.5–5 μm (micrometers; a micrometer equals 0.001 mm). The larger fibers carry impulses concerned with somatic motor function and proprioception; the smaller fibers carry impulses for pain and temperature sensations and autonomic function. In general, the larger the diameter of a nerve fiber, the faster the rate of conduction. Neurons for pain sensations are among the smaller fibers in a mixed nerve and their speed of conduction is correspondingly slow. Pain sensations travel primarily on two types of afferent fibers: thinly myelinated A delta fibers of about 5 μm diameter, which conduct at around 15 m/sec; and unmyelinated C fibers of about 1 to 2 μm diameter which conduct at approximately 1 m/sec.

Application of a painful stimulus to an area containing sensory units of both types results in two types of pain sensations: first, a sharp, well-localized, pricking or cutting sensation; followed after a brief interval by a slower, diffuse, burning or aching quality dull pain, which is poorly localized and has an unpleasant affective component. The fast sharp pain is called epicritic pain and travels mainly on the larger, faster-conducting A delta fibers; the slow dull pain is called protopathic pain and is carried primarily by the smaller slower conducting C fibers. Body parts supplied only by C pain fibers (such as some viscera), therefore, would yield only the dull slow protopathic pain when subjected to pain-producing stimuli.

All sensory nerve fibers enter the spinal cord via the dorsal roots, and the nerve cell bodies of these sensory neurons lie in the dorsal root ganglia. The peripheral processes of the neurons extend out into the structures innervated, and end in the receptors; and the central processes of the neurons enter the cord and synapse with neurons in the dorsal horn of the cord. The dorsal roots contain the nerve cell bodies of all afferent neurons and include many different types and sizes of cells, including some autonomic ganglion cells. The smaller cell bodies are those belonging to the two types of pain neurons.

Central Pain Pathways

As the central processes from cell bodies of the dorsal root ganglia approach the spinal cord, they separate into two divisions and enter the cord at slightly different locales. (1) The large diameter, fast-conducting, heavily myelinated fibers that mediate the well-localized sensations of fine touch, pressure, and kinesthetic

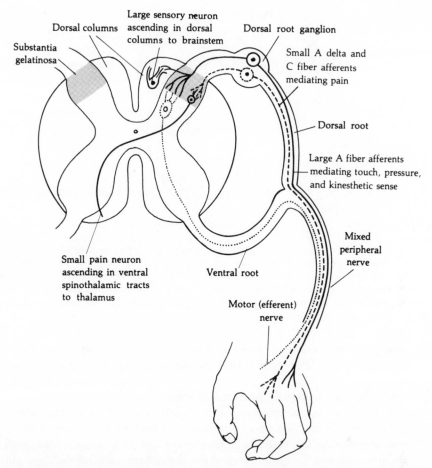

Figure 19-1. Diagram of cross section of spinal cord, showing ventral and dorsal horns; ventral and dorsal spinal roots; and a mixed motor and sensory somatic nerve. The large A sensory fibers, conveying sensations of touch, pressure, and kinesthesia, enter the cord and synapse with: 1) large sensory fibers that travel to the brainstem in the dorsal columns on the same side; and with 2) motor fibers mediating spinal reflexes. The small A delta and C pain fibers, carrying epicritic and protopathic pain impulses, respectively, synapse in the substantial gelatinosa of the dorsal horn, with sensory fibers which cross over and ascend to the thalamus in the spinothalamic tracts. A delta (epicritic) and C (protopathic) pain fibers are not differentiated in these diagrams.

sense enter the cord more medially; they synapse with large sensory neurons which ascend in the dorsal columns to the brainstem before crossing over, and with large motor (efferent) fibers which mediate spinal reflexes. This is the dorsal column or lemniscal system. The dorsal columns contain no pain fibers, but destructive lesions of the dorsal columns may cause painful stimuli to be perceived as more unpleasant and severe (see following).

(2) The smaller, slower-conducting thinly myelinated and nonmyelinated sensory fibers which mediate pain, temperature and poorly localized touch, enter the dorsal horn more laterally, pass to the substantia gelatinosa, and synapse with neurons which cross over to the ventral contralateral portion of the cord; these comprise the spinothalamic tracts—the spinal cord portions of the central

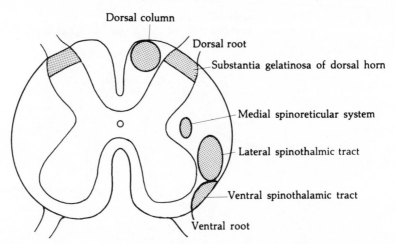

Figure 19-2. Diagram of cross section of spinal cord showing the substantia gelatinosa where incoming fibers, both large sensory and small pain, synapse; the dorsal columns, in which the large sensory fibers travel to the medulla; and the three ascending fiber tracts of the pain pathways. The dorsal columns carry sensory impulses from the homolateral side to the brain; the spinothalamic and spinoreticular tracts carry pain impulses from the contralateral side to the brain.

pain pathways. There is evidence that the level of activity in the large fast-conducting sensory fibers which form the dorsal column system has a significant influence on transmission of pain impulses in the fibers which form the spinothalamic tracts (see following: gate control theory).

Most of the central processes of the A delta and C fiber systems which mediate pain, temperature, and poorly localized touch ascend or descend the cord for a few segments on the side where they enter and then synapse with small second-order neurons in the gray matter of the dorsal horn, also on the same side. These second-order neurons then pass ventrally and cross over to the opposite side of the cord via the commissure. Directly or indirectly, these neurons arising in the dorsal horns give rise to most of the fibers of the spinothalamic tracts which comprise the central pain pathways. The spinothalamic tracts are composed mainly of thinly myelinated, relatively slow-conducting fibers of about 2 μm in diameter which have arisen in the gray matter of the dorsal horns.

The A delta and C fiber neurons, proposed to mediate epicritic and protopathic types of pain sensations, respectively, are not differentiated in the diagrams of the pain pathways. (See Figures 19-1 and 19-3).

The Lateral Spinothalamic Tracts (Neospinothalamic Tracts)

The fibers in these tracts convey sensory impulses of pain and temperature directly to the posterior ventral nuclei of the thalamus, although it is said that relatively few of the total number of fibers of the lateral tract originating in the dorsal horns actually reach these nuclei. Fibers of this system are joined in the brainstem by the trigeminothalamic tract, a group of fibers carrying sensory impulses from structures in the head.

It is reported that painful sensations produced by electrical stimulation of this tract are characterized by being sharp, clearly defined, and well localized to spe-

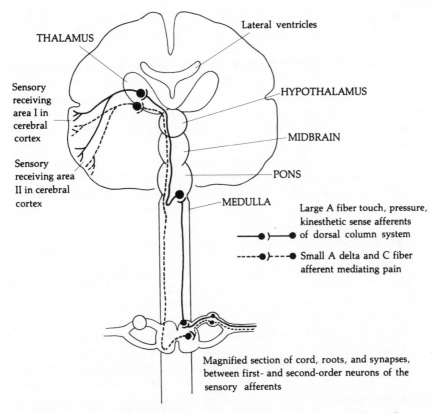

Figure 19-3. Neural pathways from the periphery to the sensory receiving area in the cerebral cortex for the large A fiber dorsal column system; and the small A delta and C fiber spinothalamic tract systems mediating pain sensations. The large A fiber system synapses in the cord, ascends in the dorsal columns of the same side to the medulla, synapses there and crosses over to the thalamus and cerebral cortex of the opposite side. The small A delta and C fiber systems synapse in the cord, cross to the opposite side, and ascend in the spinothalamic tracts to the thalamus. Here they synapse with the third order neurons to the cortex. The specific pathways of the three spinothalamic tracts are not differentiated in this diagram, but are shown as one pathway.

cific body areas; therefore, this tract would seem to be associated more with the epicritic type of pain carried by the A delta pain fibers. Third order neurons then travel from the posterior ventral nuclei of the thalamus to the sensory receiving areas of the cerebral cortex.

The Medial Spinoreticular System (Paleospinothalamic Tracts)

These tracts also originate in the dorsal horns along with the above, but they appear not to extend upward as far as the thalamus but instead terminate in the reticular formation of the medulla, pons, and midbrain. There they synapse with neurons which send fibers to the intralaminar nuclei of the thalamus, as well as to the hypothalamus. From the intralaminar nuclei of the thalamus, third order neurons project to the limbic system and limbic lobes of the cerebral hemispheres which are concerned with emotional and instinctual feelings, sensations and behavior. These are more diffuse pain pathways than the lateral spinothalamic tracts; pain pathways here consist of multiple short neuron chains with many synaptic connections throughout the brainstem, as well as numerous connections with the lateral spinothalamic tracts.

Some studies with conscious patients during brain operations indicate that stimulation of these diffuse pathways at the level of the brainstem produces vague unpleasant poorly localized bodily sensations which appear to come from the cranial, thoracic, or abdominal cavities, and emotional feelings associated with dread and other strong negative affects. Diffuse autonomic activation often accompanies such stimulation. Transmission on these pathways is slow because of the numerous synaptic delays, and the sensations tend to persist for an extended period beyond cessation of the stimulus; thus, activation of these tracts appear to be associated more with the protopathic type of pain carried by the C fibers.

The Ventral Spinothalamic Tracts

Many of the sensory impulses conveyed on these tracts are poorly localized, so-called "crude," touch and pressure, although some pain fibers are also contained within them. It appears that the fibers of this system are widely distributed throughout the ventral columns in the spinal cord and this may account in part for the lack of prolonged pain control in some patients who have had an antero-lateral cordotomy. Pain fibers in this system project to areas in the pons, midbrain, thalamus, and hypothalamus that are associated not only with pain but also with negative affect; to the brainstem reticular formation; and to specific nuclei in the thalamus.

Thalamus–Brainstem–Cortex Relationships

The second order neurons of the three spinothalamic tracts synapse in various of the relay nuclei of the thalamus with third order sensory neurons which extend to the two somatosensory receiving areas of the cerebral cortex: somatosensory area I in the postcentral gyrus, and somatosensory II along the sylvian (lateral) fissure. It is suggested that area II may be more concerned with pain perception than area I. However, the termination sites of the cortical projections from the thalamus remain something of a mystery; electrical stimulation of the sensory receiving areas in a conscious subject yields a variety of sensations: warmth, cold, numbness, a sense of movement, touch or pressure, in the body parts innervated by the specific area being stimulated. But stimulation of these areas very seldom results in sensations of pain; lesions in these cortical areas rarely cause central pain, as do lesions of the cord, brainstem, or thalamus; and partial destruction of these areas may diminish but does not abolish sensations in the body parts supplied. It has been reported that lesions in sensory receiving area I may in fact cause a kind of painful hyperesthesia resembling a central pain syndrome (see following).

Not only does the thalamus have pathways that project to the cortex, but there are also many pathways from the cortex back down to the several specific and nonspecific sensory relay nuclei of the thalamus which undoubtedly have a large influence on responses to pain.

Another significant interaction between the cerebral cortex and the deeper structures of the brain mediating pain sensation, is the arousal or alerting of the cortex from the reticular activating system. All of the spinothalamic tracts send numerous collaterals to the reticular activating system, so that painful stimuli are accompanied by marked cortical arousal (Chapter 14).

Central and Peripheral Pain

Peripheral pain may be considered to be pain which is experienced in the usual way as a result of stimulation of pain receptors, or peripheral nerves, either superficial (skin, mucous membranes), deep somatic (muscle, bones, joints, blood vessels), or visceral, by some type of noxious stimulus. On the other hand, *central pain* may be the result of some type of lesion, or abnormal neural activity, in one or more of the ascending pain pathways of the central nervous system: the lateral or medial spinothalamic tracts or the spinoreticular tracts and their tracts and nuclei in the brain. One type of central pain appears to result from a lesion in the lateral spinothalamic tract that carries sharp well-localized epicritic pain; such an impairment in the lateral tract appears to remove an inhibitory influence from the medial spinoreticular tract responsible for the burning, negative affect protopathic pain. The result is a chronic severe central protopathic pain syndrome. Lesions in the sensory thalamus such as occur in cerebrovascular lesions leading to the thalamic syndrome, or in the medulla, are also reported to cause chronic severe central pain. Central pain is unusually difficult to control and is often of the burning protopathic type associated with strong negative affect.

Phantom limb pain is another example of central pain; it is speculated that normal innervation to an appendage is associated with a tonic inflow of proprioceptive and well-localized tactile sensory information traveling on large, myelinated fast-conducting A fibers from that appendage into the sensory receiving areas of the central nervous system. This large fiber sensory input is thought to exert a tonic inhibitory influence, perhaps at some level in the brainstem reticular formation, on the small fiber somatic projection systems of the pain pathways. Following removal of the extremity, the continuous large A fiber input to the cord is removed (see above) and as a result its tonic inhibition of the small fiber pain pathways in the cord is abolished, leading to a spontaneous increase in neural activity in the central pain pathways formerly supplying the extremity. Thus the patient experiences chronic central pain which is projected by the brain to the area formerly supplied by those small fiber systems. This proposed mechanism for phantom limb pain is an outgrowth of the central gate control theory of pain modulation first proposed by Melzak and Wall (see following). Sustained neural input to the large sensory neurons by physical or electrical stimulation of another part of the body, or of the extremity proximal to the amputation, may be effective in relieving phantom limb pain, which is evidence in support of its central origin.

Referred Pain

Referred pain is defined as pain originating from one site in the body that is perceived as being localized in a different site. Pain may be referred from one somatic area to another, as from the diaphragm to the shoulder, or from a visceral site to a somatic locale, as from the heart to the precordium. There are several processes which may account for referred pain. In the first place, one nerve cell in the dorsal root may have branches or processes which supply both a deep structure, such as a muscle, as well as an area of skin over it or nearby—in other words, the same sensory unit is involved in innervating both areas. However, since the skin has more receptors than the deeper muscle, the central representation in the brain is larger from the skin than from the muscle, and so the sensation is perceived as being in the skin.

Another familiar example is the visceral referred pain of angina, in which ischemic heart muscle pain is sometimes felt as being in the precordium and left arm. In this case, although different sensory units supply the chest wall and arm, and the heart, respectively, the central processes of these nerves converge on the same pool of nerve cell bodies in the spinal cord: those supplying dermatomes T 1–5. Since the chest wall and arm have both a richer peripheral sensory supply and a larger central representation in the spinal cord, brainstem and brain pathways than does the heart, the subjective experience is often that of somatic (chest wall, arm) rather than visceral (heart) pain (Chapter 4, Figure 4-3).

Visceral Pain

Visceral pain receptors are similar to those in the skin and deeper structures, but their distribution is more sparse; visceral pain impulses are then carried on thinly myelinated processes of dorsal root ganglion cells (visceral afferents) which conduct pain stimuli from the internal organs to the spinal cord. Visceral afferents are usually type C pain fibers, they travel with the sympathetic nerve through the sympathetic ganglia without synapsing, and then reach the spinal nerves through the white ramus communicans and thence to the dorsal root ganglion. Some lower visceral pain fibers travel with parasympathetic fibers; and others from higher visceral structures enter the brainstem with certain of the cranial nerves.

In the central pain pathways, visceral pain impulses, as well as other visceral sensations, travel the same route as somatic sensations: the spinothalamic and spinoreticular systems described above and the central receiving areas for both somatic and visceral sensations appear to be the same. This is an important factor in accounting for the frequent somatic referral of visceral pain.

Modulating Influences

Increasing evidence suggests that the perception of pain depends to a large extent on the balance between neural processes which facilitate the transmission of pain impulses, and processes which inhibit their transmission. Among the mechanisms determining this balance are (1) the relative degree of neuron activation in large nonpain sensory fibers and in small pain fibers at the dorsal horn area of the spinal cord; (2) the activity of neural influences descending to the cord from the thalamus and brainstem; and (3) neural activity in higher centers: the limbic system concerned with emotions, the somatic skeletal motor control areas in the cortex, and mental "set" based on prior experience.

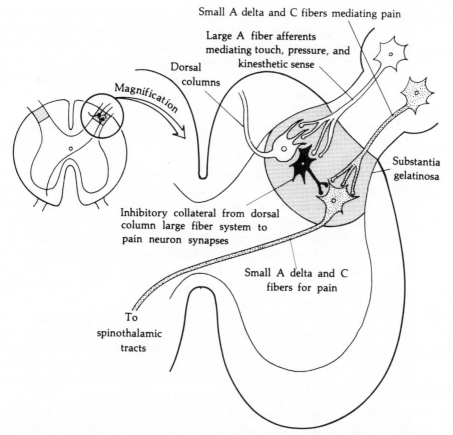

Small A delta and C fibers mediating pain

Large A fiber afferents
mediating touch, pressure, and
kinesthetic sense

Dorsal
columns

Magnification

Substantia
gelatinosa

Inhibitory collateral from dorsal
column large fiber system to
pain neuron synapses

Small A delta and C
fibers for pain

To
spinothalamic
tracts

Figure 19-4. Diagram of cross section of spinal cord showing the substantia gelatinosa of the dorsal horn and the proposed neural mechanism involved in the gate control system, by which impulses in the large A fiber dorsal column system inhibits synaptic transmission in the small A delta and C fiber spinothalamic system.

The Gate Control System

The gate control theory of Melzak and Wall proposes that the nature, intensity, and duration of pain sensations are influenced by interactions between: (1) the cells of the substantia gelatinosa (which is found at the tips of the dorsal horns); (2) the relative amount of afferent input from large sensory fibers along the dorsal column system; and (3) the central pain pathways of the three (on each side) spinothalamic tracts (Figure 19-4).

The small primary pain fibers from the periphery enter the substantia gelatinosa, as described previously, where they synapse with the second order neurons that cross over and form the spinothalamic tracts. These synapses in the substantia gelatinosa over the dorsal horns are under the influence of neural activity in the nearby large sensory fibers which form the dorsal columns and which carry touch, pressure, and proprioceptive impulses, as noted earlier. The influence of neural activity in the large sensory fibers of the dorsal columns, upon the synaptic connections of the small pain neurons in the dorsal horn, appears to be mediated by collaterals from the dorsal columns to the substantia gelatinosa (the most dorsal portion of the dorsal horn). These collaterals from the dorsal columns act as a gate which depresses synaptic transmission in the ascending pain pathways when sensory traffic on the dorsal columns is high (that is, when sensory input to the dorsal system is large). The number of incoming sensory impulses traveling on these large afferent fibers is increased markedly by vigorous simulation of the skin, subcutaneous tissues and muscles, and of the muscles and joint proprioceptors.

The skeletal muscle activity of vigorous exercise also produces a marked degree of inhibition of the small fiber pain system, because of the high amount of large A fiber traffic. This is the reason that an exercise program is an important component in the management of chronic pain which is unassociated with serious illness (chronic benign pain). Heavy impulse traffic coming into the area of the substantia gelatinosa on the large A fiber sensory system is thought to depress conduction in the synapses of the small A delta and C fiber sensory system which convey pain impulses. Conversely, increased incoming impulses on the small fiber system tend to open the gates, facilitating increased conduction at these synapses, and promoting more severe and continuous pain.

If afferent impulse traffic on the large fast fibers is high, this is believed to close the gate—that is, to suppress synaptic transmission on the small fiber pathways. The result is that incoming impulses on the small pain fibers are less effective in stimulating the ascending spinothalamic and spinorecticular pathways, and the pain is therefore decreased or blocked altogether. Conversely, if large fiber sensory input is absent from a body part (as in an amputated extremity); or diffusely reduced, as in the physical inactivity of bed rest or a markedly sedentary life style, then the inhibition to small fiber transmission is reduced or eliminated, and synaptic conduction in the pain synapses is facilitated. The resulting activation of the ascending pain pathways is correspondingly increased, and pain increases in intensity and duration. Not only does a lack of large fiber input decrease synaptic inhibition of small fiber input at the substantia gelatinosa gates, thus facilitating pain transmission, but increased small C fiber input further facilitates conduction of pain impulses into the ascending pain pathways. Therefore, large fast A fiber traffic closes the gates; small C fiber input opens them yet more. Similar gating processes in the brainstem reticular formation and the sensory relay nuclei of the thalamus have been proposed. These are the probable physiologic process which form the basis for: the dorsal column electrical stimulator, the transcutaneous electrical stimulator, the treatment of frequent brisk rubbing with a coarse terry towel for control of the pain of postherpetic neuralgia (after the skin lesions have healed, of course), vigorous massage, exercise, and other related pain-control measures.

Lesions of peripheral nerves which result in selective damage to the large A touch, pressure, and proprioceptive fibers; lesions of the spinal cord dorsal roots or the dorsal columns; damage to the brainstem and thalamic sensory nuclei; and even lesions of the epicritic A delta lateral spinothalamic pain tracts, may lead to syndromes characterized by chronic burning protopathic pain caused by failure of inhibition of the central small fiber pain pathways. Causalgia, thalamic syndrome, postherpetic neuralgia, and others, are suggested to be examples of such syndromes. This association of pathologic pain with loss of large fiber sensory input is relatively common, and such disorders have been called sensory imbalance syndomes.

Descending Pain-Inhibiting (Analgesic) System

Numerous investigations in both the human and in experimental animals in-dicate that there are areas in the thalamus, the brainstem, and spinal cord which exert a strong descending inhibitory influence on nerve impulse transmission in the central ascending pain pathways. The sites of action of this suppression ex-erted by higher centers is thought by many workers to be in the substantia gela-tinosa of the dorsal horns (which is the first site in the nervous system for the in-tegration of incoming sensory impulses—Figure 19-4) as well as at relay sites for pain impulses higher in the ascending pain pathways: certain areas of the brain-stem and the thalamus.

There is evidence that this descending pain-inhibiting system, when stimu-lated either artificially (by means of experimentally applied electrical stimulation) or naturally (in response to pain) by processes which are not yet identified, exerts its effects by secreting substances called endogenous opioids which seem to be remarkably similar to morphine. These opioids then interact with certain portions of neuron cell membranes (opiate–opioid receptors) at synapses at various levels along the pain pathways to produce active pain-inhibiting effects.

The classical concept of analgesia and the action of analgesic agents such as narcotics, has long been that these agents somehow passively block the synaptic transmission of pain impulses. However, the view of analgesia which is now emerging is that of an *active* pain-inhibiting neural system which closely in-teracts with pain pathways, but is a distinct entity having its own neural centers and pathways and neurotransmitters or neuromodulators.

Proposed Neural Pathways of the Pain-Inhibiting System

Studies with experimental animals, as well as with patients who have conditions causing severe chronic pain, indicate that the central nervous system has built-in processes that can act to ameliorate pain, and that this system is closely related in its actions to the effects of the opiate analgesics such as morphine. Electrical stimulation of certain areas of the thalamus and midbrain markedly reduces or abolishes altogether the production of pain by applied painful stimuli (in animals) and, in patients, the sensation of chronic pain caused by advanced malignancies, peripheral nerve damage, and neurologic disorders such as phantom limb. Elec-trical stimulation of these brain areas for only 15–30 min is said to produce an inhibition of pain sensations which may last for many hours. Such analgesia is blocked by naloxone and accompanied by increased CSF content of β endorphin and enkephalin-like material (see following).

The areas of the brain from which these effects are produced in animals such as rat and cat are the periaqueductal gray matter of the midbrain—the area of gray matter which lies around the aqueduct of Sylvius and the third and fourth ven-tricles. In the human experiencing intractable pain, electrical stimulation of this area (Figure 19-5a) produces strong analgesia but has a number of adverse side effects; however stimulation of areas above this level, in the diencephalon at me-dial portions of the thalamus around the third ventricle (Figure 19-5b) is re-ported to produce powerful analgesia with little emotional side effects aside from reports in some patients of feelings of relaxation and comfort. The analgesia may last far beyond the few minutes of stimulation—up to 24 hours, and occurs even

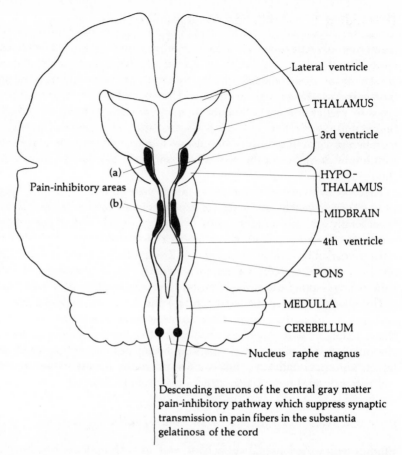

Lateral ventricle

THALAMUS

3rd ventricle

HYPO-
THALAMUS

MIDBRAIN

4th ventricle

PONS

MEDULLA

CEREBELLUM

Nucleus raphe magnus

(a)

Pain-inhibitory areas

(b)

Descending neurons of the central gray matter
pain-inhibitory pathway which suppress synaptic
transmission in pain fibers in the substantia
gelatinosa of the cord

Figure 19-5. Diagram of the central nervous system showing the proposed pain-modulating
system: the analgesia producing sites in the thalamus and midbrain, the nucleus magnus in the
medulla, and descending pain-inhibiting fibers of the dorsolateral tracts to the substantia gelatinosa. It is suggested that the endogenous opioid enkephalin is the neuromodulator secreted
as the effector substance of this analgesia system. When it is released by appropriate stimulation, it interacts with specific receptors in the cell membranes of neurons of the analgesia system to produce modulation of pain perception.

in the presence of severe pain which had been unaffected by large doses of narcotic analgesics.

One of the remarkable facts about the analgesia produced by electrical stimulation is that it is partially or completely blocked by the opiate antagonist naloxone in both humans and other animals. Therefore the assumption is that the
stimulation activates some pain-inhibiting system which operates via a narcotic-
like mechanism. And the brain sites which yield the most effective analgesia
from electrical stimulation are also those which produce most marked pain inhibition after direct injection of minute quantities of morphine directly into them.
Furthermore, analgesia produced by repeated electrical stimulation leads to tolerance in the same way that repeated morphine injections produce tolerance,
and cross tolerance develops between morphine and electrical analgesia.

The suggestion has been made on the basis of this and much additional experimental evidence that electrical stimulation of these specific brain centers pro-

duces active inhibition of impulses in the pain pathways, and resulting analgesia, by stimulating the release of an endogenous opiate-like (=opioid) factor which then interacts with opiate (opioid) receptors (see following) farther down in the central nervous system. It is postulated that these endogenous opiate-like substances may be the enkephalins (see following), that stimulation of specific brain areas causes their release from nerve terminals in specific pathways, and that they actively inhibit the transmission of pain impulses at synapses in the substantia gelatinosa of the dorsal horns of the spinal cord. In addition it is suggested that a similar inhibition of transmission of pain impulses occurs in nuclei of the lower brainstem that receive sensory fibers in the lower cranial nerves from the face, head, and viscera.

The neurons of the central gray area of the medial thalamus and midbrain which seem to be involved in the pain-inhibition system apparently do not connect directly with the cranial and spinal nerve cells which carry incoming pain impulses from the periphery to the pain pathways ascending to the brain. Instead, impulses from the central gray areas may stimulate neurons in a certain nucleus in the medulla of the brainstem—the nucleus raphe magnus—which in turn sends neural fibers down the spinal cord in the dorsolateral tracts which terminate in the substantia gelatinosa. The latter, as described above, is the area of the spinal cord dorsal horns that the first order neurons of the A delta and C fiber pain pathways enter from the periphery and make their first synapse. It is suggested that stimulation of the raphe nucleus causes the release of enkephalins in the substantia gelatinosa which blocks synaptic transmission between first and second order neurons of the pain pathways. This is but one of several proposed sites and mechanisms of action of the pain-inhibiting neural systems.

Endogenous Opioids

These substances are peptides, synthesized by certain neurons of the brain and pituitary, which have effects on the central nervous system resembling those of the opiate alkaloids and an analgesic potency comparable to morphine. These effects are exerted by means of specific interaction with opiate receptors on the cell membranes of certain neurons in the brain, brainstem and spinal cord. The endogenous opioids produced by the brain are two related chemicals called enkephalins.

Much experimental evidence indicates that the enkaphalins are neuromodulator, neuroregulator, or possibly neurotransmitter, chemicals which inhibit the firing of certain neurons involved with transmission of pain impulses. They are found concentrated in nerve terminals of axons arranged in specific neural pathways: the substantia gelatinosa of the spinal cord; the medial thalamus, which mediates the poorly localize burning protopathic pain associated with strong negative affect; the hypothalamus; and the amygdala (structures deep in the cerebral hemispheres which are part of the limbic system—that portion of the brain concerned with the emotions and with instinctual behavior). They also occur in the myenteric plexus (the intrinsic innervation) of the intestine. Enkephalins undoubtedly have other functions which are as yet unknown, but in addition they appear to participate in the integration of sensory information related to pain, the emotions, and instinctual behavior (Chapter 14).

Repeated injection of enkephalins into experimental animals produces physiologic tolerance and dependence resembling that induced by morphine; injections of enkephalin into the brains of animals induces analgesia which is as potent as that induced by morphine, and this analgesia is blocked by naloxone, an opiate antagonist. Electrical stimulation of the medial thalamus and periaqueductal gray matter of the midbrain in both humans and experimental animals releases enkephalin, and induces potent analgesia, as mentioned above, and this effect is also blocked by naloxone. Finally, a substance which resembles, and may in fact be, an enkephalin has been reported to be present in the CSF of patients with severe pain in higher concentrations than in comparable patients without such pain.

Endorphins are opioid peptides related to the enkephalins and produced by the pituitary gland; they are also present in neural tracts in the brainstem and spinal cord; the function of these substances is not known, but studies show that they are always secreted by the pituitary in increased amounts under conditions which cause the simultaneous secretion of ACTH. The condition eliciting concomitant release of endorphins and ACTH in experimental animals are physiologic stress (from pain, trauma, restraint, or other adverse influences), adrenalectomy (which is a prime stimulus for ACTH production) and ACTH-releasing factor from the hypothalamus. Conversely, administration of adrenal glucocorticoids suppresses the pituitary release of both ACTH and endorphins. The target organs and functions of pituitary endorphins are not known, but on the basis of experimental evidence it is suggested that they participate in the response of animals (and humans) to physiologic stress, pain, and danger and participate in mediating the neural and psychoemotional responses to noxious stimuli.

Opioid Receptors

Opioid receptors are specific binding sites on the cell membranes of certain neurons of the brain, brainstem, and spinal cord which presumably mediate the functions, as yet partly unknown, of the endogenous opioids. In addition they interact in a selective and specific fashion with the opiate drugs such as morphine, and appear to be the neuronal mediators of their pharmacologic actions. Opioid (or opiate) receptors in the central nervous system were discovered before the endogenous opioids were described; this created something of a mystery because (to paraphrase the words of an investigator of these receptors and the endogenous opioids) it seems illogical to assume that they evolved in the animal and human nervous system solely to mediate the effects of derivatives of the opium poppy.

Receptors are localized to specific areas of the nervous system and their occurrence closely parallels the concentration of the endogenous opioid enkephalin. They are concentrated in the medial thalamus, periaqueductal gray matter of the midbrain, substantia gelatinosa of the spinal cord, and nuclei of pain fiber-carrying cranial nerves: trigeminal, facial, glossopharyngeal and vagus, which carry pain sensations from the head and viscera; and the amygdala of the limbic system. They also are reported to occur in brainstem centers which may mediate some of the pharmacologic actions of morphine in addition to analgesia: nausea and vomiting, cough suppression, gastrointestinal hyposecretion and hypomotility, and the vasodepressor center responsible for vasodilation and hypotension.

PAIN SYNDROMES

Pain syndromes are those in which pain is the chief symptom, and may be the only one; and in which there are few, or no, associated signs. Chronic pain syndrome, and chronically recurring intermittent pain syndromes, can be classified into two basic types: those of somatic cause which originate in structures outside the nervous system, such as certain types of headache, low back pain, and muscle spasm; and those which originate in the nervous system: causalgia, thalamic syndrome, and neuralgias. Pain accompanying specific disorders is discussed in the appropriate chapters.

Headache

Headache and other unpleasant sensations from the head, which may be described as fullness, tightness, pressure, pounding, or squeezing, are probably the most common of all pains. It is often the case that, in addition to the discomfort caused by the headache itself, the patient experiences the fear and anxiety that the pain may represent a serious organic disorder, particularly brain tumor.

Assessment

Headache is one of the chief complaints in which objective signs are seldom present, and there is no disorder in which a careful and detailed history of present illness is more important in formulating an assessment and planning the management. After the patient has had the opportunity to describe his headache complaint as he experiences it, it is useful to clarify whether there is one, or more than one, type of headache being described; often muscle contraction headaches occur in patients with periodic migraines, and the qualifiers will be different in the two cases.

A history of head injury should be sought, and if present it is important to determine whether there was a loss of consciousness, hospitalization, physical examination, and skull films. Previous health history, including other neurologic manifestations, and medications taken now and in the past should be determined (especially oral contraceptive agents), as well as whether the patient has sought previous health care for the disorder, what was the opinion at that time, and the tests and treatments ordered. The most important questions relate to precipitating and palliating factors: what seems to bring it on or make it worse, what have you tried for it, and what helps relieve it or makes it go away.

Region of the head in which the pain is experienced is important to establish, as well as whether the sensations appear to spread or radiate during the course of the headache. The mode of onset, gradual vs. sudden, preceded and/or accompanied by other manifestations, during sleep or wakefulness, at work or at home, provide clues as to the nature and cause. The quality of the pain—sharp or dull, steady or pulsatile—and severity—whether the patient has to stop what he is doing and lie down, or whether it is just an annoying background type of sensation, are the attacks becoming more severe—help determine the disability the patient experiences from his headaches. At this point it is of value to ask the patient whether he has his headache now; if the answer is affirmative, yet he appears to be without distress, this is useful information.

All of the qualifiers of timing should be determined—age of first onset, frequency of occurrence, time of day, duration of each attack, becoming more or less frequent—since the different causes of headache are often associated with distinct temporal characteristics. Family history for headaches and other neurologic signs and symptoms should be explored. Associated signs and symptoms such as insomnia, pain in the muscles of the neck or back, nausea and vomiting, visual changes, diarrhea, mood alterations, weakness, or numbness and tingling, are characteristically associated with some forms of headache and not others. It is useful to conclude the history with such questions as: "How has your mood been lately?" How are things in your personal life?" and "What do you think might be causing your headaches?" The response may reveal sources of tension, anxiety, and chronic distress in the life situation; a recent loss; or evidences of depression. Often the patient will indicate at this time what he believes to be the cause of his headaches, especially in those associated with tension and adverse life circumstances.

Structures Involved in Headache and Head Pain

All extracranial tissues of the head are pain-sensitive. Chronic or recurring headache may be caused by disorders of the teeth, sinuses, nose, ears, and temporomandibular joints; the skin of face or of the scalp; the neck, scalp, and face muscles; and the extracranial blood vessels. Within the cranial cavity, pain-sensitive structures include the venous sinuses, the arteries at the base of the brain and in the dura, the basal dura itself; and the trigeminal, facial, vagus and glossopharyngeal nerves, and upper cervical nerves. The brain parenchyma, most of the meninges, and the skull (except for the periosteum) are largely pain-insensitive. Disorders affecting pain-sensitive structures above the tentorium results in head pain in the frontal, temporal, and parietal regions; the impulses are carried on various branches of the trigeminal nerve. Pain in the occipital area is carried on the glossopharyngeal, vagus, and upper cervical nerves and results from stimulation of structures below the level of the tentorium.

Types of Headache

Migraine

Although migraine has been defined as recurrent attacks of throbbing unilateral headaches, often accompanied or preceded by visual and gastrointestinal symptoms, in a person in good health between attacks, there is still much controversy as to precisely what the criteria for migraine are.

Migraine is more common in females than males and the age of onset is often before young adulthood. The headaches are periodic, the pain may be unilateral or generalized, or localized to the front, side or back of the head. The headaches often decrease in frequency and severity with advancing age. Some authors recognize two types. The classic migraine attack is said to begin with neurologic symptoms including scintillating scotoma, visual field defects, paresis or paresthesias on one side, and occasionally dysarthria. It is generally believed that these neurologic abnormalities are caused by intense vasoconstriction in the areas of the brain related to the symptoms (for example, in the occipital visual cortex during visual disturbances) during the prodromal phase. The pain begins in about 15 minutes and is unilateral and throbbing and often accompanied by nausea and vomiting and/or diarrhea. Photophobia is common. It lasts a few hours or as long as a day or two. The common migraine is described as being without neurologic symptoms, uni- or bilateral, and in other respects similar to the classic type. Both usually respond to ergotamine if given at the onset of symptoms.

There is thought to be a familial predisposition to migraine and some authors report a higher incidence of seizure disorders in migraine patients and their relatives than in a control group of patients with muscle contraction headaches. Migraine patients are said to be above average in intelligence, and studies have repeatedly failed to demonstrate psychiatric disorders or psychoneurotic traits in migrainous individuals above levels of these qualities found in control populations. Abnormalities in the EEG have been described in about a third of patients during the headache, and some, but not many, patients experience decrease in severity and frequency of attacks when given the anticonvulsant phenytoin on a maintenance basis.

During the prodromal phase of neurologic symptoms there is said to be a decrease in cerebral blood flow; then at the onset of the headache and throughout its duration there is strong vasodilation with enhanced pulsations of both extracranial and intracranial arteries, more marked on the side of the pain when it is unilateral. It is proposed by some investigators that the early vasoconstriction and subsequent vasodilation result from a release of the biogenic amines: serotonin, epinephrine, and norepinephrine, and that this release triggers the vascular responses in patients who have a genetic predisposition to vascular hyperreactivity. Plasma serotonin levels have been observed to decline markedly during the headache, and increased amounts of the metabolic degradation products of the biogenic amines are found in the urine of such patients. These amines are strong vasoconstrictors; their release in excessive amounts would produce the initial constrictive response; then when their blood levels decline there would result, in susceptible individuals, a strong reactive hyperemia. It is well known that experimentally produced dilation and pulsation of arteries of the head causes severe throbbing headache, often accompanied by nausea and vomiting. Patients with migraine headaches are said to have a generalized vascular instability and hyperresponsiveness of the arteries.

In addition to the generalized arterial dilation, it has been shown that the affected arteries and surrounding tissues become tender to palpation, swollen and edematous. Tissue fluid aspirated from this area contains a pain producing vasoactive substance called neurokinin which is a peptide related to bradykinin. This substance when injected under the skin of an unaffected area induces vasodilation, increased capillary permeability, and pain.

There are two components in the management of migraine: treating the acute attack, and reducing the frequency and severity of attacks. For acute attacks in which the headache is already established, aspirin, acetaminophen, or dextropropoxyphene may be effective and should be tried first, but when the headache is severe and unmodified by these agents, the addition of meprobamate, diazepam, or phenobarbital may increase their effectiveness. Codeine or oxycodone may be necessary for more severe pain but the danger of dependence or addiction is great. When the attacks are associated with nausea and vomiting then an antiemetic such as trimethobenzamide may be given by suppository or injection. Prochlorperazine or promethazine have combined antiemetic and tranquilizing actions, and may enable the patient to sleep, which often aborts an attack. A *single* dose of flurazepam or chloral hydrate at bedtime may also be effective in producing sleep and stopping the headache.

Ergotamine tartrate is often an effective agent if taken at the first premonitory symptom and in a readily absorbable form, sublingually, by inhalation, or rectal suppository. It is also often given by mouth in a combination with caffeine, at the first sign at the developing headache, although studies indicate that its effectiveness may be considerably reduced by oral administration. The action of ergotamine is to prevent the reactive vasodilation of the affected arteries; they are of no use once the vessels are fully dilated and their walls have become inflamed and edematous. Ergotamine is contraindicated in patients with ischemic heart disease, peripheral vascular disease, Raynaud's, Buerger's disease and other vascular disorders, and in pregnancy. Side effects are nausea, vomiting, and occasionally even in normal subjects, ischemia and gangrene.

Prevention, or reduction in frequency and severity of attacks, may be brought about by prophylactic administration of methysergide, cyproheptadine, or propranolol. Though the first two are serotonin antagonists, there is a question as to whether this is the mechanism of their action in reducing migraine attacks. Cyproheptadine also has antihistamine effects. Side effects of methysergide are nausea, vertigo and lightheadedness, and drowsiness; and the more serious retroperitoneal or pulmonary–pleural fibrosis. Propranolol has been reported to be prophylactically effective in some studies but not in others; in any event its mode of action in reducing migraine, if in fact it does, it not known. The antidepressant amitriptyline has also been proposed as an agent for reducing the frequency and severity of migraine headaches; it is not known whether this effect (if its exists) is related to its antidepressant qualities.

Cluster

Unlike migraine, which has its onset in younger individuals and is more common in females, cluster (or histamine) headaches occur more often in males, and the age of onset may be later in life. The head pain is said to be extremely severe, is steady rather than pulsatile, and is unilateral, often localized to the eye or tissues around it. The pains often occur several times in 24 hours, in clusters of many days that may last for weeks. There then may then be a complete remission for variable periods of weeks, months, or even years. The head pain, in addition to the region of one orbit, may occur in the frontotemporal region, the lower occiput, the area of the carotid, or in the cheek. It tends to remain in the same site for each cluster, but may shift from side to side with different clusters.

The onset is often two or three hours after the onset of sleep and apparently occurs during REM sleep; attacks may awaken the patient several times a night for many nights. The episodes occur less often during the daytime waking hours. Individual attacks last one or two hours, and both the onset and the cessation are abrupt. It promptly awakens the patient; unlike the migraine patient who requires to lie quietly and undisturbed during the pain, the subject with cluster headaches gets up, paces up and down and may even bang his head against a wall or threaten suicide. Accompanying signs during the periods when the headache is in progress are lacrimation, nasal congestion and rhinorrhea, flushing of the skin and injected conjunctiva; there may also be miosis, ptosis, and enophthalmos. These are manifestations of parasympathetic overactivity on the affected side.

Precipitating factors for increased frequency of individual attacks during the time a cluster is in progress are heavy meals, alcohol intake, emotional upsets, the use of nitroglycerine or organic nitrates, and a period of protracted tension or the letdown following it.

Cluster headaches are related to migraine, and are often classed with them as vascular headaches. An increase in levels of histamine in the blood is reported to occur at the onset of the headache, and injection of histamine is said to precipitate an attack. As in migraine, ergotamine may abort a cluster if taken promptly at the first sign of onset, which in some patients may be a burning paresthesia in the eye, forehead, or cheek; and ergotamine taken regularly during a cluster may control the attack until the cluster resolves. Prophylactic methysergide or cyproheptadine appear to be effective in prevention for some patients. For the attack analgesics, sedatives, and tranquilizers may be useful, and if required, adrenal glucocorticoids seem to be effective in stopping a cluster.

Muscle Contraction (Tension Headache)

This type of headache appears to be caused by sustained contraction of the muscles of the forehead, neck, and scalp. It is by far the most common headache. Characteristically it is bilateral or generalized, of gradual onset, often most noticeable in the temples and at the occiput and upper neck, and may be described by the patient as being like a tight band about the head which causes feelings of pressure, fullness, or tightness. The pain is generally of long standing, perhaps many years; it often develops soon after awakening and is present all day, becoming more severe in the late afternoon. It usually occurs every day for days, weeks, or months. Occasionally patients will describe severe sharp stabbing pains superimposed on the generalized dull ache. Electromyogram studies confirm the sustained contractions of the muscles involved. Percussion of the occipital and temporal areas, and palpation of the sternocleidomastoids, the paraspinous muscles of the neck, and particularly the trapezius muscles, will often reveal marked tenderness causing the patient to wince.

A careful history may elicit dissatisfaction with the life style, and encouraging the patient to speak freely may uncover depression, anxiety, chronic anger, and a sense of disappointment. It is remarkable how often asking the patient to describe a typical day will bring forth expressions of feeling trapped in an untenable situation to which there appears to be no solution, even though denial of all social or psychoemotional difficulties was the initial response to this line of questioning. Feelings of chronic boredom and hopelessness seem to emerge more often than affect related to a crisis state. Patients often are grateful to have the opportunity to express these feelings and the accompanying guilt which the despair engenders. Conversely, some persons strongly continue to deny, and in fact may be completely unaware of, the negative emotions which often accompany and underlie the chronic muscular bracing. It is my impression that tension headaches are often symptomatic of an adverse life style which is engendering insoluble conflicts. Often the patient encounter culminates in a request for a prescription for tranquilizers or sleeping pills (or both), a request that should be declined firmly. It is appropriate at this point to suggest that the patient might like, or be willing, to talk to a member of the mental health or psychiatric service, or accept referral to such a setting. It may then be explained to the patient that sedatives, antidepressants, and tranquilizers are psychoactive drugs and as such should be prescribed only by persons specially qualified in these areas, and used only in conjunction with ongoing therapy in the psychoemotional sphere by persons so qualified.

Studies have shown that electromyogram assessment, and biofeedback training where resting muscle tension levels are found to be high, is significantly beneficial in reducing frequency and severity of muscle contraction headaches. Many patients cannot afford this, and joining a transcendental meditation (TM) or yoga group, or learning the Jacobson progressive relaxation method is helpful to some of these. A regular exercise program including isometric neck exercises is useful. The patient is taught to clasp his hands together at the forehead and then try to bend his head forward against the counterpressure of his hands as hard as he can for a count of 60. This is repeated for lateral flexion on both sides, and hyperextension, with the hands placed appropriately to resist the movement in each case. The exercises should be done regularly three to four times a day for 10 or so minutes each time. It seems to help persons become more consciously aware of the proprioceptive impulses from sustained muscle contraction in the head and neck, and therefore to bring them under better control during the practice of deliberate relaxation.

Headaches Affecting the Elderly

Muscle Contraction Headaches.   These are the most common type of headache of the elderly as with other age groups, but with the elderly the emotional components of cause are often complicated by degenerative joint disease of the cervical spine. While many patients with osteoarthritis of the neck vertebrae do not have headaches it may predispose a person with psychoemotional tensions to headaches. Such headaches are often described as beginning with a sense of strain at the occiput and back of the neck, which then becomes painful and radiates over the top of the head to the temples or forehead. X-rays of the cervical spine may be indicated if the physical examination warrants: active range of motion of the head through flexion, extension, lateral flexion, and rotation, which is restricted and produces pain. A foam-stockinette cervical collar, aspirin, and local heat may be very helpful.

Temporal Arteritis.   This is a relatively common disorder producing head pain in the elderly which must always be considered and never missed, as it can culminate in blindness. The temporal artery is a branch of the external carotid which arises near the joint of the mandible and passes upward in front of the ear. It has numerous anastomoses with other arteries of the head, and supplies important collateral blood flow to the eyes and brain in conditions of cerebrovascular atherosclerosis. The cause of temporal arteritis is not known; it occurs almost exclusively in patients older than 50, more often in females than males, and manifests itself as a rapidly worsening headache which may be unilateral or bilateral, and is centered in the region of the scalp over the temples. The afflicted area is very tender; the artery appears prominent and tortuous, and is rigid and nodular to palpation, with diminished pulsation. There may be accompanying symptoms of myalgias, arthralgias, and fatigue; and signs of fever, mental confusion, and neurologic deficits including hemiplegia. The neurologic abnormalities may result from involvement of the internal carotid. The erythrocyte sedimentation rate is usually elevated over 50 ml/hr. Funduscopic examination may show edema of the disk and blurring of the margins, with retinal pallor. Optic nerve atrophy may develop and significant visual loss results in perhaps a third of patients. Biopsy of the artery reveals characteristic inflammatory changes. Temporal arteritis often occurs in conjunction with polymyalgia rheumatica, a disease involving a specific type of atrophy of muscle fibers. The management consists of adrenal corticosteroids begun immediately and continued, with careful tapering, for several months.

Other Causes.   Brain tumors may be a cause of headaches in the elderly; while primary tumors are rare over age sixty, metastatic tumors may occur and cause relatively mild dull steady headaches, more noticeable in the morning. The headache increases in severity as intracranial pressure elevates, as indicated by papilledema. Neurologic signs and symptoms may develop as the tumor grows.

Subdural hematoma resulting from a relatively minor head injury may manifest itself only by headache without other neurologic symptoms or signs on examination. It needs to be ruled out by special tests if other causes of headache cannot be discovered, especially if there are focal findings on the neurologic examination.

Chronic obstructive pulmonary disease with carbon dioxide retention may be a cause of headache. An elevated Pa_{CO_2} leads to chronic cerebral vasodilation sometimes marked enough to cause elevated intracranial pressure and distortion of pain-sensitive structures in the head.

Trigeminal Neuralgia (Tic Douloureux)

Trigeminal neuralgia is the most common of all the neuralgias; it is a disorder of the trigeminal nerve occurring more often in middle-aged or elderly persons and characterized by repeated searing lancinating stabs of pain in the distribution of one of the branches of the nerve supplying the lips, gums, chin, or cheek. The onset of the pain is abrupt, and paroxysms last for a few seconds or several minutes, and then subside just as abruptly. Between episodes the patient is free of signs or symptoms but lives in dread of the next attack which may occur several times a day or a few times a month. The cause is unknown and in almost all cases there is no discoverable organic disorder of the nerve or adjoining structures. There is no sensory loss in the distribution of the affected branch, and motor function is normal. The pain paroxysms are frequently initiated by touch of a trigger point which is often in the mouth, nose, or lips, or by movement of these parts, so that patients become reluctant to talk, eat or drink.

The suggestion has been made that this is an example of central pain caused by convulsive seizure-type discharge of the nucleus of the nerve in the brainstem, and there are reports of recordings made of spike discharges in that area coincident with the spasms of pain. In addition, the pain has been duplicated by electrical stimulation to the nucleus. The anticonvulsant diphenylhydantoin given intravenously is reported to abort an attack, and maintenance with this

agent is effective for many patients in reducing the frequency and severity of attacks. Carbamazepine is also often effective in controlling the disorder and may
produce a complete remission in some patients. It may be used alone or in combination with diphenylhydantoin. A large number of surgical procedures have
been advocated and performed for tic douloureux; complications of the surgery,
failure of control, or the production of anesthesias and paresthesias in the distribution of the nerve have limited their usefulness. In some cases the pain may
be relieved by a surgical procedure which protects the trigeminal nerve from
pulsations of a nearby artery at the base of the brain.

REFERENCES

Akil, H. et al: Enkephalin-like material elevated in ventricular cerebrospinal
fluid of pain patients after analgetic focal stimulation. *Science* 201:463–465,
1978.

Akil H: Enkephalin: physiological implications. In: Usdin E, Hamburg DA and
Barchas JD, editors: *Neuroregulators and Psychiatric Disorders*. New York:
Oxford University Press, 1977.

Appenzeller O, editor: *Pathogenesis and Treatment of Headache*. New York:
Spectrum, 1977.

Barchas JD, et al.: Behavioral neurochemistry: neuroregulators and behavioral
states. *Science* 200:964–973, 1978.

Beeson PB and McDermott, editors: *Textbook of Medicine*, 14th ed. Philadelphia, Pa: Saunders, 1975.

Frohlich ED, editor: *Pathophysiology*. Philadelphia, Pa.: Lippincott, 1976.

Ganong WF: *Review of Medical Physiology*, 8th ed. Los Altos, Calif.: Lange
Medical Publications, 1977.

Goldensohn ES, and Appel ES, editors: *Scientific Approaches to Clinical Neurology*, 2 vols. Philadelphia, Pa.: Lea & Febiger, 1977.

Goldstein A: Opioid peptides (endorphins) in pituitary and brain. *Science*
193:1081–1086, 1976.

Guillemin R, et al: β-Endorphin and adrenocorticotropin are secreted concomitantly by the pituitary gland. *Science* 197:1367–1369, 1977.

Guyton AC: *Textbook of Medical Physiology*, 5th ed. Philadelphia, Pa.: Saunders, 1976.

Hughes J, and Kosterlitz HW: The enkephalins: endogenous peptides with
opiate receptor agonist activity. In: Usdin E, Hamburg DA, and Barchas JD,
editors: *Neuroregulators and Psychiatric Disorders*. New York: Oxford University Press, 1977.

Hosobuchi, Y et al: Stimulation of human periaqueductal gray for pain relief
increases immunoreactive β-endorphin in ventricular fluid. *Science*
203:279–281, 1979.

Jacobson E: *Anxiety and Tension Control. A Physiologic Approach*. Philadelphia,
Pa.: Lippincott, 1964.

Lee JF, editor: *Pain Management. Symposium on the Neurosurgical Treatment
of Pain*. Baltimore, Md.: Williams & Wilkins, 1977.

LeRoy PL, editor: *Current Concepts in the Management of Chronic Pain*.
Miami, Fla.: Symposia Specialists Medical Books, 1977.

Livingston WK: *Pain Mechanisms*. New York: Plenum, 1976.

Marx JL: Analgesia: how the body inhibits pain perception. *Science*
195:471–473, 1977.

Matthews WB: *Practical Neurology*, 3rd ed. London: Blackwell Scientific Publications, 1975.

Merritt HH: *A Textbook of Neurology*, 5th ed. Philadelphia, Pa.: Lea & Febiger, 1973.

Poser CM: The types of headache that affect the elderly. *Geriatrics* 31:103–106, 1976.

Snyder SH: Opiate receptors in the brain. *N. Engl. J. Med.* 296:266–271, 1977.

Thorn GW, et al, editors. *Harrison's Principles of Internal Medicine*, 8th ed. New York: McGraw-Hill, 1977.

CHAPTER TWENTY

Parkinson's; Multiple Sclerosis; Myasthenia Gravis

The grouping of these three disorders together into one chapter in no way implies any pathophysiologic, symptomatic, or therapeutic commonalities among them. It is just that here are three fairly common, quite familiar neurologic disorders, affecting motor activity in different ways, that did not seem to fit appropriately into any of the other chapters on neurologic abnormalities.

PARKINSON'S DISEASE

Parkinson's syndrome is a common disorder characterized by muscular rigidity, akinesia and loss of postural reflexes, and tremor. The idiopathic form is a dis-

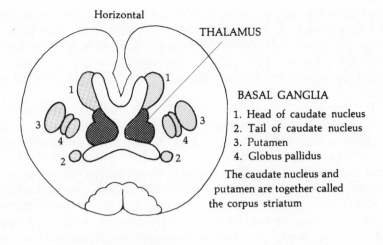

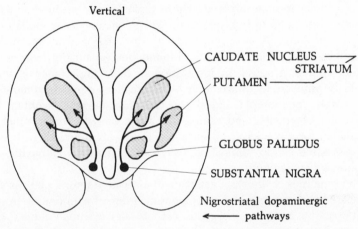

Figure 20-1. Diagrams of the brain showing the approximate structural relationships of lateral and third ventricles, thalamus, and basal ganglia.

ease of later life, it affects both sexes and all races, and, although some studies indicate a slight familial tendency, most are sporadic. It has a prolonged course with slow but inexorable progression.

Basal Ganglia (Nuclei) and Extrapyramidal System

The basal ganglia consist of three major bilateral subcortical masses of nerve cell bodies: the caudate nucleus, the putamen, and the globus pallidus. They lie on either side of the thalamus and lateral ventricles. The caudate nucleus and putamen together are called the corpus striatum. There is an additional bilateral pair of three smaller nuclear bodies just below and lateral to the six major ones, and in close association with them; they are the subthalamic nuclei, the substantia nigra, and the red nucleus. These lower nuclei are considered to be a portion of the brainstem. All twelve of the nuclear masses have complex neural interconnections not only among themselves but with the thalamus, the motor areas of the cerebral cortex, the brainstem, and the cerebellum. The term extrapyramidal system is applied to the basal ganglia themselves, the lower nuclei, and their interconnections with each other and with other brain structures. There are neural pathways connecting the substantia nigra to the caudate nucleus and putamen; these pathways are made up of dopaminergic neurons, are called the nigrostriatal system, and are of special relevance to the pathology of Parkinson's (Figure 20-1b).

The functions of the basal ganglia and their interconnecting pathways are not certain in the human, but it is thought that they may provide a stabilizing or modulating influence on movements originating in the motor areas of the cortex. Even before body movements are initiated they appear to be involved in the programming of the neural events that occur prior to the actual onset of motor activity. Voluntary physical movements that originate in the cerebral cortex are mediated through the pyramidal tracts, but they are markedly affected by reflex processes originating from various portions of the extrapyramidal system, including the basal ganglia and their interconnections. These processes regulate the general, background, stable postural adjustments upon which the voluntary motor activity is superimposed. These slower stable postural adjustments maintain the body in an upright position, provide steady accommodations to shifts in body posture and balance, and maintain sustained contraction in the large muscle groups that provide the postural foundation for smaller more rapid activity in smaller muscle groups. An illustration of their importance is the fact that it would be impossible to accomplish the smaller, rapid movements required to play tennis, for example, unless one can stand upright, maintain balance, shift the center of gravity, and change the basic body postures which provide the foundation for more localized muscle activity. Dysfunctions in the basal ganglia and associated extrapyramidal pathways affect primarily automatic positional and involuntary movements.

Abnormalities of the basal ganglia and associated neural pathways appear to be associated with two types of movement disorders: hyperkinesis, in which there is both excessive and abnormal motor activity—for example, chorea; and hypokinesis, in which motor activity is diminished and slowed. Both derangements are characteristic of Parkinson's; hyperkinesis is manifested by the 4 cps tremor, and cogwheel rigidity (see following); and hypokinesis is evident in difficulty starting the rhythmic movements of walking, absence of the associated movements of walking and talking, poverty of voluntary motion, and loss of postural reflexes.

Cause and Abnormalities

The cause is not known, and the structural abnormalities in the brain underlying the deficits are uncertain. The lesion may be a neurochemical one in the dopaminergic nigrostriatal pathways connecting the nuclear masses of the striatum with the substantia nigra, mentioned above. At autopsy in patients with Parkinson's the only consistent findings are said to be in the pigmented (melanin-containing) nerve cells of the substantia nigra and those of a closely adjacent nucleus, the locus ceruleus; the abnormalities in structure are loss of neurons, unusual cytoplasmic inclusions called Lewy bodies, and proliferation of glia. The associated neurochemical abnormality is a decreased content of the neurotransmitter dopamine.

Some authors consider there to be three categories of patients with the signs .

of parkinsonism: (1) postencephalitic parkinsonism develops subsequent to certain forms of encephalitis (encephalitis lethargica of von Economo, possibly caused by an influenza virus)—at autopsy there are degenerative changes in the basal ganglia and the substantia nigra; (2) symptomatic parkinsonism develops as a consequence of some form of brain injury from certain tranquilizers (reserpine, phenothiazines), trauma, hypoxemia, cerebral atherosclerosis, metal poisoning, carbon monoxide, and others—degenerative changes similar to the above are noted; and (3) idiopathic Parkinson's disease, in which the signs and symptoms develop in middle to late life without a known cause. The last category is by far the largest.

The relationships between the observable structural defects seen at autopsy, the biochemical deficit in dopamine content, and the signs and symptoms manifested by the patient, have not been worked out.

Assessment

Subjective

The onset of symptoms is insidious, and often takes the form of gradually increasing awareness of fatigue, weakness, and muscle stiffness, with mild diffuse myalgias, and slowing of the ability to carry out the routines of daily existence with ease. The initial symptoms may develop first in only one extremity but then are said to spread to the corresponding extremity of the same side, and then to the appendages of the opposite side. Later in the course of the disease symptoms of depression, lack of motivation, and emotional tension develop, and seem to correlate with increasing disability.

Objective

One of the common early signs is the development of the characteristic "pill-rolling" tremor in the fingers of one or both hands. The tremor is a resting one, disappears during sleep, and decreases with intentional movement of the hands. Slowing of all movements and muscle stiffness gradually increase, leading to immobile facies; loss of eyeblinking; stooped fixed posture; slowed dysarthric speech with monotonous voice; and a festinating gait—one that gives the impression of shuffling rapidly to forestall falling forward. The skin becomes oily with seborrheic dermatitis; the cause is not known. Eventually the tremor involves the hands, feet, lips and tongue, and eyelids and head. Postural abnormalities become more marked, with loss of the attempt or ability to recover equilibrium if balance is upset, either seated or standing.

Cogwheel muscle rigidity may be present on passive flexion or extension of the patient's arm or leg; the movement, instead of being smooth, occurs in a series of jerks resulting from a rigid resistance to passive movement which suddenly gives way briefly and then resumes; this rigidity may spread to muscles of the torso as the disease advances, making changes of position very difficult. Sensation and tendon reflexes remain normal. Akinesia becomes more evident, causing dressing, eating, writing, walking, and other tasks of daily life to become an increasing burden. Intellect is usually not affected; mood alterations, however, are frequent, as would be expected in a chronic progressive disorder of this nature; in addition, mental status may be markedly altered by the medications used in management of the neurologic impairments.

Laboratory values are usually normal.

Management

Physical

Management consists of three components. The first is physical measures, including a regular program of daily exercises, most effective if carried out in the context of group therapy in a physical rehabilitation setting, which offers motivation and moral support as well as exercise training. Heat and massage relieve the muscle stiffness and cramps; and gait training, walking, and other exercises help the patient maintain physical activity, self-care, and improved psychoemotional status. Taking daily long walks and remaining gainfully employed are important from both physical and mental standpoints.

Pharmacologic

Drugs should probably be reserved for patients who are unable to meet the demands of daily life without them. None slows the progression of the disease and all have undesirable side effects.

Anticholinergic Drugs

Benztropine or trihexyphenidyl may be given in gradually increasing doses to the point of side effects: dry mouth, urinary retention, visual impairment from pupillodilation, constipation, and abdominal distress; or altered mental status: confusion and impaired memory; and neurologic signs: ataxia and dysarthria. Careful titration of effectiveness of medications, as measured by relief of signs and symptoms, against their undesirable side effects, are central components of pharmacologic management.

As the disease progresses, anticholinergics, which usually give good relief for a long time, may gradually become less effective and the next step in pharmacologic management may be appropriate, namely, the addition of an antihistamine to the anticholinergic.

Antihistamines

Diphenhydramine is a commonly used antihistamine. It appears to act synergistically with the anticholinergics to relieve signs and symptoms; in addition it relieves insomnia and allays anxiety. Oversedation is a possible side effect.

This combination of drugs, again, may prove adequate indefinitely in mild to moderate disease; or for some time in more severe disease. However, with progressive incapacity additional medication may be necessary. In case the decision is made eventually to withdraw anticholinergics it should not be done other than very gradually because of the increased muscle tremor and rigidity that develops with abrupt cessation of these drugs in a patient with Parkinson's.

L-*Dopa* (L-*Dihydroxyphenylanine*)

This is the most effective of the antiparkinson drugs; it is an aromatic amino acid. Again, the dosage is started low and increased gradually to the point of onset of side effects. Maximum therapeutic benefit from this agent may not appear for weeks after starting it; and the side effects (nausea, vomiting, anorexia, postural hypotension, involuntary movements, cardiac arrhythmias) often decrease in incidence and severity with time. It may be given with a drug (carbidopa) which inhibits the enzyme dopa decarboxylase (responsible for breaking down L-dopa) and therefore it promotes maximal effects from a lower dose of L-dopa. Continuing the anticholinergic medication may produce improved control at a lower dose of L-dopa. Again, a tradeoff must be made and carefully evaluated between therapeutic and undesirable side effects. L-dopa should be given with food and antacids, since it tends to promote digestive distress if taken alone.

Amantadine

This drug, an antiviral agent, is another antihistamine which has some effectiveness as an antiparkinsonian agent, especially when combined with L-dopa.

Pharmacologic Effects of Drugs Used in Parkinson's

The basis for the anti-Parkinson effect of anticholinergics is not certain. However, it is proposed that the neurons just beyond the dopaminergic pathways (see above) from the substantia nigra to the caudate nucleus—thought to be the site of the primary deficit in this disease—are cholinergic neurons. The dopaminergic pathways exert a tonic inhibitory action on the cholinergic pathways beyond them. When the output of dopamine at the terminals of the former pathways declines as a result of degeneration of nerve cell bodies in the substantia nigra, then the tonic inhibitory effect to the cholinergic system is removed and the cholinergic pathways become hyperactive. It is suggested that the symptoms and signs of parkinsonism are those of hyperactivity of cholinergic pathways, which results in simultaneous overstimulation to both antagonist and agonist muscles of each pair. This causes immobility and stiffness; the tremor results from rapid alternation of agonist and antagonist muscle contractions. Antagonists of acetylcholine would suppress the effects of this cholinergic hyperactivity.

One suggested pharmacologic regimen said to be effective for many patients is a combination of L-dopa, the anticholinergic trihexyphenidyl, and the phenothiazine tranquilizer ethopropazine (these tranquilizers precipitate parkinsonian signs in large doses but relieve them in small doses).

The basis for the action of L-dopa in ameliorating the signs of Parkinson's is that it increases the content of dopamine in the partially degenerated nigrostriatal neurons that are responsible, in the normal, for the tonic inhibition of the cholinergic pathways lying beyond them. Dopa is the immediate precursor of, and is rapidly transformed into, dopamine. The symptoms and signs of Parkinson's are proposed to result from lack of inhibition of, and therefore excessive activity in, the cholinergic fibers, as described above.

Psychoemotional

As mentioned earlier, the major disabilities of Parkinson's are exacerbated by psychoemotional upsets, anxiety, and depression. Then as manifestations of the disease increase, daily activity level and self-dependence tend to decline, and with them so will morale and mood. So it becomes a circular situation with psychiatric complications lowering physical status and mobility, and producing worsened signs and symptoms of the disease, which then feed back to increase anxiety and depression. Patients should be reassured that most individuals with Parkinson's are able to lead reasonably satisfying and productive lives for many years after the onset of symptoms, and they should be encouraged in life-style measures which will maximize this ability. Explaining the meaning of the specific disabilities and the natural history of the disease may help alleviate anxiety for both patients and their families. A stable supportive relationship with the health care provider is a central component of management in this chronic progressive disorder.

MULTIPLE SCLEROSIS

Multiple sclerosis is a chronic, usually relapsing, but progressive disease of central (brain and spinal cord) white matter involving numerous areas of demyelination, and variable often episodic accompanying neurologic focal signs and symptoms. It is slightly more common in females than males and the age at onset is typically between 20 and 40 with a peak at 30. It is one of the most common neurologic diseases in the United States, Canada, and Europe. It occurs more frequently in cold and temperate climates than in the tropics and subtropics; it affects whites more than blacks; and it is seen more often in higher socioeconomic groups. The cause is uncertain and there is no definitive treatment.

Myelin Sheath

The gray matter of the brain and spinal cord is composed primarily of neuron cell bodies and surrounding neuroglia; the white matter, on the other hand, is made up mainly of myelinated neuron axons and neuroglia. Neuroglia functions as a supporting element; is involved in the transport of ions, metabolic substrate and end products to and from the neurons; and it participates in the formation of myelin. Neuroglia is comprised of two major cell types: the oligodendrocytes that give rise to myelin, and the astrocytes. Myelin sheaths surround the axons of white matter. Rather than being an inert substance, myelin is the living, elaborate, and metabolically active foldings of the extensive cell membranes of oligodendrocytes. The myelin sheath is about equal in thickness to the axon itself which it surrounds, and is laid down around the axon by the oligodendrocytes that are located at intervals of about 1 mm along the length of the axon. The nucleus of the oligodendrocyte is displaced to one side of the cell, while the greatly enlarged cell membrane wraps itself around the axon. The oligodendrocyte then rotates about the axon several times, depositing concentric layers of its cell membrane to form the multilayered myelin sheath.

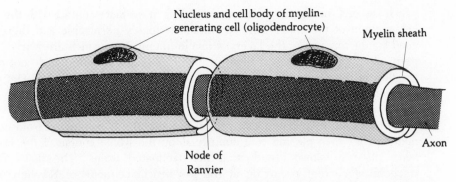

Nucleus and cell body of myelin-
generating cell (oligodendrocyte)

Myelin sheath

Node of
Ranvier

Axon

Figure 20-2. Diagram of a portion of the axon of a myelinated neuron showing oligodendrocytes which have wrapped themselves around the axon with their cell membranes forming the myelin sheath; between each two oligodendrocytes is a node of Ranvier.

Structure and Maintenance of the Myelin Sheath

Myelin is highly structured, and made up of complex molecules of several types of lipids (cholesterol, galactolipids, and phospholipids) and proteins and proteolipids. Although myelin undergoes little turnover under normal circumstances once it is laid down, studies of the O_2 consumption of white matter indicate that myelinated axons and neuroglia account for at least one fourth of the total metabolic activity of cerebral tissue. Since the myelin sheath is the cell membrane of the oligodendrocyte, both the original formation and subsequent maintenance of myelin depend on the integrity and metabolic status of the whole cell. In addition, normal function of the myelin sheath is dependent on the soundness of the axon which it invests. If the axon is damaged or destroyed by some abnormal process, the myelin sheath undergoes degeneration. Therefore, maintenance of the normal myelin system is dependent on the integrity of the oligodendrocyte of which it is a part, the neuron which it surrounds, and adequacy and normalcy of its blood supply and the blood components.

Myelin sheaths appear to be markedly susceptible to injury by a wide variety of agents and conditions, including hypoxemia, toxic chemicals, physical trauma, vascular insufficiency, and immunologic reactions. Demyelination is a common response of neural tissue to any of these adverse influences that may not yet be severe enough to result in destruction of the neuron itself. As the myelin sheath degenerates as a result of injury the membrane layers break up into small particles that undergo chemical conversion to simpler compounds and removal by blood and tissue macrophages.

Impulse Conduction in Myelinated Nerve Fibers

The myelinated axons of normal white matter conduct nerve impulses much more rapidly than nonmyelinated axons. There are several reasons for this difference, but one important one is the electrochemical effect of the myelin sheath. As mentioned above, the oligodendrocytes with their enveloping membranes that invest the axon occur at intervals of approximately 1 mm along the entire course of a myelinated axon. Between each of these cells is a node of Ranvier that is, in effect, an interruption of the sheathing and therefore a site at which the cell membrane of the axon itself is in intimate contact with the external medium of the ECF. This membrane is highly permeable and therefore a good conductor, unlike the layers of myelin membranes which are markedly impermeable and therefore excellent insulators. Myelin membranes do not permit the flow of the electrochemical current which is the nerve impulse. The movement of ions into and out of the axon, described in Chapter 17, across the axon membrane, can occur readily only at the nodes of Ranvier (Figure 20-3).

Therefore, in myelinated axons the nerve impulse is conducted from node to node, rather than passing continuously along the whole course of the fiber, as takes place in slower conducting nonmyelinated axons. The flow of electrochemical current occurring at the low-resistance node of Ranvier, as the propagated wave of excitation arrives there, passes out through the volume conduction of the surrounding ECF to the next node (and back through the axoplasm to complete the circuit) activating it; the result is a rapid direct transmission from node to node. Focal demyelination, as occurs in multiple sclerosis and other disorders that disrupt the myelin sheath, leads to impaired nerve impulse conduction: conduction delays, or partial or complete block, depending on the degree of myelin disruption. This jumping of the nerve impulse from node to node is called saltatory conduction; it not only results in a more rapid conduction of the impulse, but also conserves large amounts of oxidative energy. The reason for this is that the active transport of ions occurring during the recovery phase, which restores transmembrane resting potentials to normal levels, needs occur only at the nodes of Ranvier, rather than along the whole course of the axon membrane.

Cause

The cause of multiple sclerosis (MS) remains conjectural, although the results of epidemiologic, clinical, and laboratory studies has led to the development of a number of interrelated theories of cause that implicate geographic, climatic, socioeconomic, and other environmental factors; genetic predisposition; viral infection; and immunologic response.

In general, the prevalence of MS increases markedly with increasing latitude above and below the equator. Immigration studies indicate that the risk of developing the disease is established by some factor operating in late childhood or adolescence. Adults who move to a different geographic area retain the risk associated with the area they left, while children immigrating before about the age of 15 take on the risk associated with their new locale. There are suggestions that these risks differentials are related to factors which affect the spread of viruses: hygiene, climate, and life styles. For a number of reasons the measles (rubeola) virus, or a similar one, is suspected.

The age at which measles is contracted appears to influence the nature of possible complications; based on studies of immunity levels it is known that measles infections tend to occur in tropical and subtropical areas in early childhood, and in cold and temperate climates during later childhood. Late occurrence of measles is correlated with a higher standard of living, improved public health measures, and a more rigorous climate. Patients with multiple sclerosis had measles later in childhood than control non-MS groups matched for age, sex, and socioeconomic status. Since widespread rubeola immunizations began in about

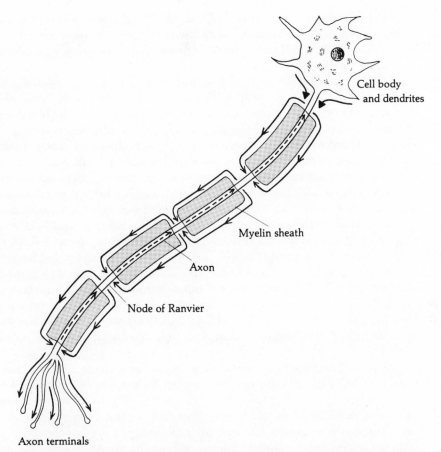

Cell body
and dendrites

Myelin sheath

Axon

Node of Ranvier

Axon terminals

Figure 20-3. Diagram of saltatory conduction in the axon of a myelinated neuron, showing pathway of current flow in the passage of the nerve impulse from node to node. Current flow is forward in the external medium and back in the axoplasm. Ionic movement across the cell membranes occurs at the low-resistance nodes.

the mid-1960s, and since there is an at least 15- to 20-year latency period between measles and the onset of early MS, if this theory is correct then incidence of MS should decline in the early 1980s.

Obviously, if the virus is that of rubeola, the vast majority of persons who contract measles do not develop MS; other studies indicate that among MS patients those who do develop it have specific genes that render them susceptible to this late complication. Certain histocompatibility antigens coded for by genes close to the immune response genes that control immunologic defense against viral infections (Chapter 22), have been shown to be present among MS patients in higher frequency than in control groups. There are some differences between various countries as to the specific histocompatibility antigens involved; in the United States and Europe, for example, HLA antigens commonly found in association with MS are HLA–A3 and HLA–B7; however, among Jewish MS patients in Israel, and Japanese with MS in Japan, these antigens are less common than in the general population of those countries. MS essentially never occurs in African blacks, and was probably introduced into the black populations elsewhere by whites; a histocompatibility antigen associated with MS in some native non-

African blacks is not found in blacks without MS. The relations between certain histocompatibility antigens and MS incidence suggests the involvement of abnormal immune system responses, perhaps to a chronic subclinical viral infection, in the cause of MS.

Many investigators have found evidence of the measles and related viruses at various locales in tissues and body fluids of most patients with MS, and higher than normal titers of antibodies to the rubeola virus occurs in the blood and CSF of many and in the brains of some who have died of MS. Since viral antibodies are rarely found in CSF and neural tissues, these findings indicate that many MS patients have had measles and that the virus became disseminated and persistent in a way that is not typical. Antibodies to many other common viruses (rubella, vaccinia, herpes, and others) have also been identified in CSF from MS patients, indicating that these individuals may have an abnormality in their immune response to viruses that results in poor control of the infection and leads to higher than normal antibody production. Other studies suggest a defect in cell-mediated immune responses as well, in which the lymphocytes that become sensitized to respond to viral infections make an inadequate defense against the invaders. Part of the impairment of the immune response to viral infections in individuals who later go on to develop MS may result from the presence of a blocking factor (Chapter 22) that inhibits lymphocytes sensitized to the measles, or other related virus antigens, from effectively destroying cells infected with the virus.

The incidence of MS is considerably higher in siblings, parents, and even cousins of MS patients than can be expected on the basis of chance. However, the incidence in monozygotic twins is no greater than in siblings. Conjugal incidence is no higher than that in non cohabiting control groups. These facts rule out a simple direct genetic determination but suggest the importance of a complex interaction between subtle genetic and environmental factors.

Abnormalities

On macroscopic examination the surface of the brain, and often that of the cord, shows no abnormalities. The brain on section reveals scattered small irregular depressed pinkish-gray lesions mainly in the white matter and periventricular areas in the cerebral hemispheres, the brainstem, the cerebellum, and the spinal cord. The diameter of the demyelinated areas is about 1.0 mm to 1.0 cm or more, and occasionally they are very large, involving the whole cross section of the cord. Microscopically the appearance depends upon the age of the lesion; recent ones show demyelinated areas most prominent around the veins supplying the white matter, degeneration of oligodendroglia, proliferation of neuroglia, and a mononuclear infiltrate. Older lesions have phagocytic infiltrates that remove the degenerating myelin and a proliferation of astrocytes; later there is deposition of fibroglial tissue which produces the characteristic appearance of sclerotic plaques. The degree of damage to the axons themselves is variable, depending on the severity of the lesion and ranges from relative intactness through moderate structural damage to complete destruction.

Assessment

In the great majority of MS patients the onset of signs and symptoms occurs between ages 20 and 40. There is no definitive diagnostic test for the disease, and since many of the manifestations are purely subjective, often of a transient nature, multiple, and variable, assessment is considered to be difficult and uncertain for extended periods following the onset of subjective complaints. Manifestations of MS are said to possess three basic characteristics; the neurologic signs and symptoms (1) are typically those resulting from abnormalities of white matter tracts (see following) rather than of gray matter nuclear masses; (2) can be explained only on the basis of multiple lesions at various sites in the central nervous system rather than on the basis of one or a few lesions; and (3) are characterized by dispersion in time, meaning that remissions and exacerbations are typical and the course is most often one of transient, variable, and episodic manifestations, superimposed on a gradual progression. The combination of anatomically disseminated manifestations is said to be the outstanding characteristic of MS.

Subjective

Ranked in order of descending frequency of occurrence, studies report that the following are the most common symptoms: muscle weakness of the extremities; visual disturbances (blind spots, double vision, visual blurring, decreased visual acuity); urinary symptoms (frequency, urgency, incontinence, retention); ataxia of gait; paresthesias (numbness, tingling, sensations of constriction, spontaneous pain, Lhermitte's sign—sensation of an electric shock radiating down the spine and into the extremities on rapid flexion of the neck—actually a symptom, not a sign); dysarthria; and altered psychoemotional status.

Objective

Frequently occurring neurologic signs include the following abnormal findings. There may be visual field defects, extraocular muscle palsies, decreased visual acuity, pupillary abnormalities, and nystagmus. Hyperactive deep tendon reflexes occur as well as muscle spasticity, plantar extensor reflexes (Babinski's sign), and absent abdominal reflexes. Dysmetria, intention tremor, impaired vibratory, temperature, position, pain, and touch sensations, and muscle weakness, including the facial muscles, are quite commonly found motor and sensory disturbances.

These signs and symptoms are often transient and may last from seconds to hours. The physiologic basis which would account for the episodic nature of the manifestations is unclear.

Laboratory values are within normal limits except for changes in the CSF: slightly increased protein content with elevation of the globulin fraction; and a moderate increase in lymphocytes. The EEG is reported to be abnormal in about half, and this may correlate with the about 50% of patients who show various kinds of psychic and emotional alterations: euphoria, depression, loss of memory, irritability, and lability of mood.

Course and Outcome

The episodic nature of the manifestations has been emphasized; nevertheless in most patients the improvements and relapses are superimposed upon a gradually progressive course during which each period of worsening leaves in its wake increased neurologic impairment correlated with the increasing number and severity of lesions. In general, about three fourths of patients survive for longer than twenty years following the onset. Perhaps of greater importance than mere survival, however, is the quality of life and degree of incapacitation. Patients who are older at the time of onset tend to have a more steady and debilitating course. In persons with initiation of symptoms at a younger age about a third are reported to be mildly to moderately impaired several years after the onset, necessitating changes in life style; another third are able to pursue their normal activities with perhaps only occasional interruptions; while the remainder become markedly disabled. Cause of death in MS is often an infection, respiratory or urinary; or, in older patients, the frequent causes of death for persons of that age group in the population as a whole: cardiovascular disease, pulmonary disorders, and cancer.

Management

Adrenal glucocorticoids or ACTH are commonly given at the earliest sign of a relapse in an effort to minimize irreversible damage to the nervous system and shorten the period of acute worsening. Initial dosage of ACTH is high and given intravenously with subsequent intramuscular injections and gradual tapering as signs and symptoms warrant. Some patients fail to respond, while others may go into remission with improvement persisting for variable periods after withdrawal of the medication. Studies have not demonstrated that the value of maintenance steroids outweighs the risks. Bed rest is indicated during exacerbations, but prolonged confinement is avoided, and a regular program of physical therapy is helpful both physically and psychoemotionally. Patients should be encouraged to remain physically and mentally active. In more severe disease the prevention of urinary and respiratory infections, decubitus lesions, contractures, and other accompaniments of severe neurologic disorders become major goals of management.

MYASTHENIA GRAVIS

Myasthenia gravis (MG) is a quite common chronic disease of unknown cause characterized by muscle weakness and abnormal fatigability. It is more common in females than males; the signs and symptoms may appear at any age but do so most commonly in the third decade of life, usually beginning insidiously. Although the weakness may be generalized, muscles supplied by the cranial nerve nuclei of the brainstem are often affected. There appears not to be a familial pattern of occurrence.

Neuromuscular Junction

The motor axons that innervate skeletal muscle fibers branch into numerous non-myelinated terminal aborizations as they approach the muscle fibers supplied by them; the axon terminals have minute enlargements, called buttons or end feet that lie in small depressions within the folds of the muscle motor end plate. These buttons contain vesicles of the cholinergic neurotransmitter acetylcholine (ACh). The muscle cell membrane is called the sarcolemma, and at the junction between nerve and muscle the membrane undergoes a special anatomic differentiation: it becomes thickened and folded upon itself to form what are called palisades. This specialized structure is the motor end plate, and it is a portion of the muscle, not the nerve. It is in the palisade on a single muscle fiber that the terminal buttons of the single axon supplying it are distributed. In spite of the intimate structural relation between nerve fiber and muscle fiber, there is a protoplasmic discontinuity that resembles the synaptic cleft occurring between pre- and postsynaptic neurons, although the space is minute. The enzyme cholinesterase (ACh-ase) is found in the postsynaptic membrance of the motor end plate and functions to degrade ACh after it has been secreted by the presynaptic terminals following arrival of the nerve impulse there.

As the propagated wave of excitation (Chapter 17) that is the nerve impulse arrives at the terminals it prompts release of the ACh stored in the end feet vesicles; ACh crosses the presynaptic membrane, diffuses into the synaptic cleft and interacts with ACh receptors in the postsynaptic membrane to increase its permeability to Na^+. Influx of Na^+ into the motor end plate results in a depolarization of that membrane called the end plate potential. This depolarization is not itself propagated directly to the muscle cell membrane, but if it is large enough to reach threshold it generates an action potential in the muscle fiber membrane which then propagates in both directions along the membrane and initiates the muscle contractile process. (In Chapter 7 the processes of muscle excitation, conduction, and contraction are described with special reference to the heart, but the mechanisms are closely similar in all muscle.)

Of the total ACh stored in the nerve terminals only a small fraction is released

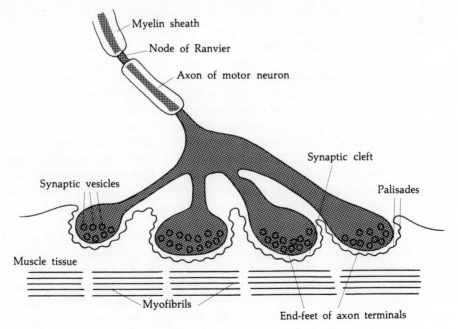

Figure 20-4. Diagram of a myoneural junction.

by the arrival of a nerve impulse; with rapid repeated stimulation of motor nerves, as occurs in normal muscle function, the amount of presynaptic ACh liberated into the synaptic cleft declines, reflecting a temporary depletion in presynaptic ACh stores. This decline results in decreased strength of the end plate potentials. With continued nerve impulses, however, more ACh is then rapidly mobilized from other storage sites in the terminal buttons and normal ACh release resumes, with a return of the end plate potentials to normal levels.

After each nerve impulse, the ACh that was bound to the postsynaptic ACh receptor dissociates from it and is hydrolyzed (inactivated) by the enzyme cholinesterase contained in the postsynaptic membranes of the motor end plate. The choline liberated by the hydrolysis undergoes reuptake by the presynaptic membrane and, with acetate, is resynthesized into ACh. This is an energy-requiring process utilizing ATP and is catalyzed by the enzyme choline acetylase.

Cause

The nature of the impairment in neuromuscular junctional transmission that is responsible for the observed muscle weakness and fatigability in MG remains uncertain in spite of much research and numerous theories. Some investigators have considered that there is a deficient amount of ACh released from presynaptic membranes into the synaptic cleft following arrival of the nerve impulse, either because of insufficiency of the synthesizing enzyme choline acetylase, defective packaging into vesicles, impaired transport of ACh into the synaptic cleft, or other defects. Other theories have suggested that there may be impaired binding of ACh to its receptor on the motor end plate membrane, or excessive hydrolytic activity of the inactivating enzyme ACh-ase. Whatever the cause, defective neuromuscular transmission is manifested in the electromyogram as a gradual decline in voltage of the muscle action potentials with continued stimulation of the motor nerve.

More recently, evidence for a postsynaptic basis for MG has come in part from studies with several species of experimental animals which have been sensitized to the antigen of the postsynaptic ACh receptor. The animals developed serum antibodies against ACh receptor antigen and demonstrated marked muscle weakness and easy fatigability; electrophysiologic studies indicate that the typical abnormalities of human MG appear in these animals. It has been shown that the antibody-containing serum from them is able to block neuromuscular transmission in other nonsensitized animals. In addition, antibodies to both motor end plate and muscle tissue, and to ACh receptor antigen, have been found in the serum of patients with MG, and it has been reported that chronic administration of serum from MG patients induces abnormal neuromuscular transmission in animals which resembles that in persons with the disease. This evidence tends to support the pathologic process as one of abnormal immune response to end plate substance.

It is proposed by some workers that abnormal binding of antibodies to the ACh receptors of the postsynaptic membrane would interfere with the normal binding of ACh to them; in effect this would constitute a partial block to neuromuscular transmission, would result in impairment of activation of muscle contraction by motor nerve impulses, and the consequence would be muscle weakness or paralysis, depending on the degree of inactivation of postsynaptic binding sites (ACh receptors) by their antibodies. A decrease in the extent of the palisades (number of postsynaptic folds) of the motor end plate has been cited as a characteristic structural abnormality in MG patients; it is proposed that this decrease may be the consequence of the action of antibodies in the serum to motor end plate substance.

Any one of the theories of the basic neuromuscular deficit in MG is consistent with the fact that cholinesterase inhibitors such as neostigmine and edrophonium ameliorate the muscle weakness. Antagonism of cholinesterase, the enzyme that hydrolyzes and therefore inactivates ACh at the motor end plate, would be expected to permit a larger buildup of ACh, facilitate its action over a longer period before it is destroyed, and allow it to act over a larger surface area of the postsynaptic membrane, thus providing larger motor end plate potentials and stronger stimulation to the excitation and contraction processes of muscle.

Abnormalities in the thymus gland are frequent in patients with MG; because of the involvement of the thymus in immune processes (Chapter 22), this fact supports the pathogenic role of the immune system in MG. Eighty percent of patients with this disorder are reported to have structural alterations of the thymus; most of these alterations (found in 70% of MG patients) take the form of thymic hyperplasia and increased numbers of germinal centers; these lymphoid follicles contain increased numbers of B lymphocytes, the cells involved with T cells in some forms of cell-mediated immune responses, and in the regulation of antibody production. About 10% of MG patients have a tumor of the thymus, a thymoma, which may be benign or malignant, but in the latter case remains confined to the mediastinum, i.e., it does not metastasize. In the remaining 20% of MG patients the thymus is histologically within normal limits.

It is said that approximately half or more of patients who undergo thymectomy show a marked relief of their signs and symptoms, in some cases amounting to a real remission. Yet in some patients the manifestations of MG do not become apparent until after removal of the thymus for a thymoma. It has been reported that the results of the operation are better in patients without thymomas. The improvement may be prompt or may not occur until months to years following the operation. As a consequence of these data, and others, some authors consider MG to be the manifestation of a disorder of the thymus resulting in the production of abnormal lymphocytes and antibodies to some components of the myoneural junction that impair neuromuscular transmission. In some centers thymectomy is recommended for essentially all MG patients able to tolerate the procedure.

Abnormalities

In addition to the abnormalities of the motor end plate, the thymus, and the serum antibodies, discussed above in the context of the cause of MG, there are some other structural and physiologic changes present in these patients. Unresolved, however, is the degree to which these changes are associated with the basic cause of MG, are the consequence of the underlying disease process, or may be the result of the various components of management of MG, perhaps prolonged treatment with anticholinesterases. Aggregates of small lymphocytes (lymphorrhages) are found around the small blood vessels of muscle tissue and adjacent to normal muscle fibers; some muscle fibers are atrophic or have degenerated and are infiltrated with or replaced by a variety of leukocytes; in muscles which are chronically paralyzed, fibers are seen to be replaced by fat or connective tissue. These changes are correlated with a more severe form of the disease. Lymphocyte infiltration is sometimes seen in other organs, and occasionally there are abnormalities in various of the endocrine glands. Heart muscle is also sometimes affected. In patients who die of MG, abnormalities of the lung include infection, atelectasis, and edema; it is suggested that these changes result from prolonged mechanical ventilation.

Assessment

Subjective

The onset of symptoms is rarely acute; subacute or insidious development of symptoms is more characteristic. Most typically the muscles involved are those supplied by the cranial nerves; therefore symptoms commonly originate from paresis of these muscles. Diplopia, transient and episodic but gradually increasing in frequency and severity, is often the first manifestation, and is caused by unequal degrees of paresis of the extraocular muscles. Eyelid ptosis is also common. Weakness of the facial, laryngeal, and pharyngeal muscles is present in many patients and leads to difficulty in chewing and swallowing and slurring of speech. Weakness and rapid fatigue of the muscles of the arms and shoulders, more than the hips and legs, is also a frequent early manifestation. Typically, regardless of whether the weakness is generalized or affects specific muscle groups, patients will complain that exercise increases it, a period of rest alleviates it, and that it tends to be more severe toward the close of the day's activities.

Objective

The neurologic signs depend on the degree and pattern of the neuromuscular deficits. The muscles of the face are commonly affected, resulting in a smooth, immobile, and expressionless appearance; eyelids ptosis is common. Paresis of the extraocular muscles may be manifested by nystagmus, disconjugate ocular movements, or unilateral ocular muscle paralysis. Testing of cranial nerve function may reveal multiple impairments of motor strength in several or all muscles supplied by brainstem nuclei. Grip strength tested by repeated trials with a dynamometer shows a gradual decline. In patients with more severe disease of longer duration muscle weakness may become more generalized and eventually muscle atrophy may develop, most commonly in the face, neck, and shoulder girdle. Deep tendon reflexes are within normal limits and sensory testing indicates no deficits.

An objective test for myasthenia, in addition to the dynamometer, is to ask the pateint to maintain upward gaze for 1 to 3 min; drooping of the eyelids occurs, increasing with time, and is relieved by rest. Injection of neostigmine (intramuscular) or edrophonium (intravenous) results in alleviation of muscle weakness. The effect begins in a few minutes and continues for about two hours in the case of neostigmine; the response to edrophonium occurs immediately and lasts several minutes. Response of the extraocular muscles to both drugs is said to be less than that of other affected muscles; the reason is not known. Routine laboratory values are within the normal range. Electromyography shows a gradual decline in the magnitude of muscle action potentials with repeated stimulation of the motor nerve. Patients with MG are said to have a higher incidence of antinuclear antibodies, rheumatoid arthritis factor, and other abnormal antibodies in their sera than control groups.

Course

The course and prognosis are said to vary according to the pattern of involvement; weakness of the muscles of the torso and appendages appears to correlate with a more benign, readily manageable course and a longer life expectancy than weakness of the extraocular muscles; the lingual, or ophanyngeal and laryngeal muscles controlling swallowing and speech; and those responsible for breathing movements. One reason for this is that, when the muscles supplied by brainstem nuclei are affected, there is a high rate of life-threatening complications: choking on and aspiration of food and liquids, respiratory infections, and episodes of ventilatory insufficiency and acute respiratory failure. These crises require hospitalization in a respiratory intensive care setting and mechanical ventilation.

Some studies have reported a 75% survival rate among MG patients followed for periods up to twenty years; the great majority of the fatalities occurred within the first ten years following the onset of signs and symptoms. Although some patients show remissions and relapses, the majority tend to run a progressive course that, without adequate management, terminates fatally in a few years.

Management

The principle component of management in MG is administration of the anticholinesterase agents neostigmine, pyridostigmine, or ambenonium. By inhibiting the action of the enzyme that degrades ACh, they permit a larger buildup of this neurotransmitter at the motor end plate, with resulting stronger end plate potentials and larger muscle fiber action potentials. K^+ and ephedrine supplements are said to improve the effectiveness of anticholinesterases. Side effects of the maintenance anticholinesterase drugs are excessive salivation, uterine cramps, gastrointestinal distress, and diarrhea; tincture of belladonna or atropine may be used to control these parasympathetic cholinergic symptoms. Some patients become refractory to the effects of anticholinesterases no matter how large the dose. Such resistance may precipitate a myasthenia crisis necessitating hospitalization in a respiratory intensive care unit and mechanical ventilation. Excessive amounts of anticholinesterase medication are also known to precipitate myasthenia crisis, and it may also be precipitated by aspiration, respiratory infections, or acute exacerbation of respiratory muscle weakness or paralysis.

Adrenal glucocorticoids are considered by many authors to be valuable components of management of MG in patients with more severe disease; in some patients they are reported to lead to significant remission, and to major improvement in signs and symptoms in others. Transient but marked increases in weakness are said to occur at the initiation of steroid administration and for this reason it may be started during a hospitalization.

As described above, thymus removal may lead to marked improvement in many patients and some workers recommend it for all MG patients.

REFERENCES

Beeson PB and McDermott W, editors: *Textbook of Medicine*, 14th ed. Philadelphia, Pa.: Saunders, 1975.

Frolich ED, editor: *Pathophysiology*. Philadelphia, Pa., Lippincott, 1976.

Ganong WF: *Review of Medical Physiology*, 8th ed. Los Altos, Calif.: Lange Medical Publications, 1977.

Goldensohn ES and Appel SH, editors: *Scientific Approaches to Clinical Neurology*, 2 vols. Philadelphia, Pa.: Lea & Febiger, 1977.

Guyton AC: *Textbook of Medical Physiology*, 5th ed. Philadelphia, Pa.: Saunders, 1976.

Matthews WB: *Practical Neurology*, 3rd ed. London: Blackwell Scientific Publications, 1975.

Maugh TH: Multiple sclerosis: genetic link, viruses suspected. *Science* 195:667–669, 1977.

Merritt HH: *A Textbook of Neurology*, 5th ed. Philadelphia, Pa.: Lea & Febiger, 1973.

Messiha FS and Kenny AD: *Parkinson's Disease*. New York: Plenum, 1977.

Stanley EF and Drachman DB: Effect of myasthenic immunoglobulin on acetylcholine receptors of intact mammalian neuromuscular junctions. *Science* 200:1285–1287, 1978.

Thorn GW et al, editors: *Harrison's Principles of Internal Medicine*, 8th ed. New York: McGraw-Hill, 1977.

CHAPTER TWENTY-ONE

Rheumatic Disorders

JOINTS

Degenerative Joint Disease (Osteoarthritis, Osteoarthrosis)

Degenerative joint disease (DJD) is one of the most frequent causes of chronic physical discomfort and disability. It appears to represent a process of wearing out of joints and is characterized by: gradual deterioration and loss of the articular cartilage of movable joints; a chronic inflammatory reaction; and the development of new bone below and at the margins of the articular cartilages and at the edges of bone, which seems to represent attempts at repair. The incidence of DJD increases with age and is so universal in various vertebrate species, in time, and in geographical distribution, that it has been considered a part of the normal aging process. The degree of subjective discomfort and disability experienced by the person with DJD is often not well correlated with the objective severity of the disorder as manifested by radiographic changes.

Types

There are two forms of DJD: primary and secondary. In the primary type there is no evidence of a predisposing injury or other prior joint abnormality, the cause is not known, the degenerative changes are more uniformly distributed among joints, and the signs and symptoms appear and progress with advancing age. This comprises the large majority of cases of DJD. In secondary DJD the accelerated degeneration of one or more joints is associated with a history of joint injury, infection, the presence of obesity, certain metabolic diseases, or congenital anatomic abnormalities. In the secondary form the deterioration begins at an earlier age and is likely to be confined to certain joints. However, in both primary and secondary forms the degenerative processes appear to be the same.

Causes and Abnormalities

The intact articular surface of a normal movable joint is comprised of a specialized type of connective tissue, cartilage, which has a perfectly smooth surface and is elastic and compressible. Its physical characteristics in permitting smooth joint movement and absorbing minor shocks occurring during musculoskeletal work depends not only on its biochemical composition, but the microscopic configuration of its components, which are collagen fibers and macromolecules of hydrated protein-polysaccharides. Studies show that normal joints subjected to a heavy load and continuous joint movement over long periods resist damage remarkably well; this freedom from frictional wear depends on the two surfaces of the articular cartilage being kept physically separated during joint movement. The physical separation is accomplished as a result of a thin fluid film which is squeezed out of the interstitial spaces of the cartilage at areas adjacent to the points of maximal pressure. The process is one in which increasing pressure on the cartilage itself squeezes out more cartilage fluid and thus produces an automatic increase in lubrication which serves to reduce friction and maintain the articular surfaces separated. As the pressure increases, the amount of fluid, and therefore the effectiveness of the lubrication, increases. This is called a "squeeze film" by some authors. At lower pressures surface lubrication by large glycoprotein molecules in the synovial fluid appears to serve a similar function.

It is suggested by some authors that it is not the static high-pressure joint stress described above, but rather the multiple small sudden shocks and jars (impulsive loads) for which the subject is not prepared by appropriate muscle bracing, and torso and extremity position, that damages cartilage and initiates and perpetuates the degenerative changes characteristic of DJD. Studies with experimental animals demonstrate that repeated impulse loading, with relatively light weight applied, leads quite rapidly to early development of cartilage fibrillation (see following) and increased numbers of chondrocytes typical of DJD.

Normally, the cartilage-forming cells, chondrocytes, are relatively sparse and are surrounded by the noncellular cartilage matrix. In the normal cartilage of the adult, chondrocytes do not synthesize new cartilage. However, damage to articular cartilage initiates activation of chondrocytes; they undergo cell multiplication, which produces clusters of chondroblasts localized to the basilar portions of articular cartilage, begin enzyme synthesis, and then initiate formation of components of new cartilage matrix. Since articular cartilage is nonvascular, the biochemical compounds necessary to supply the ingredients for this active chondrosynthesis are thought to be derived from the breakdown by enzymes of old articular cartilage. Therefore, in DJD, cartilage turnover is increased. But the newly synthesized cartilage is different in composition from the original; and cartilage damage, whether produced by physical trauma, infection, or chemical–metabolic injury, often does not heal satisfactorily. The increased quantity of hydrolytic enzymes present in affected joints initiates breakdown of the newly synthesized cartilage and eventually the rate of cartilage breakdown exceeds the rate of synthesis. Then subchondral bone becomes exposed, resulting in a narrowed joint space and promoting degenerative changes in the articular portion and margins of the bone itself.

The earliest changes in the articular cartilage appear to be microscopic flaws in its surface; whether these early defects are initiated by repeated minor joint trauma with chondral damage and release of proteolytic enzymes, or develop as a result of some more basic abnormality in the biochemistry and metabolism of articular cartilage, is unsettled. Subsequently the surface flaws become more pronounced, with softening of the cartilage, flanking and roughening of the surface, and development of irregularities called fibrillations. The latter widen into fissures which penetrate more deeply toward the bone, and eventual denudation of subchondral bone develops as the cartilage flakes off.

Changes in the articular bone are marked and include formation of sclerotic new bone with increased density; growth of bony exostoses (called osteophytes) covered by new cartilage, which occur at joint margins and in areas where ligaments and tendons attach; formation of fibrotic cysts in the bone beneath the joint surfaces; and a remodeling of the surface contours of subchrondral bone.

Eventually changes occur in the synovial membranes and tissues of the joint capsule: low-grade inflammation, hypertrophy, and fibrosis.

Assessment

Subjective

The chief complaint of patients with DJD is a steady aching pain in the affected joints which is made worse by overly vigorous physical activity and weight bearing, especially in obese persons. Increased sensations of joint stiffness on initiation of movement after a period of quiescence is characteristic; then with continuation of the movement there is a gradual "loosening up" and subjective improvement. Symptoms are relieved by aspirin, heat, rest of the affected joint, and massage. Joint ache often appears to worsen at times of cold, damp, inclement weather. As mentioned above, it should be emphasized that DJD which is not severe by objective criteria such as X-ray may be found in patients who complain of intolerable discomfort, while quite severe joint degeneration may occur in individuals who appear to be minimally symptomatic. In addition there are seemingly spontaneous episodes or exacerbation of pain and stiffness apparently unrelated to known precipitating factors, which subsequently resolve independently of management regiment or with no treatment at all.

Objective

Physical examination may reveal a reduced range of motion of affected joints; crepitation on motion; joint enlargement, change in shape, and angular deformation and malalignment; mild tenderness to palpation; small joint effusions; and atrophy of the muscles related to affected joints. In the hand, Heberden's nodes are bony protuberances at the dorsal and lateral surfaces of the base of the distal phalanges (distal interphalangeal joint; DIP); Bouchard's nodes are similar changes at the distal portion of the proximal interphalangeal joint (PIP). Findings of joint redness and increased warmth are rare in DJD.

Beyond these generalizations, the signs and symptoms of DJD depend upon the joints that are involved. Shoulders and elbows are usually spared.

Signs and Symptoms According to Specific Joint Involvement

Hip.   DJD of the hip is sometimes called coxarthrosis or malum coxae senilis. This is the most disabling form of DJD; it tends to come on later in life than some of the other joint deterioration and in half of the patients with this form it is said that some type of antecedent hip disease was present. Pain may be quite severe; it is made worse by the weight bearing and movements of walking; it is often most marked in the groin and may be referred to the medial aspect of the knee. As the disease progresses the pain is continuous and even keeps the patient awake at night. Range of motion is considerably reduced and ambulation becomes increasingly difficult.

Knees.   Involvement of the knees, common in older females (especially the obese) is also severely disabling. It is characterized by enlargement of the knee joint caused both by synovitis and effusion, and bony enlargement; reduced range of motion; increasing pain on motion; crepitations; and the deformity genu varum, where the legs bow out at the knee joint ("knock knees" is genu valgum).

Vertebral Column.   There are two types of joints in the spinal column: (1) the intervertebral joints, in which there is an intervertebral disk (composed of an inner core—the nucleus pulposus, and an outer annulus fibrosis) between the bodies of each vertebra; and (2) the posterior zygapophyseal joints, which are the articulations between the facets of the lateral area of the vertebral arches. In the cervical spine there is a third type of joint, the joints of Luschka; these are articulating surfaces between the lateral portions of adjoining vertebral bodies at either side of the intervertebral disks (Figure 21-1).

In DJD of the cervical spine it is the joints of Luschka that are most affected; the changes are formation of osteophytes and ridges of bony overgrowth that narrow the intervertebral foramina where the dorsal and ventral roots of spinal nerves and blood vessels enter and leave the cord. In DJD of the thoracic and lumbar areas it may be degeneration and herniation of the nucleus pulposus

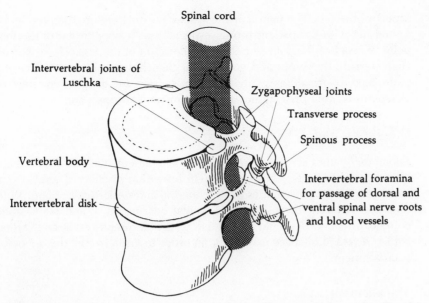

Spinal cord

Intervertebral joints of
Luschka

Zygapophyseal joints

Transverse process

Spinous process

Vertebral body

Intervertebral disk

Intervertebral foramina
for passage of dorsal and
ventral spinal nerve roots
and blood vessels

Figure 21-1. Diagram of composite vertebrae showing the sites which may be affected in degenerative joint disease of the spine.

through a portion of the annulus of the intervertebral disks, causing compression of the root of a spinal nerve that produces signs and symptoms. Other changes are displacements of the intervertebral disks, degenerative disease of the vertebral bodies themselves (spondylosis), and formation of osteophytes at the margins where the disks attach to the vertebral bodies. Degenerative changes in the zygapophyseal joints usually occur in the same areas of the spine in which disk disease is present. Spasm of associated muscles, especially the sternocleidomastoid, trapezius, and paraspinous muscles, is frequent and responsible for much of the pain.

In spine DJD the type and location of pain and neurologic signs and symptoms depend on the level of involvement. At any level, displaced disks, osteophytes, foraminal narrowing, and bony overgrowth at vertebral margins, produce their effects by compressing blood supply and nerve roots, and on occasion even the spinal cord itself. In cervical spine disease the main symptoms consist of pain on motion of the head in flexion, rotation, lateral flexion, and hyperextension, with radiation to the occiput, temples, and upper trapezius, paraspinous, and sternocleidomastoid muscles. In some patients pain in the shoulders and upper arms may be severe. Muscle atrophy, paresis, and paresthesias may occur in the upper extremities, and irritation of nerve roots may lead to painful muscle spasm.

Lumbar spine DJD is often associated with involvement of the intervertebral disks, with protrusion of the degenerated disk which then impinges on nerve roots or compresses the cord. Herniation when it occurs does so most commonly at L4–L5 and L5–S1; in most patients low back pain has been present for many years prior to the acute exacerbation. Pain may be sudden in onset following heavy lifting or twisting of the spine in some unusual exertion; sciatica may be present and may be the outstanding symptom: a sharp ache begins in the sciatic notch deep in the buttock, radiates to the thigh, and then down the lateral aspect of the leg. The pain is made worse by coughing or straining, and straight leg raising with the patient prone, especially with dorsiflexion of the foot at the point of onset of the pain (about 40° of elevation of the leg). Herniated disk pain characteristically comes and goes rather than being continuous. There may be neurologic abnormalities involving motor, sensory and deep tendon reflexes. Muscle spasm is often present and accounts for much of the pain.

Laboratory and X-Ray

Laboratory values are within normal limits in patients with DJD who are without other diseases. X-rays show osteophyte formation at affected joints, joint space narrowing, and abnormalities in subchondral and periarticular bone. When knee films are ordered, they should be weight-bearing ones; and for C-spine films, oblique projections should be added to the anteroposterior and lateral views (which reveal joint-space narrowing) in order to visualize the degree of foraminal encroachment.

Management

It is helpful to both the patient with DJD and the health-care provider to realistically acknowledge four points: (1) progression to severe deformity and disability is rare in DJD; (2) no known treatment will reverse or even arrest the progression of the disorder; (3) amelioration of signs and symptoms can be marked with a regularly followed treatment plan; and (4) signs and symptoms of the disorder are characterized by spontaneous remisssions and exacerbations which bear little or no discernible relationship to alterations in life style, management modalities, or objective status of the disease as assessed by physical or X-ray examination.

The specifics involve aspirin 0.6 gm three or five times a day on a regular, rather than a sporadic basis; this medication achieves both relief of pain and suppression of inflammatory responses, which although not a prominent feature of the disease, nevertheless are often present to some extent. Taking the aspirin with or just after meals minimizes gastric irritation. An effective liquid antacid such as Mylantan or Maalox may be added an hour after meals and at bedtime if necessary. Antiinflammatory agents having toxic effects, as they all do, should be avoided, with the possible exception of their occasional use for control of symptoms in severe disease of the hips or knees; indomethacin, ibuprofen, or others, may be used. So-called "muscle relaxants" such as methocarbamol, diazepam, and carisoprodol probably are of little or no value for the muscle spasm sometimes associated with DJD, especially that of the cervical spine. Biofeedback or progressive relaxation and other physical therapy and rehabilitation programs are more appropriate and effective where indicated. Local heat relieves muscle spasm, joint pain, and stiffness.

Maintenance of an active program of physical exercise which does not overtax affected joints, particularly weight-bearing ones, is one of the cornerstones of management. Swimming is the perfect exercise, since there is no joint strain or work against gravity involved. However, a stationary bicycle and rowing machine are also very helpful if used regularly.

Perhaps the most important component of management of DJD for many patients is the one least likely to be attained: elimination of overeating and obesity, and maintenance of a lean body weight.

Management of cervical spine disease especially, may involve certain special measures. Patients should be cautioned to avoid chiropractic manipulation of the cervical spine, and if surgery for some other disorder is necessary the anesthesiologist needs to be informed of the C-spine involvement to avoid hyperextension of the neck with possible dislocation. A cervical collar to stabilize the head and neck, and periodic cervical traction to relieve muscle spasm and nerve root compression, may be helpful. Patients should sleep flat using no pillow or only a small one, and postures involving sustained neck flexion or hyperextension should be avoided. In DJD of the lumbar spine a hard mattress or bedboard is indicated. Postural exercises to strengthen the muscles of the back should be a regular part of the patient's self-care. Some simple ones used at the University of Colorado Hospitals are illustrated in Figure 21-2.

Rheumatoid Arthritis (RA)

Rheumatoid arthritis is a chronic general systemic disease of unknown cause, involving symmetric inflammatory polyarthritis leading to joint destruction; and a number of extraarticular manifestations, especially widespread vasculitis, and characterized by apparently spontaneous remissions and exacerbations. It is more common in females than males, it may begin at any age but is more common in early middle age, and there seems to be a hereditary predisposition, though it is not marked. The course of the disease varies greatly from patient to patient as concerns the nature of the onset, the extraarticular manifestations, the course, and the patterns of involvement. In general the joint involvement tends to be symmetric, and, usually, once a joint has become affected it continues to be so intermittently, rather than the inflammatory process resolving altogether.

Cause

The cause is not known, but accumulating evidence indicates that immune processes, including both humorally (antibody-) mediated and cell-mediated responses are involved in the pathologic changes not only in the joints but also in affected tissues elsewhere. Histocompatibility antigen HLA–D4 appears to be associated with RA (Chapter 22). The factors that are responsible for initiating the immune responses are unknown, although some workers suggest that a viral or bacterial infection may trigger abnormal immune system reactions; however, there is as yet no evidence for this. It is known that in patients with RA, synovial lymphocytes and plasma cells synthesize immunoglobulin antibodies of the IgG, IgA, and IgM classes; these antibodies form immune complexes with the IgG antigen. T lymphocytes are present in synovium and synovial fluid; the antigen and IgG antibody complexes occur in synovial fluid; and deposits of immunoglobulins and components of the complement cascade are present in synovial membranes and articular cartilage. The processes concerned in the release of the mediators of inflammation (chemotactic and vasoactive responses) by activation of the complement system, and their subsequent destructive effects on tissue are discussed in Chapter 22. Additional tissue inflammation and chemical injury occur as a

Colorado General Hospital   Department of Emergency Medicine
4200 E. 9th Avenue   394-8901
Denver, Colorado 80220
399-1211

Aftercare Instructions to the Patient

-Chronic Low Back Pain-

Chronic low back pain is frequently related to poor posture and poor
muscle tone. Below are exercises long accepted as helpful in this
condition. They require a period of getting used to, so begin slowly
and work up to tolerance.

Williams' Flexion Exercises

1 & 2   3 & 4   5
Strengthening exercises.   Mobilizing exercises.   Stretching and strengthen-
Repeat each 10 times.   Repeat each 10 times   ing for low back. Repeat
Do at least 3 times   Do at least 3 times   20 times. Do at least 3
per day.   per day.   times per day.

1.   2.

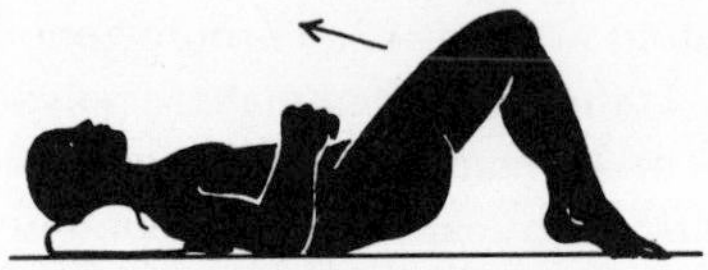

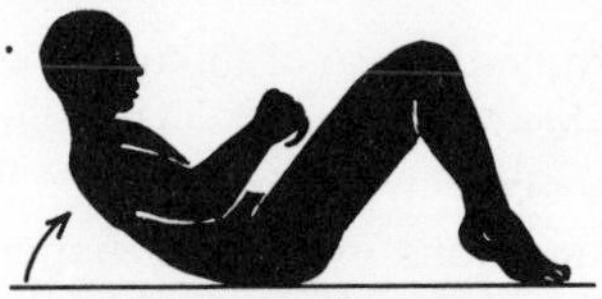

Clear shoulder blades   Keep trunk on floor

3. 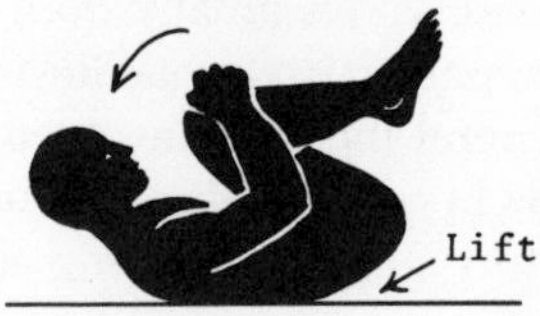   4. Keep knee
                                          straight

        Lift sacrum

                                      Force buttock towards heel

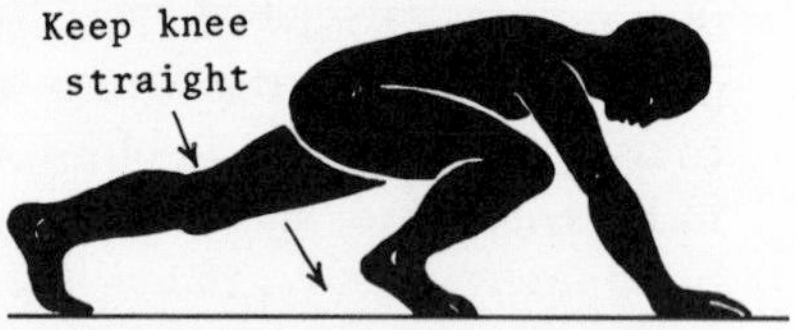

5.

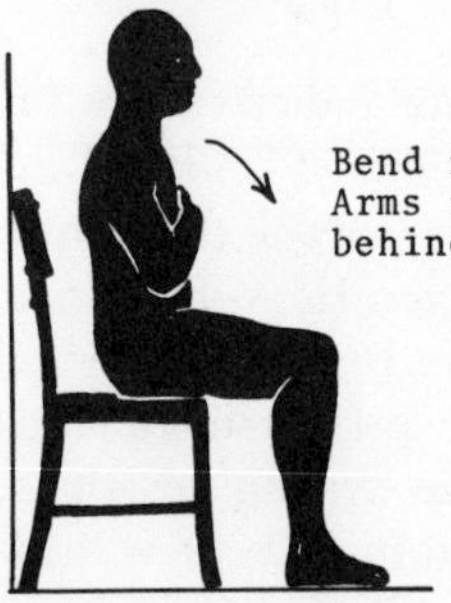

        Bend forward between knees.
        Arms folded across chest or
        behind neck.

        In addition, follow instructions stapled
        to this sheet.

Chair against wall

Figure 21-2. Simple exercises to strengthen back muscles and relieve the pain and muscle
spasm of degenerative joint disease of the spine.

result of the release of proteolytic enzymes following ingestion of antigen–antibody complexes by leukocytes attracted to the area by some of the components
of the complement system (leukotactic factors).

Finally, not only the synovial fluid but also the blood of most patients with RA
contain the so-called RA factors; these are immunoglobulin antibodies of the

classes IgM, IgG, and IgA, to IgG antigen that has been altered by some prior unknown factor. The alteration in form then causes it to act as a neoantigen for the immunoglobulins so that they synthesize antibody specific to it and form antigen–antibody complexes with it. In the test for RA factors, latex or other particles are coated with IgG antigen; if anti-IgG immunoglobulins are present in the patient's serum these will form complexes with and agglutinate the coated particles; the degree of agglutination at a given concentration is a measure of the titers of RA factor immunoglobulins. RA factors are present in about three fourths of RA patients, but occur also in some other rheumatic disorders and in some normal subjects.

The various immunologic processes lead to the formation of large amounts of chemical mediators of inflammation, influx of phagocytic white cells, and release of proteolytic enzymes, culminating in destruction of articular cartilage and bone, the joint capsule, and attaching ligaments and tendons.

Experiments with laboratory animals have shown that a disease in many respects resembling human rhematoid arthritis can be induced by infecting animals with certain pathogenic microorganisms; a chronic rheumatoid arthritis develops but by the time it is established the precipitating organisms can no longer be isolated from their tissues or body fluids. However, it is not known whether a similar situation exists in the human disease.

Abnormalities

A typical normal synovial joint is illustrated in Figure 21-3.

The synovial membrane of an affected joint shows the first changes, consisting of inflammation with vasodilation, edema and hyperemia, cellular infiltrates

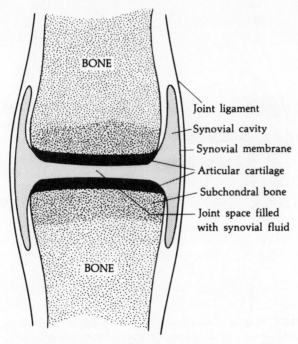

Figure 21-3. Diagram of a typical synovial freely moveable joint.

(mainly lymphocytes), formation of exudates and cellular proliferation. The cells of the synovium undergo hypertrophy and hyperplasia. The amount of synovial fluid increases and alters character, becoming less viscous and more turbid. The synovium undergoes a thickening and forms chronic granulation tissue called pannus which proliferates, spreads out over the articular cartilage, and burrows through it to the subchondral bone where it initiates a destructive process in cartilage and bone by secreting proteolytic enzymes. This in-growth begins and is most marked at the joint margins, at the junction between cartilage, bone, and the joint capsule attachments. Eventually the hypertrophied synovium replaces the destroyed articular cartilage with fibrous tissue. The cartilage is destroyed, the bone denuded, and then at the sites where the two bony articular surfaces come in contact, fusion of the bones may occur (ankylosis) through deposition of fibrous or bony tissue, leading to a reduction or total loss of joint mobility. Another characteristic joint abnormality which may result from the sum of the destructive processes is subluxation. This is a partial joint dislocation caused by the combined effect of cartilage and bone destruction, weakening of muscles, and loosening of ligaments and tendons. The result is deformity and instability of the affected joints.

As the disease progresses joints become chronically swollen with edema of the structures around the joint, effusion within it, boggy hypertrophied pannus, and fibrosis of surrounding areas. Fixed deformities occur; typical types are ulnar deviation of the phalanges and swan-neck deformity (Figure 21-5) resulting from contractures of the small muscles of the hand producing flexion of the DIP and hyperextension of the PIP joints. When the knees are affected, effusions may

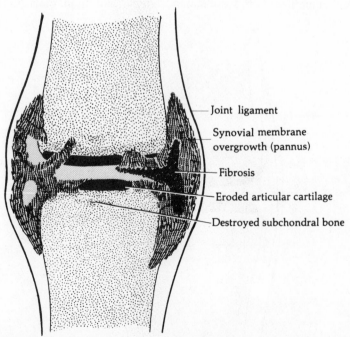

Joint ligament

Synovial membrane overgrowth (pannus)

Fibrosis

Eroded articular cartilage

Destroyed subchondral bone

Figure 21-4. Diagram showing changes in affected joint in rheumatoid arthritis: erosion of articular cartilage and subchondral bone, fibrosis, narrowing of joint space, loosening and thickening of capsule, and overgrowth of synovial membrane to form granulation tissue (pannus).

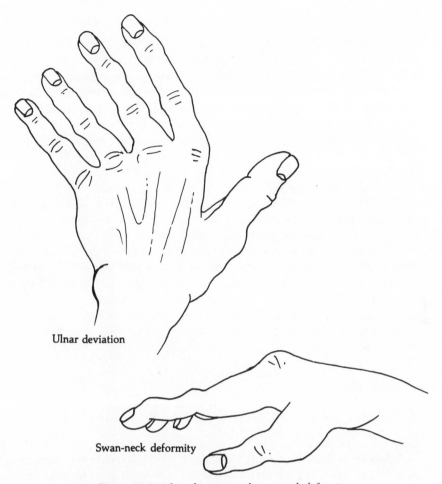

Ulnar deviation

Swan-neck deformity

Figure 21-5. Ulnar deviation and swan-neck deformity.

evolve into popliteal space cysts (Baker's cysts) which are abnormal extensions or herniations of the joint space filled with synovial fluid. These may extend down into the calf. When joints of C1 and C2 are involved subluxations at this site may cause spinal cord compression and neurologic signs and symptoms.

About one fourth of patients with RA develop subcutaneous nodules later in the course of the disease; these tend to correlate with the degree of activity of the disease, the titers of RA factor, and a poor prognosis. The most common site is the olecranon bursa of the elbow and along the lateral aspect of the forearm. They sometimes occur in the lung and other viscera. The inner zone contains cellular debris and a core of fibrinoid necrosis surrounded by macrophages, granulation tissue, and other cell types.

Other extraarticular abnormalities include rheumatoid disease of the lung with pleural effusions; granulomatous pneumonitis and diffuse interstitial fibrosis; diffuse vasculitis with thrombus formation and small infarctions in the skin; necrotizing vasculitis of the viscera and nervous system; myositis; and lymphadenopathy. Moderate anemia is a common accompaniment of RA and is said to be the consequence of inadequate bone marrow function.

Course and Prognosis

In most patients the onset of RA is insidious with constitutional symptoms of general fatigue, weakness, vague aching, and stiffness which may not be localized to specific joints. Fleeting arthralgias in the proximal finger joints are said to be a common early symptom. After a few weeks morning stiffness develops and joint inflammation (often in the wrists and metacarpophalangeal joints) with redness, warmth, swelling, tenderness, and pain. Hands and feet in a symmetrical pattern are common sites of the initial manifestations, but knees, ankles, neck and shoulders, and elbows may be involved. In less than one fifth of patients the onset may be acute with prostration and generalized joint involvement.

It is stated that approximately three fourths of patients who have had symptoms of RA for less than a year will improve and as many as a fifth may have a complete remission. Signs of a more severe course are persistence of active disease for more than one year, onset of the disease before age 30, persistence of disease without a remission, high titers of RA factor, and the presence of nodules. Half or more of patients are able to remain fully employed, although vocational retraining may be desirable or necessary for some. After ten years of the disease about half the patients are improved or at least stable; if improvement has not occurred by then, likelihood of its occuring becomes more remote with the passage of time. After an additional five to ten years about 10% of patients are severely disabled.

Assessment

Subjective

Description by the patient of the duration and severity of morning stiffness is a useful index to the activity of the disease; it may last one to two hours and be relieved only slowly during active phases by a hot tub bath, aspirin, and moving about. As improvement occurs the degree and duration of the stiffness declines. Complaints of increased difficulty accomplishing aspects of self-care and the daily routine, and increased pain and weakness, with decreased range of motion of joints, correlate with exacerbations and provide helpful data for assessing the severity of the disease and changes in the patient's level of functioning.

Objective

The complete joint survey at the time of each visit is an important component of assessment. Degree of redness, warmth, swelling, tenderness, and range of motion of each joint including the cervical, thoracic, and lumbar segments of the spine, and evidences of muscle atrophy and weakness, should be evaluated and recorded regularly. Laboratory tests in the initial assessment of RA include Westergren erythrocyte sedimentation rate, complete blood count, serum RA factors, IgM antiglobulin antibodies, serum antinuclear antibodies, and possibly synovial fluid examination (especially when a single large joint is involved) to rule out septic or other causes of a monoarthritis. It is reported that about three fourths of patients with RA have significant titers (1:80 or above) of the IgM antibodies. Initial X-ray survey may aid in diagnosis and furnish baseline information for evaluating progression of the disease; early changes may be confined to soft tissue swelling, evidence of effusion, and local osteoporosis. Later, loss of articular cartilage with narrowing of the joint space, joint malalignment and subluxation, bone erosions near the joint capsules, cyst formations, bony ankyloses, periarticular bone resorption, and secondary degenerative joint disease may develop.

Management

The primary objective in the management of RA is to enable the patient to maintain an adequate degree of function in the activities of daily life. Specific treatment measures depend on the nature of the manifestations and severity of the disease in a given patient. As the severity of disease manifestations increases, then the modalities of management require a corresponding intensification in order to meet the goal of therapy: maintenance of function. In general, escalated forms of therapy (whether pharmacologic or surgical) carry a corresponding elevated degree of risk for the patient.

Aspirin 3 to 6 gm/day in divided doses, with meals and with added antacids if required to minimize gastrointestinal irritation; and physical measures: adequate rest; heat to relieve muscle spasm, stiffness and pain; a directed regular program of moderate exercise to strengthen muscles and preserve joint stability and range of motion; and use of joint splints at night to prevent flexion contractures and delay joint deformity; remain the foundations of management in RA. Swimming is a superior form of general exercise for the RA patient. Aspirin should always be given an amply adequate trial for at least two months or more before the decision is made to use the more toxic antiinflammatory agents. Aspirin is effective not only for pain relief but importantly as an antiinflammatory agent when used in adequate doses of 4 to 5 gm/24 hr in divided doses. Toxic effects of aspirin, more marked in elderly subjects, include tinnitus and depressed hearing, pyrosis and epigastric distress, and gastrointestinal erosions and ulcerations with bleeding. The gastrointestinal effects are ameliorated by taking the aspirin with food and/or antacids such as Mylanta or Maalox. The effectiveness of aspirin in RA is suggested to be its action in inhibiting the synthesis and release of prostaglandins, which are involved in inflammatory reactions; and its action in suppressing the aggregation of platelets and release of vasoactive substances from them.

There are a number of other antiinflammatory pharmacologic agents which may be effective in management for patients who are unable to tolerate aspirin, for whom aspirin seems to be inadequately effective, or in conjunction with maintenance aspirin. Phenylbutazone and indomethacin have been used for many years and may be helpful for some patients during acute flareups or on a regular basis. Allergic skin reactions, peptic ulcer, abdominal distress, salt retention, and blood dyscrasias may occur as side effects. Ibuprofen appears to be as effective as aspirin and may have fewer gastrointestinal effects. Tolmetin is said to have relatively few side effects and to be as effective in relief of discomfort and inflammatory manifestations as aspirin. Naproxen has also been reported to be effective and well tolerated in many patients. These agents are expensive, none is markedly (if any) more effective than aspirin, and since they are relatively new, the possible toxic effects of long-term use will not be known for some time.

Antimalarial agents such as hydroxychloroquin, although they have toxic effects on the retina in large doses, are reported by some workers to be moderately effective and relatively safe in smaller amounts for some patients. Tissue accumulation of antimalarials occurs so that initial doses may be eventually tapered to low maintenance levels.

In more severe progressive disease of longer duration, where the basic components of management appear to be inadequate, intramuscular injection of the gold salts, gold thioglucose or gold sodium thiomalate, have been shown by well-controlled clinical trials to be effective in improving both subjective and objective status of RA patients when continued on a maintenance basis. It appears to reduce the number of joints involved, decrease the sedimentation rate, improve the patient's general functional level, and decrease the rate of pathologic changes in joints. The mode of action is uncertain, but it probably involves inhibition of intracellular enzymes concerned in immune and inflammatory responses. Toxic reactions include dermatitis, ulcerations of the oral mucous membranes (stomatitis), proteinuria, and occasionally blood dyscrasias including thrombocytopenia, or gastrointestinal complaints.

Systemic use of low-dose oral adrenal glucocorticoids (often prednisone) is commonly used in progressive RA and is considered to be effective in improving the patient's condition with relatively few side effects. The effects appear to be based upon the antiinflammatory actions of the steroids discussed elsewhere. Its effects appear to be additive with those of aspirin. Osteoporosis and peptic ulcerations are the most common side effects. Intraarticular injection of corticosteroids is often used on an occasional basis to control inflammation and effusion in individual joints; it appears to produce prolonged joint improvement for some patients. Aseptic necrosis of weight-bearing joints is a reported complication.

Immunosuppressive agents such as cyclophosphamide and azathioprine may be employed where the above measures have proven inadequate for control of progressive RA. Improvement in several variables such as number of joints involved and functional level of the patients has been reported in several controlled studies. Cyclophosphamide is said to be the more effective of the two. Both drugs exert a steroid-sparing effect in that with their use lower steroid doses may produce the same beneficial effects as higher ones when steroids are used alone. Toxic effects with cyclophosphamide are leukopenia, depressed ovarian function, hair loss, hemorrhagic cystitis, and in long-term use, increased incidence of various types of malignancies. The toxic manifestations of azathioprine include gastrointestinal ulcerations and bone marrow suppression. Increased incidence of infections occurs with all immunsuppressive agents including adrenal steroids.

Penicillamine (mercaptovaline) is also reported to be effective in controlling the signs, symptoms, and progression of RA. Adverse effects on the kidney (nephritis and nephrotic syndrome), thrombocytopenia, and dermatitis are toxic side effects. Consequences of long-term administration of this agent are not known. The tendency of the disease to show spontaneous remissions and exacerbations makes objective evaluation of the effectiveness of any management modality difficult.

Gout

Gout is a group of related disease of purine and uric acid metabolism and excretion, characterized by hyperuricemia and periodic acute severe arthritis resulting from deposits of sodium urate in the joints; and occasionally tophaceous deposits of urate in soft tissues. There is a strong hereditary predisposition and the prevalence is highest in adult males.

Purines are the end products of the metabolic breakdown of nucleic acids; they are derived from exogenous sources in the diet and are also synthesized endogenously from amino acids, primarily in the liver. Purines undergo metabolic breakdown in the liver to uric acid, and additional uric acid is synthesized from various other precursors. Uric acid is eliminated in the urine by the kidneys by an active transport process: all uric acid in the blood is filtered at the glomerulus; most of this is reabsorbed in the initial segment of the renal tubule; and then farther on in the tubule uric acid is actively secreted from peritubular fluid and blood back into the tubular filtrate to be removed in the urine.

Cause

Serum levels of uric acid (normal range 2.5 to 7.5 mg/100 ml) are the result of an equilibrium between the amount of uric acid produced from purines by the liver, and the quantity of uric acid eliminated in the urine by the kidneys. Therefore, hyperuricemia can be the consequence of either excess production of uric acid or inadequate elimination of uric acid, or both.

About 90% of persons with gout have abnormally high endogenous synthesis of purines; some of these patients have urinary uric acid content which is high, but most excrete uric acid only in normal quantities which, therefore, contributes to the hyperuricemia. The remaining 10% of gouty patients have not been demonstrated to have excessive purine synthesis but rather inadequate urinary elimination of uric acid. Both of these types of gout are termed primary gout. Primary gout is, therefore, said to be a *group* of metabolic disorders of purine and uric acid metabolism, because patients with gout have a variety of abnormalities in the enzyme systems and metabolic pathways concerned with purine and uric acid handling. The genetically determined metabolic deficits interact with such factors as overeating and obesity, alcohol use, pharmacologic agents, and components of the diet, to produce elevated serum uric acid.

It is reported that serum urate values are well correlated with body weight; patients with primary gout are almost all overweight, and three fourths of gouty patients also have hypertriglyceridemia, which tends to clear if the patient loses weight. Weight loss also lowers serum urate and makes gout easier to control.

Secondary gout is the term applied to manifestations of the disease associated with increased uric acid in the body fluids as a consequence of some other condition: chronic renal disease, leukemia, lead poisoning, thiazide diuretics, and others.

Abnormalities

Urate is not a toxic substance and as long as it remains in solution in the blood it causes no difficulties; however, its solubility is low and urate solutions of con-

centrations above about 7 mg% are supersaturated and crystals tend to precipitate out readily. It is apparent that serum levels at the upper limits of the
normal range approximate the solubility of the compound. However, some persons may have serum levels of 8 or 9 mg% without symptoms or signs, while
others at this level have either acute gouty arthritis or chronic tophaceous gout,
or both. The reason for this is uncertain, but it may have to do with the degree
of binding of urate to certain plasma proteins; it may be not the total uric acid
which determines supersaturation and precipitation but only the unbound fraction.

Chronic Changes: Tophaceous Gout

This form of gout was much more common prior to the use of pharmacologic
agents effective in controlling hyperuricemia, and was seen in over half of patients with gout. Deposits of sodium urate, surrounded by an inflammatory and
infiltrative tissue reaction, do not develop until the disease has been established
for several years without being effectively treated, and often only after the patient has had several attacks of acute gouty arthritis. The deposits may be found
in the synovium, subchondral bone, in joint bursae and tendons, and in subcutaneous tissue, most often the dorsal surface of the forearm and hands,
frequently over the joints. The presence of tophaceous deposits is associated
with a more severe disease and more frequent attacks of acute gouty arthritis.
They cause disruption of tissues, development of fibrosis, degeneration of cartilage, proliferation of synovium with formation of pannus and destruction of subchondral bone, especially at joint margins, and may lead to marked deformities.
Deposition of urate may also occur in the kidney, causing renal parenchymal
damage, both tubular and glomerular, and arteriosclerotic changes in the renal
vasculature with impairment of renal function.

Acute Gouty Arthritis

The initial attack typically takes the form of a rapidly developing monoarticular
arthritis, characteristically of the first metatarsophalangeal joint of the large toe;
this classical form is called podagra and is seen in 75% or more of all patients
with gout. Other sites in early attacks are the instep, ankle, heel, and knee; the
lower extremities are most commonly involved in initial phases. Later, other
frequently affected joints are the finger joints, wrist, and elbow. Shoulder and
hip joints are less commonly affected. The onset of joint inflammation is very
rapid, with severe swelling, redness, pain, and tenderness to touch evolving to
maximum within a few hours of the onset. Attacks may last from several days, if
mild, to weeks if severe. Resolution of the inflammation then occurs, with desquamation of skin, and the joint returns to normal. The patient may not have
another attack, in the same or another joint, for six months to two years.

At the cell and tissue level is has been demonstrated that during an acute attack microcrystals of Na^+ urate precipitate out from ECF supersaturated with
urate and are present in the synovial fluid and within leukocytes of the fluid. It is
suggested that the crystals initiate a cellular response with activation of the complement system, production of mediators of inflammation such as bradykinin and
the prostaglandins, and release of leukotaxins which attract phagocytic white

cells to the area. The leukocytes ingest the crystals and release lysosomal leuko-proteases into the joint fluid and tissue, and these enzymes destroy cartilage and stimulate inflammatory proliferation of synovium.

The specific factors which may account for the sudden precipitation of urate from body fluids which are chemically saturated with it are not clear. Attacks often seem to be precipitated by excess alcohol intake, overeating, unaccustomed physical exertion and fatigue, an accident involving trauma, surgery, an infection, or other systemic illness. Alcohol probably precipitates an attack by causing increased production of lactate as the alcohol is metabolized; lactate impairs renal tubular secretion of uric acid. Fasting also prompts an acute attack; decreased food intake leads to elevation in serum keto acids which worsen hyperuricemia also by decreasing tubular secretion of uric acid. The effects of alcohol and fasting are additive. Diuretics such as thiazides, furosemide, and ethcrynic acid impair tubular uric acid excretion and may initiate an acute episode of gouty arthritis.

Course

The first attack of gout occurs most often when the patient is in his fifties; in the few females with gout (5 to 10% of patients with gout) the onset is usually post-menopausal. Serum urate values tend to rise in males at puberty, so postpubertal onset is not rare, and in females at the menopause. Hyperuricemia may be present for years, in fact most patients with hyperuricemia never develop overt gout, and physiologic abnormalities seldom result from the chronically elevated urate levels. In men, however, serum urate undergoes a further elevation with increasing age over 40 which predisposes those with high baseline urate levels to an overt attack.

Following an initial acute attack there may be no further signs or symptoms for years; however, with aging the balance between urate production and elimination shifts so that hyperuricemia increases. Thus, with the passage of time there tends to be an increased frequency and severity of attacks, with increasing tendency for more than one joint to be involved, more systemic symptoms and signs such as fever, and slower resolution. Complications of gout, in addition to the pathologic changes described above, include deposition of uric acid kidney stones, nephrosclerosis, and abnormalities of kidney function leading to proteinuria, loss of renal concentrating ability, and azotemia, which is usually not severe. However, chronic renal failure is a significant cause of death in gout. Incidence of pyelonephritis is not infrequent. Arterial hypertension is significantly increased in gout: it may be a consequence of the chronic impairment in renal function.

The natural history of gout has been greatly modified by advances in pharmacologic management.

Management

Asymptomatic Hyperuricemia

The person with hyperuricemia should be advised to avoid high-purine foods; gradually decrease food intake so that he reduces to lean body weight, which may alone lower the serum uric acid and will decrease the likelihood of an acute attack; strictly avoid alcohol; and maintain a fluid intake adequate to sustain a daily urinary output of 2000 ml/24 hr. If serum urate exceeds 9 mg/100 ml treatment is probably indicated, while milder hyperuricemia without signs or symptoms probably does not warrant treatment over that suggested above. Where indicated, the prophylactic use of daily small doses of colchicine, which has no effect at all on serum or synovial fluid urate levels, will usually reduce the frequency of acute attacks. Colchicine impairs leukocyte migration and suppresses the inflammatory consequence of leukocyte phagocytosis of uric acid crystals.

Chronic Gout, Maintenance

Indications for the use of pharmacologic agents that reduce serum urate levels are said to be: hyperuricemia consistently above 9 mg/100 ml (which is thought to be associated with propensity to joint disease and formation of tophi); frequent acute attacks uncontrolled by colchicine; signs of renal impairment; a high rate of uric acid excretion (more than 800 mg/24 hr), which indicates greatly elevated uric acid production; and chronic joint involvement. The goal is to reduce serum uric acid to 6 mg/100 ml or below.

These agents are of no value in the acute attack and in fact acute attacks may increase in number during the first several months of treatment unless colchicine is given, possibly because of mobilization into the blood of tophaceous deposits, although acute attacks may occur at very low serum uric acid levels. The drugs lower the urate levels below the saturation point and therefore inhibit the deposition that produces tophi, and the crystallization that causes acute attacks. Serum uric acid determinations should be done on a regular basis to evaluate the effectiveness of the regimen.

Uricopenic Drug: Allopurinol. Allopurinol decreases the formation of uric acid by inhibiting the enzyme xanthine oxidase; the result is excretion of the precursors of uric acid, xanthine and hypoxanthine, rather than their conversion to uric acid. Uric acid is lowered in both serum and urine, which helps prevent uric acid kidney stones. The most common side effect is skin rash. This drug is very useful in patients with gouty renal insufficiency for whom the uricosuric drugs are not effective (reduced dosage are used in these patients). Allopurinol may be used concurrently with uricosurics to mobilize tophaceous deposits.

Uricosuric Drugs: Probenecid and Sulfinpyrazone. These agents impair the tubular resorption of the uric acid filtered at the glomerulus, therefore most of it stays in the tubule and is eliminated in the urine instead of being almost totally reabsorbed and then partially resecreted. A number of precautionary measures are indicated in the use of uricosuric drugs. Doses start low and are increased gradually and a large fluid intake should be maintained to keep the urine dilute; the reason is the need to avoid a too rapid increase in urate excretion and a too high concentration of it, which would lead to precipitation of crystals in the urinary system. Early in treatment urinary pH should be maintained on the alkaline side of pH 6.0 with $NaHCO_3$ or citrate solutions (which generate bicarbonate) to increase urate solubility. Side effects are gastrointestinal distress, skin rash, and headache.

The Acute Attack

Phenylbutazone or Indomethacin. Either of the two drugs may be given in appropriate doses, larger on the first day of signs and symptoms and tapering over the next two or three days, until the acute attack is aborted. With either of these agents improvement begins in 6 to 12 hr, with well-advanced resolution by 24–48 hr. The patient may then be placed on maintenance colchicine. Gastrointestinal irritation and fluid retention are major side effects, so that in peptic ulcer disease and congestive heart failure they are contraindicated.

Colchicine. This drug traditionally has been given (orally or intravenously) as the prime treatment in an acute attack; large doses are required and gastrointestinal side effects are marked so that it is less frequently used now that other effective agents are available. One useful aspect of colchicine is that, in an acute attack of monoarthritis without a prior known history of hyperuricemia or gout, essentially only gout will respond, thus ruling out other possible causes of acute monoarticular arthritis such as gonorrhea.

CONNECTIVE TISSUE

Systemic Lupus Erythematosus (SLE)

SLE is a chronic inflammatory systemic disease having widespread and diverse manifestations in a number of tissues and organ systems: the joints, skin, kidney, nervous system, blood, cardiovascular system, and serous membranes. It is characterized by remissions and exacerbations, and the cause is unknown, although increasing evidence indicates that the tissue injury results from abnormal immunologic processes perhaps induced by a combination of genetic predisposition and viral infection. Since more sensitive tests to detect its presence have been developed, it is now known that the disorder is a good bit more common than was formerly thought when only the more florid forms were recognized. The incidence is higher in negroids than caucasoids, is rare in mongoloids, occurs more frequently in females than males, and in adolescents and young adults.

Cause

Although the cause is not known, studies of the immune system abnormalities in patients with SLE, and of various pathologic processes in laboratory animals (certain types of which manifest spontaneous or acquired diseases resembling human SLE) have led to the proposal that the following sequence of events may be involved in the genesis of the disorder: (1) Certain as yet poorly understood genetic abnormalities may predispose some individuals to developing abnormal immune responses; (2) a subject with such a predisposition acquires some (usually subclinical) kind of chronic viral infection; the viruses disrupt the cells in various organs and tissues of the host, causing the release into the circulation of components of the cells' nuclei, and possibly also inducing some type of immune transformation of the antigens of the nuclei; (3) either because the nuclear components have been antigenically altered, or because the antigens were formerly "hidden" from the host's immune system, and therefore immune tolerance to them never developed (see Chapter 22), the presence of these "new" antigens in the circulation stimulates the production of antibodies to them by the host's immune system; (4) the production of these antibodies is excessive, because part of the genetic abnormalities in SLE patients is an overactivity in B lymphocytes that synthesize antibodies, and an inadequacy in suppressor T lymphocytes (those regulatory T cells that normally inhibit inappropriate synthesis of antibodies and are therefore important in the maintenance of immunologic tolerance); (5) antigen–antibody complexes (immune complexes) form between the released antigens of cell nuclei and the antibodies to them; (6) the immune complexes stimulate the activation of the complement system, and deposits of antigen, antibody and complement components occur in various tissues and organs; (7) this deposition initiates the release of the mediators of inflammation and chemotactic factors; and (8) leukocytes infiltrate the area, phagocytize the immune complexes, and release lysosomal proteolytic enzymes which cause further inflammation and tissue destruction (Chapter 22).

Abnormalities

The skin is frequently affected; the common manifestation is a symmetric erythematous rash becoming papular, maculopapular, and later scaling, in body areas exposed to sunlight. Other lesions are thickening and atrophy, hyper- or hypopigmentation, edema of the dermis and infiltration with various cell types, urticaria, hyperkeratosis and keratotic plugging, and vasculitis with focal ischemia and ulceration. Discoid lupus erythematosus is a skin lesion with central atrophy, plugging of hair follicles, and elevated red plaques which form scales; the lesion occurs over the face and neck; this form appears to be correlated with fewer systemic abnormalities and a more benign course. Alopecia is common.

Kidney involvement is a frequent and serious development in SLE. Thickening of the basement membrane and necrosis of the glomerular capillaries; parenchymal vasculitis and vascular occlusion; degeneration of renal tubules; cellular proliferation and infiltration; deposits of antigen–antibody–complement complexes and other changes; contribute to the various forms of lupus glomerulonephritis. Impaired renal function manifests as proteinuria, hematuria, casts, predisposition to pyelonephritis, and chronic renal failure with azotemia and nephrotic syndrome. Renal hypertension is a not infrequent correlate (Chapters 3 and 10).

The most common manifestation of SLE is a symmetric polyarthritis which in symptoms may resemble RA but seldom leads to destruction of articular cartilage and subchondral bone, or to permanent joint deformities. However, joint swelling, redness, warmth, pain, tenderness to palpation, and decreased range of motion are present but transitory. Myalgias and muscle atrophy are not unusual.

Serositis, especially of the pleura and pericardium, often occurs accompanied by pleurisy and pleural effusions and pericarditis. Peritonitis is somewhat less common. Pneumonitis with interstitial infiltrates and pulmonary fibrosis is also less common. Myocarditis and valvular disease develop in some patients, with tachycardia, cardiomegaly, and eventual congestive failure. Generalized nontender enlargement of the lymph nodes is common and probably represents an overactivity of the immune system.

In the nervous system a necrotizing vasculitis with formation of small infarcts may be responsible for producing a number of neurologic abnormalities: cranial nerve palsies, stroke, and seizures; and altered mental status and decreased level of consciousness.

Course and Prognosis

The disease is said often to begin with vague constitutional symptoms of fatigue, fever, weakness, anorexia, and weight loss, before the onset of more specific signs and symptoms; these may be arthritis, skin rash, lymph node enlargement, renal malfunction; or less often gastrointestinal, pulmonary, cardiac, or central nervous disturbances. Onset may involve one organ or system, or several simultaneously. Polyarthralgia and polyarthritis are said to be present in 90% of patients and often constitute the initial manifestation.

In most patients episodes of increased activity of the disease process are interspersed with longer periods of partial or complete remission. About 75% of patients have around a 5-year survival, although with marked involvement of the kidneys, heart, and nervous system life expectancy is reduced below this. The fulminating rapidly fatal course formerly seen in some patients has become much more rare now that adrenal glucocorticoids and other pharmacologic agents have come into common use for management. These agents are reported to improve life expectancy and quality of life, and reduce frequency and severity of exacerbations, in most patients with SLE.

Assessment

Aside from the clinical manifestations described above, the diagnosis, progress of the disease, and effects of the treatment regimen, are evaluated by laboratory methods. The most characteristic immune abnormality, which confirms the diagnosis of SLE, is large numbers of antinuclear antibodies to DNA and RNA, comprised of all classes of the immunoglobulins. The test is positive in essentially all patients with lupus, and the antibody titers correlate with the activity of the disease, being higher during exacerbations. Serum complement levels are also depressed during heightened activity of the disease, indicating that complement is being consumed by binding with increased numbers of antigen–antibody complexes. The erythrocyte sedimentation rate is also elevated during periods of acute worsening. Most patients are anemic, leukopenic, and have elevated serum globulins.

Tests of renal function evaluate the degree of renal impairment and its progression, and pulmonary function testing and cardiologic evaluation may be indicated in some patients. The EEG is reported to be abnormal in patients with nervous system involvement.

Management

Early diagnosis, close follow-up, and early treatment of exacerbations, appear to improve the quality of life and prolong survival. General measures include avoiding sunlight, immunizations, blood transfusions, and antibiotics where possible. Aspirin relieves muscle and joint pain, and a program of regular exercises during remission help prevent muscle atrophy and physical deconditioning. The patient should be taught to recognize early the signs and symptoms of an impending flareup: increasing fatigue and malaise, arthralgias and myalgias, ulcerations in the mouth or the mucosal surfaces, loss of weight, hair loss, or pleuritic chest pain. Frequent laboratory monitoring of serum complement; complete blood count; antinuclear antibodies; urinalysis for microhematuria, leukocytes, and protein; and tests of renal function, provide objective evaluation of the disease status and condition of the patient.

In the pharmacologic management of SLE it is important to keep in mind that the disease is characterized by spontaneous remissions and that mild disease may require little or no medication. Where the disease is more severe, involving vital organs, and for acute flareups, corticosteroids are indicated and are remarkably effective in ameliorating signs and symptoms and reducing the duration of the active phase. The dosage depends on the severity, and the degree of response to the initial amounts given. Monitoring of the serum complement levels and the antibody titers are helpful adjuncts to assessment in addition to changes in the signs and symptoms. As improvement occurs steroid dosage is slowly tapered. Some patients require continuous low-dosage steroids, while others do not.

Cyclophosphamide or azothioprine may occasionally be used where indicated, alone or in conjunction with adrenal glucocorticoids; in some patients the combination appears to be more effective than steroids alone and may permit reduction in dose of steroids required. However, there are numerous complications of use of the immunosuppressive antimetabolites: increased incidence of malignancy, hemorrhagic cystitis, and bone marrow suppression. Increased susceptibility to infection results from use of both steroids and the antimetabolites.

A recent prospective study comparing the effects of prednisone alone or with a course of cyclophosphamide on lupus nephritis indicated that in these patients there was a greater incidence of clinical nephritis in the steroid-only group. However, the proportion of 4 years survivors with adequate renal function was comparable in the two groups. Therefore the combination may not preserve renal function in the long term over that attained by steroid alone.

Scleroderma (Progressive Systemic Sclerosis)

Scleroderma is a generalized disease of connective tissue and blood vessels. Signs and symptoms of vascular insufficiency and progressive fibrosis, both of which are widespread in the skin and several organs, are the outstanding characteristics. It is much more frequent in females than males, and has its onset in middle age. It is relatively rare, appears not to have an hereditary component, and the cause is not known, although the characteristic tissue and organ abnormalities appear to be the consequence of overproduction of collagen.

Cause

Although the cause is unknown, the fact that most patients with the disorder have certain immunologic abnormalities, and scleroderma often occurs in association with other diseases having autoimmune characteristics, indicates the involvement of the immune system in the pathologic charges and possibly the cause. Antinuclear antibodies, RA factor, and hypergammaglobulinemia, are usually present. Special studies point to cell-mediated immune processes being more involved in this disease than humorally (antibody-) mediated ones, except in the case of the kidney, where deposits of immunoglobulins and complement occur. Lymphocytes from patients with scleroderma show cytotoxic activity and lymphocytes may be present in skin lesions. However, cellular infiltration is considerably less marked in scleroderma lesions (excepting the synovium) than in lesions of other autoimmune diseases.

Abnormalities

Studies indicate that the primary abnormalities occur in small arteries; there is a sequence of, first, cellular infiltration into the arterial walls; then inflammation and edema, proliferation of fibroblasts; and finally synthesis of excess amounts of collagen. The result of this process, which occurs in the skin, in joints, muscles, and tendons and in the viscera, is progressive sclerosis of the arteries themselves which become occluded causing ischemia of involved organs and tissues, as well as sclerosis of the surrounding tissues.

The skin lesion in early scleroderma is edema and generalized swelling that gradually gives way to tightening and thickening resulting from deposition of collagen bundles in the dermis, so that the skin becomes bound to deeper structures. These changes are most marked in the hands, arms, the face, and sometimes also the upper torso.

Joints, tendons, and muscles are also affected. The synovium may show inflammation and cellular infiltrates resembling those in RA. Gradually joint stiffness, synovial fibrosis, and flexion contractures develop. Resorption of distal portions of the terminal phalanges of the fingers often occurs.

The esophagus is the most commonly affected of all internal organs, and collagen deposition, smooth muscle atrophy, and muscosal erosions develop in the great majority of patients with scleroderma. Peristaltic activity declines and this and an impairment of function of the lower esophageal sphincter leads to esophageal dilation and gastroesophageal reflux. Similar muscle atrophy and fibrosis of the intestine causes dilation, hypomotility, malabsorption syndrome, and chronic constipation.

Lung involvement can be demonstrated in many patients by X-ray and pulmonary function testing, revealing interstitial and alveolar fibrosis. Pleurisy and pleural friction rubs are not uncommon.

The heart is affected, with myocardial fibrosis leading to conduction defects; right ventricular failure from the pulmonary hypertension caused by the lung disease; but more often left ventricular failure as a consequence of the cardiomyopathy itself.

Involvement of the kidney is common, serious, and a frequent cause of death; the lesions are fibrinoid necrosis, and sclerosis of the glomeruli and afferent arterioles with numerous small infarctions. Larger arteries are affected with a form of nephrosclerosis. Often these abnormalities produce a renovascular type of severe malignant hypertension, which in turn accelerates the arterial, arteriolar and glomerular disease, leading to a rapidly progressive renal failure.

Assessment

Assessment in scleroderma consists in evaluating the presence and severity of symptoms and signs resulting from the anatomic and physiologic abnormalities outlined above. Often one of the first occurrences in scleroderma is Raynaud's phenomenon, said to occur in 90% of patients. In this syndrome, there is paroxysmal vasospasm in the arterioles of portions of the fingers, precipitated by cold. It is associated with narrowing and obliteration of the capillaries in the skin from both structural changes (swelling, and intimal and basement membrane thickening) and excessive reactivity (vasospasm) leading to decreased blood flow and ischemia. Complaints of swelling, pain and stiffness of the joints, especially the fingers and knees, are frequent, and muscle atrophy is often evident.

Symptoms of gastrointestinal involvement are epigastric distress and pyrosis from esophageal reflux which causes a reflux esophagitis similar to that in hiatal hernia (Chapter 11). Delayed gastric emptying and intestinal hypomotility produce signs and symptoms of abdominal pain, bloating, feelings of distention or fullness, and copious foul-smelling stools; or constipation and fecal impaction.

Pulmonary involvement leads to shortness of breath with slight exertion and nonproductive cough, with physical findings of bibasilar rales and characteristics of restrictive lung disease (Chapter 9). Cardiac complications may produce the symptoms and signs of left ventricular or congestive heart failure (Chapter 7) or cardiac arrhythmias (Chapter 6). Hypertension, abnormal urinalysis, oliguria, and azotemia accompany the impaired renal function caused by the abnormalities listed above.

Course, Management, and Prognosis

The course of patients with scleroderma is variable, but in general there is gradual progression both in the skin and the organ abnormalities, with occasional remission or a slower progression in the minority of patients, a few of whom may survive up to 10 years from the time of onset. Prognosis is poorer in those showing early effects in heart, lung, or kidney. Most patients survive about 2 years from the beginning of symptoms.

Adrenal glucocorticoids appear not to affect the duration of survival or the course, but may lead to relief of signs and symptoms, especially early in the disease. Vasodilators used in hypertension (Chapter 3) and intraarterial injections of reserpine may relieve the vasospastic responses in the hands. The congestive heart failure is said to be poorly responsive to treatment, and the hypertension is refractory to antihypertensive medication. The reflux regimen (Chapter 11) relieves the symptoms of esophagitis, and tetracycline is reported to be effective in ameliorating the malabsorption phenomena caused by the overgrowth of flora resulting from intestinal hypomotility.

REFERENCES

Arthritis Foundation: *Primer on the Rheumatic Diseases,* 7th ed. Reprinted from *JAMA* 225, no. 5 (supplement), 1973.

Beeson PB and McDermott W, editors: *Textbook of Medicine.* 14th ed. Philadelphia, Pa.: Saunders, 1975.

Buchanan WW and Dick WC, editors: *Recent Advances in Rheumatology.* No. 1. *Underlying Mechanisms of Disease.* Edinburgh, London, New York: Churchill Livingstone, 1976.

Donadio JV et al: Treatment of diffuse proliferative lupus nephritis with prednisone and combined prednisone and cyclophosphamide. *N. Engl. J. Med.* 299:1151–1155, 1979.

Frohlich ED, editor: *Pathophysiology.* Philadelphia, Pa.: Lippincott, 1976.

Ganong WF: *Review of Medical Physiology,* 8th ed. Los Altos, Calif.: Lange Medical Publishers, 1977.

Guyton AC: *Textbook of Medical Physiology,* 5th ed. Philadelphia, Pa.: Saunders, 1976.

Hollingsworth JW: *Management of Rheumatoid Arthritis and Its Complications.* Chicago, Ill.: Year Book Medical Publishers, 1978.

Moskowitz RW: *Clinical Rheumatology: A Problem-Oriented Approach.* Philadelphia, Pa.: Lea & Febiger, 1975.

Thorn GW et al, editors: *Harrison's Principles of Internal Medicine,* 8th ed. New York: McGraw-Hill, 1977.

Wangenhaüser FJ: *Chronic Forms of Polyarthritis.* Baltimore, Md.: Williams and Wilkins, 1976.

CHAPTER TWENTY-TWO

The Immune System and Hypersensitivity

COMPONENTS AND FUNCTIONS OF THE IMMUNE SYSTEM

Organs and Tissues

The immune system is a diffuse group of organs, tissues, and cells distributed throughout various sites of the body. These structures are collectively called the lymphoreticular system and include the thymus, lymph nodes, spleen, bone marrow, liver, and Peyer's patches of the small intestine.

The thymus is considered to be the "master organ" of the immune system in that it is the first structure to produce lymphocytes during fetal life, it is essential for the differentiation of T lymphocytes (see below), and it produces a number of humoral factors (thymosin, thymic factor, thymopoietin, and others) that are required for development, control, and maintenance of immune function. Abnormalities of the thymus are associated with a number of immune deficiency, immune proliferative, and autoimmune diseases. Removal of the thymus in newborn experimental animals leads to impaired immune responses, marked decrease in numbers of lymphocytes in the blood and lymphoid organs, frequent infections, wasting, nd early death. Thymus implants, or injections of extracts of the thymus, reverse or modify most of the abnormalities resulting from removal or congenital absence of the thymus. The gland is divided into a cortex and medulla, both comprised of reticular networks of fibers containing large numbers of lymphocytes. It is large and active during childhood, reaches a peak size during adolescence, and regresses with increasing age thereafter, although it appears to be concerned with regulation of immune function throughout life by means of its secreted hormones.

Lymph nodes occur at intervals along the larger lymph vessels, mainly at areas of branching; each node has afferent and efferent lymph vessels. The nodes are made up of three areas: a central medulla, an outer cortex, and a paracortical area between the two. T cells occur mainly in the medulla and paracortical areas, while B cells are found in follicles distributed throughout the cortical areas. The lymph node is made up of a network of interlacing fibers among which occur cells with long processes; this arrangement acts as a filtering device for the lymph that flows through the node; it strains out and retains foreign cells such as bacteria, and various antigens.

Like the lymph nodes, the spleen contains masses of lymphocytes and has numerous follicles filled with B cells, and less localized areas of T cell concentration. The reticular meshwork of the spleen functions for the blood vascular system much as the lymph nodes do for the lymphocytes: a straining and trapping meshwork for removing foreign cells and antigens from the blood.

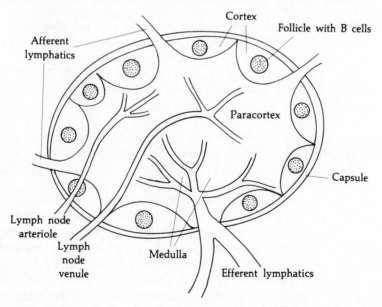

Figure 22-1. Diagram of a lymph node showing cortex with follicles containing B cells; medulla and paracortex, mainly the locale of T cells; and blood and lymph supply.

The bone marrow and the liver, as well as the spleen, contribute to the development and differentiation of lymphocytes during fetal life, and participate in immune responses, especially those of the B cell system (see following) throughout life.

Cells

The lymphocytes are the principal effector agents of the immune system. They are small migratory cells having a large nucleus and are distributed throughout the fluids and tissues of the body. Lymphocytes have the unique characteristic of immune recognition; they are able not only to distinguish cells and molecules as being either self or nonself; but are able to prevent an immune response to the cell or molecule if it is of the self, or initiate a series of processes that inactivate or eliminate it if it is foreign.

There are two major categories of immune process, involving different types of lymphocytes, operating in the normal individual. Although they possess different physiologic characteristics, nevertheless they interact at several levels in the various types of immune function. The two major divisions are B lymphocyte-dependent processes—also called antibody-mediated, humoral, or serologic immunity; and T lymphocyte-dependent processes—also called cell-mediated or cellular immunity. The B stands for bursa, from the bursa of Fabricius, a structure in birds responsible for the differentiation of B cells from their precursors; mammals (and therefore the human) have no bursa but do have evolutionally equivalent structures within lymphoreticular organs and the fetal liver. The T stands for the thymus gland in which T lymphocytes differentiate from their precursors.

B Lymphocyte Immune Responses

B cell precursors originate in the embryonic yolk sac and become stem cells which migrate into the fetal liver and spleen, remain there for further differentiation, and then transfer to sites in the bone marrow. Ultimately they populate sites in the lymphoid tissues and are also present in the blood. The probable pathways of differentiation are shown in Figure 22-2. These B cells possess microvilli on their membrane surfaces upon which are located specialized receptors for antigens. The receptors are immunoglobulins and they provide attachment sites for the binding of specific antigens. B cells also have receptors for components of the complement system (see following). Because of these specialized antigen-binding receptors, complexes comprised of antigen, antibody, and complement can bind selectively to B lymphocyte surfaces.

The first step in the initiation of a B cell-mediated immune response is recognition of a foreign (i.e., nonself) cell or molecule by a B lymphocyte. It is the immunoglobulin on the membrane of this cell that is the receptor for the foreign antigen, and binding of the antigen to the specific receptor capable of attaching to it constitutes immune recognition. All surface immunoglobulin antigen receptors present on a given B lymphocyte, or on a clone of related lymphocytes, are specific for a single type of antigen. Most surface immunoglobulin receptors are of the classes IgD or IgM (see following).

Antigens that gain entry into the ECF are carried to the regional lymph nodes

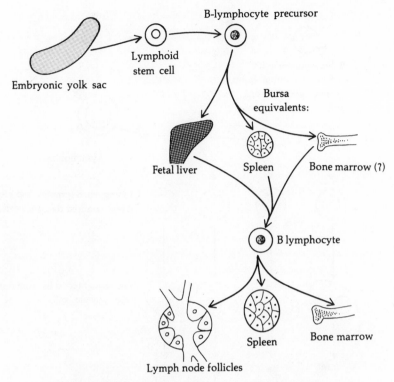

Figure 22-2. Pathway of differentiation of B lymphocytes.

(or if they enter the blood, then they are transported to the spleen) and initiate an immune response characterized by the sequence of changes described below. These changes are correlated with histologic alterations in the locally affected lymphoid tissue within a few days following entrance of the antigen: there is a cellular proliferation in the cortical follicles of the lymph nodes (or spleen). Shortly thereafter antibody production begins, collects first in the nodes, and is detectable in the blood within 10 to 14 days after antigen entry. Plasma cell development continues for several weeks. Lymphocytes sensitized to the antigen persist in the follicles for long periods or indefinitely.

Once the immunoglobulin receptors of a B cell have bound an antigen the B cell becomes activated into undergoing a special form of cell division called cloning. These processes occur primarily in the lymph nodes but also in the spleen and the tissues of the lymphoid system. First, the activated cell and its nucleus enlarge; the cell organelles increase in size and number; the cell membrane permeability increases and there is accelerated uptake of ions, glucose, and amino acids; and the rate of protein synthesis rises. The B cell becomes transformed into a lymphoblast. Then the cell divisions occur; each activated B cell ultimately gives rise to about 1000 enlarged, transformed daughter cells that are now called plasma cells. This process of differentiation then leads to the production of immunoglobulin antibodies by the plasma cells. Each plasma cell derived from the original activated B cell synthesizes immunoglobulin antibodies of a single class; the antibodies are specific to the antigen that was bound to the receptors of that original B cell. The antibodies enter the blood and contribute to the globulin

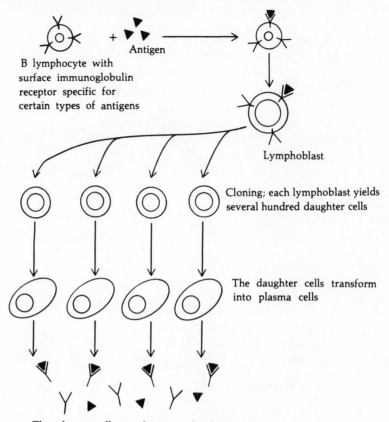

B lymphocyte with
surface immunoglobulin
receptor specific for
certain types of antigens

Lymphoblast

Cloning; each lymphoblast yields
several hundred daughter cells

The daughter cells transform
into plasma cells

The plasma cells synthesize and release
immunoglobulin antibodies that bind the stimulating antigen

Figure 22-3. Sequence of events in a humorally mediated immune response following binding of an antigen to the B cell membrane surface immunoglobulin antigen receptor.

portion of the plasma proteins. This series of events is diagrammed in Figure 22-3.

The antibodies that are synthesized and released in this way perform a number of functions. Binding of antibody to an antigen facilitates the clearance of the antigen by the reticuloendothelial system; the complexes are phagocytized by neutrophiles, macrophages, and monocytes. If the antigen is an infectious agent such as a virus, its binding by antibody decreases its virulence and ability to cause overt disease. If the antigen is a foreign cell, such as a graft or tumor cell or a microorganism, antibody can induce destruction of the cell (cell lysis) either by activation of the complement system (see following) or by a special process called antibody-dependent cell-mediated cytotoxicity. In this latter process the antibody-coated foreign cells are attacked and bound by a special subgroup of B lymphocytes called killer B cells, or by neutrophiles or monocytes, and the cells are destroyed.

B cell, or humorally mediated, antibody immune response is of major significance in physiologic defense against bacterial invaders. The bacteria or other type of antigen which is capable of eliciting an immune response must be recognized as nonself—that is, as foreign—in order for the immune response to occur;

this quality is sometimes termed immunogenicity. Entry into the body may occur via skin contact, injection, ingestion, or inhalation.

The changes outlined above that occur following exposure of the immune system to challenge by a new antigen, that is, one not previously encountered, constitute the *primary* response to the antigen. The primary response sensitizes the immune system of the subject so that when (or if) a second exposure to the antigen occurs, the immune system is able to respond more rapidly and more strongly. This is called the *secondary* response. The secondary response is dependent on a special subgroup of B cells (also T cells, see below) that possess what is called immune memory, and the cells are called memory B cells. Although the general sequence of events following a second antigen exposure are similar to the primary one, it is more effective because of the prior sensitization that is recorded and preserved in the memory B (and T) cells. Thus the secondary response is also called an *anamnestic* (=not forgotten) response. Once again the antigen enters the cortical follicles of the lymph nodes, but now there are already present a special type of antibody, called *cytophilic antibody*, formed as a consequence of memory B cell development. The cytophilic antibody is present on the macrophages of the nodes and promotes the phenomenon of *immune adherence* whereby the antigen–cytophilic antibody complex is rapidly bound to and engulfed by the macrophages, thus removing it from the ECF. In the systemic manifestations of the secondary anamnestic response the serum antibody titers increase more rapidly, more antibody is produced, and although both IgM and IgG antibodies are formed (as in the primary response) there is more IgG relative to IgM.

T Cell Mediated Immune Responses

Precursors of the thymus-dependent lymphocytes originate in the embryonic yolk sac and as primitive stem cells migrate into the fetal liver. Later in embryonic development they enter the thymus gland, which is the first lymphoid organ to develop in embryogenesis. Following a period of differentiation in the thymus, T cells populate the blood, spleen, bone marrow, and lymph nodes.

Cell-mediated immunity operates in defense against intracellular bacteria, some viruses, and fungi; it also is directed against spontaneously arising tumor cells, and against foreign tissue such as transplanted organs. T cells probably comprise the so-called immune surveillance system by which cellular mutations or malignant transformations are recognized as nonself, or foreign, and destroyed early in their development. T cells are also the producers of lymphokines (see following) which are the important mediators of most cell-mediated immune response largely by means of their actions on tissue and blood macrophages. Cellular immunity is also the portion of the immune response primarily concerned with allergic reactions of the late or delayed (type IV hypersensitivity) variety. T cells, like the Bs, also have receptors for antigens on their surface membranes, but unlike B cells their surfaces do not possess immunoglobulins, or at least not in a form which can be readily discerned by methods that are available at the present time.

There appear to be a number of subpopulations of T lymphocytes which are specialized for certain functions: (1) suppressor T cells appear to inhibit the transformation of B lymphocytes into antibody-producing plasma cells, thus act-

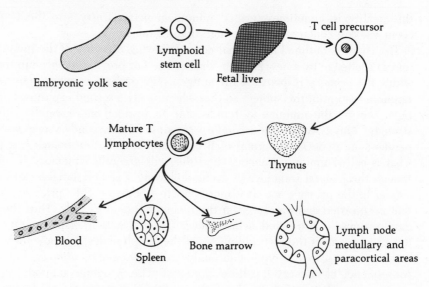

Figure 22-4. Pathway of differentiation of T lymphocytes.

ing as moderators of the humoral immune response; (2) helper T cells promote the production of certain antibody-producing plasma cells from B cell precursors, and foster some humoral immune response; (3) killer T cells attach to and exert a cytolytic and cytotoxic effect on tumor cells and upon the cells in an organ graft; (4) lymphokine-producing T cells; and (5) memory T cells that serve functions in the cell-mediated immune response similar to those served by memory B cells in humoral immunity.

The cell membrane antigen receptor of the T lymphocyte is not as well understood as is that of the B lymphocyte. It is known, however, that T lymphocytes do bind specific antigens to which they are capable of responding, but it appears that only a relatively small portion of T lymphocytes have receptors for a given antigen; and the nature of the receptor, and even whether it is an immunoglobulin (as is the case with B cells), is not known.

When T lymphocytes are activated by antigens they undergo a transformation that enables them to destroy or inactivate the antigen directly. If the antigen is that of a foreign cell such as a tissue or organ graft, certain subgroups of T cells become able to bind specifically to the cells and destroy them by a process called cell-mediated cytotoxicity. Other T cells become sensitized to different types of antigens and secrete soluble immune effector agents called lymphokines, among which are (1) chemotactic factors, that attract macrophages and neutrophiles to the area of the antigen so that it may be phagocytized; (2) interferon, that inhibit the reproduction of viruses; (3) lymphotoxin or cytotoxic factor, that kills foreign cells; (4) macrophage activating and macrophage migration-inhibiting factor, that not only makes macrophages more vigorous in engulfing antigens but also prevents their migrating from the area of the immune response; and (5) cell growth inhibitors, substances that interfere with the proliferation of foreign cells.

The T cell response to antigen challenge consists of two aspects. The first of these is in the regional lymph node supplying the area invaded by the antigen; here there is increased cell division in the medullary and paracortical areas that are the locales of T cell concentration. The lymphocytes are stimulated by the antigen to enter a phase of rapid cell growth and become transformed into immunoblasts that divide and give rise to large numbers of daughter cells (cloning), but there is no production of immunoglobulin antibodies.

The second aspect of T cell response to an antigen occurs at the site of entry of the antigen. T lymphocytes, as well as macrophages, migrate to where the antigen is localized at its site of entry. Both T cells and macrophages directly destroy the invading cells or antigenic molecules, whichever they may be. Lymphocytes engaged in this direct destruction are called cytotoxic or killer T cells. Cytotoxic T cells have a special facility for recognizing foreign antigen in the form of tumor cells, cells of grafted or transplanted organs or tissues, and the organism's own cells that have become abnormal due to the action of viruses or bacteria. The killer T cells become sensitized to the antigen, undergo activation and transformation, attach to the foreign substance, and destroy it.

Just as is the case with B cell immune responses, T cell-mediated immune responses also show a primary response upon first encounter with an antigen; then if the antigenic challenge recurs at a later time, there is a more rapid and stronger secondary T cell-mediated response. Special memory T lymphocytes, largely present in the circulation (as opposed to the B memory cells that reside mainly in the lymph nodes) are responsible for the anamnestic T cell immune response. The secondary response is characterized both by a greater degree of lymphoblastic transformation and proliferation, and a higher degree of cytotoxicity of the resulting killer T cells.

A subgroup of T lymphocytes is called the helper T cells; these specialized cells facilitate B cell humoral immune responses by releasing specific factors into the ECF that stimulate B cells to become sensitized to the antigen more rapidly and strongly, to produce larger amounts of antibody, and to do so more rapidly following antigenic challenge. The synthesis and secretion of the IgG immunoglobulin by B cells is particularly dependent on helper T cell function. It is considered that the memory T cell is a subpopulation of helper T cells that have an important function in promoting the increased speed and effectiveness of the secondary (anamnestic) immune response.

There is also a subgroup of T cells called suppressor T cells. This subgroup of T cells functions to suppress B cell (antibody-mediated) humoral responses to many antigens; it may be that they act directly by suppressing B cell immune response, or perhaps they inhibit helper T cell activity. In addition they also inhibit some forms of T cell function including cell-mediated cytotoxicity. It is speculated by some workers that it is loss of suppressor T cell function that causes the immune system to develop humoral or cell-mediated immune response against antigens of the body's own cells, resulting in the various autoimmune diseases. Conversely, excessive suppressor T cell function may lead to impaired immune response to microorganisms, tumor cells, or other antigens, and permit disease to develop because of an ineffectual immune response.

It must be emphasized that in the normal functioning of the immune system, most antigens do not evoke only a T cell or a B cell immune response but rather that both categories of response become activated. Moreover, there is increasing evidence that a normal interaction between T and B lymphocytes is crucial to the integrity of their respective kinds of responses to antigens. Normal function of the immune system is dependent on these interactions. It appears that many disorders of immune function such as hypersensitivity (allergic) reactions, autoimmune diseases, certain malignancies, and other immune abnormalities may develop as a consequence of disturbances in the equilibria among the various types of B and T cell function.

Macrophages

Tissue macrophages (=big eaters) are derived from the monocytes of the blood; the latter are formed, circulate in the blood and then enter the tissues to reside there. There is evidence that macrophages serve an important function in the preliminary processing of antigens to which T cells, and probably to some extent also B cells, respond. As described above, once antigens have entered the ECF they become localized in lymphoid tissue and here are phagocytized by the macrophages which degrade antigenic molecules and foreign cells, thus removing them from the body fluids. As is true of the lymphocytes, macrophages first must undergo a process of preliminary activation in order to become maximally effective in their function—in this case, phagocytosis. Lymphocytes that have become activated by binding antigen to their surface receptors release substances that attract macrophages to the area and increase their phagocytic actions. Antigen that has been engulfed and processed by a macrophage then becomes bound to the surface of the macrophage, and this sequence of events makes the antigen much more capable of eliciting an immune response than before. Macrophages with processed antigen bound to their surfaces in this way attract large numbers of T lymphocytes which cluster around them, attach to the antigen on the macrophage surface, and undergo differentiation and proliferation for their various immune functions as described above.

Other Cells Involved in Immune Responses

Neutrophils comprise the major cell type of the leukocytes. These cells have surface receptors for complexes between antigens and antibodies, bind to them, and then phagocytize and remove them from the ECF. Neutrophils are attracted to the area of an immune response, where there are many antigen–antibody complexes, by a leukocyte chemotactic factor secreted by activated T lymphocytes.

Mast cells are essentially tissue basophils, and bear a similar relationship to basophils that macrophages do to monocytes. These cells are among those involved in immediate hypersensitivity and anaphylactic responses. Mast cells and basophils have receptors on their membrane surfaces to the immunoglobulin IgE and therefore bind it; when an antigen to which IgE is capable of becoming sensitized binds to the IgE on a mast cell or basophil surface, this activates the latter cell to release a number of strongly bioactive molecules that produce increased capillary permeability, vasodilation, smooth muscle contraction, and in-migration of inflammatory cells. These substances cause local edema, inflammation, vascular congestion, hypersecretion of mucous membranes, gastrointestinal hypermotility, and bronchoconstriction. The substances are histamine, slow-reacting substance of anaphylaxis (SRS-A), and eosinophil chemotactic factor of anaphylaxis (ECF-A) which induces the influx of eosinophils into areas of antigen–antibody reactions. Eosinophils are actively phagocytic for antigen–antibody complexes.

Soluble Compounds

Antibodies

Structure

There are five classes of immunoglobulin antibodies that are produced by the B lymphocyte–plasma cell system in response to an antigen. The term immunoglobulin refers to serum globulins having the ability to act as an antibody in response to some antigen—that is, to form an antigen–antibody complex with it. All antibodies are made up of one or more basic units comprised of four polypeptide chains arranged into two long and two short chains. The long chains are called heavy (H) chains and the short are called light (L) chains, based on their molecular weights. The four chains are arranged in a symmetrical structure and are bound to each other by disulfide bonds. Each basic unit of an immunoglobulin consists of a Fab portion, made up of the two L chains and one end of the two H chains; and an Fc portion, made up of the other end of the two H chains (Figure 22-5).

Each of the Fc ends of the two H chains have the constituent amino acids arranged in a standard sequence; this is the portion of the immunoglobulin that binds to the surface receptors of several cell types: macrophages, lymphocytes, and neutrophils; and is able to activate the complement sequence (see following) and releases histamine, SRS-A and ECF-A from mast cells. The Fc regions of immunoglobulin molecules are much the same within each of the five classes.

The Fab portions of immunoglobulin molecules are made up of the L chains and part of the H chains. Each one is comprised of a segment in which the constituent amino acids are sequenced in a variable sequence called the V region; and a segment in which the amino acids are arranged in a constant sequence, called the C region. The V regions are the portions of the antibody molecule that constitute the antigen binding sites and confer antigen specificity upon the immunoglobulin molecule. The variable region of immunoglobulins produced by one, or all of a single clone of plasma cells, is identical; and it is different from the variable region of all immunoglobulin molecules produced by another plasma cell or clone of such cells. Since each antigen-binding site is composed of the variable region of one L and one H chain, the smallest IgG molecule has two binding sites; and the largest, IgM, made up of five basic units, has ten binding sites, although five of these are said to be not very active.

Therefore every immunoglobulin molecule has two categories of function situated at opposite ends: specific antigen binding at the Fab end, and binding to effector cells and molecules at the Fc end. The structure of a single basic unit of an immunoglobulin molecule is shown in Figure 22-5. The smallest immunoglobulin is IgG, consisting of a single unit; IgM, the largest, is comprised of a complex of five of these basic structures linked together in a symmetric array.

Classes of Antibodies

Immunoglobulin A (IgA). These antibodies are synthesized in plasma cells derived from B lymphocytes located in the secretory glands of the mucous membranes of the gastrointestinal and respiratory tracts. They are also present in the

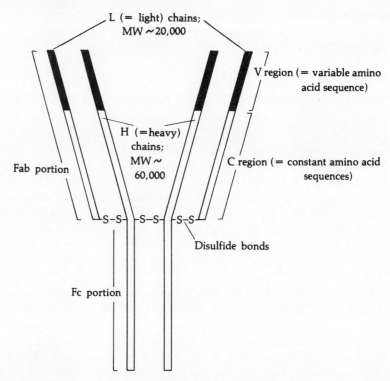

Figure 22-5. Diagram of the basic unit of an immunoglobulin, showing heavy and light chains, disulfide bonds, constant and variable regions, hinge area, and Fab and Fc portions.

salivary, lacrimal, and mammary glands and in the glands of the urinary and reproductive-genital tract. Only small amounts of IgA are present in the blood and lymph; most remains localized in the secretions of mucous membranes and other secretory surfaces. It provides an immunological barrier against pathogens originating in the environment and therefore protects the various organ systems against infection by viruses, bacteria, and fungi.

Immunoglobulin D (IgD).   This immunoglobulin is present only in very small amounts in the serum but is present in association with IgM on most B lymphocytes. Although little is known of its function it is suspected to act as a cell surface receptor and facilitate B cell recognition of specific antigens.

Immunoglobulin E (IgE).   This is also known as reaginic antibody; although it is present in only low concentrations in the sera of normal persons, some subjects with hypersensitivity (allergic) disorders have quite high titers of IgE. The plasma cells that synthesize IgE occur throughout the body but are concentrated in the gastrointestinal and respiratory tracts and their regional lymph nodes. IgE has a predilection for binding to basophiles and mast cells by the Fc portion, and the amounts bound in this way are higher in atopic individuals than in control groups. This relationship accounts for the fact that it is the antibody responsible for immediate (Type I) hypersensitivity and anaphylactic reactions. The Fab portion binds to the antigen in skin or mucous membranes to which the subject is sensitized, and the Fc portion, bound to the mast cell, activates the latter and prompts the release of histamine, SRS-A and ECF-A that are responsible for the signs and symptoms of anaphylaxis and allergy (see following). These substances are called the mediators of immediate (Type I) hypersensitivity reactions.

Immunoglobulin G (IgG). IgG is found throughout the ECF and is the immunoglobulin in highest concentration in the serum, comprising about 75%. IgG is, with IgM, the B cell surface antibody most importantly concerned with the humoral immune responses. Although it also participates importantly in the primary immune response it is the major antibody of the secondary one. Ig has several subgroups with somewhat different actions; some bind complement on their constant Fc portion, and some bind to macrophages.

Immunoglobulin M (IgM). IgM, like IgG, is present in large (though less than IgG—about 10%) amounts throughout all the body fluids, and is the major immunoglobulin for the early portions of the primary immune response, being the first one to appear following stimulus by a new antigen. It is a major immunoglobulin present on B lymphocyte surface membranes.

IgG and IgM together are responsible for physiologic functions characteristic of the humoral immune response: hemolysis, agglutination, precipitation, and opsonization. These terms are self-explanatory except for opsonization, which refers to the binding of antibody to an antigen, especially bacterial, which then promotes increased phagocytosis of the invader by macrophages or neutrophils.

Antibody Specificity

One of the remarkable characteristics of the humoral immune response is the specificity of the antibody that is formed by the plasma cells, for the antigen that elicited the response. The B lymphocyte–plasma cell system is able to synthesize an enormous number of completely different antibodies, each of which is able to bind only to a relatively small number of structurally related antigens. The degree to which an antibody is capable of binding to a group of antigens is called its binding affinity. And the binding affinity is determined by the relationship between the structural configuration of the B lymphocyte's surface antigen receptor, and the structure of the antigenic determinant on the surface of the antigen.

An antigen is defined as a molecule that can be bound by an antibody receptor. But in most cases the receptor is not large enough to encompass the entire antigen but only small portions of its surface features. The surface features of an antigen to which the antibody receptor can become affixed are called the antigenic determinants. And the ability of the antibody to bind the antigen—that is, the binding affinity—depends on the structural match between antigenic determinant and the antigen receptor of the antibody. Where the match is good, binding affinity will be high and the antibody is said to be specific for that antigen. The poorer the "fit," the lower the binding affinity, and the less the specificity. As determinant and receptor become more unlike each other in configuration, eventually no antigen–antibody binding will occur at all. As mentioned above, the ability to bind antigen is established by the Fab portion of the antibody molecule. Where a group of structurally related antigens can bind to an antibody with varying degrees of affinity, they are said to be cross-reactive.

The Clonal Selection Theory

I stated earlier that the B cell surface antigen receptor is an immunoglobulin; these receptor immunoglobulins have their Fc portion buried in the B cell membrane, and therefore the Fab portions of the immunoglobulin protrude from the surface. It is the latter which comprise the antigen receptors.

When an antigen gains entrance to the body fluids, and hence to the immune system, those B lymphocytes with antigen receptors having a good structural match to the antigenic determinants of the invader, and therefore a high binding affinity and specificity for them, bind to the antigen. This binding of the antigen by the Fab end of the B lymphocyte immunoglobulin antigen receptor, activates the B cell and leads to the cloning, differentiation into plasma cells, and antibody production, described previously. The antibody that is produced by the plasma cells has the same specificity for the antigenic determinant as did the parent

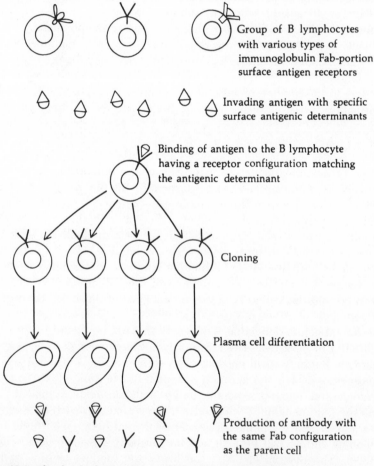

Group of B lymphocytes with various types of immunoglobulin Fab-portion surface antigen receptors

Invading antigen with specific surface antigenic determinants

Binding of antigen to the B lymphocyte having a receptor configuration matching the antigenic determinant

Cloning

Plasma cell differentiation

Production of antibody with the same Fab configuration as the parent cell

Figure 22-6. The clonal selection theory. The B cell membrane surface antigen receptor is an immunoglobulin with a specific configuration of the protruding Fab portion. It is capable of binding only with antigenic determinants of matching configuration. Encounter with an antigen having such a "fit" will permit binding and activation of the lymphocyte with production of plasma cells which secrete antibody with the same Fab configuration.

cell's surface antigen receptor. This is the process by which it is ensured that the antibodies secreted in response to an invading antigen have a high binding affinity and effective specificity for that antigen. This principle is illustrated in Figure 22-6.

Antibody Diversity

The subject of antibody diversity, that is, how such a very large number of antigens with which an individual can come into contact in a lifetime can be recognized and responded to by preformed specific B lymphocytes, has long been an area of controversy in immunology. Even granted the fact of cross-reactivity—the fact that a single B cell antigen receptor can bind several structurally related antigens, though with varying degrees of affinity; still the immune system has the capacity to respond to a huge variety of antigens by the activation of B lymphocytes with surface receptors predetermined to bind with the antigenic determinants. How does it happen that the wide range of potentially responsive and matching B lymphocytes are present prior to the initial exposure to an antigen? Basically there are two theories proposed to explain the genetic basis for this capacity: the germline theory and the somatic mutation theory.

The germline theory suggests that the diverse genetic information that codes for all of the possible antigens the organism will ever encounter is present in the genome (genetic constitution) of each individual and leads to the development of B lymphocytes possessing all the genetic material needed to respond to all possible antigens. The genetic material only has to be rearranged during cell division to produce all possible combinations of immunoglobulin variable and constant regions.

The somatic mutation theory proposes that not all of the information is innately present in the genome but rather that a few V genes are inherited and then a process of random mutation of the genes for the variable regions takes place during one of the stages of cell division, either at the cloning stage simulated by antigen–antibody binding, or at some stage in fetal development. It is suggested that the random mutations during embryogenesis could result in lymphocytes with constant and variable regions that cover the full range of antigenic possibilities, and thus be capable of synthesizing antibodies to match any antigen the organism would encounter in later life. As knowledge accumulates from more recent research these two models appear to be converging, and newer theories incorporate aspects of both the germline and somatic mutation models.

Lymphokines

Lymphokines, discussed briefly above, are the secreted products of T lymphocytes that have undergone stimulation, cloning, and differentiation. There is evidence that other sensitized lymphocytes in addition to T cells are able to produce lymphokines that have a large number of actions. Among these are: lymphokines released by both B and T cells that are cytotoxic and destroy foreign cells by lysis; lymphokines that attract macrophages and neutrophils to sites of immune reactions, increase their phagocytic capacity, and tend to hold them in the area so that they do not migrate out; and the lymphokine interferon that confers on host cells a resistance to intracellular pathogens such as viruses such that the host cells no longer accept direction of their metabolism by the viral nucleic acids.

Complement

The complement system is a group of serum proteins and enzymes that participate with the B lymphocyte–plasma cell–antibody system in humorally mediated immune responses. The components of the complement system, sometimes called the complement cascade, are normally present in the blood as inactive precursor molecules that are capable of becoming activated by certain substances. Each component of the complement chain must be activated in proper sequence by a specific stimulus in order for the cascade to proceed. There are two parallel pathways of reactions leading to activation of the last several steps in the sequence of complement reactions; it is these last six or so steps which actually produce the physiologic changes characteristic of complement function: the membrane attack mechanism. The two pathways are the classical pathway, and the properdin (or alternate) pathway. These two pathways of complement activation are set in motion by different substances and have different early steps leading to the final common sequence of the last several steps. The classical pathway appears to be more intimately involved with the immune response than the properdin because the former is activated by the binding of antigen to antibody and by immunoglobulin aggregates of the IgG and IgM classes.

The C_1 is the first component of complement and binds to the Fc portion of the antibody molecule; this reaction between complement C_1 and antibody that has bound antigen then activates the next step in the pathway: C_4. (The components of complement are not named in the order of their activation but rather in the order of their discovery.) C_4 then attaches to the antigen of the bound antigen–antibody complex. Throughout the complement cascade there is a sequential activation of a series of enzymes that catalyze successive steps in the reaction.

The activated forms of a number of the complement components have special actions in the immune response including *immune adherence*, in which macrophages and neutrophils, both of which have receptors for certain components, bind to that component by their receptors; antigen bound to this complement is then readily phagocytized and disposed of. Other reactions promote *lysis* of the antigen–antibody or foreign cell–antibody complex by causing defects to develop in the surface of the target antigen. Some complement components function as *anaphylatoxins* and cause degranulation of mast cells and basophils with release of their mediators of the immediate hypersensitivity response: histamine, SRS-A, and ECF-A as described above. Still other components exert a *chemotactic* effect for neutrophils, attracting them into the area where they are stimulated to phagocytize the antigen–antibody complexes.

Antigens

An antigen may be defined as a substance which is capable of inducing a measurable (usually specific) immune response when introduced into an animal by ingestion, injection, inhalation or body surface contact. Antigens therefore possess the property of immunogenicity, by which a substance produces humoral or cellular (or more commonly both) immune reactions. Foreignness (that is, the quality of being nonself) and a high molecular weight (greater than 10,000) are two qualities which increase the probability that a given compound will possess immunogenicity. Complex molecules of over 500,000 molecular weight with a protein or polypeptide–carbohydrate structure tend to be most effective in eliciting cellular or humoral immune responses. One important characteristic of responses elicited by antigens is their remarkable specificity to the eliciting antigen, which is of profound adaptive significance; that is, specific immune *memory* is a remarkable quality of the normally functioning immune system. The processes involved in anamnestic responses have been discussed previously.

There are several categories of antigens as concerns their relationship to the responding host. An alloantigen is an antigen present in certain individuals of a species but not in all; human histocompatibility antigens and blood group antigens are of this kind. Heteroantigens are those of a species different from the host—thus for humans, antigens of bacteria, viruses, plants, other animals. A heterophil antigen is one present in several species.

Haptens are substances which are not themselves antigens, or immunogenic, but which can become so when complexed with an appropriate other substance; they are of lower molecular weight, simpler molecular configuration and have fewer antigenic determinants than antigens. When a hapten conjugates or complexes with a suitable antigen then it becomes capable of eliciting an immune response by creating an antigenic determinant site. It is the combination of the hapten and the carrier molecule, often a protein, which elicits antigen–antibody complex formation; this is often the mechanism by which drug sensitization occurs. Such a complex is called a conjugated antigen, or a neoantigen.

HYPERSENSITIVITY

Although in general the immune system provides protection for the host against a large number of pathogenic organisms and other injurious agents, it is also the case that the immune system itself may mediate reactions that are injurious to the host. If the immune response is helpful and protective to the host, it is called immunity; if the response is damaging, then it is called a hypersensitivity reaction. The process eliciting the responses, and the components and reactions of the immune system involved in them, may be the same in the two cases: immunity and hypersensitivity. Immune reactions that result in damage to the host's tissues have been classified into four categories.

It should be emphasized that these four categories of immune system reactions, although described as separate processes, are not mutually exclusive in the intact organism, and in various hypersensitivity responses components of the four types may be present and interacting with one another.

Type I Immediate Hypersensitivity Reactions

Type I response is also called reagin-dependent or anaphylactic. Hypersensitivity reactions in this category are immunoglobulin-dependent, and the antigens are heterologous in type (heteroantigens). The response itself results from biologically active agents, called the mediators of Type I hypersensitivity, which are released from mast cells and basophils. The response may be local or systemic, or there may be elements of both. The complement system is not involved.

Immune Response

The initial exposure to the antigen or hapten usually occurs by natural means: inhalation, ingestion, dermal or mucous membrane contact or injection (bites, stings), and is not marked by any evident signs, symptoms or detectable pathologic change. Following exposure to the antigen a latent or sensitization period of about a week to ten days occurs. This period is marked by the recognition of the antigen as foreign by lymphocytes, macrophage processing of the antigen, and the production and cloning of specialized lymphocytes sensitized to that antigen, as described earlier. Evidence indicates that helper and/or suppressor T cells may cooperate in this antibody-mediated response. The culmination is the synthesis of IgE by the sensitized B lymphocyte–plasma cell system. When reexposure occurs following the sensitization period, the signs and symptoms of immediate-type hypersensitivity occur, the nature and extent of which depend on a number of factors: the magnitude of the initial (sensitizing) and subsequent dose of antigen; the genetic constitution of the subject, including both the histocompatibility (HLA) and the immune response (Ir) genes (see following); the responsiveness of the subject's autonomic nervous system; the site of antigen entry; and the individual characteristics of the subject's "shock organs"—those structures which respond most vigorously in a given individual to an antigen to which he has been sensitized. In addition, the total allergic burden (that is, the total number of different antigens to which an individual has become sensitized) appears importantly to influence the signs and symptoms; as will the overall duration of exposure to that total allergic burden.

Type I reactions may be local, systemic, or a combination depending upon the above factors. Organ system manifestations may be the skin (wheal and flare reactions); the respiratory system (bronchospasm, hypersecretion and laryngeal edema); the cardiovascular system (vasodilation, increased capillary permeability, hypovolemia, and hypotension); the gastrointestinal tract (mucous membrane edema, vomiting, diarrhea, abdominal cramping); or the urinary tract (frequency, urgency, dysuria). Many types of soluble antigens are able to produce immediate-type hypersensitivity reactions: bee and wasp venom, pollen extracts, large numbers of foods, polysaccharides, iodinated X-ray contrast compounds, therapeutic drugs (haptens) including antibiotics, many antisera, and others.

The cellular and tissue processes involved in producing the signs and systems of Type I hypersensitivity are a sequence of reactions beginning with the reaction between the antigen and antigen-specific IgE reaginic antibody which is bound to cell membranes of mast cells and/or basophils of the responding organs. The antigen–antibody reaction prompts the rapid release of the chemical mediators of Type I hypersensitivity reactions from mast cells.

Mediators of Immediate Hypersensitivity

Histamine is a vasoactive amine stored in the granules of the cytoplasm of mast cells and basophils, and is released when these cells are stimulated to degranulate. It has a rapid onset and short duration of action; the action is to increase capillary permeability, resulting in erythema and angioedema in both mucous membranes and skin.

Slow-reacting substance of anaphylaxis (SRS-A) is a compound having a gradually developing and long-sustained constricting action on smooth muscle, particularly on that of the bronchi; it therefore is an important mediator in extrinsic asthma. Its vascular and secretory glandular effects are minor. It is generated directly in sensitized lung tissue after antigen-IgE interaction.

Eosinophil chemotactic factor of anaphylaxis (ECF-A) is released in this type of response; it causes an influx of eosinophils into the site of the hypersensitive inflammatory response. The aggregated eosinophils ingest and eliminate antigen–antibody complexes. Neutrophil chemotactic factor of anaphylaxis (NCF-A) is a protein which exerts a specific attraction for neutrophils and causes them to migrate into areas where this type of immune response is proceeding; it also engulfs antigen–antibody complexes.

5-Hydroxytryptamine (5-HT, serotonin) occurs in platelets and in the mucosa of the gastrointestinal tract; it may cause vasodilation and hypotension, bronchiolar constriction, and increased intestinal motility. Platelets are attracted into areas of hypersensitivity reactions by a substance called platelet-activating factor (PAF) which causes platelet aggregation and release of their contained mediator agents.

Prostaglandins are unsaturated fatty acids of many different kinds and of wide distribution; they stimulate smooth muscle contraction and cause increased capillary permeability. They also affect smooth muscle tone of bronchi and bronchioles, and alter pulmonary vascular resistance.

The kallikrein–kinin system is also involved in immediate hypersensitivity. Bradykinin is a vasodilator polypeptide released by mast cells; it causes a slow sustained contraction of visceral muscle (vascular and bronchial), hypersecretion from mucous glands, and increased permeability of capillaries. Kinins have been found in tissue perfusates from areas undergoing Type I reactions. Kinins have the additional interesting action of directly stimulating the free nerve endings of pain-transmitting nerve fibers (Chapter 19).

Clinical Conditions of Type I Hypersensitivity

Allergic Rhinitis (Hay Fever)

Allergic rhinitis is the most frequently encountered atopic manifestation; environmental antigens such as molds, animal dander, airborne tree, grass, and weed pollen, and house dust are some common allergens; and the mucous membranes of the eyes, nose, throat, soft palate, and ears represent the shock organs. Food is an uncommon cause.

The main symptoms and signs are lacrimation, periorbital edema, itching and burning of the conjunctiva, nasal congestion and watery rhinorrhea, and itching of the soft palate and nasal mucosa resulting in paroxysmal sneezing. The conjunctivae are often erythematous, and nasal mucosa may be edematous and pale. A smear of nasal secretions shows many eosinophils, and there may be systemic eosinophilia. Symptoms and signs may be either seasonal or nonseasonal, depending on the nature of the allergen.

Patients generally give a positive family history of similar conditions and often themselves give a personal history of other allergic manifestations: hives, eczema, or asthma. The onset is generally before middle life and severity declines with aging, but usually never clears altogether.

Complications may be increased frequency of upper respiratory infections, chronic sinusitis, serous otitis media, or secondary bacterial conjunctivitis. These are the result of edema, congestion, and swelling of lacrimal ducts, turbinates, sinus ostia, and eustachian tubes which impair drainage from these structures. The complications are more common in the perennial than the seasonal types.

Assessment is based on family and personal history, complaints of symptoms, physical findings on examination, and nasal secretion eosinophilia, as described above. In addition, erythema and wheal response to injections of dilute antigens may be useful in establishing specific antigenic agents.

Other conditions that need to be considered in evaluating a patient with similar complaints are (1) rhinitis medicamentosa from excessive use of sympathomimetic nose drops or nasal sprays; (2) viral rhinitis, which can be distinguished by the immediate past health history of systemic symptoms, fever, and erythematous nasopharyngeal mucosa with polymorphonuclear leukocytes in nasal secretion smears; and (3) vasomotor rhinitis, which is perennial, without itching and sneezing, is often accompanied by postnasal discharge, and frequently shows a better response to systemic decongestants than systemic antihistamines.

The most important component of management is avoidance of the allergen, where possible; and reduction of the total allergic load by means such as a clean house and office and removal of dust traps: draperies, heavy blankets, and rugs from the rooms where the patient spends the most time; getting rid of pets; and air filters or a change of environment during periods of high pollen loads for persons with hay fever.

Pharmacologic management consists in the use of oral antihistamines, which have been shown to be the most useful drugs in these disorders. Chlor- and brompheniramine are effective and safe in regular or slow release forms. Side effects in some persons include dryness of oral mucosa because of their anticholinergic action, and drowsiness. Antihistamines should be avoided in patients with COPD because of drying of secretions. Antihistamines are specific antagonists of histamine release from mast cells. Cromoglycate spray or powder to nasal mucosa may be helpful as it prevents the release of mast cell mediators. For more prolonged effect, long-acting combinations of brompheniramine with phenylephrine and phenylpropanolamine (for local nasal decongestant action) may be useful. Combinations of triprolidine and pseudoephedrine offer shorter action but a similar combination of antihistaminic and sympathomimetic effects. Intranasal sympathomimetic amines have short duration of effect and often lead to secondary rebound nasal congestion and so should be avoided.

Immunotherapy for allergic rhinitis may be tried as a last resort if the above types of management provide inadequate relief. This approach is not without danger of systemic reactions, is expensive, slow, and time-consuming, and the results are often disappointing. The method is perennial injections of diluted allergens, following skin tests to establish what they are for a given patient. Theoretically these injections lead to the production and buildup in the patient's serum of blocking antibody, which is an IgG immunoglobulin with specificity for the injected allergen. It binds allergen probably by covering, masking, or saturating the specific antigenic attachment sites on the surfaces of the antigen molecule so that it is no longer able to combine with IgE and initiate a hypersensitivity activation of mast cells and basophils. The method appears to be effective for some patients but not for many others.

Urticaria (Hives) and Angioedema

Urticaria and angioedema are skin and mucous membrane manifestations of hypersensitivity that may appear together or separately as localized areas of edema which are nonpitting. While urticaria involves capillaries in more superficial areas of the skin, angioedema involves capillaries of the deeper skin or mucous membranes, including subcutaneous or submucous tissues. Urticarial lesions are typically well-circumscribed wheals of 1–6 cm diameter with raised erythematous margins and blanched centers; if there are many they may coalesce; itching is generally severe. They often appear on face or hands as successive groups of lesions of short duration (24—48 hr) within a few minutes of exposure to the antigenic substance; this is often oral intake of a food or drug to which the subject has been sensitized, although skin contact and inhalation may occasionally precipitate hives. Both urticaria and angioedema may be acute or chronic. In both types of manifestations emotional upsets may act as a triggering factor.

Hypersensitivity angioedema must be distinguished from the familial form which is not a manifestation of Type I hypersensitivity, but rather of a genetic disorder in which there is a failure to synthesize an inhibitor to C_1, the first component of the complement system. The lesions in both types are similar.

Assessment consists of a positive family history of allergy and a positive personal history of food allergy. The patient should be questioned carefully concerning food or drug intake and other unusual activities in the 24 hours preceding the appearance of the lesions: a change of cosmetics, soap or detergents, or some form of exposure to an unaccustomed substance. The physical sign is extreme localized swelling in the absence of either infection, tissue damage from other cause, or immediate history of trauma.

Management of the acute form consists of antihistamines: triplennamine, chlorpheniramine, or brompheniramine. Hydroxyzine may be a useful adjunct where an emotional component seems prominent, and to relieve pruritis. In the chronic form long-acting antithistamine preparations and an elimination diet may be required until symptoms disappear, at which time the eliminated foods may be cautiously reinstated, one by one, and the patient asked to observe when an item added appears to correlate with a recurrence.

Occasionally urticaria and angioedema will be produced by exposure to cold. In this case it appears that cold alters some protein constituent in the skin such that it becomes a neoantigen capable of inducing a Type I immune response.

Anaphylaxis

Anaphylaxis can be prompted by ingestion or injection of a minute quantity of antigen into a previously sensitized individual and is a life-threatening development. It is a systemic response characterized by sudden onset (within seconds or minutes) of respiratory distress, widespread vasodilation resulting in circulatory collapse, and the cutaneous manifestations such as urticaria, following intake of the allergen—often insect sting, food, or some type of drug. This Type I hypersensitivity response occurs simultaneously in several organ systems.

The signs and symptoms are airway obstruction with dyspnea, wheezing, laryngeal stridor, and hoarseness. A sensation of lump in the throat (not globus hystericus) from mucosal edema of the pharynx, and tightness in the chest may be complained of, as well as pruritis from rapidly developing urticaria. Hypotension may occur from widespread vasodilation, a generalized increased capillary permeability may permit loss of plasma into the interstitial spaces; the combination may result in hypovolemic shock. A severe bronchospastic response may occur producing acute emphysema (dilation of alveoli). Bronchi become hyperemic and edematous, and fill with mucous secretions. Eventually if the situation is not reversed, circulatory insufficiency produces decreased venous return to the right heart, with a decline in cardiac output and decreased perfusion of the brain and coronary arteries. Upper and lower respiratory tract obstruction may lead to hypoxemia and even asphyxiation.

Assessment consists of ascertaining a previous history of exaggerated hypersensitivity reactions and immediate prior history of drug or food intake, insect stings, or allergen injections, and observing the characteristic signs and symptoms, above.

Symptoms and Management

Individuals with a known severe hypersensitivity should wear a Medic Alert bracelet and be equipped with a kit for self-administration of epinephrine at the earliest sign of anaphylaxis. After an injection of any drug the subject should be under observation for 20 minutes. Prevention is the first goal.

Management consists first of early recognition. Tourniquet application if the inoculation or sting occurred in an extremity, and removal of the sting if present, with epinephrine injection into the site, is helpful where appropriate. Epinephrine may be given systemically at intervals until the situation ameliorates. For circulatory collapse intravenous volume expansion and vasopressor agents may be required. With marked respiratory distress, aminophylline, oxygen administration, and isoproterenol aerosol by nebulizer are used. Tracheotomy may be required in the presence of upper airway obstruction sufficient to produce hypoxemia. Diphenhydramine is often used for urticaria and gastrointestinal manifestations.

Type II Hypersensitivity Reactions

Most Type II reactions are cytotoxic or cytolytic ones in which antibodies of the IgM or IgG class bind to the antigenic determinants on a cell membrane. The binding initiates the activation of the complement sequence described previously, complement–antigen–antibody complex form, and the various components of complement exert their effects. The most common clinical example of the Type II reaction has been intravascular hemolysis following transfusion of incompatible blood, where the mismatch involves antibodies against major antigenic determinants. If minor determinants are involved the reaction is less intense and instead of gross red blood cell destruction, antibody binds to the red cell membrane antigen, resulting in antigen–antibody complexes on the red cells that predispose them to increase phagocytosis by the macrophages of the reticuloendothelial system, especially the spleen. Similarly, certain drugs, viruses, or bacteria are able to alter red blood cell surface antigens in such a way that they stimulate antibody formation against them causing increased red cell destruction. Type II cytotoxic reactions may also develop against white blood cells or platelets and lead to deficiencies of the affected cells.

Type II reactions also appear to be involved in a number of renal disorders (Chapter 10). Antibodies to glomerular basement membrane are deposited in and form complexes with this tissue in systemic lupus and scleroderma (Chapter 21), malignant hypertension (Chapter 3), some forms of glomerulonephritis, Goodpasture's syndrome, and other disorders.

Type III Hypersensitivity Reactions

In Type III hypersensitivity reaction there is deposition of antigen–antibody complexes in tissues; local activation of the complement system with fixation of complement to the complexes; release of leukocyte, macrophage, and platelet chemotactic factors; cell infiltration; release of lysosomal enzymes; and formation of clotting factors and kinins. The result is a marked, protracted inflammatory response.

Serum sickness is an example of Type III response and is caused by injection of a foreign (heterologous) serum such as horse serum antisera to communicable disease organisms. It is a systemic response in which there is formation of antigen–antibody complexes and activation of the complement cascade. Complexes are deposited in small blood vessels, activate complement, and cause influx of neutrophils. Drugs such as penicillin may also cause a serum sickness-type reaction.

There are a number of disorders in which antigen–antibody (immune) complexes circulate in the blood and are deposited in tissues; these disorders are called immune complex diseases and are considered to represent examples of Type III hypersensitivity. They include such diverse entities as Crohn's disease and chronic ulcerative colitis (Chapter 11), chronic aggressive hepatitis with associated cirrhosis (Chapter 12), rheumatoid arthritis and systemic lupus erythematosus (Chapter 21), glomerulonephritis (Chapter 9), and many others. Circulating immune complexes deposit out in the blood vessels, activate complement, and so on, as described above.

Immune complex disease develops when immune complexes are not cleared in the usual way by the reticulendothelial system (RES) and instead continue to circulate and ultimately deposit out in small vessels, causing a vasculitis. Ease of clearance of antigen–antibody complexes by the RES depends very much on their solubility and their size, which in turn is related to the relative amount of antigen and antibody present in the circulation. When there are excessive amounts of antigen this seems to predispose to a form of immune complexes that are poorly removed by the RES; also when large complexes are formed in the presence of approximately equal amounts of antigen and antibody, again there is impaired clearance. When the complexes deposit in blood vessels and tissues they result in tissue destruction both because of impairment of the blood supply but perhaps more because of the inflammatory reactions which they induce by the activation of complement and release of the potent biochemicals that are the mediators of the inflammatory response. The nature of the physiologic deficits induced will of course depend upon the functions of the involved organ. Therefore the abnormalities resulting from these disorders are discussed in the context of the appropriate organ systems.

Type IV Hypersensitivity Reactions

Type IV are also called cell-mediated or delayed hypersensitivity reactions. They result from the stimulation of lymphocytes that are specifically sensitized to a given antigen. The cytotoxic activity results from the release of lymphokines (see above), direct attachment and cell lysis by the sensitized cytotoxic lymphocytes, or a combination of the two. Systemic anticoagulation with warfarin impairs the skin induration (but not erythema) and production of tissue factors (mediators) but not the production of sensitized lymphocytes (transformation). Therefore the coagulation mechanism appears to be intimately involved with Type IV hypersensitivity reactions. Type IV reactions generally do not involve either production of antibody or the activation of complement. The steps involved in the sensitization and activation of cytotoxic B and T lymphocytes have been discussed previously. Clinically important examples of Type IV hypersensitivity reactions are contact dermatitis and some forms of allograft rejection.

Transplantation and Allograft Rejection

The Major Histocompatibility Complex

Almost all body cells have on their cell membranes specific protein molecules called histocompatibility antigens; these surface markers are continually being lost and then resynthesized and replaced by the cells, and are able to move readily throughout the fluid portions of the cell membrane. Histocompatibility antigens were first discovered on human leukocytes, which explains the acronym HLA—human leukocyte antigens—as a synonym for them. Cell surface antigens that differ between individuals of a single species, for example, the human, are known as alloantigens, isoantigens, or histocompatibility antigens. These antigens are the molecules responsible for eliciting the transplant rejection responses. Grafts between two persons of the same species but of different genetic constitutions are called allografts, homografts or isografts. (In an autograft, donor and recipient are the same person; in a heterograft, donor and recipient are of different species. Monozygotic twins and inbred strains of mice have identical genetic constitutions and are said to be syngeneic: grafts between such genetically identical individuals are syngenic grafts.)

The presence and specific nature of the histocompatibility antigens in a given subject are determined by clusters of genes on portions of a large genetic region of a pair of homologous chromosomes—the sixth pair. The whole region is referred to as the major histocompatibility complex and contains multiple closely linked loci and which code for many gene products that regulate immune processes. The HLA antigens are among these gene products. At present, four loci have been identified in the complex, although evidence indicates that at least one more major locus, as well as several minor ones, will yet be described. The four known loci are designated HLA-A, HLA-B, HLA-C, and HLA-D. Each

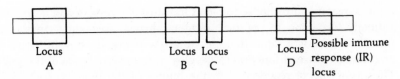

Figure 22-7. Diagram of the human major histocompatibility complex on chromosome 6, showing the major HLA loci and a possible immune response (Ir) locus.

locus has a number of alleles and each allele is identified according to the specificity of its product, which is the given HLA antigen of each class. Figure 22-7 diagrams a portion of the sixth chromosome, showing the major histocompatibility complex and probable relationships of the HLA loci, and proposed site of the Ir genes (see following).

A person inherits one of each allele of each locus from each parent; the set of four antigens inherited from each parent is called the haplotype; so each person inherits two haplotypes. Haplotypes are inherited together from a parent, usually not separate loci, indicating the fact that there is close genetic linkage between loci, and therefore crossovers are unlikely to occur. The phenotypic expression of the antigens determines the tissue type of an individual. Because of the large number of alleles occurring for each gene, the number of possible combinations of these in the general population is enormous. This, plus the fact that additional major loci and further alleles in each class remain to be discovered, helps account for the great difficulties involved in graft donor–recipient matching.

Immune Response (Ir) Genes

These genes are different from but occupy the same pair of chromosomes as the genes that control the synthesis of the HLA antigens and appear to occur in close conjunction with the HLA-D locus. They probably control not only the specific nature of an immune response but also the degree of responsiveness of the individual's immune system to a variety of specific antigens.

Immune Processes in Transplant Rejection

Rejection of a grafted tissue or transplanted kidney, when the technical procedure has been competently done, is largely the consequence of both humoral and cell-mediated reactions on the part of the recipient's immune system to the foreign histocompatibility antigens present on the cells of the donor tissue. There are three forms of allograft (=homograft) rejection involving varying rates and intensity of response, and different degrees of cooperation between antibody-mediated and cellular immune responses. Only the later delayed forms of immune rejection (acute and probably some aspects of chronic rejection) are actually Type IV hypersensitivity responses.

Immediate rejection may take one of two forms. The *hyperacute* form occurs when there are present already formed antibodies in the plasma of the recipient against some antigen(s) present in the donor tissue. Possible causes of hyperacute rejection are the presence of preformed recipient antibodies directed against the HLA antigens of the donor tissue which had been synthesized on a prior occasion as a response to blood transfusions, rejection of a prior allograft, or antibody formation to paternal antigens during pregnancy. In the hyperacute rejection there is a rapid (minutes to a few hours) decline in blood flow to the graft and a failure of function to develop in the parenchyma of the grafted organ. The major site of reaction is on the linings of the blood vessels of the grafted organ because these areas are the most fully exposed to the recipient's circulating blood. Large amounts of antigen–antibody complexes form in the graft vessels initiating the complement cascade, neutrophil invasion, and the resulting histo- and cytologic reactions discussed in a prior section. Hyperacute or immediate rejection cannot be treated with immunosuppressives and prevention by carefully screening for the presence of preformed antidonor antibodies is routine.

The second, and more usual, form of immediate graft rejection is the *accelerated reaction.* In this case the precipitating factor is once again previously synthesized circulating recipient antibody against histocompatibility antigens of the donor tissue, but the titer of such antibodies is considerably lower, hence the rejection response is slower and less vigorous. Blood flow in and function of the grafted tissue may be adequate for several hours, but gradually both decline and the graft becomes ischemic and hypoxic because of complement fixation, leukocyte infiltration, and activation of clotting processes.

Acute rejection is the second category of graft failure and in the absence of adequate immunosuppression may develop within the first few weeks following the transplant. Donor HLA antigens probably ooze out of the graft into the circulation of the recipient for long periods after the procedure; the antigens circulate to the lymph nodes and spleen and induce sensitization in the lymphocytes present there. In addition, lymphocytes of the host circulate through the graft and become sensitized to the foreign HLA antigens of the donor. This sensitization occurs rapidly and results in the migration of large numbers of lymphocytes into the graft where they undergo immunoblast transformation into cytotoxic cells. Macrophages also accumulate owing to T cell lymphokine secretion. Cell-mediated immune responses destroy capillaries and tubules of the graft; ultimately larger blood vessels undergo degeneration, and ischemic necrosis of the graft occurs. In this form of rejection, processes of humoral immunity also occur, with development of antibodies against the donor antigens; often these antibodies appear to be localized mainly within the graft itself. The presence of such antibodies is said to be correlated with poor graft function.

Chronic rejection of a grafted kidney—the third type—may develop over months to years and consists of proliferative lesions in the larger intrarenal arteries; the cause of these lesions, which impair blood flow through the kidney and therefore its function, is controversial and may represent the cumulative destruction and scarring from numerous acute rejection episodes and/or long-term deposition of immunoglobulins.

Immunosuppressive Agents

Clinically useful agents that suppress various components of the immune response have generalized immunosuppressive action and therefore not only increase the host's susceptibility to infection but also increase the incidence of malignancy. In spite of their disadvantages and dangers, however, their usefulness in preserving organ and tissue transplants, and in the management of certain autoimmune disorders such as rheumatoid arthritis and systemic lupus erythematosus, is well established.

Adrenal Corticosteroids. These are immunosuppressive agents that have a nonspecific action on lymphocytes; they have a more potent effect on T cell–mediated delayed hypersensitivity reactions than on B lymphocyte humoral immune responses. Part of the effectiveness appears to result from their action in depleting unsensitized T cells from the thymus and spleen. They also are said to suppress the action of macrophages in taking up antigen and processing it. In addition, they increase the breakdown of IgG, thus lowering the effective concentrations of specific antibodies.

Azathioprine. This drug is an antimetabolite and cytotoxic agent that appears to interfere with nucleic acid metabolism and therefore inhibits the nuclear processes required for the cell proliferation (cloning) that follows stimulation by the sensitizing antigen. It also prevents the multiplication and survival of the stimulated lymphocytes. It is said to suppress both T and B cell replication. Its main toxicity is against the bone marrow, leading to leukopenia, anemia, and thrombocytopenia. It also causes rashes, fever, nausea, vomiting, and diarrhea.

Cyclophosphamide. This is an alkylating agent, meaning that it transfers a monovalent radical to some active compound in the cells which then inactivates them. The drug ionizes, forms a carbonium ion (an organic ion with a positive charge) and this attaches to normal cell constituents interfering with various functions, including glycolysis, protein synthesis, membrane permeability, and intracellular respiration. Its most important inhibitory action is on DNA, causing it to code improperly so that it cannot replicate. Its action on the immune system is to produce atrophy of bone marrow and lymphoid tissue, in addition to destroying proliferating lymphocytes. It produces pancytopenia and hemorrhagic cystitis as unwanted toxic effects.

Antilymphocyte Globulin. This is a heterologous (different species) substance; when large animals (horses, for example) are inoculated with human lymphocytes, or thymus, spleen, or lymph node cells, the recipient animal will synthesize antilymphocyte globulins. The IgG fraction of the serum is then removed, subjected to a variety of treatments, and assayed for potency. When it is injected into another animal or human it then often induces a nonspecific decrease in lymphocyte responsiveness, and hence a depression of immune responsiveness: specifically, lymphocytopenia and decreased cell-mediated immune reactions. One mode of action may be binding to certain T cells and inducing complement-mediated cytotoxicity. It is said to be less effective in suppressing humoral immune responses, and some T lymphocytes appear not to be affected by it. There are many unpleasant side effects from the foreign protein of the horse serum including lymphomas at the injection site, deposition of immune complexes in the glomeruli, local pain and erythema, and serum sickness or anaphylaxis.

REFERENCES

Announcement: New nomenclature for the HLA system. *J. Immunol.* 116:573–574, 1976.

Barber HRK: *Immunobiology for the Clinician.* New York: Wiley, 1977.

Barrett JT: *Basic Immunology and Its Medical Application.* St. Louis, Mo.: Mosby, 1976.

Beeson PB and McDermott W, editors: *Textbook of Medicine,* 14th ed. Philadelphia, Pa.: Saunders, 1975.

Bigley NJ: *Immunologic Fundamentals.* Chicago, Ill.: Year Book Medical Publishers, 1975.

Bluestone R and Pearson CM: Ankylosing spondylitis and Reiter's syndrome: their association with HLA-B27. *Int. Med.* 22:1–19, 1977.

Cooper MD and Lawton AR III: The development of the immune system. *Sci. Am.* 231:59–72, 1974.

Cunningham AJ: *Understanding Immunology.* New York: Academic Press, 1978.

Cunningham AJ, editor: *The Generation of Antibody Diversity. A New Look.* New York: Academic Press, 1976.

Dausset J and Rapaport FT: Immunology and genetics of transplantation. *Perspect. Nephrol. Hypertens.* 6:97–137, 1977.

Edwards RL and Rickles FR: Delayed hypersensitivity in man: effects of systemic anticoagulation. *Science* 200:541–543, 1978.

Frohlich ED, editor: *Pathophysiology.* Philadelphia, Pa.: Lippincott, 1976.

Fudenberg HH et al, editors: *Basic and Clinical Immunology.* Los Altos, Calif.: Lange Medical Publications, 1976.

Ganong WF: *Review of Medical Physiology,* 8th ed. Los Altos, Calif., Lange Medical Publications, 1977.

Guyton AC: *Textbook of Medical Physiology,* 5th ed. Philadelphia, Pa.: Saunders, 1976.

Reed WP and Williams RC: Immune complexes in infectious diseases. *Adv. Int. Med.* 22:49–72, 1977.

Schmidt JR and Ferguson RM: *Immunology for the Practicing Physician.* New York and London: Plenum, 1977.

Schulof RS and Goldstein AL: Thymosin and the endocrine thymus. *Adv. Int. Med.* 22:121–143, 1977.

Seidman, JG, et al: Antibody diversity. *Science* 202:11–17, 1978.

Thaler MS et al: *Medical Immunology.* Philadelphia, Pa.: Lippincott, 1977.

Thorn GW et al, editors: *Harrison's Principles of Internal Medicine,* 8th ed. New York: McGraw-Hill, 1977.

Townes AS and Postlethwaite AE: Lymphocyte surface markers in human disease. *Adv. Int. Med.* 22:97–119, 1977.

de Weck AL and Blumenthal MN: *Monographs in Allergy II. HLA and Allergy.* Basel: Karger, 1977.

Index